MASTER DENTISTRY

VOLUME 2

Restorative Dentistry, Paediatric Dentistry and Orthodontics

Commissioning Editor: Michael Parkinson
Project Development Manager: Barbara Simmons
Project Manager: Frances Affleck
Designer: George Ajayi

MASTER DENTISTRY

VOLUME
2

Restorative Dentistry, Paediatric Dentistry and Orthodontics

Edited by

Peter Heasman BDS MDS FDSRCPS DRDRCS PhD

Professor of Periodontology
School of Dental Sciences
University of Newcastle upon Tyne
Newcastle upon Tyne

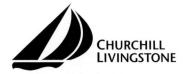

CHURCHILL
LIVINGSTONE

EDINBURGH LONDON NEW YORK OXFORD PHILADELPHIA
ST LOUIS SYDNEY TORONTO 2003

CHURCHILL LIVINGSTONE
An imprint of Elsevier Science Limited

First edition 2003

ISBN 0443 061939

British Library Cataloguing in Publication Data
A catalogue record for this book is available from the British Library

Library of Congress Cataloging in Publication Data
A catalog record for this book is available from the Library of Congress

Notice
Medical knowledge is constantly changing. Standard safety precautions
must be followed, but as new research and clinical experience broaden our
knowledge, changes in treatment and drug therapy may become necessary
or appropriate. Readers are advised to check the most current product
information provided by the manufacturer of each drug to be administered
to verify the recommended dose, the method and duration of
administration, and contraindications. It is the responsibility of the
practitioner, relying on experience and knowledge of the patient, to
determine dosages and the best treatment for each individual patient.
Neither the Publisher nor the author assumes any liability for any injury
and/or damage to persons or property arising from this publication.

 your source for books,
journals and multimedia
in the health sciences
www.elsevierhealth.com

The
publisher's
policy is to use
**paper manufactured
from sustainable forests**

Printed in Spain

Contributors

Craig W Barclay BDS FDSRCPS DRD MRD MPhil PhD
Consultant in Restorative Dentistry
University Dental Hospital of Manchester

Stewart C Barclay BDS FDSRCPS DRD MRD RCS
Consultant in Restorative Dentistry, Dental Hospital,
Newcastle upon Tyne

Peter Heasman BDS MDS FDSRCPS DRDRCS PhD
Professor of Peridontology, School of Dental Sciences,
University of Newcastle upon Tyne

Douglas Lovelock BDS MSc MDS FDSRCS DDRRCR
Head of Department of Radiology, Newcastle upon Tyne
Dental Hospital and School; Consultant in Oral Surgery and
Radiology, Newcastle upon Tyne Hospitals NHS Trust;
Honorary Senior Lecturer, University of Newcastle upon Tyne

Philip J Lumley BDS FDSRCPS MDentSci PhD FDSRCS
Senior Lecturer and Honorary Consultant in Restorative
Dentistry, University of Birmingham

Declan Millett BDSc DDS FDSRCPS DOrthRCS MOrth RCS
Senior Lecturer in Orthodontics, University of Glasgow
Dental School; Honorary Consultant in Orthodontics
Glasgow Dental Hospital and School, North Glasgow
University Hospitals NHS Trust

Nigel D Robb PhD, BDS, FDSRCSEd, FDS(Rest Dent), ILTM
Senior Lecturer in Sedation in Relation to Dentistry and
Honorary Consultant in Restorative Dentistry, Glasgow
Dental Hospital and School

Philip Preshaw BDS FRSRCS PhD
Lecturer in Restorative Dentistry, School of Dental Sciences,
University of Newcastle upon Tyne

Richard Welbury MBBS BDS PhD FDSRCS FDSRCPS
Professor of Paediatric Dentistry, Glasgow Dental Hospital
and School

Acknowledgment
We would like to thank John Brown, Dental Technician in
Orthodontics at Glasgow Dental Hospital, for his assistance
with the orthodontics chapters

Contents

Contents

Using this book

Philosophy of the book

Most students need a textbook that will provide all the basic facts within a discipline and that also facilitates understanding of the subject. This textbook achieves these objectives and also provides test questions for the student to explore their level of knowledge. It is also important for students to achieve a 'feel for the subject' and learn communication skills.

The book is designed to provide basic information necessary to pass an undergraduate examination in restorative, paediatric and orthodontic dentistry. It also expands on the core curriculum to allow the motivated student an opportunity to pursue the subject in greater detail. The information is presented in such a way as to aid recall for examination purposes but also to facilitate understanding of the subject. Key facts are highlighted, and principles of diagnosis and management emphasised. It is hoped that the book will also be a satisfactory basis for postgraduate practice and studies.

Do not think though that this book offers a 'syllabus'. It is impossible to draw boundaries around the scientific basis and clinical practice of dentistry. Learning is, therefore, a continuous process carried out throughout your career. This book includes all that you *must* know, most of what you *should* know, and some of what you *might* already know.

We assume that you are working towards one or more examinations, probably in order to qualify. Our purpose is to show you how to overcome this barrier. As we feel strongly that learning is not simply for the purpose of passing examinations, the book aims to help you to pass but also to develop *useful* knowledge and understanding.

This introductory chapter aims to help you:

- to understand how the emphasis on self-assessment can make learning easier and more enjoyable
- to use this book to increase your understanding as well as knowledge
- to plan your learning.

Layout and contents

Each chapter begins with a brief overview of the content and a number of learning objectives are listed at the start of each subsection. The main part of the text in each chapter describes important topics in major subject areas. We have tried to provide the essential information in a logical order with explanations and links. In order to help you, we have used lists to set out frameworks and to make it easier for you to put facts in a rational sequence. Tables are used to link quite complex and more detailed information. Techniques used in various procedures are listed in boxes.

You have to be sure that you are reaching the required standards, so the final section of each chapter is there to help you to check your knowledge and understanding. The self-assessment is in the form of multiple choice questions, case histories, short notes, data interpretation, possible viva questions and picture questions. Questions are designed to integrate knowledge across different chapters and to focus on the decisions you will have to take in a given clinical situation. Detailed answers are given with reference to relevant sections of the text; the answers also contain information and explanations that you will not find elsewhere, so you have to do the assessments to get the most out of this book.

How to use this book

If you are using this book as part of your examination preparations, we suggest that your first task should be to map out on a sheet of paper three lists dividing the major subjects (corresponding to the chapter headings) into your strong, reasonable and weak areas. This will give you a rough outline of your revision schedule, which you must then fit in with the time available. Clearly, if your examinations are looming, you will have to be ruthless in the time allocated to your strong areas. The major subjects should be further classified into individual topics. Encouragement to store information and to test your ongoing improvement is by the use of the self-assessment sections – you must not just read passively. It is important to keep checking your current level of knowledge, both strengths and weaknesses. This should be assessed objectively – self-rating in the absence of testing can be misleading. You may consider yourself strong in a particular area whereas it is more a reflection on how much you enjoy and are stimulated by the subject. Conversely, you may be stronger in a subject than you would expect simply because the topic does not appeal to you.

It is a good idea to discuss topics and problems with colleagues/friends; the areas that you understand least well will soon become apparent when you try to explain them to someone else.

Effective learning

You may have wondered why an approach to learning that was so successful in secondary school does not always work at university. One of the key differences between your studies at school and your current learning task is that you are now given more responsibility for setting your own learning objectives. While your aims are undoubtedly to pass examinations, you should also aim to develop learning skills that will serve you throughout your career. That means taking full responsibility for self-directed learning. The earlier you start, the more likely you are to develop the learning skills you will need to keep up with changes in clinical practice.

We know that students learn in all sorts of different ways, and differ in their learning patterns at different stages in a given course. You may intend to do as little work as you can get away with, or you may do the least that will guarantee to get you through the examinations; however, the students who gain most are usually those who take a deep and sustained interest in the subject. It will be worth the effort to start out this way, even if good intentions flag a little towards the end.

You will also get more out of your course by participating actively. Handouts, if given, may help, but they are rarely a satisfactory substitute for your own lecture notes. Remember that timetabled teaching sessions are not the only opportunities for effective learning. It is safer to regard lectures, practicals and tutorials as a guide to the core material that you are expected to master. Greater depth and breadth to this core knowledge must be achieved by reference to more detailed texts. Well-organised departments will provide a set of learning objectives and a reading list early in the course. Many lecturers will give more detailed learning objectives, either in their handouts or verbally at the start of a lecture. If not, paragraph headings can be used as a rough guide to the teacher's expectations. An active approach to learning does not necessarily mean being highly individualistic or over competitive. Many students gain a broader and deeper understanding of the subject by working in small informal groups. This may be particularly helpful when it comes to revision.

The final run up to examinations should require little more than a tying up of loose ends, and a filling of learning gaps. An effective way of doing this is to work through a steady stream of self-assessment questions and to keep a daily note of points that need clearing up. In other words, concentrate on what you do not know and strengthen the links with what you already know. By this time, the value of pigeonholing factual information within a framework should be self-evident.

Approaching the examinations

The discipline of learning is closely linked to preparation for examinations. Many of us opt for a process of superficial learning that is directed towards retention of facts and recall under examination conditions because full understanding is often not required. It is much better if you try to acquire a deeper knowledge and understanding, combining the necessity of passing examinations with longer-term needs.

First you need to know how you will be examined. Does the examination involve clinical assessment such as history taking and clinical examination? If you are sitting a written examination what are the length and types of question? How many must you answer and how much choice will you have?

Now you have to choose what sources you are going to use for your learning and revision. Textbooks come in different forms. At one extreme, there is the large reference book. This type of book should be avoided at this stage of revision and only used (if at all) for reference, when answers to questions cannot be found in smaller books. At the other end of the spectrum is the condensed 'lecture note' format, which often relies heavily on lists. Facts of this nature on their own are difficult to remember if they are not supported by understanding. In the middle of the range are the medium-sized textbooks. These are often valuable irrespective of whether you are approaching final university examinations or the first part of professional examinations. Our advice is to choose one of the several medium-sized books on offer on the basis of which you find the most readable. The best approach is to combine your lecture notes, textbooks (appropriate to the level of study) and past examination papers as a framework for your preparation.

Armed with information about the format of the examinations, a rough syllabus, your own lecture notes and some books that you feel comfortable in using, your next step is to map out the time available for preparation. You must be realistic, allow time for breaks and work *steadily*, not cramming. If you do attempt to cram, you have to realise that only a certain amount of information can be retained in your short-term memory. Cramming simply retains facts. If the examination requires understanding, you will undoubtedly have problems.

It is often a good idea to begin by outlining the topics to be covered and then attempting to summarise your knowledge about each in note form. In this way your existing knowledge will be activated and any gaps will become apparent. Self-assessment also helps to determine the time to be allocated to each subject for examination preparation. If you are consistently scoring excellent marks in a particular subject, it is not very effective to spend a lot of time trying to achieve the 'perfect' mark.

In an essay, it is many times easier to obtain the first 50% of the marks than the last. You should also try to decide on the amount of time to assign to each subject based on the likelihood of it appearing in the examination.

The main types of examination

Multiple choice questions

Most multiple choice questions test recall of information. The aim is to gain the maximum marks from what you can remember. The common form consists of a stem with several different phrases that complete the statement. Each statement is to be considered in isolation from the rest and you have to decide whether it is 'True' or 'False'. There is no need for 'Trues' and 'Falses' to balance out for statements based on the same stem; they may all be 'True' or all 'False'. The stem must be read with great care and, if it is long with several lines of text or data, you should try and summarise it by extracting the essential elements. Make sure you look out for the 'little' words in the stem such as *only*, *rarely*, *usually*, *never* and *always*. Negatives such as *not*, *unusual* and *unsuccessful* often cause marks to be lost. *May occur* has entirely different connotations to *characteristic*. The latter generally indicates a feature that is normally observed, the absence of which would represent an exception to a general rule, e.g. regular elections are a characteristic of a democratic society. Regular (if dubious) elections may occur in a dictatorship but they are not characteristic.

Remember to check the marking method before starting. Most employ a negative system in which marks are lost for incorrect answers. The temptation is to adopt a cautious approach answering a relatively small number of questions. This can lead to problems, however, as we all make simple mistakes or even disagree vehemently with the answer favoured by the examiner! Caution may lead you to answer too few questions to pass after the marks have been deducted for incorrect answers.

Essays

Essays are not negatively marked. Relevant facts will receive marks as will a logical development of the argument or theme. Conversely, good marks will not be obtained for an essay that is a set of unconnected statements. Length matters little if there is no cohesion. Relevant graphs and diagrams should also be included but must be properly labelled.

Most people are aware of the need to 'plan' their answer yet few do this. Make sure that what you put in your plan is relevant to the question asked, as irrelevant material is, at best, a waste of valuable time and, at worst, causes the examiner to doubt your understanding. It is especially important in an examination based on essays that time is

managed and all questions are given equal weight, unless guided otherwise in the instructions. A brilliant answer in one essay will not compensate for not attempting another because of time. Nobody can get more than 100% (usually 70–80%, tops) on a single answer! It may even be useful to begin with the questions about which you feel you have least to say so that any time left over can be safely devoted to your areas of strength at the end.

Short notes

Short notes are not negatively marked. The system is usually for a 'marking template' to be devised that gives a mark(s) for each important fact (also called criterion marking). Nothing is gained for style or superfluous information. The aim is to set out your knowledge in an ordered, concise manner. The major faults of students are, first, devoting too much time to a single question thereby neglecting the rest and, second, not limiting their answer to the question asked. For example, in a question about the treatment of periodontal disease all facts about periodontal disease should not be listed, only those relevant to its treatment.

Picture questions

Pattern recognition is the first step in a picture quiz. This should be coupled with a systematic approach looking for, and listing, abnormalities. For example the general appearance of the facial skeleton as well as the local appearance of the individual bones and any soft tissue shadows can be examined in any radiograph. Make an attempt to describe what you see even if you are in doubt. Use any additional statements or data that accompany the radiographs as they will give a clue to the answer required.

Case history questions

A more sophisticated form of examination question is an evolving case history with information being presented sequentially; you are asked to give a response at each stage. They are constructed so that a wrong response in the first part of the question still means that you can obtain marks from the subsequent parts. Patient management problems are designed to test the recall and application of knowledge through an understanding of the principles involved. You should always give answers unless the instructions indicate the presence of negative marking.

Viva

The viva examination can be a nerve-wracking experience. You are normally faced with two examiners (perhaps including an external examiner) who may react with irritation, boredom or indifference to what you say. You should try and strike a balance between saying too little and too much. It is important to try not to go off the topic. Aim to keep your answers short and to the point. It is worthwhile pausing for a few seconds to collect your thoughts before launching into an answer. Do not be afraid to say 'I don't know'; most examiners will want to change tack to see what you do know.

In many centres, vivas are offered to candidates who have either distinguished themselves or who are in danger of failing. Interviews for the two types of candidate vary considerably. In the 'distinction' setting, the examiner may try to discover what the candidate does *not* know and may also be looking for evidence of knowledge of the current literature. A small number of topics will usually be considered in depth. In the pass/fail setting, the examiner will try to cover many topics, often quite superficially. She/he will try to establish whether the candidate did badly in the written examination because of ignorance in just a couple of areas, or whether ignorance is wide ranging.

Remember also that the examiners may have your written paper in front of them; if you have done particularly badly in one topic, they may well take this up in the viva. This is not an attempt to be unpleasant, but a chance for you to redeem yourself somewhat, so be prepared.

Conclusions

You should amend your framework for using this book according to your own needs and the examinations you are facing. Whatever approach you adopt, your aim should be for an understanding of the principles involved rather than rote learning of a large number of poorly connected facts.

1 Periodontology

Overview

A healthy or a stable periodontium is an important prerequisite both for the maintenance of a functional dentition and to ensure a long-term, successful outcome of restorative dental treatment. In view of the high prevalence of gingivitis and chronic periodontitis in the population, all dental patients should undergo periodontal screening, although more thorough clinical and radiographic examinations are essential before a definitive periodontal diagnosis is confirmed and a treatment plan formulated. These examinations, together with medical, dental and social histories may also reveal predisposing and risk factors that increase an individual's susceptibility to, and the subsequent rate of progression of, periodontal disease.

The intensive oral hygiene phase of treatment and the patient's compliance with a personalised plaque control regimen are of major importance in stabilising the disease and improving the long-term prognosis for an affected dentition. Scaling and root planing are frequently indicated to debride tooth surfaces of plaque, calculus and necrotic cementum.

Additional adjunctive treatments that may be indicated are periodontal surgery, guided tissue regeneration, systemic or locally delivered antimicrobials and the management of localised problems such as furcation defects, mucogingival problems, periodontal–endodontic lesions and loss of attachment that has been exacerbated by a traumatic occlusion.

1.1 Healthy periodontium

Learning objectives

You should

- know the clinical and radiographic features of healthy periodontal tissues in adults and in children
- be familiar with the histological structures of the periodontium.

The diagnostic skills required to identify periodontal diseases, particularly in the early stages, are based upon a sound knowledge of the clinical appearance of healthy tissues.

Clinical features

The gingiva is pink, firm in texture and extends from the free gingival margin to the mucogingival line. The interdental papillae are pyramidal in shape and occupy the interdental spaces beneath the contact points of the teeth. Gingiva is keratinised and stippling is frequently present. The gingiva comprises the free and the attached portions.

The free gingiva is the most coronal band of unattached tissue demarcated by the free gingival groove, which can sometimes be detected clinically. The depth of the gingival sulcus ranges from 0.5 to 3.0 mm.

The attached gingiva is firmly bound to underlying cementum and alveolar bone and extends apically from the free gingival groove to the mucogingival junction. The width of attached gingiva varies considerably throughout the mouth. It is usually narrower on the lingual aspect of the mandibular incisors and labially, adjacent to the canines and first premolars. In the absence of inflammation, the width of the attached gingiva *increases* with age.

The mucogingival line is often indistinct. It defines the junction between the keratinised, attached gingiva and the oral mucosa. Oral mucosa is non-keratinised and, therefore, appears redder than the adjacent gingiva. The tissues can be distinguished by staining with Schiller iodine solution; keratinised gingiva stains orange and non-keratinised mucosa stains purple/blue. This can be used to determine clinically the width of keratinised tissue that remains, for example, in areas of gingival recession.

Radiographic features

The crest of the interdental alveolar bone is well defined and lies approximately 0.5–1.5 mm apical to the cementoenamel junction (Fig. 1). The periodontal membrane space, often identifiable on intraoral radiographs taken using a paralleling technique, is approximately 0.1–0.2 mm wide. This accounts for the minimal tooth mobility that is observed when lateral pressure is applied to a tooth with a healthy periodontium.

Histology

Epithelial components **include (Fig. 1):**

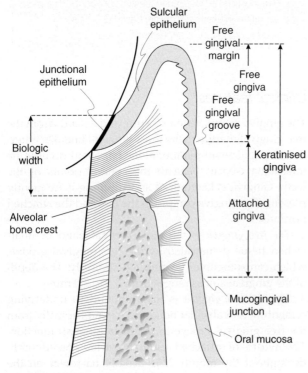

Fig. 1 Diagrammatic representation of the epithelial and connective tissue attachments of the gingiva.

- junctional epithelium cells: non-keratinised and attached to the tooth surface by a basal lamina and hemidesmosomes
- sulcular epithelium: non-keratinised and lines the gingival crevice
- oral epithelium: keratinised and extends from the free gingival margin to the mucogingival line.

Gingival connective tissue core contains ground substance, blood vessels and lymphatics, nerves, fibroblasts and bundles of gingival collagen fibres (dentogingival, alveologingival, circular and trans-septal). The combined epithelial and gingival fibre attachment to the tooth surface is the *biologic width*, which is typically 2 mm, not including the sulcus depth (Fig. 1).

Periodontal connective tissues comprise alveolar bone, periodontal ligament, principal and oxytalan fibres, cells, ground substance, nerves, blood vessels and lymphatics, and cementum.

Periodontal tissues in children

The gingiva in children may appear red and inflamed. Compared with mature tissue there is a thinner epithelium that is less keratinised, greater vascularity of connective tissues and less variation in the width of the attached gingiva.

During tooth eruption, the gingival sulcus depths may reach 5 mm and gingival margins will be at different levels on adjacent teeth. Following tooth eruption a persistent hyperaemia can lead to swollen and rounded interproximal papillae, thus giving an appearance of gingivitis.

Radiographic features

In the primary dentition, the radiographic distance between the cementoenamel junction (CEJ) and the alveolar crest is 0–2 mm. Greater variation (0–4 mm) is observed at sites adjacent to erupting permanent teeth and exfoliating primary teeth. The periodontal membrane space is wider in children because of the thinner cementum, immature alveolar bone and a more vascular periodontal ligament.

Gingival crevicular fluid

Gingival crevicular fluid (GCF) is a serum exudate that is derived from the microvasculature of the gingiva and periodontal ligament. The 'preinflammatory' flow of GCF may be mediated by by-products from subgingival plaque that diffuse intercellularly and accumulate adjacent to the basement membrane of the junctional epithelium. This creates an osmotic gradient; consequently, GCF flow can be regarded as a transudate rather than an inflammatory exudate.

GCF is, in some ways, similar to serum but also contains components from microbial sources, interstitial fluid and locally produced inflammatory and immune products of host origin. The proportions of these components are dependent upon:

- the presence and composition of subgingival plaque
- the rate of turnover of gingival connective tissue
- the permeability of epithelia
- the degree of inflammation.

Several techniques have been developed for collecting GCF from the gingival sulcus:

- absorbent paper strips
- microcapillary tubes
- gingival washing.

The fluid can then be analysed for specific mediators of the immunoinflammatory response (for example cytokines) and breakdown products of connective tissues, both of which have been associated with ongoing periodontal destruction.

1.2 History and examination

Learning objectives

You should

- understand the importance of obtaining thorough histories (medical, social and presenting complaint) from patients who attend for treatment

- know those medical conditions that impact upon periodontal diseases and therapy

- be familiar with the diagnostic procedures and special tests to be used when evaluating patients with periodontitis.

From the periodontal viewpoint, the aims of history-taking and the clinical examination are to establish the extent of periodontal destruction and to evaluate the effects of disease on the remaining dentition. It is also important to evaluate the individual patient's susceptibility to periodontal disease and, as far as possible, identify the sites that appear to be associated with active or ongoing destruction and need to be considered a priority for treatment.

Presenting complaint

One of the principal features of periodontal diseases is that their onset and progression occur very often in the absence of pain. This means that the onus for detection rests firmly with the clinician, and the importance of regular examinations must be impressed upon the patient, with emphasis placed on prevention rather than cure. The well-informed patient who is a regular dental attender should be able to detect some of the signs or symptoms that are associated with the early stages of plaque accumulation. Unfortunately, many patients are irregular dental attenders and only present with complaints that are the consequence of oral neglect. When gingivitis and periodontal inflammation do cause symptoms, the chief complaints are usually 'bleeding gums', 'bad taste or breath', 'localised pain' and teeth that have 'changed position' or 'become loose'. Details of when such problems started, the frequency of pain or discomfort, and any associated symptoms should be recorded. The expectations of the patient with regard to the outcome of treatment should also be discussed at this stage.

Gingival bleeding

Bleeding gums is perhaps the most common complaint of patients with periodontal disease. The bleeding is usually noticed during, or following, toothbrushing or eating. When bleeding occurs spontaneously, a patient may complain of tasting blood on awakening in the morning. The severity of the haemorrhage does not necessarily relate to the severity of disease, as a marginal gingivitis can be associated with quite profuse bleeding. Gingival bleeding is exacerbated by the use of certain drugs (anticoagulants, antithrombotics and fibrinolytic agents). Symptoms of relatively recent and sudden onset should be investigated thoroughly during the taking of the medical history.

Drifting of teeth

Drifting of anterior teeth and the appearance of spaces between teeth are often the first signs of an underlying periodontal problem. When teeth begin to drift it is because their periodontal support has been compromised to such an extent that the teeth are no longer in equilibrium with forces from occlusion and the adjacent soft tissues. In some instances, this position of equilibrium is so finely balanced that the destruction of only crestal bone and the coronal periodontal fibre groups will precipitate changes in tooth position. Furthermore, the pressures exerted on the teeth by gingiva that are swollen through oedematous or fibrous change can also induce tooth movement. Drifting of anterior teeth may also be a consequence of an occlusal interference in the posterior segments, which leads to a forward slide of the mandible during its arc of movement from the retruded contact position to the intercuspal position.

Loose teeth

When periodontal disease remains untreated, attachment loss is progressive and teeth become increasingly mobile. The degree of mobility that some patients accept before attending for treatment is remarkable and many patients still believe that increasing tooth mobility and, ultimately, tooth loss is a natural consequence of the ageing process. An increase in mobility also occurs when a tooth is subject to increased or abnormal occlusal forces, particularly those of a 'jiggling' nature. Mobility may be the first signs of an advanced stage of periodontitis or perhaps a rapidly progressive, or aggressive, type of disease.

Bad taste and halitosis

Altered sensation of taste can accompany the halitosis that is associated with

- necrotising ulcerative gingivitis (NUG)
- purulent exudate from a periodontal abscess
- poor oral hygiene/accumulated food debris from packing beneath open contact points, in furcations, beneath overhanging or leaking restorations, and associated with dentures
- excessive bacterial growth on the dorsal surface of the tongue.

Pain

Acute and often quite severe pain is a feature of necrotising ulcerative gingivitis and herpetic gingivostomatitis. Pain, particularly on eating, is also a symptom of an acute periodontal abscess and/or a periodontal–endodontic lesion. Gingival recession with exposure of root surfaces can also precipitate pain if dentine is exposed as a result of toothbrush abrasion. This pain is characterised as sharp and transient, with a sudden onset that is precipitated by extremes of temperature. Pain is not typically a feature of chronic periodontitis, however.

Dental history

The dental history provides an indication of the patient's overall attitude to dental care. Lengthy intervals between appointments and attendance for only symptomatic treatment suggest a low priority on dental health and a patient who is unlikely to appreciate comprehensive periodontal care.

The reasons for previous loss of teeth should be established and a record made of previous and recent dental treatment. Information (including radiographs) relating to previous dental treatment should, whenever possible, be sought by written request from a previous dentist, and the written response incorporated in the patient's notes. Another criterion sometimes used to assess dental behaviour is the frequency with which a patient brushes (or claims to brush!) his or her teeth. It is more important to assess the efficiency of the method of toothbrushing rather than to place too much emphasis on frequency. An individual who brushes once a day for 4–5 minutes is often able to maintain a superior standard of oral hygiene than a patient who brushes several times a day, but ineffectively and for only short periods of time.

In young patients in particular, a note should be made of previous orthodontic treatment. Extended periods of fixed appliance therapy can cause loss of crestal alveolar bone partly from tooth movements and partly from the periodontal inflammation that is a consequence of limited access to cleaning interproximally and subgingivally. More importantly from the diagnostic viewpoint, teeth that have been tipped rather than moved bodily through bone often have an angular alveolar crest on the mesial and distal surfaces. Such topography gives the appearance of the lesions often seen in localised aggressive periodontitis.

Social history

Details of the patient's occupation, marital status, diet and consumption of alcohol and tobacco should be noted. Periodontal status appears to be linked to social class as defined by occupation. Generally, those with non-manual occupational backgrounds tend to have healthier gingiva and less calculus than those from unskilled, manual backgrounds. When an occupation involves considerable social contact (e.g. teachers, shop assistants and lawyers), there may be a greater awareness of small changes of tooth position and appearance.

Stress induced by examinations, divorce, or change of employment should also be noted as they may promote bruxism and aggravate existing tooth mobility from periodontal disease. Stress has been shown to be associated with osteoporosis of alveolar bone, reduced osteoblastic activity, the formation of periodontal pockets, delayed wound healing of connective tissue and bone, and necrotising ulcerative gingivitis (NUG). As most patients have some element of stress in their lives, the potential influence of this on bone metabolism and periodontal disease should be appreciated. A lack of ability to cope with stress, and particularly financial strain, has been implicated as a specific risk factor in periodontal disease.

Smoking is a known risk factor for periodontal disease and is considered in Section 1.6. The frequency and duration of smoking should be established and the detrimental effects of smoking on periodontal health must be conveyed to the patient before any treatment is started.

It should now be apparent that much of the information that can be derived from a thorough personal and dental history has a bearing on establishing the susceptibility of an individual to periodontal disease. When potential risk factors are established, it is often not possible to determine their individual effects on the disease process, as many of the factors are inter-related. For example, an individual who has job insecurity and is under financial strain may be also a smoker and a poor dental attender.

Medical history

A thorough medical history must be recorded and updated at each visit. The patient's perception of their present health status is also a valuable indicator of their psychological make-up and potential compliance with treatment.

A patient with a history of rheumatic fever, congenital cardiac defects or prosthetic heart valves may require antibiotic prophylaxis before periodontal probing and treatment. Whenever possible, this should be confirmed by the patient's general medical practitioner or consultant. Patients who have received prosthetic joint implants do not routinely require antibiotic prophylaxis. Patients with cardiac pacemakers also do not need prophylaxis but ultrasonic scalers and other dental electromagnetic devices should not be used as they may interfere with normal function of the pacemaker.

Diabetic patients are at particular risk of periodontal breakdown, especially when poorly controlled. A positive family history should be noted and vigilant periodontal monitoring undertaken. The HIV-positive patient is also at risk from very extensive and aggressive periodontal breakdown.

Patients with particular food fads or unusual diets should be questioned as part of an overall dietary analysis to evaluate their vitamin and protein intake. Nutritional deficiencies may modify the severity and extent of periodontal disease by altering the host resistance and potential for repair although such deficiencies are rare in Westernised societies.

Gastric hyperacidity and reflux from hiatus hernia and gastric ulceration predispose to erosion and root caries if there is existing gingival recession. Pregnant patients should be monitored carefully during the second and third trimesters as endocrine changes may lead to marked gingival inflammation and the development of epulides. Radiographic assessment of periodontal disease should be avoided during pregnancy.

Current medications must be noted, especially dosage and types of medication: particularly anticoagulants, steroids, analgesics and sedatives. When a patient is receiving anticoagulant therapy, the general medical practitioner or patient's physician must be consulted with a view to modifying the anticoagulant dosage to coincide with invasive periodontal treatment, thus reducing the risk of postoperative haemorrhage. Some drugs such as phenytoin, ciclosporin and nifedipine can cause gingival overgrowth, which may compromise good oral hygiene leading to aesthetic problems. Antimicrobials often used in the treatment of periodontal diseases are contraindicated for certain patients for whom the unwanted effects of the drugs may be enhanced, or because of a potential interaction with drugs that the patient is already taking.

Examination

Extraoral examination

A careful extraoral examination may reveal important signs that are associated with periodontal problems. A severe periodontal abscess can lead to facial swelling and a regional lymphadenopathy. The temporomandibular joints should be palpated routinely, noting joint pain, noise or limitation of opening. The location in the opening cycle (recorded as millimetres of opening and closing) at which crepitus or clicking occurs is recorded and freedom of mandibular movement in function evaluated. A mandibular displacement on closing can be a consequence of a traumatic occlusion, which may have periodontal sequelae.

Prominent maxillary incisors make a lip seal difficult to achieve, which may aggravate an existing gingivitis. The drying effect on exposed gingiva produced by mouthbreathing leads to enlarged and erythematous gingiva, particularly in the maxillary anterior region. Mouthbreathing does not inevitably lead to increased plaque accumulation and gingivitis but should be regarded as a predisposing factor in a susceptible patient.

Intraoral examination

A record should be made of local factors that predispose to the accumulation of plaque, for example, restorations with overhanging margins, poorly contoured and deficient restorations, and partial dentures.

A quick and simple method of assessing the level of oral hygiene is to score, after disclosing, the number of plaque-covered smooth tooth surfaces as a percentage of all smooth surfaces. On each surface, plaque is recorded as being either present or absent (a dichotomous scoring method). Patients are informed of their scores and realistic targets can be set for the patient to achieve at future visits. This method gives a useful overall assessment of plaque control as well as identifying tooth surfaces that are difficult to clean. These occur typically at interproximal sites and on the lingual smooth surfaces of mandibular molars.

In epidemiological studies, it is easier and quicker to select six teeth/subject to be representative of the entire dentition when scoring plaque. The so-called Ramfjord teeth are $\frac{6}{4}\frac{/1}{1/}\frac{4}{6}$; if any one tooth is missing, then the distal neighbouring tooth should be used. A significant number of indices are now available for scoring plaque, oral debris and calculus on a quantitative basis (Table 1). These indices can be applied to a full dentition or to the selected Ramfjord teeth and may be used to monitor plaque control in the individual patient and/or to use in clinical trials and epidemiological studies.

Periodontal diseases and gingivitis occur in all patients regardless of age. Chronic periodontitis is prevalent in adults and gingivitis is extremely common in children. Furthermore, children and young adults are also at risk from the more aggressive, early-onset diseases. It is, therefore, imperative that all dental patients undergo a screening examination to provide a rapid, basic assessment of periodontal status. The basic periodontal examination (BPE) has evolved from the Community Periodontal Index of Treatment Needs (CPITN) and is a quick method for assessing a patient's periodontal status. The examination involves the use of a specially designed periodontal probe with a 0.5 mm diameter ball end and a coloured band extending 3.5–5.5 mm from the tip (Fig. 2). The dentition is divided into sextants; each tooth is probed circumferentially and only the highest score in each sextant is recorded. The score codes are used as a guide to determine the need for periodontal treatment (Table 2). If the results of the screening examination indicate the presence of periodontal disease (code 4) then a detailed periodontal examination should be undertaken.

Gingiva

Visual examination of the gingiva may reveal colour changes of the tissues, gingival swelling (generalised or localised), ulceration, suppuration and gingival recession. Where there is gingival enlargement, the tissues should be probed gently to assess consistency and texture. Oedematous tissues are soft and may have a tendency to bleed spontaneously or following pressure and gentle manipulation. Conversely, fibrous tissue is usually quite firm and resistant to pressure.

The width of attached gingiva should be assessed and measured as the distance from the free gingival margin to the mucogingival line minus the depth of the gingival crevice (in health) or periodontal pocket (when disease is present). Sites with minimal or no apparent attached gingiva should be noted together with the inflammatory condition of the associated marginal tissues. At such sites, the attached gingiva can be dyed with Schiller iodine solution so that the border between

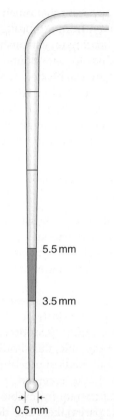

5.5 mm

3.5 mm

0.5 mm

Fig. 2 Colour-coded probe for the basic periodontal examination. (WHO probe – World Health Organization probe.)

the keratinised (orange) and non-keratinised (dark blue) epithelium (mucogingival junction) is seen and the actual width of keratinised tissue becomes more readily apparent. Sites of gingival recession are recorded by measuring from the CEJ to the free gingival margin of the affected site. Sensitivity of associated exposed root surfaces should also be recorded.

The presence of a prominent labial frenum may effectively reduce the width of attached gingiva, although the precise role of a frenal attachment as a predisposing factor to gingival recession is disputed. A prominent frenum can, however, reduce sulcus depth and restrict access for toothbrushing; it can thus lead to the development of local periodontal problems.

Periodontal probing

Periodontal probing should be undertaken systematically on each tooth to determine the probing depth, the presence of bleeding after probing and the extent of attachment loss. The probe should be moved gently around the sulcus to avoid trauma. A force of approximately 0.25 N is recommended, but this is difficult to achieve consistently without the use of a pressure-sensitive probe. An attempt should be made to probe along the contour of the root surface although interproximally it is necessary to angle the probe slightly

Table 1 Indices for scoring oral debris, plaque and calculus

Index	Deposit	Scoring system	Score
Plaque index (Silness and Löe, 1964)	Plaque	0 no plaque 1 film of plaque seen with disclosing solution or by running probe along surface 2 moderate accumulation seen with naked eye 3 abundance of plaque in pocket and on tooth surface	Record on four surfaces of tooth. Divide total by number of surfaces scored
Plaque index (Quigley and Hein, 1962)	Plaque	0 no plaque 1 separate flecks at cervical margin 2 continuous band of plaque ≤1 mm wide at cervical margin 3 band of plaque ≥1 mm wide but covering <1/3 of coronal tooth surface 4 plaque on >1/3 but <2/3 of coronal surface 5 plaque on >2/3 of coronal tooth surface	Record scores on four surfaces of each tooth. Divide total by number of surfaces scored
Oral hygiene index (Greene and Vermillion, 1960)	Scores debris and calculus as separate components	0 no deposits 1 not covering more than 1/3 of exposed tooth surface 2 coronal deposits >1/3 but <2/3 of tooth surface; individual flecks of subgingival calculus 3 deposits on >2/3 tooth surface; continuous band of subgingival calculus	Scores made on facial and lingual surfaces. Record worst score/sextant. Index = total scores number of sextants
Volpe–Manhold index (VMI 1969)	Calculus	The height and width of calculus is measured with a graduated probe along three planes on the lingual surfaces of six lower anterior teeth	Any calculus scores 0.5 mm; Index is the sum of the individual measurements divided by the number of scores made
Calculus surface severity index (CSSI) (Ennever et al., 1961)	Calculus	0 no calculus 1 calculus <0.5 mm in width and/or thickness 2 calculus not exceeding 1.00 mm in width and/or thickness 3 calculus exceeding 1.0 mm in width and thickness	The scale is used to measure quantitatively the presence of calculus on each of four surfaces of the mandibular incisors

Ennever J, Sturzenberger O P, Radike A W 1961 The Calculus Surface Index method for scoring clinical calculus studies. J Periodontol 32: 54–57
Greene J C, Vermillion J R 1960 The oral hygiene index: a method for classifying oral hygiene status. J Am Dental Assoc 61: 172–179
Quigley G A, Hein J W 1962 Comparative cleaning efficiency of manual and power brushing. J Am Dental Assoc 65: 26–29
Silness J, Löe H 1964 Periodontal disease in pregnancy. II. Correlation between oral hygiene and periodontal condition. Acta Odont Scand 24: 747–759
Volpe A R, Manhold J H 1962 A method of evaluating the effectiveness of potential calculus inhibiting agents. N Y State Dental J 28: 289–290

Table 2 The Basic Periodontal Examination (BPE)

Code[a]	Probing	Treatment needs
0	Coloured area of the probe is completely visible; no calculus detected; no gingival bleeding on probing	No need for periodontal treatment
1	Coloured area is completely visible; no calculus detected; bleeding on probing	Oral hygiene instruction (OHI)
2	Coloured area is completely visible; supra- or subgingival calculus detected, or overhanging restorations	OHI; elimination of plaque-retentive areas; scaling and root planing (SRP)
3	Coloured area is partly visible, indicating probing depth	OHI; Elimination of plaque-retentive areas; SRP
4	Coloured area completely disappears, indicating probing depth of greater than 3.5 mm but less than 5.5 mm	Complex treatment in addition to OHI and SRP; referral to a specialist may be necessary

[a]The symbol (*) should be added to score when furcation involvement is evident or when the pocket depth and gingival recession is 7 mm or greater.

Periodontology

to reach the site directly beneath the contact area. This site should be probed from the buccal and the lingual aspects since deep pockets frequently develop here.

A number of factors may lead to errors in measuring probing depths

- thickness of the probe
- contour of the tooth surface
- angulation of probing
- pressure applied
- presence of calculus deposits.

The extent of inflammation is also important. A probe will more easily penetrate the pocket epithelium and the adjacent connective tissues when there is a prominent inflammatory cell infiltrate. A probing depth measurement is influenced by the position of the gingival margin and the integrity of the tissues at the base of the pocket, and these factors are dependent upon the extent of inflammation in the tissues. Attempts have been made to reduce probing errors by using constant pressure probes and, more recently, electronic probes. In addition, computer-assisted probes have been developed for automatic recording of probe measurements or to allow voice-activated data entry. These probes have a high degree of resolution, measuring with a precision of 0.1–0.2 mm, but their accuracy and repeatability still depends upon angulation and positioning of the probe.

A more precise assessment of the degree of periodontal destruction is made by measuring from the CEJ to the base of the pocket. This gives an approximation of the loss of connective tissue attachment to the root surface. The loss of attachment is easier to measure when there has been gingival recession and the CEJ is visible. When patients are being monitored longitudinally before and after treatment, sequential attachment level measurements can be made relative to a fixed point, for example an incisal edge or cusp tip. The differences between successive measurements then give an estimate of the *change* in attachment level, which is often used to assess the success or failure of a particular treatment.

About 20–30 seconds after probing, each site is re-evaluated to determine the presence or absence of bleeding from the base of the pocket. Bleeding is simply a consequence of the trauma caused by probing the epithelial pocket lining and connective tissue. Gingival bleeding after probing has been implicated as an *indicator* of active disease. Longitudinal clinical trials, however, suggest that bleeding has a low sensitivity for disease progression. Conversely, absence of bleeding is a good indicator of periodontal health or inactivity. Any site with a probing depth of less than 4 mm that does not exhibit bleeding on probing is not likely to require treatment beyond supragingival scaling and polishing.

Furcation involvement

A curved explorer is used to determine the topography of the furcation lesion in multi-rooted teeth, allowing accurate classification into three groups.

Class I has initial involvement. The tissue destruction does not exceed more than 3 mm (or not more than one third of the tooth width) into the furcation.

Class II includes cul-de-sac involvement. The tissue destruction extends deeper than 3 mm (or more than one-third of the tooth width) into the furcation but does not completely pass through the furcation.

Class III has through-and-through involvement. The lesion extends across the entire width of the furcation; consequently, an instrument can be passed between the roots to emerge on the other side of the tooth.

Tooth mobility

Mobility is assessed by applying a labio-lingual, horizontal force to each tooth in turn using the handles of dental mirrors. Movement is scored according to a simple index such as:

0 normal, physiological mobility (<0.3 mm)
1 horizontal mobility >0.3 to 1.0 mm
2 moderate horizontal mobility exceeding 1.0 mm
3 severe mobility exceeding 2.0 mm in horizontal plane or vertical movements.

Diagnostic investigations

Radiographic evaluation

Radiographic selection criteria for periodontal disease should take into account the diagnosis made from the clinical examination and the overall state of the patient's dentition. The panoramic radiograph is an acceptable alternative to full-mouth periapical radiography on the basis of diagnostic yield of clinically unsuspected patterns of bone loss. The panoramic view is useful for screening but rarely provides the detail of periodontal status seen on full-mouth periapical films. It is often necessary, therefore, to supplement the panoramic radiograph with individual, non-geometrically standardised films, which are simple to take and provide a better visual interpretation of bone topography. In the posterior segments, vertical bitewings are often a useful supplement if a panoramic view suggests bone loss localised to this region.

Features that can be identified on full-mouth, periapical films are:

- pattern of bone loss: horizontal/vertical, localised/generalised
- furcation involvement
- variation in root anatomy
- subgingival calculus

- widening of the periodontal membrane space
- periapical infection (periodontal–endodontic lesions)
- overhanging restorations.

A decreased alveolar bone height on a radiograph is only a historical record of previous periodontal involvement and gives little, if any, information on recent or current activity. Standardised, sequential radiographs have been used in association with computerised techniques to evaluate bone loss or gain over intervals as short as 6 months. The images of successive films are digitised and then subtracted to identify changes in bone height of as little as 0.1 mm and bone mass changes of about 1.0 mg. Longitudinal studies suggest that digital subtraction radiography has considerable potential for the sensitive detection of bone changes in clinical trials, although the expense of the basic apparatus precludes this technique from use in the General Dental Services.

Microbial sampling

Some species of periodontal pathogens can be identified by sampling directly from the periodontal pocket and growing colonies of the organisms under suitable conditions on culture media in the laboratory. This method has the advantage that antimicrobial sensitivity testing can be undertaken to identify antimicrobials that may be valuable as part of the treatment. Unfortunately, finding a service laboratory that has experience in culturing periodontal samples is likely to be a problem for many general practitioners. Furthermore, a number of species that are strictly anaerobic will fail to survive unless special sampling methods are adopted.

A number of other methods have been used for identification of bacteria (or their products) in subgingival plaque. Some of these have been developed into tests for use at the chairside so the clinician can determine more immediately the presence or absence of certain pathogens. One bacterial test is an immunological assay that detects surface antigens of three species of bacteria associated with periodontal disease: *Actinobacillus actinomycetemcomitans*, *Porphyromonas gingivalis* and *Prevotella intermedia*. The kit is designed for use at the chairside and incorporates a colorimetric detection system to define a positive antigen–antibody reaction for each of the three species. Enzymatic methods identify specific bacteria through their production of specific enzymes. This method has been developed as another chairside diagnostic test for detecting bacteria which produce any trypsin-like enzyme that hydrolyses a naphthylamide (BANA) substrate, forming a positive blue colour reaction on a diagnostic strip.

The application of molecular biology to diagnostic periodontics has led to the development of DNA and RNA probes to identify species-specific sequences of nucleotide bases in periodontopathic organisms. This is the basis of an off-site screening service where samples are mailed to a laboratory for analysis. A chairside detection system involves lysis of organisms from subgingival plaque, releasing DNA. This is then processed automatically through a hybridisation reaction using specific probes to target nucleic acids, which are detected colormetrically on a probe analysis card.

The detection of active disease

Ideally, it is important that the clinician should be able to determine current, or predict future, disease patterns rather than just record previous periodontal destruction. A considerable amount of research has, therefore, been targeted towards the identification of immunoinflammatory mediators and products of tissue destruction at disease sites that could be used as predictors or markers of attachment loss. Conceptually, it may be possible to identify periodontal activity as a biochemical lesion before it progresses to clinical destruction and in this way the biochemical mediator would have a *predictive* value rather than just being associated with the disease. Association, rather than prediction, is the limitation of many of the clinical measurements such as bleeding on probing, which are often erroneously regarded as markers of disease activity or progression. Identification of biochemical risk factors would augment the clinical examination and be used for patient evaluation and for therapeutic decisions. They would help the clinician to

- distinguish between active and stable sites
- assess prognosis
- determine treatment strategies
- monitor the outcome of therapy
- establish maintenance schedules.

Some potential markers have been incorporated into in vitro diagnostic tests for use at the chairside. In the long term, however, the success of such tests will depend upon whether or not they provide accurate data that can be used reliably to determine treatment approaches.

1.3 Gingivitis

Learning objectives

You should

- know the differential diagnosis of the various forms of gingivitis

- be able to provide appropriate therapy.

In this section we describe the clinical features of the chronic and acute forms of gingivitis. The treatment of gingivitis and periodontitis is discussed in Section 1.12 although specific aspects of treatment are also noted in this section (and Section 1.4). The microbiology and pathogenesis of gingivitis are discussed in Section 1.5.

Chronic gingivitis

Chronic gingivitis is a plaque-induced, inflammatory lesion of the gingiva. Accumulation of dental plaque in the gingival sulcus initiates the development of an inflammatory lesion (subclinical) that, after 10–20 days, is detected clinically as an established chronic gingivitis.

Gingivitis occurs in 26% of 5-year-olds, 62% of 9-year-olds and 52% of 15-year-olds (Children's Dental Health Survey, UK, 1993). There has been no reduction in the prevalence of gingival inflammation in children over the 20-year period between 1973 and 1993. Indeed, in 1993 approximately 10–15% more children aged 6–12 years had gingivitis compared with 1983 (Fig. 3). It is clear that the reduction in the prevalence of caries over the same period has not been accompanied by an improvement in gingival inflammation.

Clinical features

The gingiva become red, shiny, swollen, and soft or spongy in texture. Sulcus depths increase (false pockets) as a result of the tissue swelling from inflammatory oedema. Bleeding occurs after gentle probing. The interdental papillae and marginal gingiva are initially involved before inflammation spreads to the attached gingiva.

Treatment

- instruction in toothbrushing
- use of interdental cleaning aids

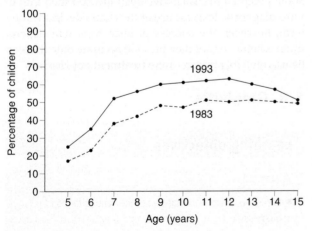

Fig. 3 Prevalence of gingival inflammation in UK children aged 5–15 years (1983–1993).

- supragingival scaling
- elimination of plaque-retentive factors
- subgingival scaling and polishing.

Pregnancy gingivitis

An increase in circulating levels of oestrogen, progesterone and their metabolites aggravates a pre-existing or subclinical gingivitis. The hormones and their metabolites effect an increase in gingival vasculature and the permeability of the capillary network. A similar increase in the severity of an established gingivitis may also be seen at, or around, puberty, during hormone-replacement therapy and with long-term use of oral contraceptives.

Clinical features

Pregnancy gingivitis is a generalised, marginal, oedematous inflammation. The extent of gingival enlargement is variable but an increase in gingival bleeding is a common complaint. The severity of the gingivitis tends to increase from the second to the eighth month of pregnancy. There is often some resolution during the final trimester and after parturition. A local gingival overgrowth – pregnancy epulis – may result from chronic irritation or mild trauma to the soft tissues.

Treatment

A preventive regimen is preferred whenever possible. Otherwise a conventional treatment approach including oral hygiene instruction (OHI) and scaling should be undertaken.

Plasma cell gingivitis

Plasma cell gingivitis is a contact hypersensitivity reaction most frequently attributed to cinnamon flavoured chewing gum. Cinnamon, mint and herbal flavoured toothpastes are also implicated. Microscopically, the epithelium is atrophic and there is a massive infiltrate of plasma cells in the connective tissues.

Clinical features

In plasma cell gingivitis, the gingiva are fiery red in appearance with varying degrees of swelling. The lesion extends to involve the entire width of attached gingiva. The reaction may affect other areas such as the tongue, palate and cheeks. Lips can be dry and desquamative with an angular cheilitis. The principal symptom is extreme soreness of the affected areas.

Treatment

Identification and withdrawal of the causative allergen. If toothbrushing is painful during the acute stage, chlorhexidine mouthrinse can be given for chemical plaque control.

Desquamative gingivitis

Desquamative gingivitis is not a discrete clinical entity but rather a term used to describe a gingival manifestation common to plasma cell gingivitis and mucocutaneous disorders including:

- benign mucous membrane pemphigoid
- lichen planus
- pemphigus vulgaris.

The fiery-red, desquamative lesions affect the entire width of keratinised gingiva and may be localised or generalised throughout the mouth.

Necrotising ulcerative gingivitis

NUG is an acute condition that has characteristic signs and symptoms and a tendency to recur. In Europe and the USA the incidence is 0.5–7.0% in the 16–30-year-old age group. In African countries, a more severe, aggressive form of NUG is found in children as young as 1–2 years.

Clinical features

'Punched out' ulcers occur covered with a yellow-grey pseudomembranous slough. The tips of interdental papillae are affected first but spread to the labial and lingual marginal gingiva can be rapid. NUG is very painful and accompanied by a distinctive halitosis. A pre-existing or long-standing chronic gingivitis is usually present. Fever and regional lymphadenopathy are associated only with severe disease.

Aetiology

A fusiform–spirochaetal complex is traditionally associated with NUG. Gram-negative anaerobic species are also implicated: *P. gingivalis* and *Veillonella* and *Selenomonas* spp. A viral aetiology has been suspected because certain aspects of the condition are similar to those of known viral infections, for example the restriction of NUG to children and young adults and the frequency of recurrence.

Pathology

Ulceration of the gingival epithelium occurs with necrosis of connective tissues. Superficially, deposits of fibrin are intermeshed with large numbers of dead and dying cells: epithelial cells, neutrophils and bacteria. Deeper tissues demonstrate a dense infiltrate of neutrophils characteristic of non-specific inflammation.

It is possible that all of the predisposing factors act through the common pathway of lowering the patient's cell-mediated immune response. The nature of the disease and the likelihood of recurrence with incomplete treatment must be explained carefully to the patient.

Risk factors

Pre-existing gingivitis confirms a poor standard of plaque control.

Smoking favours the development of an anaerobic Gram-negative flora and depresses the chemotactic response of neutrophils.

Mental stress, producing high plasma levels of corticosteroids, predisposes to NUG and is a possible explanation for epidemics in college students or army personnel.

Malnutrition and debilitation predispose to infection and severe NUG in underdeveloped countries.

Treatment

Reduce cigarette consumption. Oral hygiene instruction and ultrasonic scaling. A soft, multi-tufted brush should be recommended if a medium (or hard) textured brush is too painful to use. If mechanical therapy is painful, or if fever/regional lymphadenopathy are present, then a 3 day course of systemic metronidazole, 200 mg three times a day is indicated. Oxygenating mouthrinses (hydrogen peroxide, sodium hydroxyperborate) cleanse necrotic tissues. Subgingival scaling and prophylaxis are essential to prevent recurrence. Incomplete treatment leads inevitably to recurrence and loss of gingival contour. A long-standing necrotising gingivitis may progress to a chronic necrotising ulcerative periodontitis.

Primary herpetic gingivostomatitis

Primary herpetic gingivostomatitis is an acute, common and highly infectious disease caused by herpes simplex virus. Most adults have neutralising antibodies to the virus, indicating that an acquired immune response developed in childhood. Circulating maternal antibodies provide immunity in the first 12 months. Transmission of the virus is predominantly by droplet infection and the incubation period is about 5–10 days. Primary infection occurs most frequently in young children between 2 and 5 years but the disease can affect young adults.

Clinical features

The clinical features and history are so specific that diagnosis of the disease is not difficult.

Symptoms are fever, pyrexia, headaches, general malaise, mild dysphagia and regional lymphadenopathy.

Signs are of the onset of an aggressive marginal gingivitis and formation of fluid-filled vesicles with a grey membranous covering on the gingiva, tongue, palate and buccal mucosa. The vesicles burst after only a few hours to leave painful, yellow-grey ulcers with red, inflamed margins. The ulcers heal without scarring after about 14 days.

Treatment

Treatment is mainly palliative: bed rest, soft diet and maintain fluid intake. Paracetamol suspension is given for pyrexia and severe disease is treated with acyclovir, 200 mg as suspension to swallow, five times daily for 5 days. In young children, plaque can be controlled with chlorhexidine spray two or three times a day.

Complications

In immunocompromised patients, the disease can be very severe and run a protracted course. Other complications like aseptic meningitis and encephalitis are very rare.

Latent herpes viruses dormant in host's sensory ganglia are reactivated by exposure to sunlight, stress, nutritional deficiency, malaise, or systemic upset. The clinical features are an attenuated presentation of the primary infection. Herpes labialis presents as a 'cold sore' at the mucocutaneous borders or commissures of the lips. The cold sores may be managed with topical acyclovir cream (5%), five times a day, for 5–7 days.

1.4 Periodontal diseases

Learning objectives

You should

- know the important clinical features of periodontal diseases
- be able to differentiate between chronic periodontitis and aggressive periodontal diseases
- understand the rationale for adjunctive therapies.

Chronic periodontitis

Chronic periodontitis is bacterially induced inflammation of the periodontium. Approximately 54% of adults have some 4 mm pockets present and 5% have pockets of 6 mm or greater (Adult Dental Health Survey, UK, 1998).

Clinical features

Pocket formation

Periodontal pocket formation is one of the most important clinical signs of periodontitis. A pocket is defined as a pathologically deepened sulcus. Pockets can be classified as *true* pockets, which result from apical migration of the junctional epithelium following loss of connective tissue attachment to the root surface, or *false* pockets, which result from gingival enlargement with no alteration in the position of the junctional epithelium. Additionally, pockets can be *suprabony*, in which case the junctional epithelium remains entirely coronal to the alveolar crest, or *infrabony*, in which case the junctional epithelium extends apically beyond the alveolar crest (Fig. 4).

Bleeding

Bleeding on probing occurs at inflamed sites where thin and ulcerated junctional and pocket epithelia are not resistant to penetration by the probe tip.

Alveolar bone resorption

Alveolar bone resorption occurs concurrently with attachment loss and pocket formation. Two distinct patterns of bone destruction are recognised radiographically. *Horizontal* bone loss occurs when the entire width of interdental bone is resorbed. *Vertical* bone defects are

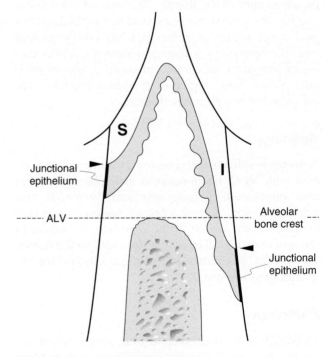

Fig. 4 Supra- and infrabony pockets.

produced when the interdental bone adjacent to the root surface is more rapidly resorbed, leaving an angular, uneven morphology. Frequently, both patterns of bone resorption are seen at different sites in the same patient. Infrabony defects are also classified according to the number of remaining base walls; 1-, 2- or 3-walled defects (Fig. 5). Such observations can only be confirmed by direct vision during flap surgery.

Tooth mobility
Tooth mobility can be either physiological or pathological.

Physiological mobility allows slight movements of a tooth within the socket to accommodate masticatory forces, without injury to the tooth or its supporting tissues.

Pathological mobility is increased or increasing mobility as a result of connective tissue attachment loss. Its extent depends upon the quantity of remaining bony support, the degree of inflammation in the periodontal ligament and gingiva, and the magnitude of occlusal or any jiggling forces (Section 1.9) that may be acting upon the teeth. A reduction in mobility follows successful treatment and resolution of inflammation. A scale for the assessment of tooth mobility is given in Section 1.2.

Migration of teeth may occur following attachment loss or gingival overgrowth. Frequently, maxillary incisors drift labially, resulting in increased overjet and diastemata. Affected teeth also have a tendency to over-erupt.

Gingival recession
Gingival recession is localised or generalised.

Localised recession is associated with factors such as toothbrush trauma, high frenal attachment and factitious injury, superimposed upon anatomical factors such as bony dehiscences or thin alveolar bone plates.

Generalised recession occurs when the gingival margin migrates apically as a result of ongoing periodontal disease or following resolution of gingival inflammation and oedema, as a consequence of successful periodontal treatment.

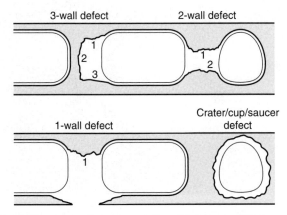

Fig. 5 Diagrammatic representation of infrabony defects.

Furcation lesions
Furcation lesions (see also Section 1.2) arise when attachment loss occurs vertically and horizontally between the roots of multirooted teeth. Lesions are detected using

- direct visualisation
- a furcation probe
- radiographic examination.

Acute periodontal abscess
Acute periodontal abscess is an acute suppurative inflammatory lesion within the periodontal pocket or gingival sulcus, which usually arises from:

- an acute exacerbation of chronic periodontitis
- trauma to the pocket epithelium (from instrumentation, toothbrush bristles, food impaction)
- orthodontic movement of teeth through untreated, periodontally compromised tissues.

The clinical signs and symptoms of a periodontal abscess are:

- Gingival erythema
- Swelling of the overlying gingivae
- Discharge of pus from the gingival margin
- Pain from the affected site made worse by biting
- Unpleasant taste
- Tenderness to percussion
- Acute pain on probing, with discharge of pus and blood.

Treatment

The basic treatment of chronic periodontitis is discussed in detail in Section 1.11 and invariably includes:

- oral hygiene instruction: systematic toothbrushing technique and interproximal cleaning aids (dental floss, mini-interdental brushes, interspace brushes)
- scaling and root planing to remove subgingival plaque, calculus and necrotic cementum
- re-evaluation to assess the response to treatment, reinforce oral hygiene instruction and provide further instrumentation if necessary.

Treatment of a periodontal abscess

- incision if drainage cannot be achieved through the pocket
- subgingival instrumentation and irrigation with chlorhexidine
- warm saline mouthrinses to encourage further drainage
- systemic antimicrobials when there is evidence of spread of infection and involvement of regional lymph nodes: metronidazole 400 mg three times a day for 5 days is effective against anaerobes; penicillins may also be prescribed
- re-evaluation to assess response to treatment and prognosis of the affected tooth.

Aggressive periodontitis

Aggressive periodontitis is characterised by rapid attachment loss, rapid bone destruction and familial aggregation. Except for the presence of periodontitis, patients are otherwise clinically healthy. The term 'aggressive periodontitis' is used to denote those conditions that were previously referred to as the early-onset periodontal diseases (which comprised prepubertal periodontitis, juvenile periodontitis and rapidly progressive periodontitis).

Aggressive periodontitis can be localised or generalised. Very aggressive forms of periodontal disease may also be seen in children in association with certain syndromes and medical conditions (see Section 1.10), some of which are very rare. The clinical features of aggressive periodontitis associated with systemic disease are discussed below, followed by a description of the features of localised and generalised aggressive periodontitis.

Aggressive periodontitis associated with systemic disease

This condition may be clinically detected soon after the primary teeth erupt. It can be localised or more generalised. In generalised forms, the gingiva are fiery red, oedematous, swollen and haemorrhagic. Granular or nodular proliferations of the gingiva precede the formation of gingival clefts and multiple sites of recession. Bone loss is generalised and affects most teeth, which can be lost as early as 3–5 years of age. Patients often suffer from more general infections, particularly of the upper respiratory tract and middle ear. By comparison, in localised forms of the disease, the gingival changes and plaque deposits are minimal with only mild inflammation of the marginal tissues. Bone loss has a typical incisor–molar distribution, and the disease progression is slower than that of the generalised form.

A number of very aggressive periodontopathogens are associated with these conditions: *Actinobacillus actinomycetemcomitans*, *Porphyromonas gingivalis*, *Fusobacterium nucleatum*, *Eikenella corrodens*.

Treatment
Localised forms of aggressive periodontitis associated with systemic disease may respond well to conventional treatment: oral hygiene instruction, scaling and root planing. Antimicrobials are indicated if infection persists or the disease is refractory to conventional treatment. Extraction of teeth may help to restrict the condition to the primary dentition, though this is a contentious treatment strategy.

Localised aggressive periodontitis

Classically localised aggressive periodontitis affects the permanent dentition and has its onset around puberty.

Prevalence in developed countries is about 0.1% but is somewhat higher in developing countries (0.5%). In the UK, prevalence is higher in certain ethnic groups: Asians (0.2%), Afro-Caribbeans (0.8%). There is no predilection for either sex.

Localised aggressive periodontitis is characterised by pocketing, bleeding on probing and loss of attachment (BPE 4) localised to the incisor and first molar regions. There is rapid bone and soft tissue destruction. The gingiva can appear healthy where there are low levels of supragingival plaque. The radiographic pattern of bone loss is distinctive, with bilateral angular defects around first molars and horizontal loss around incisors (Fig. 6). Up to two other permanent teeth may also be affected within the definition of localised aggressive periodontitis.

Analysis of the subgingival flora will typically reveal greatly elevated levels of *Actinobacillus actinomycetemcomitans* and also *Porphyromonas gingivalis*. There is often a robust serum antibody response to the infecting agent. Patients with localised aggressive periodontitis may have abnormalities of neutrophil and macrophage chemotaxis and phagocytosis. Such defects are probably transmitted as an inherited trait, which may partly explain the familial aggregation of aggressive periodontitis.

Increased levels of *Actinobacillus actinomycetemcomitans (Aa)* are found in over 90% of localised aggressive periodontitis cases (and this species is usually absent in health). *Aa* has the ability to invade epithelial cells and connective tissues and produces a number of very potent virulence factors:

- leukotoxin (kills PMNs and macrophages)
- epitheliotoxin (toxic to epithelial cells)
- collagenase (degrades collagen)
- fibroblast inhibiting factor (impairs fibroblast function).

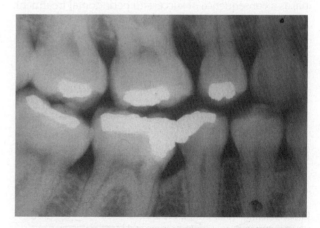

Fig. 6 Radiograph showing distinctive bone loss in localised aggressive periodontitis.

Treatment

The ability of *Aa* to invade the gingival tissues represents a reservoir of infection that is difficult to eradicate by scaling and root planing alone. Conventional treatment is frequently combined with systemic tetracycline therapy (250 mg four times a day for 2 weeks), to which *Aa* is particularly susceptible. Ideally, however, the antimicrobial regimen should be based on the results of culture and sensitivity testing of samples from pockets. An antimicrobial regimen can also be used in conjunction with periodontal surgery. Long-term maintenance is essential. Family studies show that localised aggressive periodontitis is a heritable trait with an autosomal recessive pattern. It is, therefore, important to screen siblings and (eventually) offspring of affected individuals wherever possible.

Generalised aggressive periodontitis

The age of onset of generalised aggressive periodontitis is usually less than 30 years, but it may affect older individuals. The disease is characterised by marked gingival inflammation, deep pocketing (BPE 4), bleeding (after probing, but sometimes spontaneous), purulent exudate and periodontal abscess formation. Bone resorption is very rapid, generalised and irregular, with a combination of vertical and horizontal defects (Fig. 7). Tooth loss is almost inevitable if the disease is untreated. The most common presenting complaints are drifting and spacing of teeth, or marked displacement (or exfoliation) of a tooth following a relatively minor traumatic episode.

The subgingival flora comprises loosely adherent, Gram-negative, anaerobic periodontopathogens: *Actinobacillus actinomycetemcomitans*, *Capnocytophaga* sp., *Prevotella intermedia*, *Porphyromonas gingivalis* and *Eikenella corrodens*.

There is typically a poor serum antibody response to the infectious agents, and defects in neutrophil function (chemotaxis and phagocytosis). Also, defects in cell-mediated immunity may be present, with altered $T_{helper}/T_{suppressor}$ cell ratios. Affected individuals typically produce high levels of destructive, pro-inflammatory mediators, such as prostaglandin E_2 (PGE_2), interleukin-1β (IL-1β) and tumour necrosis factor-α (TNF-α), in response to the presence of bacteria.

In some instances, the disease may eventually become quiescent or may convert to a more slowly progressing chronic periodontitis.

A differential diagnosis of periodontitis associated with insulin-dependent diabetes (Section 1.10) must be considered. An enquiry about family history of diabetes is prudent. A glucose tolerance test may reveal subclinical or early stages of diabetes.

Treatment

Teeth that have a hopeless prognosis are extracted. Conventional non-surgical management or surgical therapy can provide better access for root planing at sites of deep pockets. Systemic antimicrobial therapy (see localised aggressive periodontitis) should also be considered when multiple abscesses occur.

Again, systemic antimicrobial therapy should be based upon culture and sensitivity testing. A combination of metronidazole 400 mg plus amoxicillin 250 mg three times daily for 1 week, with concurrent full-mouth root planing, may sometimes be used in severe cases.

1.5 Microbiology and pathogenesis of periodontal diseases

Learning objectives

You should

- understand the key steps involved in the accumulation and maturation of dental plaque

- know the microbiology associated with different periodontal conditions and to understand why certain specific pathogens are important in periodontitis

- understand the histological changes that occur during the development of gingivitis and periodontitis, and how these changes relate to the clinical signs of disease

- understand the importance of the interactions between plaque bacteria and host defence mechanisms in the pathogenesis of periodontitis

- be familiar with specific destructive mechanisms in periodontal disease progression.

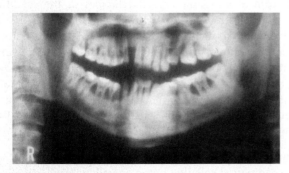

Fig. 7 Radiograph showing the irregular bone loss with both vertical and horizontal defects in generalised aggressive periodontitis.

Microbiology of periodontal diseases

Dental plaque

Dental plaque is an accumulation of bacteria and intercellular matrix that forms the biofilm that adheres to the surfaces of teeth and other oral structures in the absence of effective oral hygiene. Accumulation of plaque is the key aetiological factor in the pathogenesis of periodontal diseases. Plaque is generally classified as being *supragingival* or *subgingival*.

Supragingival plaque

Supragingival plaque is located on the clinical crowns of the teeth, at or above the gingival margin. It forms as a soft, yellow-white layer on the tooth surface. It accumulates primarily at the gingival margin and also other regions (grooves, pits, under overhanging restorations) where there is protection from the mechanical cleaning effect of the oral soft tissues. The rate of plaque formation varies among individuals and is influenced by oral hygiene, dietary composition and salivary flow rates. Small amounts of plaque may not be visible to the unaided eye but may be detected by running a periodontal probe around the gingival margin, or by the use of disclosing solutions.

Subgingival plaque

Subgingival plaque is found within the gingival sulcus or periodontal pocket, below the gingival margin. It develops from the downgrowth of supragingival plaque into the gingival sulcus or periodontal pocket; it cannot be seen directly unless the overlying gingiva is retracted. The composition of subgingival plaque differs from that of supragingival plaque as a result of the unique conditions that exist in the gingival sulcus, which favour colonisation and growth of anaerobic bacteria. In the sulcus, there is an altered redox potential, protection from cleansing mechanisms within the oral cavity and GCF supplies a ready flow of nutrients to the bacteria.

Composition and formation of plaque

Plaque consists of microorganisms (accounting for approximately 75% of the plaque volume) suspended in an extracellular matrix. More than 300 bacterial species have been identified in dental plaque. Some non-bacterial organisms that are also found in plaque include yeasts, *Mycoplasma* spp. and viruses. The extracellular matrix consists of organic and inorganic components derived from plaque bacteria, saliva and GCF. Organic components include extracellular polysaccharides secreted by plaque bacteria (which have storage and anchorage roles), salivary glycoproteins (which are important in the initial adherence of bacteria to the tooth surface), desquamated oral epithelium cells and defence cells. The inorganic component primarily comprises calcium and phosphorus from saliva.

Following professional tooth cleaning, plaque formation occurs in a predictable sequence of events.

1. *Acquired pellicle formation* (immediately after cleaning). Salivary glycoproteins selectively adsorb onto the tooth surface. The acquired pellicle functions as a protective, lubricating layer, but it also allows for bacterial adherence.
2. *Early colonisation* (0–7 days after cleaning). The tooth surface is initially colonised by Gram-positive cocci, predominantly *Streptococcus* spp. Over the next 7 days, the numbers of all bacterial types increase, although their relative proportions alter. Gram-positive rods, particularly *Actinomyces* spp., become more prevalent, as do Gram-negative cocci (e.g. *Veillonella* spp.) and rods (e.g. *Capnocytophaga* spp.). As the bulk of the plaque increases, an oxygen-deprived environment develops within the deeper layers of the biofilm and conditions begin to favour the growth of anaerobic organisms like *Fusobacterium* spp. (Gram-negative rods) and *Prevotella intermedia*.
3. *Late colonisation and maturation* (>7 days after cleaning). If undisturbed, the plaque mass matures through further growth of species already present and the appearance of late colonising species. Late colonisers do not attach to clean tooth surfaces and are often virulent organisms that have been implicated as specific periodontal pathogens. *Porphyromonas gingivalis*, motile Gram-negative rods and spirochaetes are important examples of late colonising organisms.

Dental calculus

Calculus is a hard, mineralised substance that forms on the surfaces of teeth and other solid structures in the oral cavity following the prolonged accumulation of dental plaque. Calculus is plaque that has become mineralised by calcium and phosphate ions from saliva. Inorganic calcium phosphate crystals grow within the plaque matrix and enlarge until the plaque is mineralised. The mixture of inorganic crystals changes as the calculus ages. Brushite ($CaHPO_4.2H_2O$) forms first, and is followed by octocalcium phosphate ($Ca_8(HPO_4)_4$). Mature calculus contains predominantly crystals of hydroxyapatite ($Ca_{10}(PO_4)_6.OH_2$) and tricalcium phosphate ($Ca_3(PO_4)_2$). Calculus crystals grow into close contact with the tooth, gaining mechanical retention in surface irregularities. The outer surface of calculus remains covered by a layer of unmineralised plaque.

Supragingival calculus

Supragingival calculus forms as yellow-white calcified deposits located at, or just coronal to, the gingival margin and is frequently stained brown by tobacco and certain foods and drinks. The mineralisation of plaque to form calculus is influenced by salivary gland secretions and consequently, the greatest deposits of calculus are found in close proximity to the duct openings of major salivary glands, in particular the buccal surfaces of maxillary molars, and the lingual surfaces of mandibular anterior teeth.

Subgingival calculus
Subgingival calculus forms apical to the gingival margin, particularly at interproximal sites, as tenacious dark brown-black deposits on the root surface. If the gingival margin is dried, the dark colour of subgingival calculus may be seen through the marginal soft tissues. A fine calculus probe is used to detect deeper subgingival calculus, and interproximal deposits may be seen on radiographs. Direct vision of subgingival calculus may be achieved using a gentle stream of air to reflect the gingival margin, or following gingival recession, or during periodontal surgery.

Calculus itself is not a primary cause of periodontitis and is always covered by a layer of unmineralised plaque. However, calculus does form a plaque-retentive surface, keeping plaque in close proximity to the tissues; it also impairs the ability of the patient to remove plaque.

Specific periodontal conditions

Gingival health
Total recovery of organisms from the gingiva is low and mainly comprises Gram-positive species, particularly streptococci and Actinomyces (e.g. S. sanguis, S. mitis, A. naeslundii, A. viscosus). The predominance of these species may exert a protective influence for the host by preventing the colonisation or proliferation of more pathogenic organisms (for example, S. sanguis produces H_2O_2, which is toxic to Actinobacillus actinomycetemcomitans). Pathogenic species may be isolated from healthy sites but probably represent a transient component of maturing plaque.

Chronic gingivitis
A more complex bacterial flora develops in chronic gingivitis comprising a mixture of Gram-positive and Gram-negative species, and aerobic and anaerobic organisms. Gram-positive organisms include the Streptococcus and Actinomyces spp. found in health; Gram-negative organisms include Prevotella intermedia, Fusobacterium nucleatum, Eikenella corrodens and Capnocytophaga spp.

Chronic periodontitis
Microorganisms most often identified in sites exhibiting chronic periodontitis include Porphyromonas gingivalis, Actinobacillus actinomycetemcomitans, Bacteroides forsythus, Prevotella intermedia, Actinomyces naeslundii, Campylobacter rectus, Eikenella corrodens, Fusobacterium nucleatum, Treponema and Eubacterium spp.

Aggressive periodontitis
Actinobacillus actinomycetemcomitans is strongly implicated in localised aggressive periodontitis and may comprise more than 90% of cultivable bacteria at affected sites. Other organisms associated with localised aggressive periodontitis include Porphyromonas gingivalis, Prevotella intermedia and Capnocytophaga spp. Generalised aggressive periodontitis is associated with increased prevalence of Porphyromonas gingivalis, Actinobacillus actinomycetemcomitans, Bacteroides forsythus, Prevotella intermedia and Eikenella corrodens.

Putative periodontal pathogens

The microbial composition of subgingival plaque varies between patients, and not all subgingival bacteria are important in the onset and progression of periodontitis. Periodontitis is usually caused by several microbial species rather than one single organism. Periodontopathogens may be divided into endogenous and exogenous sources of origin.

Endogenous infections are caused by indigenous organisms present in health that are non-pathogenic under normal circumstances but overgrow and reach harmful levels after changes in the conditions of the local environment (commensal organisms). Accumulation and maturation of plaque creates an environment that favours the selective growth of anaerobes, leading to gingival inflammation. Most forms of gingivitis and mild periodontitis are associated with bacteria that are part of the oral flora in health.

Exogenous infections are acquired from outside the oral cavity (primary pathogens). Porphyromonas gingivalis and Actinobacillus actinomycetemcomitans may be regarded as true infectious agents in periodontal disease. Both exhibit low prevalence in health and gingivitis, both are risk factors for periodontal destruction, both provoke a marked immune response, and there is evidence that both species may be transmitted between family members.

Virulence factors
Virulence factors assist bacteria in achieving access to, and colonising, sites.

Adherence. Bacteria must first adhere to teeth via surface fimbriae, which attach to components of the acquired pellicle, or to other bacteria. Adherence allows bacteria to accumulate and to withstand the mechanical cleansing effects of the oral soft tissues, and salivary and GCF flow.

Invasion. Certain species have the ability to invade the gingival soft tissues, in particular Actinobacillus actinomycetemcomitans and Porphyromonas gingivalis, which allows for the direct delivery of toxic bacterial products to the tissues. Additionally, bacteria that have invaded the tissues represent a reservoir of organisms that are not easily eradicated from the local environment by scaling and root planing, and adjunctive antimicrobial therapy may be indicated during treatment.

Tissue damage and evasion strategies. Many by-products of bacterial metabolism are damaging to the host tissues, including NH_3, H_2S and fatty acids, such as butyric acid. Additionally, many bacteria produce enzymes such as proteases and collagenases. *Actinobacillus actinomycetemcomitans* possesses many virulence factors that help the organism to evade host defence mechanisms, including collagenase, endotoxin, proteases, epitheliotoxin and leukotoxins (which inhibit polymorphic mononuclear cells (neutrophils) and T and B lymphocyte functions). *Porphyromonas gingivalis* also possesses collagenase, endotoxin and immunoglobulin-degrading proteases and it is encapsulated, which protects it from phagocytosis. These organisms, therefore, have the ability to destroy connective tissues, inhibit host defence mechanisms, induce a marked inflammatory response, and prevent attempts at repair.

Pathogenesis of periodontal diseases

Pathogenesis is the sequence of events leading to the occurrence of a disease. In periodontology, the pathogenesis of gingivitis and periodontitis are related but tend to be described separately, and although the clinical and histological changes that occur are well known, the details of specific pathogenic mechanisms are less clearly defined.

Gingivitis

Pathogenesis
As plaque bacteria accumulate at the gingival margin, bacterial products (e.g. metabolic by-products, H_2S, endotoxin, proteases) cross the junctional epithelium and invoke an inflammatory response in the gingival tissues. This response is characterised by increased vascular permeability, vasodilatation and leakage of fluid into the tissues and gingival sulcus. Neutrophils migrate from the blood vessels into the tissues and the gingival sulcus. Collagen fibres around blood vessels and apical to the junctional epithelium are degraded. After several days, lymphocytes (particularly T cells) and macrophages accumulate. Fibroblasts show morphological changes and have a reduced ability to form collagen. Ultimately, plasma cells become the predominant inflammatory cell type in the gingival tissues, collagen depletion continues, and the junctional epithelium proliferates. The chronic gingivitis inflammatory lesion is confined to the tissues adjacent to the junctional and sulcular epithelia.

Histopathology
For descriptive purposes, the inflammatory changes occurring during the development of gingivitis can be described as the *initial*, *early* and *established* gingival lesions, although there are no clear boundaries between these stages histologically.

The initial inflammatory lesion develops after 0–4 days of plaque accumulation and is characterised by:

- vascular dilatation and increased vascular permeability, leading to leakage of fluid from vessels, and increased GCF flow
- migration of neutrophils out of vessels into the tissues, through the junctional and sulcular epithelia, and into the gingival sulcus
- breakdown of collagen fibres around blood vessels.

The early inflammatory lesion develops after approximately 4–7 days of plaque accumulation. It is characterised by:

- continued vascular dilatation and increased permeability, with increased fluid exudation, and migration of neutrophils into the tissues
- increased breakdown of collagen subjacent to the junctional epithelium
- accumulation of lymphocytes (particularly T lymphocytes) and macrophages
- cytotoxic changes in fibroblasts, resulting in a reduced capacity for collagen formation
- proliferation of the cells of the junctional epithelium.

The established inflammatory lesion is apparent after approximately 14–21 days of undisturbed plaque growth and coincides with the clinical diagnosis of chronic gingivitis. Histopathological changes include:

- further engorgement of blood vessels, leading to venous stasis and the superimposition of a dark blue tinge over the erythematous gingiva
- migration of plasma cells into the gingival connective tissues to become the predominant inflammatory cell type
- continued collagen depletion
- continued proliferation of the junctional epithelium, forming epithelial ridges with widened intercellular spaces.

By definition, the inflammatory changes occurring in gingivitis are confined to the gingiva and do not involve alveolar bone or result in apical migration of the junctional epithelium. *The advanced inflammatory lesion* occurs when the inflammation extends beyond the gingiva. Extension beyond the gingival tissues is coincident with the clinical diagnosis of periodontitis (see below).

Initiation of gingivitis

Plaque is essential for the initiation of gingivitis. Accumulation of plaque leads to gingivitis; as plaque matures, the subgingival environment alters to favour the growth of Gram-negative organisms. The inflammatory lesion in the gingiva leads to increased GCF flow, and products from the tissues are utilised as nutrients by pathogenic organisms. The inflammatory changes in the tissues lead to increased permeability of the junctional epithelium, allowing bacterial products to penetrate the tissues more easily. The host responds to the bacterial challenge by continuing to mount an immune inflammatory response, such that neutrophils, lymphocytes and macrophages are activated to combat the growth and spread of bacteria. As a result, a chronic inflammatory state develops in which there is a balance between the host and the bacteria, and there are continued attempts at healing in the presence of continued inflammation and destruction.

Periodontitis

Pathogenesis

Chronic gingivitis may persist indefinitely, and very little is known about the factors that influence a shift from gingivitis to destructive periodontitis. An alteration in the balance between the bacteria and the host response may be important in determining disease progression. The acquisition of a more pathogenic microflora, or an impaired host response (e.g. as a result of altered immune function, psychological stress or smoking) may tip the balance in favour of disease progression.

In this chronically inflamed state, putative periodontal pathogens tend to predominate that possess specific virulence factors which can contribute to destructive processes and/or impair host defences. The host-derived immuneinflammatory response also results in the destruction of periodontal hard and soft tissues, leading to the clinically observed signs of periodontitis. There are a number of host-derived mechanisms of destruction.

Neutrophils spill lysosomal enzymes and granule contents (including lysozyme, elastase, collagenase, proteases, myeloperoxidase) during phagocytosis or following cell death, resulting in damage to the surrounding tissues.

Stimulation of neutrophils results in a sudden increase in oxygen consumption by the cells (the 'respiratory bust'), which is utilised to oxidise NADPH (reduced nicotinamide adenine diphosphate), leading to the production of superoxide radical (O_2^-), and H_2O_2 (hydrogen peroxide), which in turn is converted by the enzyme myeloperoxidase to hypochlorous acid, all of which are destructive oxidants for both bacteria and host tissues.

Collagenases from neutrophils and fibroblasts destroy connective tissue fibres of the periodontal ligament.

Proliferation of the epithelial cells of the junctional epithelium follows the destruction of collagen fibres in the periodontal ligament; the epithelial cells migrate apically along the root surface, resulting in pocket formation. This allows for downgrowth of subgingival plaque into the protected environment of the periodontal pocket, favouring the growth of pathogenic anaerobes and resulting in a perpetuating cycle of destructive changes.

Osteoclasts are stimulated to resorb alveolar bone by cytokines and inflammatory mediators released by neutrophils and macrophages, including interleukins and prostaglandin E_2 (PGE_2).

Role of immune cells Neutrophils represent the first cellular host defence mechanism against plaque bacteria and predominate in the gingival sulcus and the junctional epithelium. Neutrophils possess a formidable array of antimicrobial weaponry. If they do not control the pathogen, then monocytes are recruited from the blood. These infiltrate the gingival connective tissues and develop into macrophages, which either digest the antigen completely or present the antigen to lymphocytes. Neutrophils, therefore, are involved in the initial acute response, whereas macrophages and lymphocytes characterise a more long-standing or chronic inflammatory response and are activated in response to deeper penetration of bacteria and their products. The response of these cells to bacterial antigens appears to be primarily genetically determined in terms of the balance between the protective antibody response and the destructive inflammatory response. Differences in periodontal disease expression between individuals are probably a consequence of different response traits of the immuneinflammatory cells. For example, macrophages in disease-susceptible subjects are believed to secrete higher levels of PGE_2 (resulting in inflammation and bone resorption) in response to the bacterial challenge compared with secretion in disease-resistant individuals. If activation of macrophages and lymphocytes contains the bacteria, disease progression is halted. If the host defences are compromised, then disease can recur. This model of disease progression requires a pathogenic flora and evasion of neutrophils to initiate disease; the individual's host response subsequently has a key role in modulating the severity of disease expression. It is clear that patients with defective defences (for example, those with neutrophil defects or HIV infection) are at significantly greater risk for periodontal disease than those with normal immuneinflammatory responses.

Histopathology

The transition from established gingivitis to periodontitis constitutes the development of the *advanced* inflammatory lesion (Fig. 8), which is characterised by:

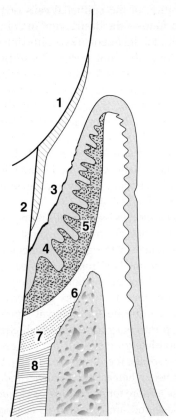

Fig. 8 Histopathological development of the advanced inflammatory lesion. 1 = dental plaque; 2 = plaque front; 3 = ulcerated pocket epithelium; 4 = epithelial ridges; 5 = cellular infiltrate (neutrophils, macrophages, plasma cells and invading bacteria); 6 = resorbed alveolar bone; 7 = connnective tissue fibre destruction; 8 = intact ligament fibres.

- vascular proliferation and vasodilatation; vessels becoming engorged with blood
- plasma cells and B lymphocytes in the connective tissues
- the pocket epithelium being very thin, frequently ulcerated and permeable to bacterial products, inflammatory mediators and defence cells
- connective tissues exhibiting signs of degeneration and foci of necrosis
- fibres of the periodontal ligament apical to the junctional epithelium being destroyed by collagenases
- the junctional epithelium proliferating in an apical direction
- exposed cementum adsorbing bacterial products and becoming soft and necrotic
- osteoclast bone resorption, driven by plaque and host-derived mediators such as endotoxin, prostaglandins, interleukins and tumour necrosis factor (TNF), becoming evident.

Specific pathogenic mechanisms
The tissue destruction observed in periodontitis arises partly from direct injury sustained from factors pro-

duced by plaque bacteria, but primarily it arises from the resultant activation of the local inflammatory/immune response, and the release of inflammatory mediators.

Direct injury by plaque bacteria Many periodontopathogens produce substances that have potentially harmful effects on the periodontal tissues, including enzymes such as proteases, collagenases and hyaluronidase, and metabolic waste products including NH_3, H_2S and butyric acid. Organisms such as *Porphyromonas gingivalis* and *Actinobacillus actinomycetemcomitans* also posses virulence factors that have direct cytopathic effects, including the destruction of host tissues and inhibition of defensive mechanisms. Whereas bacteria are essential for the initiation of periodontal diseases, however, the signs of destructive periodontitis result predominantly from the activation of host inflammatory and immune processes in response to the presence of bacterial products in the tissues.

Injury via inflammation The host tissues produce certain endogenous mediators during the inflammatory response to bacteria and their products.

Histamine is present mainly in mast cells and basophils, particularly around blood vessels. Mast cells degranulate, releasing histamine, in response to many stimuli, including the binding of complement proteins and binding of antigen to IgE-sensitised mast cells. Histamine causes changes in the vascular plexus subjacent to the junctional epithelium, vasodilatation and increased vascular permeability.

The Complement system comprises a series of over 20 proteins that are present in inactive form in serum and are activated in gingival inflammation. The system has three functions, (i) targeting phagocytic cells to microorganisms (opsonisation), (ii) recruiting immune cells to sites of inflammation (chemotaxis) and (iii) bacterial destruction. There are two pathways of activation of the complement cascade. The classical pathway is activated by antigen (e.g. a bacterial cell or fragment) binding to immunoglobulin M or G (IgM or IgG). The alternate pathway is initiated by various substances, including endotoxin. Complement activation causes various proinflammatory events, including leukocyte chemotaxis, opsonisation of microorganisms, stimulation of the respiratory burst ('killing phase') in neutrophils and mast cell degranulation. Activated complement proteins can directly damage bacterial or host cells by binding to cell membranes and causing osmotic lysis.

Kinins are peptides produced as a result of activation of kallikrein in inflammatory conditions. Bradykinin is one such peptide; it causes increased vascular permeability and leukocyte emigration from blood vessels.

Arachidonic acid metabolites include the prostaglandins and leukotrienes. Prostaglandin levels are increased in the gingival tissues at inflamed sites and cause vasodilatation and increased vascular permeability. Prostaglandins also modulate lymphocyte function and stimulate osteoclastic bone resorption. Leukotriene B_4 is a leukotriene that causes increased vascular permeability, is chemotactic for neutrophils and increases adhesion of neutrophils to endothelial cells.

Oxygen free radicals are produced during the respiratory burst in neutrophils when reduced NADPH traps O_2, reducing it via O_2, H_2O_2 and OH to H_2O. Free radicals are essential for the bactericidal activity of neutrophils but can be spilled into the surrounding tissues during phagocytosis or following cell necrosis. Oxygen radicals not only kill bacteria but also damage host defence cells, fibroblasts, endothelium and connective tissue matrix. They also activate latent collagenases present in the extracellular environment.

Matrix metalloproteinases (MMPs) are a family of enzymes capable of degrading extracellular matrix macromolecules including collagens, elastin, fibronectin and proteoglycan core protein. Matrix metalloproteinases have a zinc ion at the active site, are secreted in latent form and are activated by proteolytic activity or reactive oxygen radicals once outside the cell. MMPs are produced by neutrophils, macrophages, fibroblasts and keratinocytes. MMP-8 is a collagenase produced by neutrophils; it is rapidly released and is the predominant collagenase in GCF sampled from periodontitis sites.

Cytokines are bioactive polypeptides produced by a variety of cells and are subdivided into lymphokines (produced by lymphocytes) and monokines (produced by monocytes/macrophages). Cytokines include the interleukins, tumour necrosis factors and interferon-γ. **Interleukin-1 (IL-1)** appears to have a central role in the regulation of immuneinflammatory responses and exists in three related forms: IL-1α, IL-1β and an IL-1 receptor antagonist that binds to the IL receptor and inhibits IL-1α, and IL-1β. Macrophages are the predominant source of IL-1α and IL-1β, which have similar proinflammatory effects, including enhancement of bone resorption, inhibition of bone formation, stimulation of prostaglandin synthesis, increased collagenase production, proliferation of fibroblasts and potentiation of neutrophil degranulation. II-1 is a very potent bone resorbing agent and stimulates the proliferation of mature osteoclasts and osteoclast precursors. **TNF-α** and **TNF-β** are proinflammatory mediators produced by macrophages (TNF-α) and lymphocytes (TNF-β). TNF-α induces the formation of collagenase, PGE_2 and interleukins. TNF-α induces bone resorption and inhibits bone formation, although is less potent in this effect than IL-1. **Interferon-γ** is produced by activated T cells and is a potent inhibitor of IL-1, TNF-α, and TNF-β; it also has an inhibitory effect on bone resorption, suggesting a protective role in the pathogenesis of periodontitis.

Patterns of progression of periodontitis

Early studies investigating the progression of periodontitis concluded that there is continuous, linear loss of attachment over time, although the rate of progression varied according to the population studied. However, longitudinal monitoring of patients reveals that many periodontal sites do not change over long periods, and destruction at a site may arrest and progress no further. Periodontitis is thought to progress by *bursts* of destructive activity. The *random burst model* of disease progression states that:

- certain sites remain free of destruction throughout life
- some sites demonstrate a brief burst of destruction that may last an undefined period of time before becoming quiescent
- sites that experienced destruction may never demonstrate an active burst again, or may be subject to one or more bursts later
- the burst are random with regards to time and previous episodes of destruction.

An extension of this theory is the *asynchronous multiple burst theory*, in which multiple sites show breakdown within a short period of time, with prolonged periods of remission.

1.6 Risk factors and predisposing factors

Learning objectives

You should

- know what is meant by the term 'risk factor'
- understand the important risk factors for periodontitis
- understand the problems that iatrogenic plaque-retentive factors can create, and know how to avoid and correct them.

Risk factors

Risk factors can be defined as characteristics, behavioural aspects or environmental exposures that are associated with a specific disease; the association may, or may not, be causal. A number of specific criteria must be met before a risk factor for a disease can be identified:

- the factor must be associated with the development of the disease
- the factor must precede the occurrence of the disease
- the observation or association must not occur through any source of error (such as a design flaw in a clinical trial).

Several risk factors have been associated with the onset and/or progression of periodontal disease. These include:

- poor access to dental care
- a history of periodontitis
- stress
- systemic disease (such as diabetes)
- genetic factors
- smoking.

Conversely, it has been suggested that periodontal disease may be a risk (or associated) factor for systemic events, notably coronary heart disease and pre-term, low birth-weight infants. In this section, we explore the potential association of periodontal disease and risk factors using two examples mentioned above; smoking and coronary heart disease.

Tobacco smoking

Smokers have a significantly higher prevalence of periodontal disease (pocket depths, attachment loss, bone loss) than non-smokers and this observation cannot only be explained by lower levels of oral hygiene and/or socio-economic factors. Observations from numerous clinical studies suggest that smoking increases, in a dose-dependent manner, the risk of

- periodontal destruction by 3–6-fold
- generalised aggressive periodontitis in adolescents
- infection with causative microorganisms
- tooth loss and edentulism
- recurrence of periodontitis and the risk of 'refractory' periodontitis
- soft tissue and osseointegration problems with implants.

Smoking also reduces the magnitude and predictability of the success of periodontal treatment. The rate of progression of periodontitis and the rate of tooth loss are reduced in ex-smokers when compared with current smokers. This, together with the evidence that implicates smoking as a significant risk factor for periodontitis, suggests that

- an assessment of smoking status must be made during history taking
- the dentist and hygienist must take an active part in encouraging all patients who are smokers to quit as part of an oral health care strategy.

Coronary heart disease

An association between periodontal disease and coronary heart disease has been explained on the basis that chronic infection has been implicated as a risk factor for atherogenesis. Susceptible individuals may have hyper-

inflammatory monocytes, which, under bacterial challenge, release high levels of destructive cytokines (PGE_2, IL-1, TNF-α). Consequently periodontal infections (diseases) may directly enhance the development of atherosclerosis and the subsequent risk of thromboembolic events by providing a chronic challenge to the host from bacterial lipopolysaccharides and host potent, inflammatory cytokines. Furthermore, the activity of these hyperinflammatory monocytes may be upregulated by high-fat diets. Of course, it is also possible that the apparent association between coronary heart disease and periodontitis is because the diseases share risk factors such as tobacco smoking, stress, ageing, ethnic origin, genetic predisposition and socioeconomic status.

Predisposing (plaque-retentive) factors

Overhanging restorations

Poor technique when restoring teeth can result in amalgam overhangs; these occur frequently at interproximal sites and are avoided by ensuring that matrix bands are closely adapted to the tooth surface when packing amalgam. Overhangs render interproximal cleaning impossible and result in plaque-induced inflammation, loss of attachment and alveolar bone destruction.

Treatment
It is best to remove any overhang.

- where access permits, remove overhang with a fine diamond bur or a flat diamond stone in a horizontally reciprocating handpiece (Eva^R handpiece) placed interproximally
- replace restoration if necessary
- OHI (interproximal cleaning), scaling, root planing.

Defective crown margins

Supragingival crown margins are easy to clean but may compromise appearance. Subgingival margins are generally indicated at aesthetically important sites but care must be taken not to compromise the biologic width of attachment. Crown margins should not 'interrupt' the normal contour of the tooth surface. A *positive* defect, or ledge, is one in which the crown margin extends beyond the intended margin of the prepared tooth. A *negative* defect finishes short of the margins of the preparation.

Defective margins inevitably result in plaque accumulation even if the overall standard of oral hygiene is high. Gingival tissues are erythematous and oedematous and bleed readily on probing.

Treatment

- At try-in, reject crowns with defective margins and take new impressions

- Small positive defects may be corrected with fine diamond burs and polishing stones
- Replace the defective crown.

Bridge pontics

Bridge pontics must be carefully designed to facilitate cleaning and minimise plaque accumulation. This is achieved by ensuring the pontics are clear of the gingival tissues. A compromise between aesthetics and cleansibility is usually necessary. Pontics should have smooth surfaces, be convex in all directions and have minimal, light contact on the buccal surface of the edentulous ridge. This allows for self-performed cleaning with superfloss and is aesthetically pleasing. Pontics that impinge on the soft tissues increase plaque accumulation and inflammation. Aesthetics are compromised as a result of poor soft tissue appearance.

Treatment
- Replace bridge
- OHI (superfloss) and scaling.

Partial dentures

Removable prostheses encourage plaque accumulation in the absence of effective oral hygiene. Acrylic dentures with interproximal collets 'gum strippers' cause plaque-induced inflammation, destructive periodontitis and recession of the gingival tissues. Framework components and clasps of cobalt–chrome dentures positioned too close to the gingival margin aggravate plaque-induced inflammation and, occasionally, cause direct trauma.

Prevention
- Utilise tooth support in preference to mucosal support
- Ensure adequate clearance of the gingival tissues by saddles, major and minor connectors and clasps
- Avoid interproximal collets
- Simplify denture design where possible.

Treatment
- Replace poorly designed dentures
- OHI and denture hygiene (clean denture with a toothbrush and water; leave denture out at night).

Orthodontic appliances

Fixed and removable appliances encourage plaque accumulation. Fixed appliances require considerable effort to keep brackets, bands, wires, elastics and tooth surfaces plaque free. Removable appliances can be taken from the mouth to be cleaned and allow toothbrushing. Plaque-induced gingivitis in the region of the appliance is very likely.

Prevention
- Appliances should not be provided to patients who are unable to practice good oral hygiene
- Ensure adequate clearance of the gingival tissues
- Simplify appliance design.

Treatment
- OHI with mini-interdental and interproximal brushes, superfloss.

1.7 Furcation and periodontal–endodontic lesions

Learning objectives

You should

- understand the significance of furcation involvements in periodontitis

- be able to diagnose and classify furcation lesions

- be familiar with the indications for, and techniques of, treatment of furcations

- be able to differentiate between the different types of periodontal-endodontic lesion and plan treatment accordingly.

Furcation lesions

The loss of attachment that occurs with periodontitis eventually reaches the furca of multirooted teeth. Attachment loss then continues both in vertical and horizontal directions, frequently giving rise to lesions with complex bone topography. The management of furcation lesions depends, to some extent, upon the severity of the defect at diagnosis. The early detection of incipient lesions improves the long-term prognosis of the tooth involved. A detailed knowledge of furcation anatomy is, therefore, fundamental to the management of teeth with furcation involvement.

Furcation anatomy

Root anatomy

There are numerous concavities, convexities and grooves associated with root surfaces (Fig. 9). The roots of the mandibular molars are typically broad and flattened mesiodistally. Concavities are found on the furcal aspects of mandibular first molar roots, with those on the distal surfaces of mesial roots being the most accentuated. The roots of the mandibular second and third molars demonstrate similar anatomy, although the roots are closer together and may be fused.

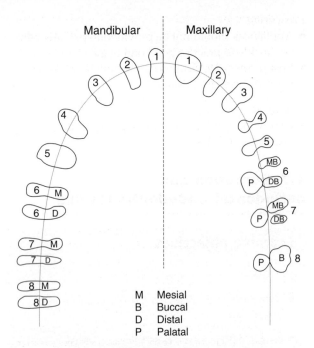

Fig. 9 Typical root morphology seen at horizontal cross-sections made at half root lengths.

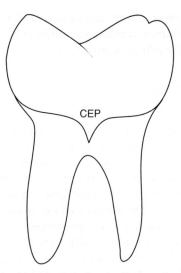

Fig. 10 Cervical enamel projection (CEP) or spur.

The maxillary first molar usually has three separate roots: mesiobuccal, distobuccal and palatal. The two buccal roots are flattened mesiobuccally and the broader, mesiobuccal root has a groove on its distal surface. The palatal root is conical and may be fused to the distobuccal root. The flattened contour of the mesiobuccal root means that the mesiopalatal entrance to the furca of maxillary first molars is accessible to probing. The second and third maxillary molars have the same basic root anatomy as that of the first molar. The roots tend to be less divergent and fused roots are more prevalent. The maxillary first premolar has two roots (buccal and palatal) in about 50% of individuals. The second maxillary premolar may also have two roots, although more commonly the root is single with pronounced grooves on the mesial and distal surfaces. Mandibular incisors, canines and premolars can all have multiple roots, and supplemental roots are common on maxillary and mandibular molars.

Furcation entrance dimensions vary significantly between teeth. On the upper first molar, the mesial and distal furcal entrances are usually sufficiently wide to accommodate periodontal instruments. The buccal entrance is narrower and approximately the width of a Gracey curette. The furcal dimensions on second molars are narrower than the corresponding widths on the first molar. The buccal and distal openings are often accessible to only narrow ultrasonic instruments. In the mandible, the buccal and lingual furcal dimensions of molars are virtually identical. Entrances on the second molar are narrower than those on the first and are approximately the same width as the blade of a Gracey curette.

Cervical enamel projections (Fig. 10) (CEPs) or enamel spurs are pointed, extensions of enamel that arise from the cervico-enamel junction and extend apically, towards and occasionally into the furca of molar teeth. Localised periodontal defects are associated with CEPs in about 90% of patients. Periodontal attachment to CEPs is epithelial in nature; consequently, the distance from the base of the gingival crevice to the point of root bifurcation is effectively reduced. Examination of dry skull material often shows early bone loss, some cratering, or small notch-like lesions adjacent to CEPs.

Intermediate furcation ridges run mesiodistally, in the midline across the bi-and trifurcations of molars. When situated buccally or lingually, they form an exaggerated arch at the entrance of furca. Furcation ridges have a core of dentine but are composed predominantly of cellular cementum, which increases in thickness with age. Ridges are natural obstructions to both plaque control procedures and professional debridement of furcation lesions. Cementum ridges can be recontoured relatively easily during the instrumentation of affected furca.

Accessory root canals are a common finding in the furca of molar teeth. They provide pathways through which inflammation can spread, either from the pulp to the periodontal ligament or, more rarely, from a deep periodontal pocket or abscess to the pulp. Furcation involvement may, therefore, be of pulpal origin, and an assessment of tooth vitality should confirm the diagnosis. When a furcation lesion is of both pulpal and periodontal origin, then complete resolution will only follow combined periodontal and endodontic treatments.

Enamel pearls are isolated 'droplets' of enamel that are found predominantly on the root surfaces of molars and premolars. They form when small islands of Hertwig's epithelial root sheath are retained on dentine during root development. Enamel pearls have no periodontal fibre insertions and occasionally retain a connection with the cementoenamel junction. Pearls are a further potential obstruction to instrumentation of root surfaces.

Distribution of furcation lesions

Epidemiological studies show that the prevalence and severity of furcation lesions increase with increasing age, as the severity of periodontal disease increases. In one study of more than 600 molars, furcation lesions were observed much more frequently in maxillary than in mandibular molars. One possible explanation for this is the position of the furcal openings in the upper and lower teeth. Maxillary molars have mesial and distal furcation entrances that, being sited interproximally (from where plaque is more difficult to remove), are at increased risk of periodontal destruction. Mandibular molars have only buccal and lingual entrances to furcation and these sites are more accessible to oral hygiene practices. The third molars in both jaws have less furcation involvement than first or second molars, principally because the roots are smaller, less divergent and very often fused to form a single tapering root.

Classification and diagnosis

Classification of the severity of furcation involvements is based upon the degree to which a periodontal probe will penetrate the defect. Specially designed furcation probes facilitate the examination of lesions and measurements are made from an imaginary line that crosses the furcation opening, tangential to the contour of the adjacent roots. A 4-point (0–3) scale is frequently used to assess loss of attachment in a horizontal plane (Section 1.2). The vertical loss of attachment at a furcation entrance should also be assessed by measuring from the roof of the furcation to the base of the adjacent pocket. In the absence of gingival recession, clinical probing of furcations is restricted by the soft tissues, with the probe tip coming to rest in the inflamed connective tissues. Measuring a furcation lesion thus gives an indication of horizontal probing depth, rather than of actual attachment loss, or bone resorption.

Intraoral, periapical radiographs taken using the paralleling technique are a useful adjunct to furcation diagnosis. In the maxilla, superimposition of palatal roots of molars and premolars on the furcation makes radiographic interpretation of bone levels difficult. A general assessment of the height of alveolar bone, the presence of vertical bone defects and a reduction in radio-opacity of intraradicular bone may suggest a furcation lesion. The mesial and distal location of roots of mandibular molars usually enables a clear radiographic view of furcation anatomy.

Radiographs of teeth with advanced furcation involvement frequently show vertical bone defects that extend to, or around, a root apex. Vitality testing should be undertaken as an aid to establishing pulpal involvement and to confirm, or exclude, a periodontal–endodontic lesion. The presence of periapical disease is an important factor to take into consideration when assessing the prognosis of a furcation-involved tooth.

Treatment

The basic aims of treatment are to eliminate disease, to provide an environment that the patient is able to clean using home care oral hygiene measures, and to establish a maintenance regimen to prevent reinfection and disease recurrence in the long term. Better access and direct vision for root debridement can be achieved by raising flaps, which also facilitates identification of anatomical irregularities. The surgical approach also allows root anatomy to be modified as well as osseous recontouring, and the creation of an improved morphology of the soft tissues.

Traditionally, the more radical and complex methods of treatment have been used for treatment of the more severe defects (Table 3). Such a guide is clearly very useful, although it is important to assess each patient carefully before deciding upon a definitive treatment plan.

Oral hygiene and preventative measures
Many aspects of treatment aim to provide improved access for self-performed oral hygiene. Patients, therefore, require very careful monitoring to ensure that plaque can, and is, being removed from *all* aspects of the treated furcation. For this purpose certain oral hygiene aids are essential. The single tufted, interspace brush is

Table 3 Treatment of furcation lesions

Grade	Treatment options
1	Oral hygiene Scaling, root planing Furcoplasty
2	Oral hygiene Scaling, root planing with or without surgical access Root resection Guided tissue regeneration
3	Oral hygiene Scaling, root planing, with or without surgical access Root resection Hemisection Tunnel preparation Extraction

indicated for cleaning shallow cave entrances of grade I lesions, as well as more accessible areas such as those created following root resection. An interdental brush is indicated for cleaning between roots, for example in tunnels where the brushes can be used immediately postoperatively to clean subgingivally. Superfloss and floss threaders are also useful in these circumstances. Irrigation of furcation sites using water in a monojet syringe is helpful to loosen food debris or to remove loose deposits of materia alba. A stream of water cannot remove plaque, however, so irrigation devices should not be used as substitutes for mechanical cleaning methods. Root surface caries is a concern at all furcation-treated sites, but particularly at those at which it is very difficult to maintain a plaque-free surface. A daily rinse with a sodium fluoride solution should be included in the immediate postsurgical schedule. Thereafter, regular applications of a fluoride varnish to the root and furcation surfaces are advisable as part of a maintenance recall programme.

Scaling and root planing

Scaling and root planing are often the only treatments required for incipient lesions. Curettes, reciprocating and rotating instruments are not always able to remove calculus from areas such as the furcation roof and the concave distal surfaces of mesial roots. The finer tips of ultrasonic scalers may improve efficacy of debridement.

Flap surgery

With grade 2 and 3 lesions, root surface debridement is likely to be more effective following the elevation of mucoperiosteal flaps. The exact topography of the defect is assessed after the removal of any granulation tissue, and the remaining bone support of individual roots can be evaluated. At this stage, it is useful to compare the actual severity of the lesion with the grade that was given at the initial examination, when, because of the presence of soft tissues, a degree of underestimation of severity is likely. Flaps are replaced and sutured to achieve a gingival architecture that is conducive to effective, home care oral hygiene measures. This is not always attainable, however, without undertaking some modification of the tissues within, or adjacent to, the furcation entrance.

Furcoplasty

The aim of furcoplasty is to produce a healthy gingival papilla in the furcation entrance, which should be accessible to self-performed plaque control. In addition to root surface debridement, furcoplasty comprises two tissue modification procedures.

Odontoplasty is the removal of tooth substance to widen a narrow entrance to the furcation. To prevent postoperative dentine sensitivity, only very limited removal of tooth tissue should be carried out.

Osteoplasty is the recontouring of the adjacent bone of the buccal, lingual or palatal alveolar plates that provide no tooth support.

Tunnel preparation

In deep grade II and grade III defects, the inter-radicular osteoplasty should be more radical to create a tunnel through the furcation. This procedure can be undertaken on any multirooted tooth, although mandibular first and second molars, with their long and well-separated mesial and distal roots, are the favoured candidates. Closure of the mucoperiosteal flaps through the furcation is achieved using an inter-radicular suture and the patency of the tunnel in the immediate postoperative period is maintained by placing a small surgical dressing in the tunnel. Nevertheless, proliferation of soft tissues in the tunnel is common, leading to postsurgical pocketing of 2–3 mm. Furthermore, the tunnel that has been created remains a very difficult area to achieve meticulous plaque control, and caries of root surfaces in the furcation is a potential complication.

Bone regeneration

Regenerative techniques using non-resorbable and resorbable membranes have been applied successfully to the treatment of furcation defects (Section 1.11).

Root amputation

In some cases it is possible to improve the prognosis for a multirooted tooth with furcation involvement by surgically amputating one (or more) of its roots. This procedure effectively eliminates the most periodontally compromised root, and the furcation is made more accessible for cleaning. If a single root is amputated from a maxillary molar, the entire crown can be maintained in occlusion but the remaining furcation should be relatively uninvolved (grade I), thus providing support for the retained natural crown. When both furcations are affected, it may be necessary to divide the roots to assess the precise involvement and mobility of each root separately before deciding which can be retained and which should be removed. In such cases, function can only be restored by coronal restoration. If the mesial or distal root of a mandibular molar is resected, preoperative analysis of the occlusion is recommended to determine whether or not the remaining single root is likely to withstand the loads transmitted by the entire occlusal surface. Where there is doubt, a hemisection is the procedure of choice, removing the involved root and its coronal half of crown. Subsequent coronal restorations are almost always indicated.

Maxillary molars When a single root amputation is planned, a pulpectomy is undertaken and the other roots are filled with gutta-percha before periodontal surgery. Amalgam is condensed into the root to be removed at the level of the planned section to ensure an effective seal at the cut surface (Fig. 11). A final decision regarding which root to resect may not, however, be possible until flaps have been elevated, granulation tissue curetted and the severity of the furcation lesion examined directly. In such cases, the root canals can be filled with a non-setting calcium hydroxide cement. This saves time and expense by obviating the need to prepare and fill unnecessarily a canal in a root that will ultimately be removed.

Very occasionally, root resection may not have been previously contemplated until surgical access has been gained and the severity of involvement appreciated. In these circumstances, a vital root resection is an option. The pulpal exposure at the cut root surface is irrigated with cold saline to control both infection and haemorrhage. A rapid-setting calcium hydroxide lining is applied to the exposed pulp and a glass ionomer restoration is placed over the entire cut section of the root stump. The long-term vitality of the pulp can be maintained if bacterial contamination is prevented at surgery, this being more likely with narrow canals and a small pulpal exposure. If vitality is lost, root canal treatment of the remaining roots is carried out.

When a single root of a maxillary molar has been targeted for amputation, the procedure can be undertaken without raising flaps providing the level of resection is supragingival. Surgical access has the advantages of:

- better vision of the surgical site
- direct evaluation of bone in the remaining furcations
- improved access for recontouring the cut root surface and adjacent post of the crown
- reducing the likelihood of soft tissue trauma
- eliminating soft tissue defects when repositioning flaps.

Mandibular molars A decision regarding which root to retain and which to resect in mandibular molars can nearly always be made prior to surgery. Candidate roots for resection include:

- those with excessively curved root canals that would complicate endodontics
- those that are associated with more extensive bone loss
- those with radiographic evidence of periapical infection.

When a hemisection is indicated on a last standing first (or second) mandibular molar, and there is an intact segment in front of the affected tooth, then the mesial half of the hemisected tooth should be retained to maintain an intact occlusal segment without the need to resort to bridges.

A gutta-percha filling is placed in the root to be retained and an amalgam restoration placed in the

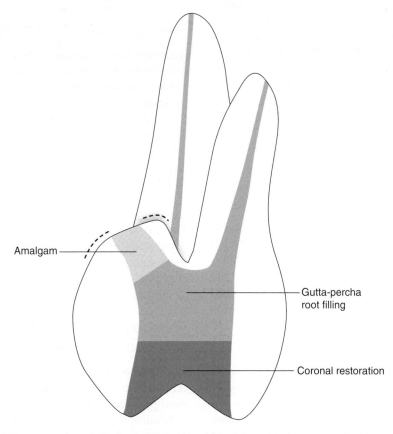

Fig. 11 Root resection on a previously root-filled maxillary molar. Note the rounded contours of cut/resected surface (- - -).

Amalgam

Gutta-percha root filling

Coronal restoration

access cavity down to the level of the planned section. Full thickness mucoperiosteal flaps are raised to maximise vision and improve access, and the tooth is divided. After extraction of the condemned root, the retained part is examined carefully and any irregular edges, or spicules of enamel, dentine or bone, are removed. Redundant soft tissue is excised, before the mucoperiosteal flaps are repositioned and sutured.

Extraction

Grade III furcation involvements of several multirooted teeth are a common finding in patients with advanced periodontal disease. Increased tooth mobilities in both horizontal and vertical directions can severely compromise function, and it may be in the operator's and the patient's best interests to extract teeth with hopeless prognoses so that a concerted effort is targeted to managing the teeth that have a more favourable chance of being retained. If function is not compromised, however, and the patient is free of associated symptoms, then a conservative approach of furcation debridement and instruction in oral hygiene measures at regular intervals may slow the progression of disease. In this way, a functional dentition can be maintained intact for many years.

It is essential to evaluate a number of important general criteria before deciding upon whether a tooth with a furcation lesion should be treated and restored, or extracted. The patient must be committed to receiving the proposed treatment and be able to achieve, and maintain, a high standard of oral hygiene. The involved tooth must also be a valued part of the dentition. For example, it may maintain the integrity of the arch or provide an abutment for a proposed bridge or partial denture. Furthermore, the time and the number of visits needed for treatment, and the expense likely to be incurred should not be overlooked. All should be discussed with the patient before a definitive treatment plan is formulated.

Prognosis

Clearly, the outcome of the procedure is dependent upon the experience of the clinician, not only in carrying out the treatment, but also in case selection and determining the most appropriate treatment. Generally, the treatment that is selected depends predominantly upon the degree of furcation involvement at diagnosis. Molars with tunnel preparations have been shown to have a poor prognosis because of their susceptibility to root caries.

Observations suggest that very few failures occur during the first 5 years after root resection. The 10-year follow-up studies of root resections show a success rate of 60–70%. Further, a high proportion of failed cases result from non-periodontal causes such as caries, root fractures, periapical infection, as well as problems with crowns and bridges (recurrent caries, cement washout, loss of retention). The long-term outcome is, therefore, dependent upon the overall restorative management of the patient as well as the standard and selection of periodontal care.

Five- and 10-year studies of buccal class II furcation defects that have been treated using resorbable and non-resorbable membranes confirm that these techniques improve the prognosis for the affected teeth.

Periodontal–endodontic lesions

Periodontal–endodontic lesions are inflammatory reactions originating in either the pulp or the periodontal ligament with the potential to spread from one site to the other via a number of pathways: apical foramina, lateral and furcation accessory root canals, exposed dentinal tubules, and root defects caused by caries, fractures or perforations during operative procedures.

There are five types of lesion based upon pathogenic interactions of pulpal–periodontal disease:

- primary endodontic
- endodontic with secondary periodontal involvement
- primary periodontal
- periodontal with secondary endodontic involvement
- combined lesions.

Primary endodontic lesions

Infection from a necrotic pulp drains into the periodontium to produce a periapical abscess. This remains localised, drains coronally through the periodontal membrane and gingival sulcus, or tracks through the alveolar bone to leave a swelling and a sinus opening in the attached gingiva. There is no periodontal aetiology.

Clinical features involve persistent discomfort rather than frank pain and a negative response of the tooth to a vitality test. Periapical radiolucency can be seen on radiograph, which may show evidence of spread coronally. There is no loss of alveolar bone height on mesial and distal alveolar crest. Furcation bone loss between molar roots suggests spread of infection via accessory furcation canal.

Treatment of the root canal is indicated.

Endodontic lesions with secondary periodontal involvement

Untreated or inadequately managed endodontic lesions can become a persistent source of infection to the marginal periodontium (Fig. 12a).

Clinical features are similar to those of primary endodontic lesions. Gingival inflammation, increased

(a)　　　　　　　　(b)　　　　　　　　(c)

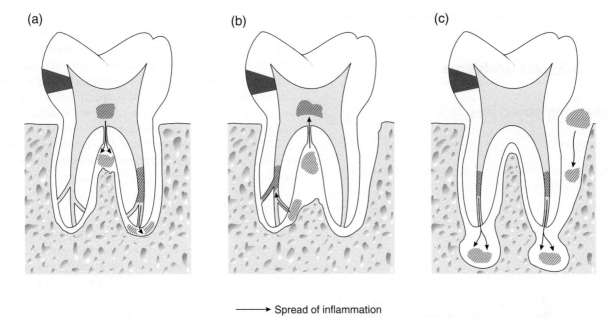

⟶ Spread of inflammation

Fig. 12 Periodontal–endodontic lesions. (a) An endodontic lesion with secondary periodontal involvement in the furcation. (b) A periodontal lesion with secondary endodontic involvement. (c) A combined lesion with both primary pulpal and periodontal origins.

probing depth, bleeding or pus on probing may be evident. Subgingival plaque and calculus can be detected. Radiographs show periapical radiolucency and some resorption of crestal alveolar bone.

Treatment involves root canal treatment and replacement of a previous, unsatisfactory root filling, OHI, scaling and prophylaxis. Extraction should be considered in the case of an extensive lesion.

Primary periodontal lesions

Periodontal infection that spreads to involve the periapical tissues is a primary periodontal lesion. It may be associated with a local anatomical defect such as a radicular groove on a maxillary lateral incisor.

Clinical features include localised, long-standing pain or discomfort and a positive response of the tooth to a vitality test. Gingivitis occurs, and localised deep pocketing is seen, with pus and bleeding following probing or application of pressure to the gingiva. Radiographs show localised bone resorption, which can appear as horizontal, vertical or furcation defects. Anatomical predisposing factors may occasionally be detected.

Treatment includes OHI, scaling and root planing. Surgical treatment to improve access for instrumentation or to eliminate anatomical factors may be indicated. Locally delivered antimicrobials can be considered if infection persists. Consider extraction in the case of an extensive lesion.

Periodontal lesions with secondary endodontic involvement

Secondary endodontic involvement is seen when infection spreads from the periodontium to the pulp, causing pulpitis and necrosis (Fig. 12b).

Clinical features are similar to those of primary periodontal lesions but the tooth gives a negative response to vitality testing. Radiographic appearance may be identical to teeth with periodontal involvement only, although bone loss is generally more extensive. Conversely, narrow, tortuous defects can be associated with grooves on the root surface.

Treatment involves root canal therapy, OHI, scaling and root planing. Local antimicrobials should be considered if infection persists. Surgery can facilitate access to deeper pockets/anatomical defects or allow regenerative procedures. Extraction should be considered in an extensive lesion.

Combined lesions

In combined lesions, the periodontal infection 'coalesces' with a periapical lesion of pulpal origin. There are two distinct origins: periodontal and periapical (Fig. 12c).

The clinical features and management of combined lesions are the same as for periodontal lesions with secondary endodontic involvement. The remaining periodontal attachment is often minimal; consequently, tooth mobility is usually quite pronounced. Root amputation or hemi-section may be indicated but the prognosis is often very poor.

1.8 Gingival problems

Gingival recession

When gingival recession occurs, the width of attached gingiva is reduced or eliminated. However, a narrow or absent width of attached gingiva is compatible with health and the width of attached gingiva alone should not be regarded as the only 'risk factor' for gingival recession.

Gingival recession can affect any site in the mouth and, depending upon aetiological factors, may be localised or generalised.

Aetiology

There is often an element of trauma that can be identified as a contributing factor, particularly to localised recession:

- excessive toothbrushing force, incorrect technique or use of a particularly abrasive dentifrice
- traumatic incisor relationships
- habits such as rubbing the gingiva with a finger nail or the end of a pencil.

Generalised recession occurs when the gingival margin migrates apically as a consequence of ongoing periodontal disease or following resolution of inflammation after successful periodontal treatment. Localised or generalised recession may also be a complication of orthodontic treatment when teeth (roots) are moved labially through an existing dehiscence or very thin labial alveolar plate.

An exposed root surface on an anterior tooth is often aesthetically unacceptable. Exposure of dentine may cause extreme sensitivity and root surfaces are susceptible to caries. Sibilant speech may result from widened interdental spaces.

Clinical features

Apical migration of the gingival complex exposes the root surface. Wear cavities on root surfaces are indicative of toothbrush abrasion as an aetiological factor.

Stillman's cleft (Fig. 13) is an incipient lesion, a narrow, deep and slightly curved cleft extending apically from the free gingival margin. As the recession progresses apically, the cleft becomes broader exposing the cementum of the root surface. When the lesion reaches the mucogingival junction, the apical border of oral mucosa is usually inflamed because of the difficulty in maintaining good plaque control at this site.

McCall's festoon (Fig. 13) is a rolled, thickened band of gingiva usually seen adjacent to canines when recession approaches the mucogingival junction.

Predisposing factors

Dehiscences (clefts) or fenestrations (windows) are natural defects in labial alveolar plates that are often, but not exclusively, associated with prominent roots or teeth that are crowded out of the arch. Such defects need not necessarily initiate recession but rather increase its rate of progression once established.

(a)

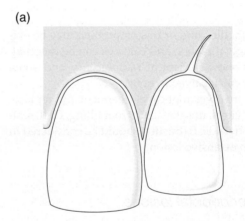

(b)

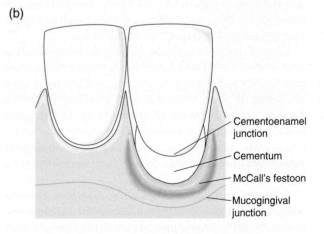

Cementoenamel junction

Cementum

McCall's festoon

Mucogingival junction

Fig. 13 Mucogingival lesions. (a) Stillman's cleft. (b) McCall's festoon in which a rolled, fibrous 'curtain' of gingiva occurs.

Treatment

- Record the magnitude of recession (clinically or on study models) on a regular basis to assess progression or stability
- Eliminate aetiological factors
- OHI
- Topical desensitising agents/fluoride varnish
- Gingival veneer to cover exposed roots/embrasure spaces
- Crown teeth (after diagnostic wax up) but exercise extreme caution to prevent exposure of coronal pulp at level of radicular preparation.
- Mucogingival surgery (Section 1.11)

Gingival enlargement

Gingival enlargement may occasionally be the first presenting sign of an underlying systemic disorder. A full medical history should always be taken, and clinicians must be alert for additional signs and symptoms to confirm the diagnosis. A systematic approach will reveal the medication history, haemorrhagic tendencies, abdominal and gastrointestinal upset, or any respiratory problems. Careful extraoral and intraoral examinations are necessary to determine the nature and extent of the lesion, additional signs and predisposing or traumatic factors. Referral to a specialist centre for additional investigations may be appropriate.

Gingival fibromatosis

Gingival fibromatosis is an uncommon condition with autosomal dominant inheritance pattern. There is generalised fibrous enlargement of the gingiva as a result of the accumulation of bundles of collagen fibres. It is frequently associated with fibrous enlargement of the maxillary tuberosities.

Treatment is usually not required, unless access for cleaning is impaired or aesthetics are compromised. It tends to recur following surgical excision.

Chronic hyperplastic gingivitis

Chronic hyperplastic gingivitis may occur following prolonged accumulation of dental plaque. It is frequently associated with concomitant systemic medications, though predisposing factors may not be identifiable. There is firm, pink gingival enlargement, particularly at interdental sites, although an inflammatory component may also be present. The gingiva may partially cover the crowns of teeth, resulting in aesthetic problems and cleaning difficulties.

Treatment is oral hygiene instruction, scaling and gingivectomy.

Drug-associated gingival overgrowth

Phenytoin, ciclosporin and the calcium-channel blockers (notably nifedipine) are all associated with the unwanted effect of gingival overgrowth.

Incidence

The incidence varies between the different drugs; it affects approximately 50% of patients taking phenytoin, 30% taking ciclosporin and 20% taking nifedipine. Prevalence is increased in children and adolescents. It predominantly affects the anterior gingival tissues.

Clinical features

Overgrowth commences within the interdental papillae, which enlarge until they coalesce, involving all of the attached gingivae. Overgrowth extends coronally and may interfere with speech, occlusion and mastication. Aesthetics are severely compromised. The colour varies from pink to deep red-purple, depending on the degree of inflammation in the tissues. Occasionally it can present in the edentulous.

Histopathology

The epithelium is parakeratinised and acanthotic, often with long, slender, elongated rete ridges. Fibrous tissue forms the bulk of the overgrowth, featuring a proliferation of fibroblasts and increased collagen content. Inflamed tissues are highly vascularised and contain collections of inflammatory cells. Plasma cells predominate, although lymphocytes and macrophages are also present.

Pathogenesis

The precise mechanism of overgrowth is uncertain and involves complex interactions between the drug, fibroblasts, plaque-induced inflammation and genetic factors. Subpopulations of fibroblasts exist that synthesise increased quantities of collagen, the relative proportions of which are genetically determined. Plaque-induced inflammation is a prerequisite for overgrowth; in inflamed tissues, high-activity fibroblasts may become sensitised to the effects of systemic drugs. A drug-related increase in the metabolism of certain hormones (e.g. androgens) by fibroblasts may explain the increased incidence observed in adolescents. Human lymphocyte antigen (HLA) expression may be associated with fibroblast phenotype and could act as a marker for overgrowth.

Treatment

A strict programme of OHI and plaque control must be implemented. Overgrown tissues should be surgically excised.

Crohn's disease

Crohn's disease is a chronic granulomatous disorder of unknown aetiology affecting any part of the gastrointestinal tract.

Oral manifestations include oedema, hypertrophy and fissuring of the buccal mucosa ('cobblestone appearance'), swelling of the lips and cheeks, mucosal tags, oral ulceration and angular cheilitis. An erythematous granular enlargement of the entire width of the attached gingiva may be evident.

Treatment is OHI, scaling and root planing.

Orofacial granulomatosis

Orofacial granulomatosis is not a discrete clinical entity but describes the common clinicopathological presentation of a variety of disorders including Crohn's disease and some topical hypersensitivity reactions.

Acute leukaemia

Malignant proliferation of white blood cells and their precursors results in increased numbers of circulating leukocytes and infiltration of tissues by leukaemic cells giving several periodontal manifestations.

Gingival enlargement results from infiltration of the gingival connective tissues by leukaemic cells. It gives impaired plaque control and further inflammatory oedema.

Gingival bleeding results from the thrombocytopenia that accompanies the leukaemia and may be spontaneous.

Acute periodontal abscesses can develop from an acute exacerbation of pre-existing periodontitis.

Treatment
OHI and effective mechanical plaque control are essential but are impaired by enlarged, bleeding tissues. Chemical antiplaque agents (e.g. chlorhexidine) should be prescribed and acute infections managed with systemic antimicrobials.

Sarcoidosis

Sarcoidosis is a systemic chronic granulomatous disorder of unknown aetiology typically affecting the lungs, lymph nodes, liver, skin and eyes.

Oral lesions are rare, but reported periodontal manifestations include a hyperplastic granulomatous gingivitis. Altered lymphocyte and neutrophil function may (rarely) lead to rapid periodontal destruction.

Wegener's granulomatosis

Wegener's granulomatosis is a systemic disease characterised by necrotising granulomas of the respiratory system and kidneys, and necrotising vasculitis of small arteries.

There is a characteristic hyperplastic gingivitis with petechiae and an ulcerated 'strawberry' appearance.

Gingival condition improves when systemic drug therapy (prednisolone and cyclophosphamide) is initiated.

Epulides

Epulides are localised hyperplastic lesions arising from the gingiva.

Aetiology
Trauma and chronic irritation from plaque and calculus invoke a chronic inflammatory response in which continued inflammation and attempts at repair proceed concurrently. Excessive production of granulation tissue results, forming the epulis.

Clinical features
Fibrous epulis is a firm, pink, pedunculated mass that may be ulcerated if traumatised. Histologically, it comprises chronically inflamed, hyperplastic fibrous tissue, which may be richly cellular or densely collagenous. Metaplastic bone and/or foci of dystrophic calcification are common.

Vascular epulis (pyogenic granuloma and pregnancy epulis) is a soft, purple/red swelling, frequently ulcerated, which bleeds readily. Histologically, a proliferation of richly vascular tissue is supported by a fibrous stroma with a thin, often extensively ulcerated epithelium. A pregnancy epulis is a pyogenic granuloma occurring in a pregnant female. Vascular and fibrous epulides probably represent different phases of the same inflammatory process.

Peripheral giant cell granuloma (GCG) involves a dark reddish/purple, ulcerated swelling, frequently arising interdentally and often extending buccally and lingually. It may cause superficial erosion of crestal alveolar bone. Radiographs are essential to differentiate from a central GCG that has perforated the cortex to present as a peripheral swelling. Histologically, GCG contains multiple foci of osteoclast-like giant cells supported by a richly vascular and cellular stroma.

Treatment
Surgical excision is the treatment of choice. Haemostasis may be problematic when removing pregnancy epulides. These can be left until after parturition as they then tend to reduce in size and become increasingly fibrous. Excision during pregnancy generally results in recurrence.

Iatrogenic gingival enlargement

Denture induced enlargement
Chronic trauma from ill-fitting dentures, particularly when associated with poor oral hygiene, can result in hyperplasia of the underlying gingival tissues. Frequently this is associated with prostheses supported by mucosa only, with inadequate gingival clearance and poor stability. The tissues may be oedematous, erythematous and bleed readily; they can become increasingly fibrous in the long term.

Treatment is with OHI, denture hygiene, scaling and root planing, and replacement of defective prostheses.

Orthodontically induced enlargement

Orthodontic movement of teeth occasionally results in the 'heaping-up' of gingival soft tissues in the direction of tooth movement. This occurs more frequently when teeth are repositioned with removal appliances (tipping movement) than when using fixed appliances (bodily movement).

The gingiva 'accumulates' in the direction of tooth movement. It frequently affects the palatal gingiva adjacent to maxillary incisors when these are being retracted. The enlargement tends to resolve on completion of orthodontic treatment.

OHI and appliance hygiene are usually the only treatment needed.

Cystic lesions

Gingival cysts account for less than 1% of cysts of the jaws. More common in neonates, these tend to resolve spontaneously in early life. In adults, they are generally chance findings in histological sections from gingivectomy specimens and are typically asymptomatic. Cystic lesions are probably odontogenic in origin, arising from remnants of the dental lamina.

Developmental lateral periodontal cysts may present with expansion of alveolar bone, but most are incidental findings on radiographs. They resemble gingival cysts if arising near the alveolar bone crest. Radiographically, they appear as a radiolucency with well-defined bony margins.

Treatment is by surgical excision.

1.9 Trauma and the periodontium

Learning objectives

You should

- be alert to the possibility that certain traumatic injuries to the periodontium may be self-inflicted

- be aware of the potential relationships that exist between trauma from occlusion and periodontal disease

- be able to classify traumatic incisor relationships.

The periodontium has an inherent capacity to adapt to physiological or traumatic forces that occur during normal function or hyperfunction. In some cases, the trauma exceeds the adaptive nature of the tissues and pathologic change and injury result.

Self-inflicted trauma

Factitious gingivitis

A minor form of self-inflicted trauma is seen in young children. Food packing or local inflammation provides a locus of irritation and the child picks or rubs the area with a finger nail, pencil, or abrasive food such as crisps or nuts. If untreated, ulceration and inflammation persist and gingival recession may ensue. The lesion usually resolves when the habit is corrected.

The lesions of the major form are more severe and widespread both intra- and extraorally. They present as ulcers, abrasions, gingival recession or blisters, which may be blood filled. Trauma can be inflicted subconsciously, or purposely in an attempt to deceive clinicians into diagnosing organic disease. Outlines of lesions provide clues as to the object used to produce them. The lesions are remarkably resistant to conventional treatment and may reflect an underlying psychological problem. Referral to a psychologist/psychiatrist is advised but rarely welcomed by patients or relatives.

Oral hygiene practices

Used incorrectly and without instruction, toothbrushes and interproximal cleaning aids can cause irreversible trauma to both periodontal tissues and teeth. Injudicious toothbrushing causes gingival abrasions, clefting and recession, which can be localised or generalised. Excessive toothbrushing force also produces typical V-shaped abrasion cavities. Localised defects can be caused by mini-interdental brushes, incorrect use of floss and dental woodpoints.

Iatrogenic trauma

Dental procedures and components of poorly designed restorations or appliances can cause direct local irritation/trauma to the gingiva. Examples include:

- injudicious use of rotary, ultrasonic, and scaling instruments
- placement of excessive gingival retraction cord or leaving remnants of material in the gingival sulcus after taking an impression
- spillage of caustic chemicals used in dental treatments
- components of fixed/removable orthodontic appliances
- components of removable partial dentures
- extension of a palatal denture base into the interproximal areas to rest upon the gingival papillae.

In the short term, traumatic lesions of the soft tissues are reversible when the stimulus is removed. More persistent chronic irritation can lead to gingival recession.

Occlusal trauma

Glickman's hypothesis

In 1965, Irving Glickman suggested that, in order to understand fully the role of trauma from occlusion in periodontal disease, the periodontium should be considered as two zones:

- the zone of irritation comprises the marginal and interdental gingiva, which are susceptible to plaque-induced inflammation
- the zone of co-destruction comprises the periodontal ligament, alveolar bone and cementum, which become involved when marginal gingival inflammation spreads in the alveolar crest.

Glickman's hypothesis was that excessive occlusal force, in the presence of gingivitis, acts as a co-destructive factor, altering the pathway of inflammation so that it spreads directly into the periodontal ligament (Fig. 14). The presence of inflammation was crucial in reducing the adaptive capacity of the healthy periodontium to occlusal forces, the consequence being the development of vertical, infrabony defects around affected teeth. This hypothesis is almost certainly an oversimplification of the interaction between periodontal inflammation and occlusal trauma. Nevertheless, it provided a basis from which subsequent animal model experiments were developed.

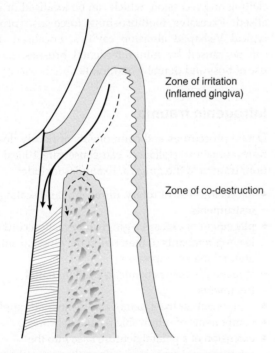

Fig. 14 Glickman's occlusal trauma hypothesis. Gingival inflammation in the presence of occlusal trauma spreads into the periodontal ligament (solid arrows) to produce a vertical bone defect, rather than through the channels in the alveolar bone (dotted arrow).

Zone of irritation (inflamed gingiva)

Zone of co-destruction

Jiggling forces

Jiggling forces act successively, in opposite directions, thus preventing the tooth from moving orthodontically away from the forces and subjecting the periodontium to alternating phases of pressure and tension. Such forces may originate from the components of removable prostheses or appliances. Observations made from animal experiments suggest that the teeth subjected to jiggling forces show an accelerated progression of experimental periodontitis compared with controls. Tooth mobility increases progressively as affected sites display both horizontal and vertical bone loss, with the latter being similar to that described by Glickman.

These observations have led to a number of important conclusions:

- traumatic occlusal forces initiate neither periodontitis nor connective tissue attachment loss in a healthy periodontium
- jiggling forces may predispose to some loss of alveolar bone height and density as the healthy periodontium adapts to the increased forces placed upon it; tooth mobility increases and radiographically there is widening of the periodontal membrane space
- when jiggling forces and periodontitis act as co-destructive factors to increase the rate of disease progression, tooth mobility may reduce when the forces are removed but periodontal stability and/or regeneration will occur only when the inflammatory component is resolved
- treatment of periodontal inflammation, consequently, is of paramount importance.

Occlusal interferences

Occlusal interferences or premature occlusal contacts can arise when the occlusal morphology and/or position of teeth are altered, for example, following placement of restorations or after orthodontic therapy.

Clinical features

Occlusional trauma can give rise to pain, fracture or faceting of cusps, attrition, bruxism, increased tooth mobility and temporomandibular joint symptoms. Widening of the periodontal membrane space can be seen in radiographs and suggests tissue remodelling as an attempt to adapt to the interference. Potentially, the most damaging interferences result from premature contacts in retruded contact position (RCP) or non-working contacts in lateral mandibular excursion. In the presence of periodontal inflammation, a persistent interference with increased occlusal loading can produce localised, infrabony defects, which may jeopardise the survival of the tooth.

Treatment

The periodontal inflammation must be resolved and the interference identified. It can be confirmed by mounting study models in retruded contact position on a semi-adjustable articulator. Occlusal adjustment is then undertaken.

Traumatic incisor relationships

The Akerly classification identifies the relationship between the maxillary and mandibular incisors, and the nature of complete overbite (Fig. 15).

- *Class I*: lower incisors impinge upon the palatal mucosa
- *Class II*: lower incisors occlude on the palatal gingival margins of the maxillary teeth
- *Class III*: a deep, traumatic overbite (class II division 2) exists with shearing of the mandibular labial and maxillary palatal gingiva
- *Class IV*: lower incisors occlude with the palatal surfaces of upper incisors; evidence of tooth wear owing to attrition can be seen and there is minimal, if any, effect upon supporting tissues.

Aggravating factors include inherent development of a severe, class II division 2 incisor relationship; injudicious orthodontic or restorative treatment; gradual loss of posterior support with distal movement of premolars and canines and the presence of powerful lip musculature.

Treatment

Interventive treatment is possible for developmental cases in childhood. In adults, it is important to establish periodontal health, to protect tissues temporarily with a soft acrylic splint and to restore posterior dimension. More complex relationships may require orthodontic therapy, orthognathic surgery and segmental or full mouth rehabilitation, with or without the use of Dahl and overlay appliances.

1.10 Syndromes and medical conditions associated with aggressive periodontitis

Learning objectives

You should

- understand the periodontal implications of certain rare, and sometimes life-threatening, hereditary conditions
- be aware of the reasons for the increased risk of progressive periodontitis in uncontrolled diabetics.

Aggressive periodontitis (Section 1.4) may also be a manifestation of several rare, but well-recognised, heritable syndromes. Many of these syndromes are associated with profound abnormalities of neutrophil function, which predispose these patients to their periodontal problems.

Papillon–Lefevre syndrome

Papillon–Lefevre syndrome is a rare condition transmitted as an autosomal recessive trait with an estimated incidence of 1–4 per million births. A history of consanguinity between parents is found in about 30% of affected individuals.

Clinical features

The syndrome is characterised by a diffuse palmar–plantar hyperkeratosis and an aggressive periodontitis, with an onset of about 2 years of age. The child may be edentulous by 5–6 years. Progressive periodontal destruction usually also affects the permanent dentition, with patients becoming edentulous by the age of 20. The clinical presentation may show wide variation, and

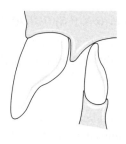 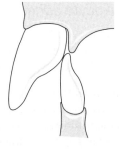 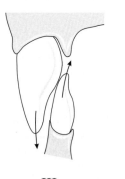 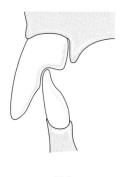

| I | II | III | IV |

Fig. 15 The Akerly classification of traumatic incisor relationships. (I) Palatal trauma. (II) Trauma at the gingival crevice. (III) Shearing trauma of the class II division 2 overbite. (IV) Palatal attrition.

occasionally the skin and periodontal lesions present on their own as distinct clinical entities. Variations in periodontal presentation include those affecting only the primary dentition and a late-onset disorder where the primary dentition remains unaffected. Defects in neutrophil adhesion, chemotaxis and phagocytosis have been observed in some patients.

Treatment

Intensive periodontal therapy includes OHI, chlorhexidine rinses, scaling, and prescription of antimicrobials (metronidazole and amoxicillin) to control acute phases. Severely involved teeth must be extracted. The loss of teeth is almost inevitable, even with a high degree of patient compliance. A more realistic aim is to maintain alveolar bone height to support eventually removable or implant-retained prostheses.

Ehlers–Danlos syndrome

Ehlers–Danlos syndrome is as an autosomal dominant or recessive trait with the primary defect being related to the synthesis and extracellular polymerisation of collagen molecules. Ten types have been described.

Clinical features

The main features are excessive mobility of joints and increased extensibility of skin, which is also susceptible to bruising and scarring following superficial wounds. In types I and IV, the oral soft tissues are prone to bruising and haemorrhage because of defective support of the lamina propria. Gingival bleeding may occur after toothbrushing. The type VIII variant appears especially associated with advanced periodontal disease.

Pathology

Lesions are characterised by massive proliferation of Langerhans cells (resembling histiocytes), with varying numbers of eosinophils and multinucleate giant cells. Histopathological changes of teeth have been detected: enamel hypoplasia, abnormalities of dentine and an increased incidence of pulp stones.

Treatment

Conventional treatment for periodontal disease is undertaken but extreme caution must be taken because of the fragility of the soft tissues and their susceptibility to trauma.

Oral lesions are accessible for biopsy to confirm a diagnosis. Local excision and curettage of bone lesions is often successful, although the prognosis is poor when soft tissues become widely involved. When a patient presents with oral lesions, a complete radiographic screening or bone scan is needed to detect or exclude multifocal involvement.

Diabetes mellitus

Diabetes mellitus is a metabolic disorder that is associated with an intolerance to glucose. In type I insulin-dependent diabetes mellitus, there is a sudden onset in predominantly young adults. Type II is non-insulin dependent and has a gradual onset in middle age. The general symptoms are thirst, hunger, polyuria and weight loss. The incidence is about 2%.

Generally, the well-controlled diabetic is at no increased risk from periodontal disease. A poorly controlled diabetic with complications (nephropathy, retinopathy) is at risk from aggressive forms of periodontal disease. Multiple periodontal abscesses or suppurating pockets are a feature.

Aetiology

The subgingival microflora in diabetic patients contains recognised periodontopathogens: *Actinobacillus actinomycetemcomitans, Capnocytophaga* sp., *Prevotella intermedia, Campylobacter recta* and *Porphyromonas gingivalis*. Several factors may contribute to the disease pathogenesis. Impaired neutrophil function includes reduced chemotaxis, phagocytosis and intracellular killing. Well-recognised vascular changes that accompany diabetes (thickening and hyalinisation of vascular walls) appear to have little, if any, bearing on the periodontal status. Recent evidence suggests that, in diabetics, hyperglycaemic episodes glycate body proteins forming advanced glycation end-products (AGE) which, in turn, induce phagocytes to release TNF-α, IL-1 and IL-6. The elevated levels of cytokines could exacerbate inflammatory responses.

Treatment

Extraction of hopelessly involved teeth is followed by conventional non-surgical or surgical therapy. Systemic antimicrobials (amoxicillin and metronidazole) are indicated for persistant or recurrent infections. In view of the susceptibility of diabetics to general infections, antibiotic prophylaxis should be considered prior to periodontal surgery.

Leukocyte adhesion-deficiency syndrome

The leukocyte adhesion-deficiency (LAD) syndrome is a single gene defect with an autosomal recessive pattern of inheritance.

Clinical features

Delayed separation of the umbilical cord occurs at birth and there is impaired wound healing and severe, often life-threatening bacterial infections. Aggressive periodontitis is present with an acute gingivitis, profuse bleeding and suppurating pockets. The permanent dentition is also affected. In mild variants, symptoms can be mild and the disease appears stable over long periods, only for an acute phase to develop and the patient to deteriorate very rapidly. The syndrome is usually fatal by about 30 years.

Pathology

Impaired adhesion of neutrophils to vessel walls occurs as a result of restricted expression of cell surface integrins.

Treatment

Palliative treatment is used for periodontal disease, which is frequently regarded as being of secondary importance to the life-threatening infections which occur.

Langerhans cell histiocytosis

The Langerhans cell histiocytosis was previously known as histiocytosis X. It is a triad of conditions characterised by widespread proliferation of foci of histiocytic cells with features of Langerhans cells. The acute form, Letterer–Siwe disease, is usually fatal in infancy. Eosinophilic granuloma (unifocal) and Hand–Schuller–Christian disease (multifocal) are closely related.

Clinical features

Single or multiple osteolytic lesions involve the pituitary fossa and the frontal, orbital and sphenoid bones of the skull. Progressive involvement may cause diabetes insipidus and exophthalamus (Hand–Schuller–Christian disease). Other bones involved include the ribs, pelvis, clavicle, femur and humerus. Osteolytic involvement of alveolar bone is more common in the mandible and presents as an aggressive periodontitis with a generalised and irregular pattern of bone resorption. Involved bone shows radiolucencies of considerable size. Pain and excessive tooth mobility are common early symptoms. Recurrent acute periodontal abscess formation is also common and the gingiva can be swollen, oedematous, necrotic and ulcerated.

Down syndrome

Down syndrome is a common autosomal chromosome abnormality: trisomy of number 21. It occurs in about 1 in 700 births. The incidence increases with age of the mother.

Clinical features

Affected children have increased susceptibility to aggressive or advanced types of periodontitis. Institutionalised patients have a greater prevalence of dental and periodontal problems than those cared for at home. Local clinical factors that predispose to accumulation of dental plaque and restrict access for its removal include:

- class III malocclusion with crowding
- anterior open bite
- lack of lip seal leading to drying of plaque
- reduced salivary flow
- high frenal attachments
- tongue thrusting.

Treatment

A good standard of plaque control is difficult to achieve because of lack of dexterity and motivation. Use of anti-microbial mouthrinse helps to reduce plaque deposits between regular visits for scaling and prophylaxis.

Hypophosphatasia

Hypophosphatasia is an inborn error of metabolism with autosomal recessive and dominant patterns of inheritance. There is a deficiency of the liver/kidney/bone isoenzyme of alkaline phosphatase, which is crucial for the mineralisation of hard tissues.

Clinical features

Juvenile (childhood) hypophosphatasia has an age of onset around 2 years. The bone defects can lead to mild bowing of the legs, proptosis and a delay in closure of the fontanelles. Aplastic or hypoplastic cementum leads to premature loss of the primary dentition through extensive root resorption or bone loss as a result of a weakened periodontal attachment and disuse atrophy. The gingiva can appear quite healthy. In the adult form, which presents during middle age, the periodontal changes are localised to the incisor region.

Treatment

When primary teeth are lost it is important to maintain space for their permanent successors, which erupt prematurely.

1.11 Treatment of periodontal disease

Learning objectives

You should

- understand the importance of effective plaque control in determining the success of periodontal therapy
- know how plaque control may be achieved in individual patients
- know the instruments and techniques required to perform scaling and root planing
- understand the principal indications for various surgical treatments
- be familiar with the basic procedures involved in periodontal surgery.

Mechanical plaque control

Plaque control refers to the removal of plaque from the tooth surface and gingival tissues, and prevention of new microbial growth. Effective plaque control results in resolution of gingival inflammation and is fundamentally important in all periodontal therapy. Periodontal treatment performed in the absence of plaque control is certain to fail, resulting in disease recurrence. Mechanical plaque control is performed using toothbrushes, toothpaste and other cleaning aids. Plaque-control programmes should be tailored to the requirements of individual patients. Motivation of patients to change their behavioural habits is a great challenge and patients must be educated so they understand the importance of their contribution to maintaining health and preventing disease.

Powered toothbrushes

The brushheads of powered (electric) toothbrushes tend to be more compact than those of their manual counterparts; this feature facilitates interproximal brushing and cleaning of the less accessible posterior teeth. Bundles of bristles are arranged in rows (similar to manual brushes) or in a circular pattern mounted in a round head. Some brushes have single, compact tufts, which are specifically designed for interproximal cleaning. The traditional design of brushhead operates with a side-to-side or back and forth motion. The circular heads have an oscillating motion and the single tufted heads also operate with a rotary action.

Traditionally, powered toothbrushes have been considered advantageous for handicapped/special needs patients, patients with fixed orthodontic appliances and those who are hospitalised or institutionalised and who may need a careworker or nurse to carry out oral hygiene.

Numerous studies have confirmed that, for most patients, powered toothbrushes are slightly more effective than manual brushes. This may be because of better mechanical cleaning per se, although the 'novelty effect' of using a powered toothbrush is a likely contributing factor.

Toothbrushes

Toothbrushes vary in design and size, and the type of brush used is a matter of personal preference. Bristles are generally made of nylon, which is relatively flexible, resistant to fracture and does not become saturated with water. Bristles are arranged in tufts, and rounded bristles cause fewer scratches on the gingiva than do flat-ended bristles. Softer bristles have greater flexibility and have been shown to reach further interproximally and subgingivally. Hard bristles are more likely to result in gingival trauma. However, the technique and the force applied when brushing are more important determinants of plaque-removal capability and likelihood of gingival trauma than the hardness of the bristles themselves. With use, toothbrushes begin to show signs of excessive wear and flattening of bristles, generally, they should be replaced approximately every 3 months.

Toothpastes

Toothpastes are used as aids for cleaning tooth surfaces and contain abrasives (e.g. silica), water, preservatives, flavouring, colouring, detergents and therapeutic agents (e.g. fluoride). Abrasives (approximately 20–40% of the paste) enhance plaque removal but may result in damage to the tooth surface if there is overzealous brushing. Smokers' toothpastes and tooth powders contain significantly higher proportions of abrasives and their use is not recommended. Chemotherapeutic agents (e.g. chlorhexidine) may be added to toothpastes and are discussed in more detail below.

Toothbrushing techniques

The majority of patients use a 'horizontal scrub' technique, which frequently does not clean effectively around gingival margins and can lead to tooth wear. When brushing, a systematic approach is essential, and all accessible surfaces of all teeth should be cleaned thoroughly. The Bass technique is useful for the majority of patients with or without periodontal disease. The Charters technique is useful for gentle gingival cleaning, particularly during healing immediately after periodontal surgery.

Bass technique

- The toothbrush is placed at the gingival margin, with bristles orientated at 45° to the long axis of the tooth, pointing in an apical direction
- Short vibratory strokes are applied to the brush so that the bristles are not dislodged (this forces the bristles interproximally and approximately 1 mm subgingivally, resulting in gingival blanching)
- After about 20 strokes, the brush is repositioned to clean the next group of teeth.

Charters technique

- The toothbrush is placed on the tooth with the bristles orientated at 45° to the long axis of the tooth, pointing in a coronal direction, such that the sides of the bristles are against the gingiva
- A short back and forth motion is applied so that the sides of the bristles flex against the gingiva.

Interproximal cleaning aids

Interproximal areas are particularly susceptible to plaque accumulation. Toothbrushing does not effectively remove plaque from these surfaces and additional cleaning aids are required.

Dental floss

Floss is usually made from nylon and is available as a twisted or untwisted multifilament, with or without a coating of wax (wax facilitates passage beyond the contact point), as a thread or in tape form. Floss made from expanded polytetrafluoroethylene (Teflon) materials that do not fray is also available. The plaque-removal capabilities of different types of floss do not vary significantly. Floss should be wrapped around the fingers then stretched tightly between the thumbs, or thumb and first finger, of each hand so that it can be eased carefully past the interproximal contact point. The floss should be moved carefully up and down the proximal surface of each tooth, from just below the contact point to just below the gingival margin. Floss holders, which stretch the floss between two plastic arms, may be useful for patients with limited manual dexterity.

Interspace brushes

Interspace brushes (ISBs) look like toothbrushes that contain just one tuft of bristles. These are especially useful for cleaning:

- interproximal surfaces of teeth when adjacent teeth are absent
- distal surfaces of the most posterior remaining tooth
- the lingual surfaces of mandibular teeth
- around orthodontic appliances
- areas of gingival recession
- areas of crowding with instanding teeth that are missed by a regular toothbrush
- tooth/root concavities and incipient (class I) furcation lesions.

Mini-interdental brushes

Mini-interdental brushes (MIBs) are conical or tube-like brushes ('bottle brushes') made of bristles mounted on a twisted metal wire handle. They are used by patients with periodontitis to clean:

- interproximally, particularly in locations where there is loss of the interdental papillae and there is sufficient room for the brush to be placed
- in class II and class III furcations
- around implant restorations (wire handle should be plastic coated to prevent scratching of the titanium surface).

Chemical plaque control

Chemical agents have been incorporated into mouthrinses and toothpastes with the objective of inhibiting the formation of plaque and calculus. Antiplaque agents may also have a significant clinical effect of resolving an established gingivitis.

Cationic agents

Chlorhexidine digluconate

Chlorhexidine is frequently used as a mouthrinse (0.2% or 0.12% w/v). The compound can also be applied as a gel and has been incorporated into chewing gum, slow-release devices and periodontal packs.

At low concentrations, chlorhexidine is bacteriostatic; at high concentrations, it is bactericidal. The mode of action of chlorhexidine in killing bacteria is dependent upon the drug having access to cell walls. This is facilitated by electrostatic forces, since chlorhexidine is positively charged, while the phosphate and carboxyl groups of bacterial cell walls carry negative charges. Binding causes disruption of the osmotic barrier and interference with membrane transport.

Rinsing with chlorhexidine reduces the number of bacteria in saliva by between 50% and 90%. A maximum reduction of 95% occurs around 5 days, after which the numbers increase gradually to maintain an overall reduction of 70–80% at 40 days.

An important property of chlorhexidine is its substantivity, that is, the retention in the mouth and subsequent release from oral structures. After a 1 minute oral rinse of 10 ml chlorhexidine 0.2%, approximately 30% of the drug is retained; within 15 seconds of rinsing, half will have bonded to receptor molecules.

Chlorhexidine mouthrinses and gels are beneficial

- after periodontal surgery
- in the management of periodontal problems in the mentally handicapped
- for preventing phenytoin-induced gingival overgrowth
- in the management of HIV gingivitis and periodontitis
- for patients wearing fixed orthodontic appliances or an intermaxillary fixation device.

The main unwanted effects are staining of the teeth, restorations and the tongue, and taste disturbances.

Quaternary ammonium compounds

Quaternary ammonium compounds (QACs) include cetylpyridinium chloride (often combined with domiphen bromide), benzalconium chloride and benzethonium chloride. These substances have a net positive charge, which reacts with the negatively charged phosphate groups on bacterial cell walls. The walls are disrupted, resulting in increased permeability and loss of cell contents.

Studies suggest that cetylpyridinium chloride 0.05% (with or without domiphen bromide) and benzethonium chloride cause a reduction in plaque of between 25 and 35%, but with less obvious effects on gingival inflammation. Cetylpyridinium chloride (0.1%) is also marketed as a prebrushing rinse.

Pyrimidine derivatives

Hexetidine is a hexahydropyridine derivative that has antibacterial and antifungal activity. It inhibits the rate of ATP synthesis in bacterial mitochondria by uncoupling oxidative phosphorylation. Increasing the concentration from 0.1 to 0.14% increases the antiplaque activity of hexetidine to that obtained with 0.2% chlorhexidine. The frequency of desquamative lesions increases correspondingly.

Phenols

Phenols exert a non-specific antibacterial action that is dependent upon the ability of the drug, in the non-ionised form, to penetrate the lipid components of bacterial cell walls. Phenolic compounds also exhibit anti-inflammatory properties, which may result from their ability to inhibit neutrophil chemotaxis, the generation of neutrophil superoxide anions and the production of prostaglandin synthetase.

Listerine

An over-the-counter antiplaque agent that contains thymol (0.06%), eucalyptol (0.09%), methyl salicylate (0.06%) and methanol (0.04%) in 16.9% alcohol. Listerine is not as effective as chlorhexidine (0.2%) in reducing plaque and gingivitis. Twice daily rinsing with 20 ml Listerine as a supplement to normal oral hygiene produces a 35% reduction in plaque and gingivitis.

Triclosan

Triclosan is a bisphenol, non-ionic germicide with a broad spectrum of activity against Gram-positive and Gram-negative bacteria and fungi. The compound adsorbs onto the lipid portion of the bacterial cell membrane. At low concentrations, triclosan interferes with vital transport mechanisms in bacteria. A concentration of 0.1–0.2% is suitably efficacious with minimal side-effects. Activity is enhanced when the compound is combined with zinc citrate or incorporated into a copolymer of methoxyethylene and maleic acid. The copolymer increases the substantivity of triclosan and acts as a reservoir.

Sanguinarine

Sanguinarine is a benzophenathridine alkaloid structure obtained by alcoholic extraction from the blood root plant *Sanguinaria canadensis*. The antibacterial properties of sanguinarine are thought to result from its ability to suppress the activity of intracellular bacterial enzymes, possibly through oxidation of thiol groups. The extract has been incorporated into a mouthrinse and toothpaste; 0.03% is the most frequently used concentration. The antiplaque efficacy is low compared with that of chlorhexidine. The main advantage of sanguinarine over chlorhexidine is the relative absence of unwanted effects. A mild-to-moderate burning sensation in the mouth and mild sloughing of the oral mucosa have been reported.

Heavy metal salts

Salts of zinc, tin and copper inhibit the growth of dental plaque and impede calculus formation.

Zinc salts

Zinc salts possess antiplaque activity, although generally less than that of chlorhexidine. Zinc citrate and chloride are frequently incorporated into toothpaste. Zinc salts exhibit good substantivity, with 30% of zinc retained in the mouth after toothbrushing with a 0.5% zinc citrate toothpaste. The activity of both zinc citrate and triclosan is enhanced when the products are used in combination.

Tin salts

The suggested antibacterial mechanisms of tin ions are thought to be mediated through their ability to bind to lipoteichoic acid present on the surfaces of Gram-positive bacteria. The net surface charge of the organism is, therefore, reversed and the adsorption of the bacteria on the teeth is reduced. The accumulation of tin in bacteria may alter their metabolism and other physico-chemical characteristics. Stannous salts cause staining of the teeth and the tongue, although the stain is easily removed using prophylaxis paste.

Enzymes

Lactoperoxidase–hypothiocyanite

Certain oral bacteria are known to produce hydrogen peroxide (H_2O_2) by the oxidation of $NADH_2$ by $NADH_2$ oxidase. This H_2O_2 oxidases another $NADH_2$ molecule or is inactivated by the enzyme catalase. When the level of H_2O_2 in saliva is increased, it assists lactoperoxidase in the oxidation of thiocyanate (SCN^-) to produce the hypothiocyanite ion ($OSCN^-$). The latter interferes with the redox mechanisms of bacterial cells by upsetting the $NADH_2^- NADPH_2$ balance. This production is achieved by introducing a further enzyme system, involving amyloglycosidase and glucose oxidase. This system is the basis for the production of the commercially available toothpaste Zendium (Oral B, UK). In addition to amyloglycosidase (1.2% w/w) and glucose oxidase (1.0% w/w), Zendium contains potassium thiocyanite (0.2% w/w) and sodium fluoride (0.26%).

Surfactants

Surfactants or 'wetting agents' provide an alternative method of plaque inhibition. Agents with low surface tension and lipophilic–hydrophilic properties interfere with plaque growth without affecting the ecological balance of oral flora.

Amino alcohols
Substituted amino alcohols have comparatively low antibacterial properties. They also have a lower surface tension than that of the tooth surface; consequently, the low antimicrobial effect may be compensated by a high local concentration on the enamel surface. Delmopinol 1% has a plaque inhibitory effect of 75%. Twice daily rinsing with a 0.2% solution of delmopinol has an equivalent effect upon gingival bleeding and plaque indices as 0.2% chlorhexidine applied with the same frequency. It is likely that delmopinol disrupts the interbacterial matrix, causing the plaque to be more loosely adherent to the tooth.

The unwanted effects of amino alcohols include a minor local anaesthetic effect on soft tissues, a slightly bitter taste and light-brown staining of the teeth.

Plax
Plax is a mouthrinse with surfactant properties. The rinse is a combination of anionic and ionic surfactants including sodium lauryl sulphate and polysorbate 20. These ingredients act upon already formed plaque to loosen and remove deposits. Use of the rinse is recommended before daily brushing. The efficacy of Plax has been increased by the addition of triclosan 0.3% and a 0.125% copolymer of methoxyethylene and maleic acid to the rinse.

Scaling and root planing

Non-surgical management (NSM) of periodontal diseases comprises OHI and scaling and root planing (SRP):

- scaling is the removal of plaque and calculus from the tooth surface
- root planing is the removal of subgingival plaque, calculus and necrotic cementum to leave a hard, smooth root surface.

SRP is generally undertaken with various hand instruments and/or ultrasonic scalers. As a result of OHI and SRP, plaque bacteria are reduced and there is resolution of the inflammatory lesion in the periodontium. This leads to shrinkage of the gingival soft tissues (as oedema resolves), increased resistance to probe tip penetration by the tissues at the base of the pocket (as inflammation resolves) and the formation of a long junctional epithelium at the base of the pocket. All these mechanisms contribute to the reduction in probing depths observed after effective NSM, although gingival shrinkage and resolution of inflammation have the most significant effects on pocket reduction.

Clinical research has shown that effective OHI alone can reduce mean probing depths by approximately 0.5 mm, and SRP results in additional reductions of about 1.0–1.5 mm. There is no initial probing depth above which NSM does not confer a benefit to patients. However, root planing performed at sites with minimal or no pocketing is detrimental rather than beneficial. Root planing of shallow sites with initial probing depths ≤3 mm results in loss of attachment to the root surface as a result of mechanical trauma from instrumentation.

Periodontal instruments

There are a number of instruments required to perform effective SRP.

Periodontal explorers are used to detect subgingival calculus deposits and root surface roughness. A variety of shapes and designs are available; generally, all are very light instruments (to improve tactility) with fine curved tips to reach subgingivally.

Sickle scalers are strong, heavy instruments used to remove supragingival calculus deposits. They have two cutting surfaces that converge in a sharp tip. They should not be used subgingivally as they will traumatise the gingiva. They are inserted under ledges of calculus and used with a pull stroke to remove the calculus from the tooth surface.

Curettes are fine instruments used for subgingival SRP. They are designed to adapt to the root surface and provide good access to deep pockets without causing significant trauma to the soft tissues. Curettes have a spoon-shaped blade with a rounded tip, and there are cutting edges on both sides of the blade. Curettes can be area-specific: different curettes are designed to adapt to specific anatomical areas of the dentition and are used to instrument specific root surfaces. Universal curettes have cutting edges that afford access to the root surfaces by altering their position and angulation. Curettes were originally designed to achieve *curettage*, in which the epithelial lining of the periodontal pocket was removed at the same time as was subgingival plaque and calculus. Curettage was undertaken in the belief that it enhanced healing, but later research has shown this not to be the case. Indeed, curettage is associated with significant tissue damage and pain and is no longer undertaken as a specific aim of periodontal therapy.

Periodontal hoes are used for removal of ledges of calculus, primarily from broad, flat root surfaces. They are inserted into the pocket, placed against the tooth surface and pulled coronally to remove calculus. They should not be used in furcations as they will score the cemental surface in this anatomically complex region.

Chisels are used to clean the interproximal surfaces of teeth that are too closely positioned to permit access to other scalers, particularly mandibular anterior teeth.

They are inserted from the buccal aspect and pushed lingually while maintaining contact against the interproximal surface of the tooth.

Ultrasonic scalers are used for SRP. An electrical generator delivers energy to a handpiece in the form of high-frequency (ultrasonic) vibrations such that the tip vibrates at between 20 000 and 50 000 Hz, depending on the machine. A variety of inserts (tips) are available for instrumentation. Water cooling is essential to dissipate the heat generated by the vibrations; ultrasonic scalers should be operated in a wet field and kept in motion (to prevent heat build-up and also gouging of the tooth surface). The vibrating tip shatters cementum adhering to the tooth surface. Within the water spray mist, tiny vacuums develop that quickly collapse, releasing energy (cavitation). The cavitating water spray also helps to flush calculus debris and plaque from the periodontal pocket. Ultrasonic scalers are **contraindicated** in patients with cardiac pacemakers, as the electromagnetic field generated by the scaler can interfere with the operation of the pacemaker. Because of the water spray generated by the scaler, proper barrier infection control measures should be employed. Finally, care should be employed around adhesive and porcelain restorations as these can be damaged or removed by the scaler.

Polishing instruments are rubber cups used with polishing pastes to clean and polish the tooth surface. Rubber cups are used in the slow handpiece and are disposed of after use. Overzealous use of a rubber cup, particularly if combined with a coarse or abrasive paste, can result in abrasion of the tooth surface. Rubber cups are used in preference to bristle brushes as the latter can traumatise the gingival soft tissues and, therefore, should not to be used close to the gingival margin.

Techniques

For effective instrumentation, the operator should be comfortably seated, the patient should be supine in the dental chair and there should be good illumination. An assistant should retract the oral soft tissues, where necessary, and maintain a clean operating field through the use of an aspirator. The operator should have a good knowledge of dental anatomy and root morphology, and appropriately selected, sharp instruments should be used. The *modified pen grip* is preferred, in which the instrument is held by the thumb, index finger and middle finger in the same way as a pen is held. However, the index finger is bent so it can be positioned well above the middle finger on the instrument handle. In this way, a triangle of force is applied to the instrument, and this tripod effect allows for stability and tactility during use. The fourth finger (ring finger) is used as a *finger rest* to stabilise the hand and reduce the likelihood of uncontrolled movements and injury. The finger rest also acts

as a fulcrum for working movements of the instrument. Finger rests may be on tooth surfaces in the immediate vicinity of the working area, they may be cross arch (on tooth surfaces in the other side of the same arch), opposite arch or extraoral.

Calculus should be identified prior to SRP. Supragingival calculus can be seen with good lighting and a dry field. The dark colour of subgingival calculus may be visible through thin overlying gingival tissues. An air syringe to retract the gingiva may also reveal subgingival calculus. Interproximal calculus may be visible radiographically. An explorer should be used subgingivally to check for calculus, grooves, furcations and other anatomical structures.

Scaling instruments should be *adapted* to the tooth surface, which means that the cutting edge of the instrument conforms to the anatomy of the root surface. This results in maximal efficiency during scaling and minimal damage to the adjacent tissues. The cutting edge should be *angled* at between 45 and 90° to the root surface: less than 45° and the instrument will not engage the calculus, more than 90° and subgingival curettage will be achieved instead. Instruments should be placed apical to the calculus and *pulled* coronally with firm, controlled strokes to remove the calculus. Increasing *lateral pressure* may need to be applied to remove particularly tenacious deposits. Following SRP, debris should be flushed from the pocket with an irrigating solution (for example, chlorhexidine) in a syringe with a blunt needle.

Scaling and root planing are not separate procedures and both aim to restore gingival health by removal of plaque and calculus. Scaling is indicated for removal of plaque and calculus from enamel surfaces. On root surfaces, however, calculus and plaque grow in surface irregularities of cementum, and this thin layer of cementum may need to be removed during root planing. Furthermore, bacterial products, such as endotoxin, penetrate into the cementum surface, and removal of a superficial layer of cementum promotes healing. It is not necessary, however, to remove extensive amounts of cementum and/or dentine, and to do so can cause dentine hypersensitivity, pulpitis and, at extremes, render the tooth susceptible to fracture.

Although the definition of root planing specifies that the root surface be left hard and smooth, there is debate as to the relative hardness and smoothness that must be achieved. More importantly, SRP aims to remove plaque, calculus and toxins so that the host–parasite balance is tipped in favour of the host to promote healing. The pockets should not be probed sooner than 4–6 weeks after SRP as this may interfere with the healing process. Post-treatment evaluation of the healing response to SRP should be considered together with patient plaque-control capabilities and motivation prior to embarking on further treatments, such as additional SRP, adjunctive antimicrobial usage or periodontal surgery.

Antimicrobials

The use of systemic antimicrobials in the management of periodontal disease should be restricted to the following conditions:

- severe necrotising ulcerative gingivitis
- multiple or severe periodontal abscesses with involvement of regional lymph nodes
- some cases of aggressive periodontitis.

Routes of administration

The aim of using antimicrobials as part of a treatment regimen is to achieve, within the periodontal environment, a concentration of the drug that is sufficient either to kill (bactericidal) or arrest the growth (bacteriostatic) of pathogenic microorganisms. The most effective and reliable method of achieving these concentrations is by systemic administration, whereby the drug enters the crevicular fluid and is then able to bathe the subgingival flora. Systemic therapy may be capable of eliminating pathogens, not only from periodontal lesions but also from the oral cavity. Such an action may have considerable prophylactic benefits and reduce the risk of reinfection of the periodontal sites.

Antimicrobials have also been incorporated into formulations that can be applied locally into periodontal pockets. Advantages of this route of administration are

- lower doses of antimicrobials are administered
- high local concentrations of the drugs are achieved locally in periodontal pockets
- incidence of adverse reactions is reduced
- administration is not dependent upon patient compliance
- placement is site specific
- there is prolonged duration of action when the matrix (vehicle) biodegrades to release the drug (slow-release device).

The placement of local delivery systems can be time-consuming when the treatment of multiple sites is indicated. The extent to which the drug penetrates the connective tissues may be less predictable than when systemic dosing is undertaken.

Choice of antimicrobial agent

The choice of antimicrobial agent depends upon the presence and sensitivity of so-called periodontopathogens and the risks of adverse reactions that can arise from antimicrobial usage. The tetracyclines and metronidazole are the drugs that have been evaluated most extensively.

Tetracyclines

Tetracyclines are a group of related bacteriostatic antimicrobials. They provide a 'broad spectrum' of activity against both Gram-positive and Gram-negative microorganisms. Tetracyclines are effective against most spirochaetes and many anaerobic and facultative bacteria. Additional properties of tetracyclines that may be valuable in the management of periodontal diseases are

- inhibition of collagenase
- anti-inflammatory actions
- enhancement of fibroblast attachment to root surfaces
- inhibition of bone resorption.

In chronic periodontitis, systemic tetracycline has little advantage when used as an adjunct to these procedures.

Systemic tetracyclines are valuable in the management of localised aggressive periodontitis and refractory periodontitis. In localised aggressive periodontitis, the prime pathogen is *Actinobacillus actinomycetemcomitans*, which is very susceptible to tetracyclines. This microorganism is difficult to eliminate from patients with aggressive periodontitis by mechanical debridement alone, presumably because of its ability to invade the gingival connective tissues. A 3–6 week course of tetracycline of 1 g per day will halt the progression of aggressive periodontitis, although it is more usual to give the tetracycline in a 2-week course as an adjunct to non-surgical or surgical management. Tetracycline medication should be continued for 1 week after obtaining negative culture results for *Actinobacillus actinomycetemcomitans* as this minimises the chance of recolonisation.

Tetracycline has been incorporated into slow-release devices for adjunctive local treatment following SRP. Monolithic ethylene vinyl acetate fibres are efficacious in achieving prolonged delivery of the drug from the entire length of the fibres. The concentrations of tetracycline in crevicular fluid achieved by controlled local delivery are up to 100 times those obtained from system dose (1500 versus 15 μg/ml). These high local concentrations increase the chance of complete suppression of bacterial growth.

Minocycline and doxycycline have also been available as proprietary controlled release systems for local application.

Metronidazole

Antibacterial activity against anerobic cocci, Gram-negative and Gram-positive bacilli has led to the use of metronidazole in the treatment of periodontal disease. The microbial effects of the drug depend upon its selective reactivity, which is achieved through the actions of electron transport proteins of susceptible bacteria. Once in the cell, metronidazole binds to DNA, leading to cell death. This process results in rapid killing of anaerobic microorganisms.

In periodontal treatment, metronidazole has been used systemically; common dosage is 200 mg three times a day for 3–5 days. For more severe infections the dose is increased to 400 mg twice daily for 3–5 days. Metronidazole is effective in controlling necrotising ulcerative gingivitis. Gingival ulceration, bleeding, pain and halitosis usually resolve rapidly within about 48–72 hours of starting therapy. The dosage and duration of metronidazole therapy used will depend upon the severity of the disease. Most respond to a 200 mg dose three times a day for 3–5 days.

Systemic metronidazole appears to be useful as an adjunct to non-surgical management in advanced or refractory periodontitis. Metronidazole has been found to be very effective when combined with amoxicillin in the treatment of refractory aggressive periodontitis that has not responded to conventional periodontal treatment or tetracycline therapy. A 7-day regimen of both drugs three times a day, combined with further subgingival debridement, results in almost total elimination of *Actinobacillus actino-mycetemcomitans*. Efficacy studies of a commercially available 25% metronidazole gel suggest that two applications of the gel (1 week apart) are as effective as conventional non-surgical management in reducing probing depths and bleeding on probing. Furthermore, the clinical benefit of such local drug application is evident at 6 months after treatment.

Host modulation

The realisation that the destructive host immuneinflammatory response to the presence of plaque bacteria in the periodontal pocket is the primary cause of periodontal breakdown has led to the concept of adjunctive host modulation using systemic medication. The tetracycline family of antibiotics has an additional therapeutic benefit, namely inhibition of collagenase. At doses of 20 mg twice daily, doxycycline has been shown to inhibit collagenases in GCF and reduce the breakdown of collagen. Twenty milligrams is a subantimicrobial dose, exerting no influence on the flora found in various body compartments. Subantimicrobial dose doxycycline (SDD), when used as an adjunct to SRP, has been shown to improve the clinical response by 30–50% above that observed following SRP alone. The use of SDD has not been associated with the development of bacterial antibiotic resistance.

Surgical treatment

The major limitation of closed SRP (non-surgical treatment) is that root surfaces cannot be visualised directly, and access for removal of subgingival plaque and calculus may be limited. Periodontal therapies (both surgical and non-surgical) are aimed at the removal of all plaque and calculus, and while this is seldom achieved, improvements in periodontal health are observed nonetheless. Therefore, while total elimination of causative factors is an appropriate goal for periodontists, reduction of plaque and calculus below a certain threshold acceptable to the host may be a more realistic aim. This tips the balance between the host and bacteria in favour of the host, allowing reduction in the signs of inflammation and improvements in clinical parameters.

It is typical, therefore, for patients to receive a course of non-surgical therapy and then to be monitored. For those sites that do not respond favourably to treatment (e.g. because of complicated local anatomy such as grooves or furcation involvements), then a decision may be taken to expose the area surgically for further treatment. The majority of periodontal surgery is undertaken to improve access to the root surface for cleaning, generally via a flap procedure, although there are also several indications for specific surgical procedures too. *It is fundamentally important that a high level of oral hygiene is maintained before and after surgery; surgical treatments will fail if plaque is not adequately controlled.*

Other indications for periodontal surgery:

- crown lengthening to increase clinical crown length
- gingivectomy for the removal of overgrown gingival tissues
- guided tissue regeneration (GTR) to regenerate periodontal supporting structures
- mucogingival surgery for correction of mucogingival and aesthetic defects.

Flap surgery

Following flap procedures, and the removal of plaque, calculus and chronically inflamed granulation tissue, healing occurs by the formation of a long junctional epithelium. This leads to reduced probing depths, which are easier to maintain in the maintenance phase of periodontal therapy. A new connective tissue attachment may form following flap procedures, although this cannot be predicted with certainty. The long junctional epithelium that forms following periodontal surgery is more susceptible to plaque-induced breakdown than the original connective tissue attachment, and, consequently, postoperative plaque control must be of a very high standard.

Flap procedures can be classified as involving *replaced flaps* or *apically repositioned flaps*, with or without bone removal (Boxes 1–3).

Replaced flap, no bone removal

A replaced flap is one that is replaced at (or very close to) its presurgical position and is not apically repositioned. The modified Widman flap is an example of a replaced flap (Box 1).

Indications
- access to root surface for root planing
- elimination of deep pockets.

Box 1 Technique for replaced flap procedure (Fig. 16)

1. Inverse bevel incision (first incision) (approximately 0.5 mm from the gingival margin) to the level of the alveolar bone.
2. Crevicular incision (second incision) from the base of the pocket to the bone crest.
3. Full thickness mucoperiosteal flap is raised, to expose alveolar bone crest and the remaining inflamed pocket epithelium and connective tissue are removed with a horizontal incision (third incision).
4. The crest of the alveolar bone is exposed and the root surface is debrided by scaling and root planing.
5. The flap is replaced at the original level and sutured. Simple interrupted sutures may be used, although vertical mattress sutures, which position the tissues more coronally, often provide better aesthetics. A surgical pack may be placed if there is continued bleeding but is often not necessary if the flaps are well adapted.

Box 2 Technique for apically positioned flap

The procedure is similar to that for the replaced flap except:

1. Initial incision may be made further from the gingival margin to thin the tissues and allow for better adaptation to the tooth and bone during suturing.
2. Flaps are raised to a greater extent.
3. Flaps are apically repositioned during suturing so that they just cover the bone crest. Trimming of the flaps may be necessary to conform to the shape of the alveolar bone and teeth.
4. Interrupted sutures are placed to hold the tissues in their new position.

Box 3 Technique for apically repositioned flap with bone removal (Fig. 17)

Identical to the apically repositioned flap procedure described previously, except that bone is removed using burs and saline irrigation to eliminate infrabony defects. Bone removal can be classified as being either *osteoplasty* in which bone is recontoured without removing alveolar bone proper, or *ostectomy* in which alveolar bone proper is removed, together with associated connective tissue attachment.

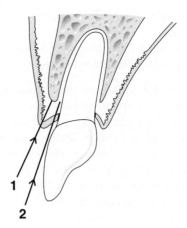

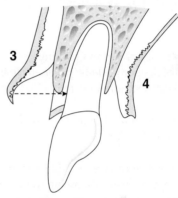

Fig. 16 A replaced flap with no bone removal (modified Widman flap). 1 = inverse bevel incision; 2 = crevicular incision; 3 = a full thickness flap is raised and the remaining inflamed pocket epithelium and connective tissue are removed with a horizontal incision or a sharp curette; 4 = the crest of the alveolar bone is exposed and the root surface is accessible for debridement.

Advantages
- good access to root surface
- replacement of flap at presurgical location minimises problems of aesthetics and root hypersensitivity

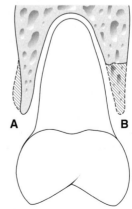

Fig. 17 Techniques for bone removal. (A) Osteoplasty. (B) Ostectomy.

• width of keratinised gingiva is maintained

Disadvantages

• deep, infrabony pockets may not be eliminated
• long junctional epithelium is formed.

Apically repositioned flap, no bone removal

The procedure involving an apically repositioned flap is very similar to the replaced flap procedure, except that the flap is elevated to a greater distance, exposing more alveolar bone, and is then apically repositioned and sutured just coronal to the alveolar bone crest (Box 2). This procedure is not recommended for anterior teeth, where apical repositioning of the flaps leads to aesthetic problems. However, at posterior sites where aesthetic concerns are not as great, this technique is preferred over the replaced flap as it results in greater pocket reductions.

Indications

• access to root surface for root planing
• elimination of deeper pockets, particularly in areas where aesthetics are not important

Advantage

• greater probing depth reduction as a result of apical repositioning of the flap

Disadvantage

• apical repositioning can create problems of aesthetics and dentine hypersensitivity owing to root exposure.

Apically repositioned flap, with bone removal

The procedure used for the eradication of deep pockets involves the loss of some alveolar bone and connective tissue attachment (Box 3).

Indications

• deep, infrabony pockets in areas where aesthetics are not a concern
• adequate remaining bony support for the tooth once procedure (including bone removal) is completed

Advantage

• good reductions in pocket depths

Disadvantages

• removal of alveolar bone and connective tissue attachment to the root surface
• problems of aesthetics and hypersensitivity as a result of root exposure.

Crown lengthening

Crown lengthening procedures are essentially apically repositioned flaps with bone removal, usually undertaken to increase clinical crown height prior to placement of restorations in order to maximise retention and preserve the *biologic width*. The concept of biologic width states that it is important to maintain a distance of approximately 2–2.5 mm between the margins of a restoration and the alveolar bone crest. This space is required for the epithelial and connective tissue components of the soft tissue attachment to the root surface (Fig. 1). If restorations are placed that encroach upon this space, inflammation and uncontrolled attachment loss may occur.

Indications for crown lengthening

• Short clinical crowns requiring increased retention for the placement of full coronal restorations (including cases of gross tooth wear requiring full mouth rehabilitation)
• Deep, subgingivally located crown preparation margins, resulting in difficulty finishing margins and taking impressions, and also encroachment on the biologic width
• Subgingival caries
• Root fractures or root resorption in the cervical third of the tooth root
• Aesthetic improvement of anterior teeth with short clinical crowns and a high lip line.

Gingivectomy

Gingivectomies are primarily used to remove excess gingival tissue in gingival overgrowth (for example, resulting from drug-induced gingival hyperplasia) (Box 4).

Guided tissue regeneration

Following periodontal surgery, the newly instrumented root surface is rapidly colonised by gingival epithelial cells that migrate apically to form a long junctional epithelium. This prevents the formation of new connective tissue attachment to the root surface, the ultimate goal of periodontal therapy. Guided tissue regeneration (GTR) aims to manipulate the repopulation of the wound such that pluripotential cells from the periodontal ligament proliferate and migrate into the healing area. These cells have the capability to differentiate into fibroblasts, cementoblasts and osteoblasts and thus can produce new periodontal ligament fibres, cementum

---

Box 4 Technique for gingivectomy (Fig. 18)

1. Pockets are probed, and probing depths are marked on the gingival tissues with a sharp probe (Fig. 18a).
2. A 45° bevelled incision is made apical to the points marking the base of the pockets and directed coronally to the base of the pocket (Fig. 18b).
3. The excised gingival tissues (including the pocket wall) are removed.
4. Remaining granulation tissue is excised and the root surface is debrided.
5. A surgical pack is placed to protect the healing area. Healing occurs by secondary intention.

(a)

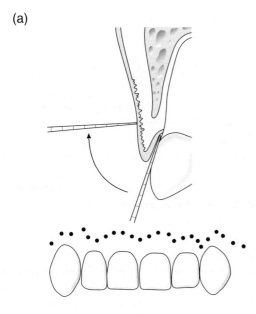

(b)

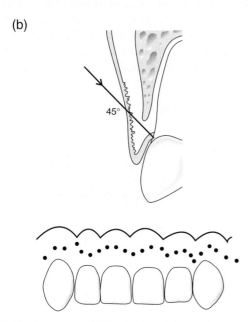

45°

Fig. 18 Gingivectomy. (a) The depths of the pockets are marked on the gingival surface using pocket-marking tweezers or a pocket probe. (b) A bevelled 45° incision contacts the tooth surface at the base of the pocket.

and bone to regenerate the lost connective tissue attachment to the root surface.

GTR is achieved by placing barrier membranes over periodontal defects to exclude gingival epithelium and connective tissues, and to create a space into which proliferating cells from the periodontal ligament and bone can migrate (Fig. 19). Key aspects of GTR include exclusion of epithelium, preservation of space under the membrane into which cells can migrate and formation of a stable blood clot under the membrane. Membranes

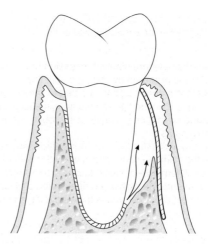

Fig. 19 Guided tissue regeneration. A barrier membrane is placed over the bone defect to exclude epithelium and to create a space for blood clot and migration of pluripotential cells of the periodontal ligament (arrow).

are either *non-resorbable* (e.g. expanded polytetrafluoroethylene, ePTFE), which require removal 4–6 weeks after placement, or *resorbable* (e.g. polylactic acid membranes, collagen membranes) which biodegrade within the tissues over 1–2 months and do not require a second surgical procedure for removal. Non-resorbable membranes can also be reinforced with titanium so that the membrane can be 'tented' to create space for the development of a blood clot. Membranes may also be placed over implants and in conjunction with bone grafts in an attempt to increase the quantity of available bone.

GTR produces most predictable results in class II furcations and in 2- and 3-walled osseous defects (Box 5). Improvements may be gained in class III furcations, although complete bone fill is rare. Complications include infection, perforation of the flap (sharp corners on the membrane must be trimmed prior to placement), sloughing of the flap and gingival recession (1–2 mm recession may occur following GTR procedures).

Box 5 Technique for guided tissue regeneration (Fig. 20)

1. A full thickness mucoperiosteal flap is raised.
2. The root surface is thoroughly debrided of plaque, calculus and granulation tissue.
3. Membrane is selected and trimmed to extend approximately 3 mm beyond the margins of the osseous defect, then it is sutured against the tooth with a sling suture.
4. Flaps are replaced and sutured, ensuring the membrane is fully covered.
5. A periodontal pack is placed if necessary.
6. If the membrane is non-resorbable, a second surgical procedure is undertaken after 4–6 weeks to remove the membrane.

Box 6 Technique for a free gingival graft

1. Recipient site where gingival recession has occurred (Fig. 21a) is prepared by raising a split thickness flap to generate a connective tissue bed to receive the graft (Fig. 21b). The flap (primarily epithelial tissue) is discarded so that only a layer of immobile connective tissue remains.
2. Epithelium and a thin layer of connective tissue is harvested from the donor site, usually the palatal mucosa. A template of sterile aluminium foil may be used to ensure the graft is the right shape and size for the recipient site. The graft is trimmed to fit, and any glandular tissue is removed.
3. The graft is placed, connective tissue side down, onto the recipient site (Fig. 21c). Any clot or debris must be removed from the recipient site to ensure the graft is closely adapted to the underlying connective tissues.
4. The graft is sutured in place, and a periodontal dressing applied.

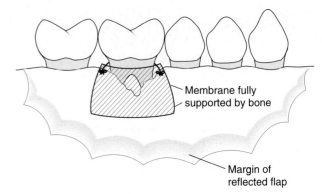

Fig. 20 Guided tissue regeneration.

Mucogingival surgery

Surgical procedures for the correction of mucogingival defects are varied and range from simple gingivectomies or crown lengthening procedures (e.g. to increase the clinical crown length if there is a 'gummy' smile with a high lip line) to complex gingival grafting procedures (Boxes 6–8). In patients with bone defects, GTR and bone grafting may also be employed to increase the bulk of available alveolar bone. Grafting procedures generally aim to cover exposed roots, to increase the width of keratinised gingiva, and to prevent further gingival recession. Grafting procedures include the *free gingival graft*, the *pedicle sliding graft* and the *subepithelial connective tissue graft*. The donor site heals by secondary intention.

(a)   (b)   (c)

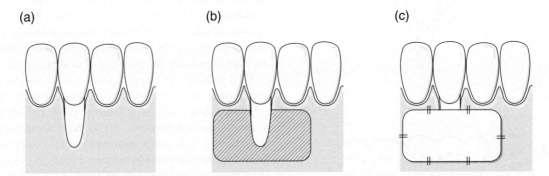

Fig. 21 Free gingival graft. (a) Gingival recession. (b) Recipient site prepared by raising a split thickness flap. (c) Graft from palate placed over recipient site and sutured. Some coverage of the root is achieved but the principal aim is to limit further recession by increasing the width of keratinised tissue.

(a)   (b)

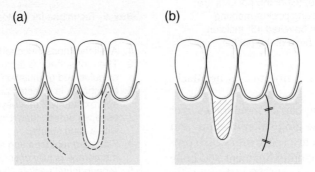

Fig. 22 Pedicle sliding graft. (a) Gingival margin around the exposed root is excised and a split thickness flap raised. (b) The flap is rotated laterally to cover the defect. The donor site heals by secondary intention.

Box 7 Technique for pedicle sliding graft

1. Pedicle flap is raised by split thickness dissection from keratinised tissues adjacent to a narrow recession defect (Fig. 22a). A split thickness flap is preferred because it results in more rapid healing of the donor site.
2. Gingival margins around the exposed root are excised (Fig. 22a)
3. The flap is repositioned laterally to cover the root and sutured, and a periodontal dressing is placed (Fig. 22b).

Box 8 Technique for a subepithelial connective tissue graft

This procedure to deal with a recession defect (Fig. 23a) is similar to the free gingival graft procedure, except:

1. A split thickness flap is raised at the recipient site to beyond the mucogingival junction (Fig. 23b).
2. A wedge of connective tissue and overlying epithelium is harvested from the palate (Fig. 23c).
3. The graft is placed with the strip of epithelium located at the cementoenamel junction and sutured (Fig. 23d).
4. The flap is repositioned coronally to cover the graft and sutured.

This technique, which requires a split thickness graft, has the advantage that the graft receives a blood supply from two sources: the overlying flap, and the underlying connective tissues and periosteum.

(a)   (b)   (c)   (d)

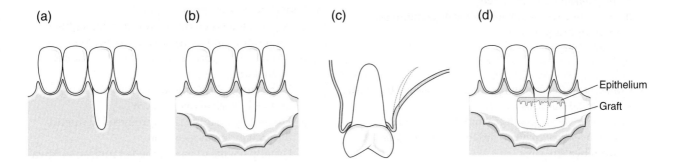

Fig. 23 Subepithelial connective tissue graft. (a) Recession defect. (b) A split thickness flap is elevated. (c) A 'wedge' of epithelium and connective tissue is dissected from the palate. (d) The graft is sutured over the defect with the band of epithelium at the cementoenamel junction, the flap is then sutured over the graft.

References

Adult Dental Health Survey: Oral Health in the UK 2000 London: HMSO, Government Statistical Service 2000
Children's Dental Health in the UK (O'Brian M) 1993 London: HMSO

Self-assessment: questions

Multiple choice questions

1. Dental calculus:
   a. Is a causative agent in periodontitis
   b. Forms on the coronal aspects of teeth only
   c. Is plaque that has become mineralised with ions from gingival crevicular fluid
   d. Contains predominantly crystals of hydroxyapatite when mature
   e. Does not contain bacteria

2. *Porphyromonas gingivalis*:
   a. Is one of the first bacterial species to colonise a newly cleaned tooth surface
   b. Has the ability to invade gingival soft tissues
   c. Is generally encapsulated
   d. Is a causative organism for localised aggressive periodontitis
   e. Is an obligate aerobe

3. Concerning the following organisms associated with periodontal diseases:
   a. *Porphyromonas gingivalis* and *Actinobacillus actinomycetemcomitans* are frequently isolated from healthy sites
   b. *Streptococci* and *Actinomyces* spp. are early colonising organisms
   c. *Fusobacterium nucleatum* is an anaerobic motile rod implicated in chronic periodontitis
   d. *Actinobacillus actinomycetemcomitans* is effectively removed from periodontally involved sites by scaling and root planing
   e. *Actinobacillus actinomycetemcomitans* is an indigenous component of oral microflora

4. The established inflammatory lesion of gingivitis:
   a. Is recognisable histologically within 2–4 days of plaque growth
   b. Represents the transition between gingivitis and periodontitis
   c. Is dominated by a T lymphocyte infiltrate
   d. Is associated clinically with increased flow of gingival crevicular fluid (GCF)
   e. Can be diagnosed clinically by the presence of gingival erythema and oedema

5. Polymorphonuclear leukocytes (neutrophils):
   a. Are not found in the gingival sulcus
   b. Secrete matrix metalloproteinase (MMP) type 1
   c. Contribute to the destruction of the periodontal tissues during periodontitis
   d. Represent the first line of cellular defences against periodontal pathogens
   e. Are almost always found in the gingival tissues

6. Guided tissue regeneration (GTR):
   a. Is indicated in class I furcation defects
   b. Is dependent on the formation of a stable blood clot for best results
   c. Typically results in clinical improvements in probing depths, attachment levels and gingival recession
   d. Requires the use of a non-resorbable membrane (e.g. ePTFE) for best results
   e. Results in osseointegration

7. Periodontal flap surgery:
   a. Is indicated when non-surgical treatment is contraindicated owing to poor plaque control
   b. Results in the formation of a long junctional epithelium
   c. Is the surgical treatment of choice for drug-induced gingival overgrowth
   d. Frequently results in compromised aesthetics through gingival recession
   e. Usually results in loss of the keratinised gingiva

8. Regarding alveolar bone destruction in periodontitis:
   a. Vertical bony defects have a better prognosis than horizontal defects following non-surgical treatment
   b. Fenestrations and dehiscences predispose sites to periodontal breakdown
   c. Three-walled vertical defects are well suited for treatment by guided tissue regeneration
   d. Radiographs provide an accurate representation of sites undergoing active bone loss
   e. Osteoclasts are stimulated to resorb bone by interferon-γ

9. Regarding periodontal surgery:
   a. The gingivectomy incision should commence at the level of the base of the pocket
   b. One major goal of guided tissue regeneration (GTR) is to exclude epithelial cells from the healing area
   c. Split thickness flaps are raised when repositioning flaps apically
   d. Plaque control is less critical than when considering non-surgical treatment
   e. Gingivectomy wounds heal by granulation

10. A traumatic occlusal force acting on a tooth with a healthy periodontium will likely cause:
    a. Gingivitis
    b. Periodontal disease
    c. Radiographic widening of the periodontal membrane space
    d. Increased tooth mobility
    e. Gingival recession

11. Vertical, infrabony defects are frequently seen on radiographs:
    a. In patients with localised aggressive periodontitis
    b. Adjacent to a tooth which has 'tipped' into an extraction space
    c. Adjacent to an overhanging restoration
    d. On teeth that serve as abutments to partial dentures
    e. On teeth that serve as abutments for bridge retainers

12. In periodontal health:
    a. The width of keratinised gingiva is the same through the mouth
    b. The alveolar bone crest is at the same level as the cementoenamel junction
    c. Gingival crevicular fluid (GCF) is absent
    d. Teeth show no mobility
    e. There are no periodontal pockets

13. The aim of root planing is to:
    a. Remove calculus deposits and necrotic cementation
    b. Remove the entire cementum layer to expose dentine
    c. Remove the ulcerated epithelial pocket wall
    d. Facilitate healing by formation of a long junctional epithelium
    e. Obtain a new connective tissue attachment to the root surface

14. Chlorhexidine gluconate:
    a. Is a phenolic compound
    b. Demonstrates substantivity
    c. Is bactericidal only against streptococci
    d. Is available in the UK as mouthrinses of both 1.2 and 0.2%.
    e. Only stains teeth in patients who smoke

15. The Basic Periodontal Examination (BPE):
    a. Should be undertaken using a Hu–Friedy periodontal probe
    b. Was designed as a screening tool to assess treatment need
    c. Records only the maximum scores in each quadrant
    d. Does not identify furcation involvement
    e. Does not identify mobile teeth

16. Clinical measurements of probing depths are likely to be influenced by:
    a. Subgingival calculus
    b. Probing force
    c. Dimensions of the probe
    d. Inflammatory infiltrate at the base of the pocket
    e. Angulation of the probe

17. Drugs that are known to cause gingival overgrowth include:
    a. Ciclosporin
    b. Nifedipine
    c. Insulin
    d. Metronidazole
    e. Tetracycline

18. Localised aggressive periodontitis:
    a. Is highly prevalent in adolescents
    b. Can affect any teeth in the permanent dentition
    c. Is typically characterised by *Actinobacillus actinomycetemcomitans* infection
    d. Commonly runs in families
    e. Is associated with neutrophil defects

19. Necrotising ulcerative gingivitis (NUG):
    a. Is a viral infection
    b. Is characterised by vesicles that break down to form yellow-grey ulcers with a red 'halo' of inflammation
    c. Is a painful condition
    d. Is likely to recur in the absence of long-term maintenance
    e. Should always be treated using metronidazole as the first line of treatment

20. Advantages of locally delivered antimicrobials for treatment of periodontal disease include:
    a. Prolonged duration of action of the antimicrobial
    b. High local concentrations of the antimicrobial are achieved
    c. Patients themselves are able to insert the antimicrobial at the appropriate site
    d. The need for patient compliance is eliminated
    e. Incidence of adverse reactions is reduced

21. Powered toothbrushes:
    a. Are more effective in removing plaque than manual toothbrushes
    b. Have brushheads that are designed specifically for patients with fixed orthodontic appliances
    c. Have a 'novelty effect' associated with their use
    d. Are generally cheaper than manual toothbrushes
    e. Should be used with the Bass toothbrushing technique

22. Mandibular first molars with grade I furcation involvement:
    a. Demonstrate horizontal mobility of >1.0 mm
    b. Are almost certainly non-vital
    c. Have horizontal attachment loss of <1/3 the width of the tooth
    d. Should be managed using a tunnel preparation
    e. May be managed using guided tissue regeneration (GTR)

23. Features associated with periodontal disease that may be identified on intraoral periapical radiographs are:
    a. Pattern of alveolar bone loss
    b. Extent of alveolar bone loss
    c. Overhanging restorations of interproximal tooth surfaces
    d. Subgingival calculus
    e. Furcation involvement

24. A localised acute periodontal abscess:
    a. Is almost certainly associated with a non-vital tooth
    b. Should be managed initially using systemic antimicrobials
    c. Often tracks through the alveolar bone, resulting in a buccal sinus opening
    d. Is usually painful when the associated tooth is percussed
    e. Should be managed initially using locally delivered antimicrobials

25. According to the random burst model of periodontal disease progression:
    a. Bursts of disease activity are random with respect to previous episodes of destruction
    b. Multiple sites break down within a finite time period
    c. Some sites remain free of disease throughout the life of the patient
    d. Sites of previous disease may remain quiescent indefinitely
    e. Disease activity is present only at sites that bleed

Case history

> A 25-year-old healthy female presents to your surgery complaining of gum recession adjacent to one of her mandibular lower incisors. Apparently, this has developed during the previous 3 months and she is very worried that the tooth might have to be extracted. The tooth is free of symptoms.

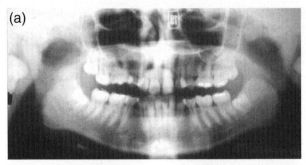

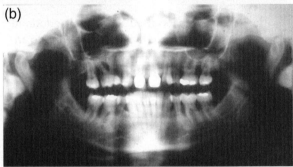

Fig. 24 Radiographs of a patient at (a) 19 years and (b) 34 years of age.

1. Describe how you would assess the problem clinically
2. How would you advise the patient?
3. Discuss your management of the case.

Picture questions

Picture 1

Study the two radiographs (Fig. 24) which are of the same patient at (a) 19 years and (b) 34 years of age.

1. What is the most likely periodontal diagnosis at 34 years of age?
2. What does the initial phase of treatment involve?
3. The patient has a sister who is 29 years old. What advice might you offer?

Picture 2

Study the position of the probe in the pocket (Fig. 25).

1. What type of probe is this?
2. What is the 'score' for the pocket?
3. What does the 'score' infer regarding the extent of attachment loss?

Picture 3

This 23-year-old patient (Fig. 26) complains of extremely painful gums and a foul taste, both of recent onset.

1. What is the most likely diagnosis for this characteristic presentation?

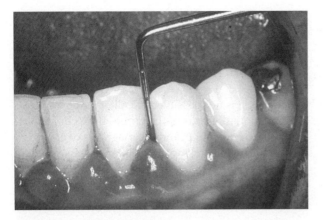

Fig. 25 Probe within a pocket.

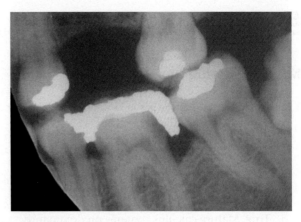

Fig. 27 Intraoral radiograph.

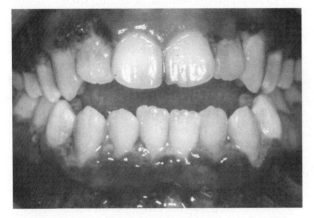

Fig. 26 Mouth of a patient with painful gums.

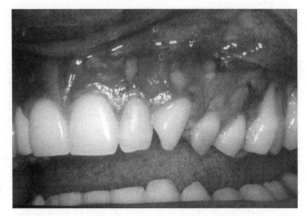

Fig. 28 A 20-year-old female with painful ulcers.

2. Identify possible risk factors for this condition.
3. Outline your management strategy.

Picture 4

Figure 27 is an intraoral radiograph taken for a 20-year-old female who was complaining of an acute, aching pain from her lower left molar teeth.

1. What is the most likely cause of the pain?
2. Identify the radiographic findings on this film
3. What is the differential diagnosis for the appearance of the bone defect on the distal aspect of the first molar?

Picture 5

This 20-year-old female complains of severe pain from the ulcers on her gums, mainly in the upper jaw (Fig. 28). The history of their onset is extremely vague.

1. Apart from the gingival and mucosal ulceration, what other significant periodontal feature(s) can be identified from the photograph?
2. Consider your differential diagnosis for these ulcers.

Short note questions

Write short notes on:

1. *Actinobacillus actinomycetemcomitans*
2. long junctional epithelium
3. random burst model of periodontal disease progression
4. tooth mobility
5. virulence factors of periodontal pathogens
6. dental calculus
7. collagenases.

Self-assessment: answers

Multiple choice answers

1. a. **False**. Dental plaque is the key aetiological factor in periodontitis (although calculus is always covered by a layer of unmineralised plaque).
   b. **False**. Calculus forms both supra-and subgingivally.
   c. **False**. Plaque is mineralised by calcium and phosphate ions from saliva.
   d. **True**. Mature calculus contains predominantly crystals of hydroxyapatite and tricalcium phosphate.
   e. **False**. Calculus contains (non-viable) plaque bacteria that have become mineralised.

2. a. **False**. *Porphyromonas gingivalis* is an example of a late colonising species, typically found in mature subgingival plaque.
   b. **True**. *P. gingivalis* invades and also replicates within gingival epithelial cells.
   c. **True**. Most strains of *P. gingivalis* are encapsulated, which inhibits phagocytosis of the organism.
   d. **False**. *Actinobacillus actinomycetemcomitans* is the organism most strongly implicated in localised aggressive periodontitis.
   e. **False**. *P. gingivalis* is an anaerobic non-motile rod.

3. a. **False**. These organisms are associated with periodontally diseased sites.
   b. **True**. These Gram-positive species are amongst the first to colonise a newly cleaned tooth surface.
   c. **True**. *Fusobacterium nucleatum* is associated with chronic periodontitis.
   d. **False**. *Actinobacillus actinomycetemcomitans* invades the gingival soft tissues and, therefore, is not totally eradicated by scaling and root planing. Adjunctive antimicrobial therapy or surgery may be indicated.
   e. **False**. *A. actinomycetemcomitans* is a true infectious agent, with low prevalence in health but associated with aggressive forms of periodontitis.

4. a. **False**. The established lesion is apparent after 2–3 weeks of undisturbed plaque growth.
   b. **False**. The established lesion is confined to the gingival tissues.
   c. **False**. Plasma cells are the predominant inflammatory cell type in the established lesion.
   d. **True**. Increased vascular permeability, vasodilatation and an increasingly permeable junctional epithelium all lead to increased GCF flow.
   e. **False**. It is not possible to evaluate the histological status of the tissues from clinical appearance alone, and the diagnosis of gingivitis is made solely using clinical parameters. Furthermore, there are no clear boundaries between the histological changes occurring during the development of gingivitis.

5. a. **False**. Neutrophils cross the junctional epithelium in response to chemotactic stimuli from subgingival plaque bacteria.
   b. **False**. The main collagenase produced by neutrophils is MMP-8. MMP-1 is produced by fibroblasts.
   c. **True**. Lysosomal enzymes, granule contents and products of the respiratory burst can all be spilled into the surrounding tissues from neutrophils, leading to tissue damage.
   d. **True**. Neutrophils are involved in the intial acute response to plaque, cross the junctional epithelium and form a 'leukocyte wall' between plaque bacteria and the underlying tissues.
   e. **True**. Neutrophils can be identified histologically even in clinically healthy gingival tissues. They are present to combat bacteria present in the gingival sulcus, even in the absence of clinically diagnosed gingivitis.

6. a. **False**. GTR is primarily indicated in class II furcation defects. Scaling and root planing (with or without flap elevation) is the treatment of choice for class I furcations.
   b. **True**. The space under the membrane must be filled with clot, which acts like a scaffold for the migration of colonising cells from the periodontal ligament.
   c. **False**. Although probing depths reduce and gains in attachment are seen, there is usually an increase in recession of 1–2 mm following GTR.
   d. **False**. Many resorbable membranes produce results equivalent to those seen when using a non-resorbable membrane.
   e. **False**. Osseointegration refers to the intimate contact observed between alveolar bone and the titanium surface of implants.

7. a. **False**. Plaque control is of paramount importance before and after surgery, and surgery will fail if oral hygiene is not of the highest standard.
   b. **True**. The long junctional epithelium that forms is more at risk for subsequent plaque-induced

breakdown; plaque control must, therefore, be of the highest standard.

c. **False**. Gingivectomy is the preferred surgical treatment option for hyperplastic gingiva.

d. **True**. Recession, leading to poor aesthetics and also dentine hypersensitivity, is common after flap procedures, particularly when flaps are apically repositioned.

e. **False**. The width of keratinised gingiva can be maintained in flap procedures.

8. a. **False**. Vertical bony defects are harder to treat and maintain; therefore, the prognosis is worse.

b. **False**. Providing oral hygiene is good, sites with dehiscences or fenestrations are not more at risk for periodontitis.

c. **True**. Three-walled defects are easier to isolate from the epithelium with a membrane than 1-and 2-walled defects, and the prospects for bone infill are, therefore, enhanced.

d. **False**. Radiographs provide a historical representation of which sites have already lost bone and do not provide reliable information regarding active bone resorption.

e. **False**. Osteoclasts are stimulated by cytokines such as prostaglandins and interleukins. Interferon-γ has a more protective role in periodontal pathogenesis, inhibiting bone resorption.

9. a. **False**. The gingivectomy incision should start apical to the base of the pocket and be angled at 45° towards the base of the pocket.

b. **True**. The prevention of downgrowth of epithelial cells to form a long junctional epithelium is the main aim of GTR.

c. **False**. Full thickness flaps are raised when apically repositioning.

d. **False**. Plaque control is of paramount importance in promoting healing following both surgical and non-surgical periodontal treatment.

e. **True**. Gingivectomy wounds heal by secondary intention – there is no primary closure.

10. a. **False**. Occlusal forces do not initiate an inflammatory response.

b. **False**. Forces may exacerbate an existing lesion but will not cause periodontal disease.

c. **True**. An adaptive response of the periodontal membrane.

d. **True**. The mobility results from the widened membrane space.

e. **False**. Recession represents attachment loss which is not precipitated by occlusal trauma alone.

11. a. **True**. They are typically associated with first permanent molars.

b. **True**. The cementoenamel junction to bone crest dimension tends to remain constant. An angular alveolar bone crest is usually evident.

c. **True**. Local bone loss associated with plaque accumulation, which results from an inability to clean beneath the 'ledge'.

d. **False**. Occurs, only occasionally, if those abutments are subject to jiggling forces and there is pre-existing periodontitis.

e. **False**. Occurs, only very occasionally, if the occlusal scheme has not been planned and overloading/jiggling of the abutment occurs in the presence of pre-existing periodontitis.

12. a. **False**. The width of keratinised gingiva can show considerable variation throughout the mouth.

b. **False**. Bone crest is usually at least 1 mm below the cementoenamel junction.

c. **False**. There is always a flow of GCF, even in health.

d. **False**. Tooth mobility in periodontal health is minimal but detectable by the naked eye.

e. **True**. A pocket is defined as a pathologically deepened crevice, which excludes their presence in the healthy state.

13. a. **True**. Although it is difficult to assess when all the necrotic cementum has been removed.

b. **False**. This may occasionally occur but should not be the aim of treatment.

c. **False**. Epithelium is inevitably damaged during instrumentation but its removal is not an aim.

d. **True**. A long junctional epithelium may form as part of the healing response.

e. **False**. Epithelium downgrowth will preclude new connective tissue attachment.

14. a. **False**. Chlorhexidine is a bisbiguanide antimicrobial.

b. **True**. Retention in the oral cavity is one of the most important properties of this agent.

c. **False**. Chlorhexidine is a broad-spectrum antimicrobial.

d. **False**. The concentrations are 0.12% and 0.2%.

e. **False**. Chlorhexidine stains teeth independently of whether the patient smokes.

15. a. **False**. The examination should be undertaken using the specifically designed WHO (CPITN) probe.

b. **True**. The screening examination should be supplemented by a detailed periodontal investigation in cases where scores of 4 are recorded.

c. **False**. Trick. The record is the maximum score in each *sextant*.
d. **False**. The asterisk (*) denotes furcation involvement.
e. **True**. The BPE has no facility to record the mobility of teeth.

16. a. **True**. Calculus acts as a physical barrier to probing.
 b. **True**. A number of 'pressure-sensitive' probes are available to control the degree of pressure (force) used when probing pockets.
 c. **True**. Many designs of probe exist with variation in length, thickness and dimension of probe tip. To minimise variation in probing depth, measurements in one patient at different visits should be made using the same type of probe.
 d. **True**. The inflammatory infiltrate will facilitate penetration of the probe through both epithelial and connective tissues at the base of the pocket.
 e. **True**. The probe should be maintained, as far as possible, parallel with the vertical root length. The probe tip should then approximate the base of the pocket. Probing depth can be overestimated when the probe is placed at an angle to the vertical root length.

17. a. **True**. Ciclosporin is a potent immunosuppressant used in the field of organ transplantation.
 b. **True**. Nifedipine is a calcium-channel blocker used for the management of hypertension and angina.
 c. **False**. However, remember that both type I and type II diabetics appear to be at increased risk from periodontal disease.
 d. **False**. This drug is indicated for the *treatment* of some periodontal conditions.
 e. **False**. This drug is indicated for the *treatment* of some periodontal conditions.

18. a. **False**. Prevalence is <1%.
 b. **False**. There is a localised first molar and incisor presentation with no more than two other teeth affected (if more teeth than this are affected, the diagnosis is generalised aggressive periodontitis).
 c. **True**. Microbial analysis typically reveals elevated levels of this organism.
 d. **True**. Studies show that localised aggressive periodontitis is a heritable trait.
 e. **True**. Patients with localised aggressive periodontitis may have abnormalities of neutrophil chemotaxis and phagocytosis.

19. a. **False**. Traditionally, the condition has been associated with a fusobacterial–spirochaetal complex, although aspects of the disease are characteristic of viral involvement, for example the relatively narrow age range affected and the tendency to recur. As yet, however, no specific virus has been identified as causal.
 b. **False**. These signs are characteristic of acute herpetic gingivostomatitis. Vesicle formation does not occur in NUG.
 c. **True**. NUG is one of the few periodontal conditions that is associated with acute pain.
 d. **True**. If predisposing factors are not removed, the disease is very likely to recur.
 e. **False**. Metronidazole is indicated in severe, acutely painful disease and when there is involvement of regional lymph nodes. In less severe disease, mechanical debridement under local anaesthesia and hygiene phase therapy are of primary importance and antimicrobial therapy is not indicated.

20. a. **True**. The antimicrobials are released slowly as the vehicle matrix biodegrades/breaks down.
 b. **True**. Placement is site specific so the entire dose of the antimicrobial is targeted to the site where it is required.
 c. **False**. All products have to be placed by the clinician.
 d. **True**. As the product is placed by the clinician, there is no need for patient compliance. Furthermore, the majority of products now available in the UK have a biodegradeable matrix so the products do not have to be removed at a follow-up visit.
 e. **True**. The incidence of adverse reactions will be reduced by avoiding the systemic route of drug administration.

21. a. **True**. The vast majority of clinical trials have shown powered toothbrushes to be as, if not more, effective for removing plaque than conventional manual brushes. Most of these observations are short term and may well be the result of a 'novelty' effect of using a new brush rather than as a consequence of better mechanical cleaning per se.
 b. **True**. Some powered units have brushheads that are designed specifically for cleaning fixed appliances.
 c. **True**. See (a) above
 d. **False**. Powered brushes are more expensive.
 e. **False**. Instructions for use of powered brushes are provided by the manufacturers. Generally, the brushes should be guided around the dental arches with the knowledge that the movement of

the brushhead itself is generated by the powered unit.

22. a. **False**. This is a possibility but the classification of furcation involvement is not linked with tooth mobility.
    b. **False**. A periodontal–endodontic lesion might be present, but the classification does not imply vitality or non-vitality of a tooth.
    c. **True**. The horizontal attachment loss refers to the progression of the disease at the furcation site. Don't forget that pocketing/vertical loss of attachment will also have occurred but is not identified in the grading of furcation involvement.
    d. **False**. A grade I lesion will, by definition, have considerable remaining intraradicular bone and attachment. This must be preserved, so tunnelling is certainly contraindicated.
    e. **True**. Most class I lesions should be managed conservatively with oral hygiene, scaling and root debridement. Studies have shown, however, that these defects can be managed predictably and successfully using GTR.

23. a. **True**.
    b. **True**.
    c. **True**.
    d. **True**.
    e. **True**.

    All of these features may be seen on radiographs. The important word in this answer is *may*. Overhanging restorations, calculus and furcation involvement (particularly class I) can sometimes only be detected clinically while not being apparent on radiographs.

24. a. **False**. The tooth may be non-vital if there is a combined periodontal–endodontic lesion. If the infection is primarily of periodontal origin, the tooth will very likely still be vital.
    b. **False**. Local debridement of the site should be the primary treatment. Periodontal abscesses usually drain through the pocket opening, thus reducing the need for systemic antimicrobials.
    c. **False**. A sinus opening on the attached gingiva is usually associated with a *periapical* infection that tracks along the path of least resistance from the apex of the tooth.
    d. **True**. A periodontal abscess is one of the relatively few periodontal conditions that is painful.
    e. **False**. Drainage and local debridement are the first lines of treatment. The purulent exudate

and localised bleeding are likely to restrict the efficacy of local antimicrobial therapy.

25. a. **True**.
    b. **False**. This is consistent with the asynchronous multiple burst theory/model.
    c. **True**.
    d. **True**.
    e. **False**. This is not a criterion for the random burst model, nor is it a true statement in itself.

Case history answer

1. Record the extent of the gingival recession by measuring the vertical distance from the cementoenamel junction to the free gingival margin. Study models or an intraoral photograph are useful permanent records to which reference can be made at a later date to establish whether the lesion is progressing. Note whether the gingival soft tissues adjacent to the recession are inflamed and whether there are plaque and calculus deposits on the exposed root surface. Record the mobility of the tooth (if any). Identify any factors that might predispose to the gingival recession. For example, an incisor which is displaced labially from the arch may have only very thin or completely absent labial alveolar support. A very prominent midline or labial frenal attachment may restrict access for toothbrushing. It is also important to measure the width of attached/keratinised gingiva adjacent to the affected tooth. When this tissue is compromised, the ability of the soft tissues to resist masticatory and toothbrushing forces is reduced and the depth of the labial sulcus is also affected. The width of keratinised tissue can be identified more clearly by using an iodine solution, which preferentially stains keratinised tissue bright orange and non-keratinised oral mucosa a deeper purple colour.

2. For gingival recession, a history of the presenting complaint is not always accurate. It is possible that the recession has occurred over a very short period of time. In many cases, however, the lesion may have been present for many months (if not years) before the patient first noticed it. In the absence of tooth mobility, the patient should be reassured that the prognosis for the tooth remains good provided that any plaque-induced inflammation is resolved and stability of the lesion can be achieved. It is also worth mentioning to the patient that gingival recession that affects mandibular incisor teeth is often covered by the lower lip. When patients become aware of this they do not usually consider the appearance of the recession to be a major problem.

3. In the first instance the lesion should be managed conservatively. Any causative factors, such as an injudicious toothbrushing technique, should be corrected. Oral hygiene instruction should be given and localised toothbrushing using a single tufted, interspace brush might be indicated when access for a conventional toothbrush is compromised. Deposits of plaque and calculus should be removed from the root surface, although excessive root planing should be avoided to reduce the chance of exposing dentine and the root surface becoming sensitive to hot and cold. Topical desensitising agents, such as a fluoride varnish, should be applied frequently to reduce both the likelihood of sensitivity and the development of root caries in the longer term. Surgical widening of the keratinised gingiva might be indicated in the long term if the patient is unable to practise good oral hygiene procedures because of local mucogingival morphology and reduced sulcus depth. Progression of the recession despite the removal of causative factors and establishment of good plaque control might also be an indication for a surgical procedure to increase the width of keratinised tissue.

Picture answers

Picture 1

1. Generalised aggressive periodontitis. The severity of bone resorption and the radiographic absence of signs of resorption at 19 years preclude a diagnosis of chronic periodontitis.
2. Initially conventional cause-related treatment is instigated: instruction in toothbrushing and use of adjunctive aids for interproximal and subgingival cleaning, scaling and root planing, prophylaxis. Ultimately, treatments such as surgery and the adjunctive use of antimicrobials might be indicated, but conventional treatment is first in line.
3. Periodontal screening and radiographic examination. There is evidence that certain subjects are at high risk from developing aggressive periodontitis and this risk may be under genetic control. Siblings should be screened and affected individuals with children warned that early signs may develop from around puberty onwards.

Picture 2

1. World Health Organization (WHO) or BPE probe. The black band extends from 3.5–5.5 mm from the tip.
2. Part of the band remains visible above the gingival margin giving a score of 3.

3. Nothing at all. The score of 3 tells you that the pocket is greater than 3.5mm but less than 5.5 mm. This could be a false pocket or a true attachment loss. Both situations require treatment and, therefore, the BPE score gives you an indication of treatment need.

Picture 3

1. The clinical appearance of 'punched-out', yellow-grey ulcers of the interdental and marginal gingivae is characteristic of necrotising ulcerative gingivitis (NUG).
2. Risk factors are:
   - poor oral hygiene
   - pre-existing chronic gingivitis
   - smoking
   - malnutrition
   - stress.
   A persistent NUG is associated with immunocompromised patients and the possibility of HIV infection must be considered in such cases.
3. Management involves:
   - reduce cigarette consumption
   - oral hygiene advice
   - mechanical debridement, ultrasonic scaling (under local anaesthesia).
   - oxygenating mouthrinse (for example hydrogen peroxide) to irrigate and cleanse the necrotic tissues and superficial debris
   - if general symptoms (regional lymphoadenopathy) are present, treatment with systemic metronidazole (200 mg three times a day)
   - long-term follow-up must include regular visits to reinforce oral hygiene measures and so reduce the likelihood of recurrence.

Picture 4

1. Recurrent caries beneath the distal aspect of the MOD restoration in ⌐6.
2. Findings include:
   - recurrent caries ⌐6
   - missing ⌊6
   - overhanging restoration MOD⌐6
   - mesio-angular impaction ⌐8.
3. Angular bone defects may be associated with overhanging restorations, when difficult access for cleaning leads to stagnation and an environment in which predominantly Gram-negative anaerobic pathogens will flourish. Such defects are also found on the *mesial* surfaces of teeth that have tipped into an adjacent edentulous space and on periodontally involved teeth that have been subject to excessive occlusal loading or jiggling forces.

In this case, the most obvious causal factor appears to be the overhanging restoration. However, the patient suffers from localised aggressive periodontitis and identical vertical bone defects were found on the contralateral first molars, neither of which were restored. There is also another clue to this diagnosis, in that 6⌋ has already been lost.

Picture 5

1. The gingival recession adjacent to the maxillary molars is very severe for a 20-year-old patient.
2. Gingival ulceration may occur in a number of conditions: necrotising ulcerative gingivitis; herpetic gingivostomatitis; mucocutaneous diseases such as erosive lichen planus, benign mucous membrane pemphigoid and pemphigus vulgaris; and squamous cell carcinoma affecting the gingiva. Recurrent aphthae tend to appear on the more labile oral mucosa rather than on the immobile gingival tissue. In this case, the lesions were self-inflicted, with the diagnosis being factitious gingivitis. Eventually, lesions appeared in contralateral quadrants, on the palate, the lips and extraorally on the face. The lesions did not respond to simple treatment measures including protective dressing and at no time did the patient admit to knowing the cause of the lesions. Eventually, the patient was referred for a psychiatric opinion.

Short note answers

1. *Actinobacillus actinomycetemcomitans* is a Gram-negative anaerobic rod that is strongly linked to localised aggressive periodontitis. *A. actinomycetemcomitans* has been isolated in up to 97% of patients with localised aggressive periodontitis and appears to be associated particularly with progressing periodontal lesions. It is a virulent organism and produces collagenase, leukotoxin, endotoxin, proteases and toxins. These factors are important in the evasion of host defence mechanisms and the destruction of periodontal tissues, including connective tissues and bone. Transmission between family members is common and may constitute a source of re-infection following therapy. *A. actinomycetemcomitans* has the ability to invade gingival soft tissues and replicate within epithelial cells. This means that the organism is difficult to eradicate by scaling and root planing alone. Adjunctive antimicrobial therapy (amoxicillin 250 mg + metronidazole 400 mg three times a day for 7–14 days) prescribed to coincide with root planing typically results in good improvements clinically. Surgical treatment may be required to allow for improved access to the root surface and excision of infected soft tissues.

2. Following efficacious periodontal therapy, the newly cleaned root surface is rapidly colonised by the downgrowth of gingival epithelial cells to form a long junctional epithelium (JE). Attachment of the long JE to the tooth surface occurs via hemidesmosomes. Rapid downgrowth of the gingival epithelial cells prevents colonisation of the tooth surface by cells migrating from the gingival connective tissues, which would otherwise result in root resorption or ankylosis. In this way, the integrity of the epithelial barrier is maintained, preventing ingress of bacteria into the tissues. However, pluripotential cells from the periodontal ligament are also prevented from colonising the root surface, and there is no opportunity for the generation of new connective tissue attachment to the root. Providing there is a high standard of oral hygiene, the long JE is maintained and probing depths are reduced compared with pretreatment measurements. However, the long JE is susceptible to plaque-induced breakdown and if plaque accumulates, apical migration of the JE will occur, resulting in increased probing depths.

3. Early studies that investigated patterns of progression of periodontitis concluded that there is linear, progressive loss of attachment (LOA) over time, although the rate of progression may vary according to the population studied. This suggests that, once initiated, periodontal disease progresses relentlessly throughout life. However, the use of more sophisticated probes and statistical models for assessing disease progression revealed that (i) rates of LOA in some individuals can be too slow/fast to fit a linear model, (ii) many sites do not change over long periods (which is inconsistent with the linear progression model), and (iii) destruction at a site may arrest and progress no further. Therefore, the random burst model was suggested in which certain sites do not exhibit periodontal destruction at all and other sites exhibit bursts of destruction that may last for an undefined period of time. Those latter sites subsequently may become quiescent or may exhibit one or more bursts of disease activity in the future. The bursts are random with regards to time and previous LOA.

4. Tooth mobility may be either physiological or pathological. Physiological mobility allows slight movement of the tooth within the socket to accommodate masticatory forces without injury to the tooth or its supporting structures. Pathological mobility is increased or increasing mobility as a result of connective tissue attachment loss. Pathological mobility is dependent on the quantity of remaining bony support, inflammation in the periodontal ligament and the magnitude of any

occlusal or jiggling displacing forces that may be acting on the tooth. Tooth mobility is measured by displacing the tooth with a rigid dental instrument and a moderate force and is classified according to horizontal (class I <1 mm, class II >1 mm, class III >2 mm) and vertical (class III) mobility.

5. Virulence factors enable bacteria to cause disease. In periodontitis, virulence properties can be broadly divided into factors that enable bacteria to adhere to and invade host tissues, and factors that enable bacteria to cause host tissue damage (either directly or indirectly). Adherence to the tooth surface, the soft tissues or other plaque bacteria is generally via surface fimbriae. Adherence represents a critical step in colonisation and bacterial invasion. Bacteria may enter the tissues through ulcerated sulcular and pocket epithelia, and they proliferate in the intercellular spaces of the gingival tissues. Certain species (for example, *Porphyromonas gingivalis, Actinobacillus actinomycetemcomitans*) have the ability to invade host cells directly. Bacterial invasion is strongly associated with diseased sites, and bacteria in the tissues are ideally placed to deliver toxic molecules and enzymes to the host cells. Furthermore, bacteria in the tissues may enable persistence of the infection by providing a reservoir for recolonisation. Many periodontopathogens also possess mechanisms for the evasion of host defences, including proteases to degrade immunoglobulins (and thus inhibit opsonisation), toxins that suppress or kill leukocytes and lymphocytes, collagenases, and harmful metabolic by-products such as ammonia and butyric acid.

6. Dental calculus is plaque that has become mineralised by calcium and phosphate ions from saliva. It forms as a hard substance on the tooth surfaces and requires professional removal. Calculus is covered by a layer of unmineralised plaque and prevents effective oral hygiene at the gingival margin. Calculus that forms at, or coronal to, the gingival margin is termed supragingival calculus, is generally yellow in colour and is often stained by food, drinks or tobacco. The greatest quantities of supragingival calculus are typically found close to the openings of the parotid and submandibular salivary glands. Subgingival calculus forms on the root surface apical to the gingival margin as dark brown/black deposits. A fine calculus probe may be required for detection of subgingival calculus, although larger deposits may also be seen radiographically.

7. Collagenases are enzymes that degrade collagen. Collagen degradation requires special enzymes because its cross-linked molecules resist most proteinases. The enzymes that degrade collagen (and also other matrix molecules) comprise a family of enzymes called matrix metalloproteinases (MMPs). All have a zinc ion at the active site and are synthesised and secreted as inactive precursors. Conversion to the active form occurs outside the cell and requires activation by proteinases, such as plasmin and trypsin, or reactive oxygen species. Production of MMPs is regulated by growth factors and cytokines, such as interleukin-1 (increases MMP synthesis) and transforming growth factor-β (decreases MMP synthesis). Inhibitors of MMPs exist in the serum (α_2-macroglobulin) and in the tissues (TIMPs, or tissue inhibitors of metalloproteinases). MMPs are produced by fibroblasts (MMP-1), keratinocytes, macrophages, and neutrophils (MMP-8).

Endodontics

Overview

The field of Endodontology has experienced rapid growth over recent years. In particular there has been a dramatic evolution in the technology available to help in treatment. These developments have however not changed the fundamental reasons for treatment, that is pulpal and periradicular disease which is principally bacterial in origin. The aim of treatment therefore is to eliminate these bacteria from within the complex anatomy of root canal systems and seal the canal space to prevent re-entry.

The section on Endodontology initially provides an overview of pulpal and periradicular disease and the methods used in its diagnosis. This is followed by a review of both traditional and some of the more recent treatment developments that have proved useful in day to day practice. Root canal treatment is not always successful, thus there is a requirement for knowledge of re-root canal treatment procedures and periradicular surgery. The section concludes with a review of some of the key aspects of restoration of the endodontically treated tooth.

2.1 Pulpal and periradicular pathology

Learning objectives

You should

- be able to recognise conditions that may affect the dental pulp

- understand the relationship between pulpal diagnosis and appropriate treatment.

Pulpal or periradicular inflammation results from irritation or injury usually from bacterial, mechanical or chemical sources.

Bacteria

Bacteria, usually from dental caries, are the main sources of injury to the pulpal and periradicular tissues and these enter either directly or through dentine tubules. The link between bacteria and pulpal and periradicular disease is well established as periradicular pathology does not develop in the absence of bacteria. Modes of entry for bacteria other than caries include periodontal disease (dentine tubules, furcal canals, lateral canals), erosion, attrition and abrasion (dentinal tubules), trauma with or without pulpal exposure, developmental anomalies and anachoresis (the passage of microorganisms into the root canal system from the bloodstream).

Mechanical irritants

Examples of mechanical irritation include trauma, operative procedures, excessive orthodontic forces, subgingival scaling and overinstrumentation using root canal instruments.

Chemical irritants

Pulpal irritation may result from bacterial toxins or some restorative materials/conditioning agents. Periradicular irritation may occur from irrigating solutions, phenol-based intracanal medicaments or extrusion of root canal filling materials.

Pulp disease

Irritation from any of the above sources causes some degree of inflammation. The response of the pulp depends on the severity of the insult and may result in a transient (reversible) inflammatory response or an irreversible one, which will eventually proceed to pulp necrosis.

Classification of pulp disease

There is an inconsistent correlation between clinical symptoms and histological findings in pulpal disease. Diagnoses are, therefore, usually based on patient symptoms and clinical findings. Pulpal disease may result in changes to both the soft and hard tissues.

Soft tissue changes

Reversible pulpitis Reversible pulpitis is a transient condition that may be precipitated by caries, erosion, attrition, abrasion, operative procedures, scaling or mild trauma. The symptoms are usually:

- pain does not linger after the stimulus is removed
- pain is difficult to localise (as the pulp does not contain proprioceptive fibres)
- normal periradicular radiographic appearance
- teeth are not tender to percussion (unless occlusal trauma is present).

Treatment involves covering up exposed dentine, removing the stimulus or dressing the tooth as appropriate. Reversible pulpitis may progress to an irreversible situation.

Irreversible pulpitis Irreversible pulpitis usually occurs as a result of more severe insults of the type listed above; typically, it may develop as a progression from a reversible state. The symptoms are, however, different:

- pain may develop spontaneously or from stimuli
- in the latter stages heat may be more significant
- response lasts from minutes to hours
- when the periodontal ligament becomes involved, the pain will be localised
- a widened periodontal ligament may be seen radiographically in the later stages.

Treatment involves either root canal therapy or extraction of the tooth.

Hyperplastic pulpitis Hyperplastic pulpitis is a form of irreversible pulpitis and is also known as a pulp polyp. It occurs as a result of proliferation of chronically inflamed young pulp tissue. Treatment involves root canal therapy or extraction.

Pulp necrosis Pulp necrosis occurs as the end result of irreversible pulpitis; treatment involves root canal therapy or extraction.

Hard tissue changes

Pulp calcification Physiological secondary dentine is formed after tooth eruption and the completion of root development. It is deposited on the floor and ceiling of the pulp chamber rather than the walls and with time can result in occlusion of the pulp chamber. Tertiary dentine is laid down in response to environmental stimuli as reactionary or reparative dentine. Reactionary dentine is a response to a mild noxious stimulus whereas reparative dentine is deposited directly beneath the path of injured dentinal tubules as a response to strong noxious stimuli. Treatment is dependent upon the pulpal symptoms.

Internal resorption Occasionally, pulpal inflammation may cause changes that result in dentinoclastic activity. Such changes result in resorption of dentine; clinically, a pink spot may be seen in the later stages if the lesion is coronal. Radiographic examination reveals a punched out outline that is seen to be continuous with the rest of the pulp cavity. Root canal therapy will result in arrest of the resorptive process; however, if destruction is very advanced extraction may be required.

Classification of periapical disease

Acute apical periodontitis

Causes of acute apical periodontitis include occlusal trauma, egress of bacteria from infected pulps, toxins from necrotic pulps, chemicals, irrigants or over instrumentation in root canal therapy. Clinically, the tooth is tender to biting. Widening of the periodontal space may be seen on a radiograph. Treatment depends on the pulpal diagnosis; it may range from occlusal adjustment to root canal therapy or extraction.

Chronic apical periodontitis

Chronic apical periodontitis occurs as a result of pulp necrosis. Affected teeth do not respond to pulp sensitivity tests. Tenderness to biting, if present, is usually mild; however some tenderness may be noted to palpation over the root apex. Radiographic appearance is varied, ranging from minimal widening of the periodontal ligament space to a large area of destruction of periapical tissues. Treatment involves root canal therapy or extraction.

Condensing osteitis

Condensing osteitis is a variant of chronic apical periodontitis and represents a diffuse increase in trabecular bone in response to irritation. Radiographically, a concentric radio-opaque area is seen around the offending root. Treatment is only required if symptoms/pulpal diagnosis indicate a need.

Acute apical abscess

An acute apical abscess is a severe inflammatory response to microorganisms or their irritants that have leached out into the periradicular tissues. Symptoms vary from moderate discomfort or swelling to systemic involvement, such as raised temperature and malaise. Teeth involved are usually tender to both palpation and percussion. Radiographic changes are variable depending on the amount of periradicular destruction already present; however, usually there is a well-defined radiolucent area, as in many situations an acute apical abscess is an acute exacerbation of a chronic situation. One well-recognised event is that of a phoenix abscess, which refers to an acute exacerbation of a chronic situation during treatment. Initial treatment of an acute apical abscess involves removal of the cause as soon as possible. Drainage should be established either by opening the tooth or incision into a dependent swelling. An antibiotic may need to be prescribed, depending on the patient's condition. Once the acute symptoms have subsided, then root canal therapy or extraction may be performed.

Chronic apical abscess

In a chronic apical abscess, the abscess has formed a communication through which it discharges. Such communications may be through an intraoral sinus or, less commonly, extraorally. Alternatively the discharge may be along the periodontal ligament; such cases mimic a periodontal pocket. Usually these communications or tracts heal spontaneously following root canal therapy or extraction.

Lesions of non-endodontic origin visualised radiographically

Although lesions noted on radiographs are usually of endodontic origin, this is not always the case. Other causes may be normal anatomic structures, benign or malignant lesions. (The following list is not exhaustive and readers should refer to an appropriate text on oral pathology.)

Certain normal anatomic structures may mimic radiolucencies (e.g. maxillary sinus, mental foramen, nasopalatine foramen). In these situations, the associated teeth will respond normally to pulp sensitivity tests and a radiograph taken from a different angle will reveal that the lesion is not so closely related to the root.

Benign lesions that may mimic endodontic pathology include cementoma, fibrous dysplasia, ossifying fibroma, primordial cysts, lateral periodontal cyst, dentigerous cyst, traumatic bone cyst, central giant cell granuloma, central haemangioma and ameloblastoma. Usually in such situations, the lamina dura will be intact around the teeth and final diagnosis relies on appropriate biopsy.

Malignant lesions to be aware of include squamous cell carcinoma, osteosarcoma, chondrosarcoma and multiple myeloma. These lesions are usually associated with rapid hard tissue destruction.

2.2 Patient assessment

Learning objectives

You should

- be able to recognise the need for following a structured approach in history taking
- understand the relevance of special tests
- appreciate the importance of patient-specific treatment planning.

Successful endodontic diagnosis requires a systematic approach to the history and clinical examination, followed by the use of appropriate diagnostic aids. Finally, careful planning of the treatment strategy is essential.

The most common cause of orofacial pain is pulpal or periradicular disease. However, it should be remembered that the periodontium, sinuses, TMJs, muscles of mastication, ears, nose, eyes and blood vessels may also be affected by lesions that can mimic pain of pulpal origin.

History

Presenting complaint

The aim of this stage is to record the patient's symptoms or problems, preferably in their own words.

Medical history

An up-to-date medical history should be taken for each new patient or be updated for previously registered patients, dated and signed.

Dental history

The purpose of the dental history is to summarise current and past dental treatment. Such information may provide clues as to the source of the patient's complaints. It is also an opportunity to establish the patient's attitude towards dental health and treatment as these findings may affect treatment decisions/planning (Section 1.2).

Pain history

Initially, information on pain is obtained by asking questions regarding the current problem(s). This examination is subjective, frequently asked questions include:

- *Location*. Occasionally a patient may identify the location of the pain; however, one must be cautious as pulpal pain may be referred to a different area. Pain may be felt in any of the orofacial structures.
- *Type and intensity of pain*. The patient may describe pain in many ways. Examples include sharp, dull,

throbbing, stabbing, burning, electric shock like, deep or superficial. The more the pain disrupts the patient's lifestyle because of its intensity, the more likely it is to be irreversible in origin.

- *Duration.* For how long after removal of the stimulus does the pain continue? The longer the pain continues after the stimulus, the more likely it is to be irreversible.
- *Stimulus.* Many different stimuli may initiate the pain, for example hot, cold, sweet, biting, posture. Alternatively the pain may be spontaneous. Special tests may be selected on the basis of what causes the main complaint.
- *Relief.* Pain-relieving factors, especially type and frequency of analgesics, antibiotics, sipping cold drinks.

Provisional diagnosis

The history and identification of signs and symptoms may help the clinician to reach a provisional diagnosis. The clinical examination gathers the information necessary to confirm or modify this diagnosis.

Clinical examination

Extraoral examination

The patient's general appearance and well-being are assessed. A note is made of any swelling, redness or extraoral sinuses. Lymph nodes are palpated for enlargement and/or tenderness. Muscles of mastication and TMJs are also palpated for tenderness and a note made of the degree of mouth opening.

Intraoral soft tissues

The oral mucosa and gingival tissues are examined for discoloration, inflammatory change and sinus tract formation. A basic periodontal examination (BPE) is performed (Section 1.2).

Intraoral hard tissues

Teeth are examined for caries, large restorations, crowns, discoloration, fracture, attrition, abrasion, erosion and restorability.

Special tests

All special tests have their limitations and require care in the way they are performed and interpreted. The objective is to find the tooth that is causing the discomfort. In general, healthy (control) teeth are tested first.

Percussion

Percussion refers to gently tapping or pressing the occlusal or lateral surface of a tooth. A painful response indicates periradicular inflammation.

Mobility

A mirror handle is placed on one side of the tooth and a note made of the degree of movement: up to 1 mm scores 1, over 1 mm scores 2 and vertically mobile teeth score 3.

Occlusal analysis

It is important to examine suspect teeth for interferences on the retruded arc of closure, intercuspal position and lateral excursions. Interferences in any of these positions could result in a degree of occlusal trauma and institute acute apical periodontitis.

Pulp sensitivity tests

Pulp sensitivity tests determine the response to stimuli and may identify the offending tooth. It is usual to try to mimic the stimulus that initiates the pain. Pulp sensitivity testing may help to distinguish between an infection of endodontic or periodontal origin when an endodontal–periodontal communication is present. Thermal tests are usually the most useful as they give an indication not only as to whether the pulp is alive but also how healthy it is.

Cold test Ethyl chloride spray on a cotton pledget, ice or dry ice sticks may be used to mimic cold stimuli.

Hot test Hot gutta-percha or hot water after the application of rubber dam may be used to mimic hot stimuli.

Electric pulp test

Electric instruments can provide an indication as to whether or not there is vital nerve tissue in the tooth; they do not give an indication of different stages of degeneration.

Sinus tract exploration

Where a sinus tract is present, it may be possible to insert a small gutta-percha point. A radiograph is then taken to see which root the tract/point leads to.

Transillumination

Transillumination with a fibre optic light can be useful in the diagnosis of cracks in teeth.

Periodontal probing

Detailed periodontal probing around suspect teeth may reveal a sulcus within normal limits. However, on occasions deeper pocketing will be noted. A narrow defect may be an indication of a root fracture or an endodontic lesion draining through the gingival crevice. Broader-based lesions are usually an indication of disease of periodontal origin.

Radiographs

Radiographs should be taken using film holders and a paralleling technique and be viewed using an appropriate viewer with magnification as necessary. They will not show early signs of pulpitis as there is no periodontal widening at this stage of pulpal degeneration. Radiographs may provide much important information to help to confirm a diagnosis, but they should not be used alone. Radiographic findings may include the loss of lamina dura (laterally or apically) or a frank periradicular radiolucency indicative of pulp necrosis. Alternatively, radiographs may show pulp chamber or root canal calcification, which may explain reduced responses to pulp sensitivity testing. This emphasises the need for considering using more than one test. More rarely, radiographic examination may reveal tooth/root resorptive defects.

Checklist for radiographic assessment All the following can be assessed:

- periodontal bone support
- caries
- crown shape and size
- proximity of restorations to pulp chamber
- quality of restorations, including coronal seal
- the size of the pulp chamber +/– calcifications
- crown root ratio
- the number of roots
- root anatomy
- canal anatomy
- canal calcification
- root end proximity to important structures
- presence of lesions of endodontic origin periradicularly or furcally
- root fractures
- extra root canals
- resorptive defects
- quality and effectiveness of previous treatment
- root filling materials used
- iatrogenic complications
- presence of pins/posts.

Test cavity
Occasionally, as a last resort, an access cavity is cut into dentine without local anaesthesia as an additional way of sensitivity testing.

Selective anaesthesia
Selective anaesthesia can be useful in cases of referred pain to distinguish whether the source of pain is mandibular or maxillary in origin. It is less useful for distinguishing pain from adjacent teeth, as the anaesthetic solution may diffuse laterally.

Diagnosis

Following this systematic approach to history taking and the application of appropriate special tests, it will usually be possible to make a diagnosis of the pulpal or periradicular problems. Such diagnoses have been covered in Section 2.1 and include reversible pulpitis, irreversible pulpitis, pulp necrosis, resorptive changes, acute apical periodontitis, chronic apical periodontitis and acute and chronic apical abscesses.

After taking thorough history and performing appropriate special tests, the clinician may be unsure as to whether the pain is of dental origin. Endodontic treatment should not be performed on an ad hoc or 'hit and miss' basis. In cases of difficult diagnosis, a referral to an orofacial pain clinic, a neurosurgeon or an eye, nose and throat specialist may be considered.

Cracked tooth syndrome
Cracked teeth appear to be an increasing clinical problem. Cracks may not be visible initially and the use of a piece of rubber dam between the teeth may aid diagnosis. A plastic bite stick (tooth sleuth) has been introduced to allow each cusp tip to be checked in turn; typically, the pain occurs on release of biting pressure. Small cracks may be treatable, although communications through the floor of the pulp chamber usually result in tooth loss.

Case selection and treatment

Once a diagnosis has been reached, a plan needs to be formulated as to how to deal with the problem. The fact that an endodontic procedure is feasible is not sufficient justification for performing it. Endodontic treatment must be considered as part of an overall treatment plan in such a way that it represents the patient's best interests and wishes. The past dental history will have provided much information as to the patient's attitude towards treatment. Good endodontic treatment takes time, requiring a commitment from both clinician and patient.

Treatment planning

Sequencing of treatment involves the management of pulpal or periodontal pain as a priority, and the extraction of unsaveable teeth. Large carious lesions should be stabilised and a preventive regimen including periodontal therapy instituted. Endodontic and restorative procedures can then be performed in a healthier environment and more predictable results can be obtained.

Indications for root canal therapy

Pulpal and periradicular disease
The most common indication for root canal therapy is pulpal or periradicular pathology. Elective root canal therapy may be performed for endodontic reasons: for example, teeth for which extensive restorative dentistry is planned and the subsequent tooth preparation would

further stress a pulp of dubious prognosis. Alternatively, radiographs may show progressive calcification of the pulp space. This itself is not an indication for root canal therapy. However, such treatment may be performed if it is thought likely the pulp space will be required for restorative purposes.

Restorative requirements

Occasionally, it may be decided to root treat a tooth electively for restorative reasons. Such situations include teeth that have fractured at the gingival level and for which post space is required for their restoration, and teeth that are going to be used as overdenture abutments.

Periodontal disease

If the periodontal lesion is of primary endodontic origin then reattachment will usually occur provided the lesion has not been longstanding. If resolution is only partial, then periodontal therapy will be required if a successful result is to be obtained. In cases of advanced periodontal disease, one or more roots may require resection after root canal therapy (Chapter 1).

Re-root treatment

Re-root treatment is an increasing clinical problem and is considered in detail in Section 2.7.

Contraindications to treatment

General factors

The patient's medical history or general well-being may preclude treatment. If there is an indication for antibiotic cover, then it should be given because even if the instrumentation does not cause a bacteraemia the placement of a rubber dam most likely will. Lack of patient interest or restricted opening may preclude endodontic treatment. Access to posterior teeth may be difficult, with a minimum of two fingers opening being required. Remember that any degree of opening may reduce as the patient's jaw muscles become fatigued.

Restorative factors

The clinical examination may have revealed the tooth to be unrestorable, to be of little functional use or to have a hopeless periodontal prognosis. Such situations preclude root canal therapy. Other forms of pathology may be present, such as extensive internal or external resorption. Although internal resorption will cease once the pulp is removed, consideration must be made as to the strength of the remaining root in function.

Trauma

Root fractures may be present either horizontally or vertically. Horizontal root fractures in the middle to apical third can have quite a good prognosis as the apical segment frequently remains vital with root canal therapy only being necessary to the fracture line. Fractures involving the gingival crevice, however, rapidly become infected as there is a continuation of the fracture line and the periodontal space. This includes vertical root fractures and many oblique fractures resulting from trauma.

Complex internal or external anatomy

Other contraindications include anatomy that is too complex to treat. Such variations may be internal (dens in dente) or external (root grooves). Palatal root grooves on upper incisors have a poor prognosis, as again there is a continuum along the root side that like a root fracture, cannot be adequately cleaned and represents a constant nidus of infection.

2.3 Root canal morphology

Learning objectives

You should

- understand the complexity of root canal morphology
- appreciate the importance of adequate access in root canal therapy.

Radiographs give some idea of basic root canal anatomy, although the reality is far more complex. Studies of cleared extracted teeth have shown that all roots enclose at least one root canal system, which frequently consists of a network of branches. Communications with the periodontal ligament also exist either in the furcation (furcal canals) or laterally (lateral canals). In addition, the root canal may frequently terminate as more than one opening with an array of accessory canals forming an apical delta. These furcal, lateral and apical communications have been termed 'portals of exit' from the root canal system. Furcal, lateral and accessory canals are created during tooth formation either when there is a break in the sheath of Hertwig or the sheath grows around an existing blood vessel. On occasions, such canals can be as large as the apical constriction. Their significance is not fully understood; however, it would seem sensible to use a preparation technique that aims to clean as much of the root canal system as possible.

The pulp chamber and root canal orifices may be reduced in size as a result of the deposition of secondary and tertiary dentine. If the irritation is severe with extensive destruction of pulpal cells then further inflammatory changes involving the rest of the pulp will take place and could lead to pulp necrosis. Such pulpal degeneration starts coronally and progresses apically. Necrotic pulpal breakdown products may leach out of the root canal system to form lesions of endodontic origin around the portals of exit. Frequently these changes in the periodontium will be visible lateral to the root before they are apparent apically. It is, therefore, extremely important to examine roots periradicularly as opposed to periapically as such examination may provide an early indication of pulp degeneration.

Important general considerations of pulpal anatomy

Shape. The shape of the coronal pulp and the outline of the canals is a reflection of the outline of the crown and root surfaces (Fig. 29).

Pulp morphology. This alters with age, irritants, attrition, caries, abrasion and periodontal disease.

Root anatomy. Over 90% of roots are curved. The only roots that rarely, if ever, contain two canals are maxillary anteriors, maxillary premolars with two roots and the distobuccal and palatal roots of maxillary molars. All other (note this includes all mandibular) roots may contain two canals.

Apical anatomy changes with age. The apical constriction is variable and usually cannot be detected by tactile sense, especially early in preparation, as dentine laid down in the coronal third of root canals will frequently cause files to bind coronally before they reach the apical third of the root canal.

Planes of curvature. Radiographs from a labial/buccal projection show only two planes of curvature. Many curvatures are towards or away from the film.

Access

Access to the root canal system involves both coronal access to the pulp chamber and radicular access to the root canals.

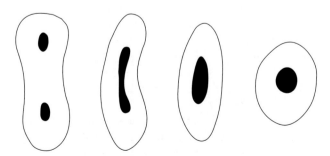

Fig. 29 Cross-sections of root canal anatomy showing the relationship between pulpal and radicular shape.

Coronal access

The coronal access preparation in root canal therapy serves several important functions:

- provide an unimpeded path to the root canal system
- eliminate the pulp chamber roof in its entirety
- be large enough to allow light in and enable examination of the pulp chamber floor for root canal orifices or fractures
- have divergent walls to support a temporary dressing between visits
- provide a straight line path to each canal orifice.

The ideal access cavity will achieve the above objectives but will preserve as much sound coronal and radicular tissue as possible. Occasionally, however, it may be necessary to enlarge and deflect the access to enhance the preparation of roots that are especially curved in their coronal thirds. In these situations, access preparation is dynamic, developing as instrumentation progresses.

Radicular access

The principle of straight line radicular access cannot be overemphasised as it allows instruments to flow down the cavity line angles into the apical third of the root canal system without interruption and provides maximum tactile feedback whilst instrumenting the most delicate apical portion of the root canal. Adequate straight line access reduces the angle of curvature in the coronal third of the root canal where it exits from the floor of the pulp chamber and thus reduces the overall canal curvature. Further advantages will be discussed later.

Access to the root canal system is aided by examination of:

- coronal anatomy
- tooth position and angulation
- external root morphology
- the preoperative radiograph (or preferably more than one taken at different angles).

Examination of the tooth will provide guidance as to the position, size and angulation of the access cavity as many teeth are tilted in one or more planes relative to the arch and adjacent teeth.

Examination of the radiograph affords information on:

- the size of the pulp chamber +/− calcifications
- the distance of the chamber from the occlusal surface (overlay the access bur to determine the maximum safe depth)
- the angle of exit of root canals from the floor of the pulp chamber; this provides an indication of the amount of coronal third root canal modification required to obtain straight line access
- the number of roots, degree of root curvature and canal patency.

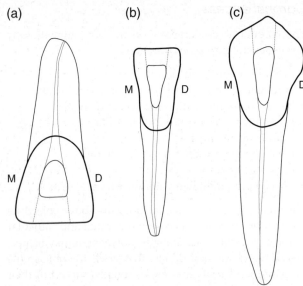

Fig. 30 Access cavity outline for the anterior teeth. (a) Upper incisor. (b) Lower incisor. (c) Canine teeth. M = mesial; D = distal.

Endodontic access openings

Incisor and canine teeth

The access cavities for maxillary central and lateral incisors are similar and generally triangular in shape (Fig. 30). Access cavities for maxillary and mandibular canines are almost identical and more ovoid in shape (Fig. 30). Access for mandibular central and lateral incisors are triangular in shape and a second canal may be present in 40%. In general, extend the access in anterior teeth towards the incisal edge and under the cingulum (Fig. 30).

Premolar teeth

The maxillary first premolar in most individuals contains two canals and is extended more buccolingually than in single-rooted premolars. Approximately 5% may have a third root/canal placed buccally. In such situations, the access will be triangular in outline with the base towards the buccal side (Fig. 31).

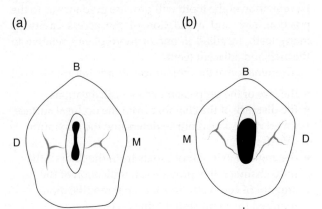

Fig. 31 Access cavity outline for (a) upper and (b) lower premolar teeth. M = mesial; D = distal; P = palatal; B = buccal.

The maxillary second premolar and both the mandibular first and second premolars usually have one centrally located root canal. However, if the canal appears to be situated under either the buccal or lingual cusp, look carefully for a second canal under the opposite cusp. The opening is a narrow oval in shape. The maxillary second premolar access is centred over the central groove. Access for mandibular premolars is buccal to the central groove (Fig. 31).

Maxillary molars

The maxillary molar access is generally triangular in shape with the base to the buccal and the apex to the lingual. Usually one palatal and two buccal canals are identified. However, two canals may be present in the mesiobuccal root in 70% of cases (Fig. 32).

Mandibular molar

The mandibular molar access is more trapezoid in shape with its base to the mesial and apex to the distal sides. They usually have two roots with two canals in the mesial root and one in the distal root. There is a possibility of a second canal in the distal root (33%) (Fig. 32).

Access: prior considerations

A number of steps should be taken to prepare for access (Box 9).

Rubber dam

The rubber dam is essential for root canal treatment and affords the following advantages:

- improved visibility
- soft tissue protection
- confinement of excess irrigant
- prevention of saliva contamination
- reduced liability in the medicolegal sense.

On occasions it may be deemed appropriate to initiate access prior to placement of rubber dam as this

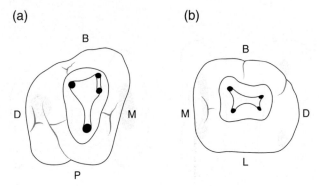

Fig. 32 Access cavity outline for (a) upper and (b) lower molar teeth. M = mesial; D = distal; P = palatal; B = buccal.

Box 9 Technique to prepare for access to root canals

- Remove as much restoration as necessary prior to entering the chamber in order to reduce the likelihood of filling material entering the canal system.
- Remove all temporary materials when feasible. Remove crowns when feasible.
- Only restore broken down teeth with amalgams, bands or temporary crowns when it is not possible to isolate them with rubber dam. It may be preferable to perform crown lengthening.
- Remove all caries prior to entering the pulp chamber.
- Full-coverage crowns are frequently not oriented to the original tooth anatomy.
- Study radiographs carefully prior to commencing access to see if the tooth may be rotated, also check external root anatomy.

Box 10 Technique for producing access to a root canal

1. The access cavity is outlined provisionally on the tooth and progress is directed pulpally, constantly being mindful of the depth of bur penetration into the tooth. A round-ended bur is to be preferred as flat-ended ones tend to gouge the access cavity walls. It is wise to compare depth of penetration of the bur to the apparent pulp chamber depth on the preoperative radiograph. If there is vital pulp tissue (haemorrhage), remove the coronal pulp with an excavator and/or radicular pulp with broaches and irrigate with sodium hypochlorite as good visibility is important.
2. Stop and take radiographs if the canal(s) cannot be readily located. Place an endodontic explorer in the hole you have prepared, ask the patient to bite on it and take radiographs from two different angles. It is useful to remember that dentine is yellow/brown in colour, the floor of the pulp chamber is grey.
3. Once the pulp chamber has been identified, it is deroofed using a slow speed round bur (long neck bur if necessary) directed coronally. The walls can then be smoothed and flared using a tapered bur in the air turbine.
4. The pulp chamber space should now be thoroughly irrigated with sodium hypochlorite solution and canal orifices identified using a straight probe or DG16 endodontic explorer. Knowledge of dental anatomy and undulations in the floor of the pulp chamber in multirooted teeth are used as a guide. Magnification and coaxial lighting are particularly useful in helping to identify small root canal openings and to refine access.
5. Further refinement of the access may now be performed to enable straight-line access to the canals (Fig. 33). In addition, troughing may be performed using a small long-neck bur or ultrasonic inserts to remove dentine overlying canal orifices, especially in the MB2 region of upper molar teeth. Early progress into such canals is frequently hindered by an abrupt exit from the pulp chamber. Careful removal of overlying dentine permits easier access to these canals, which prior to coronal enlargement may only allow small files to pass for 2 mm before impacting on the outer canal wall. The concept of initial canal enlargement will be discussed further below.

allows better appreciation of external root contour and tooth position. Rubber dam should be placed as soon as the pulp chamber is identified for the above reasons.

Access technique

Box 10 describes the technique used to achieve access.

2.4 Root canal preparation

Learning objectives

You should

- understand the technical procedures involved in combating root canal infection
- appreciate some of the problems that may be encountered in root canal preparation
- appreciate some of the technological advancements that have made root canal preparation more predictable.

Any root canal preparation technique should be simple, safe and predictable. Many techniques have been described over the years. In principle these can be split into methods of instrument manipulation (reaming and filing) and preparation philosophies, the most recent one being a crown-down approach with apical preparation being developed throughout the procedure and completed at the end. New developments extend or facilitate the process.

Reaming infers rotating the root canal instrument clockwise, this motion draws the instrument into the canal and cuts dentine. Filing infers a linear motion of the instrument in a push–pull manner. Filing may be performed around the perimeter of a root canal especially if it is oval or dumbell shaped; such instrument manipulation is termed circumferential filing.

Root canal preparation has both biological and mechanical objectives. The biological objectives are to eliminate the pulp, bacteria and related irritants from the root canal system. The mechanical objectives are directed at producing a continuously tapering preparation with the original anatomy and foramen position maintained. The apical foramen should also be kept as small as practical.

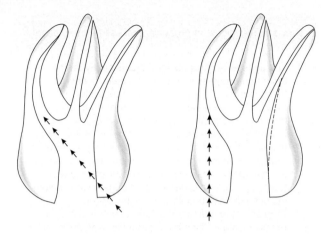

Fig. 33 Modification of coronal and radicular access to create straight-line access.

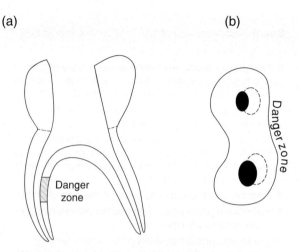

(a) (b)

Danger zone

Fig. 34 The danger zone where care needs to be taken in order to avoid strip perforation. (a) Lateral view. (b) Cross-sectional view.

In summary the aim of root canal preparation is to debride the pulp space, rendering it as bacteria free as possible, producing a shape amenable to obturation. This apparently straightforward task is complicated by the anatomy of root canal systems, which is complex and makes cleaning them in their entirety a clinical challenge.

Current trends in canal preparation

Current thinking on canal preparation emphasises the development of shape in a crown-down manner removing infected dentine as it is encountered. Further cleaning of the canal is provided by correct choice and use of root canal irrigants (in particular sodium hypochlorite because of its antimicrobial and tissue-dissolving properties), with the combination being termed chemomechanical debridement.

Instrument manipulation

The two most commonly used motions are watchwinding and balanced force.

Watchwinding refers to the gentle side-to-side rotation of a file (30° each way). This motion is useful for all stages of canal preparation especially initial negotiation and finishing the apical third.

Balanced forces (in many ways a development from watchwinding) involves rotating the instrument 60° clockwise to set the flutes and then rotating it 120° anticlockwise while maintaining apical pressure sufficient to resist coronal movement of the file. Balanced forces is an efficient cutting motion and has been shown to maintain a central canal position even round moderate curvatures while allowing a larger size to be prepared apically (compared with other hand instrumentation techniques).

Coronal interferences influence the forces a file will exert within a canal. This is of particular importance in curved canals where files may prepare more dentine along the furcal (danger zone), as opposed to the outer canal wall. It is important to be aware of this, to limit the size of enlargement in curved canals and direct files away from the furcal wall to avoid a strip perforation (Fig. 34).

Irrigation

Irrigating solutions are usually delivered using a syringe with a 27 or 28 gauge needle. Care should be taken to ensure that the needle does not bind in the canal and that irrigating solution does not pass into periapical tissues. The role of the irrigant is to remove debris and provide lubrication for instruments. Specifically, an irrigant such as sodium hypochlorite will dissolve organic remnants and, most importantly, also has an antibacterial action. It may be used in a range of concentrations from 0.5 to 5.25%, 2.5% being popular. It is important that the irrigant is changed frequently; ideally irrigation should be performed between each file, at least every two to three files being the minimum. If removal of the smear layer is desired, then an irrigation solution containing ethylenediamine tetraacetic acid (EDTA) should be used. There is no clinical consensus as to whether or not the smear layer should be removed.

A most effective way of delivering irrigating solutions is through an ultrasonic handpiece. Ultrasonic agitation (acoustic microstreaming) has been shown to be effective at removing debris from canals.

Canal preparation

Several methods of canal preparation exist. The method described here encompasses current thought:

- canal exploration
- pre-enlargement (when necessary)
- straight-line radicular access
- length determination
- apical third preparation.

Canal exploration

Root canals are infinitely variable in their shapes and sizes. Larger canals allow easy placement of instruments and irrigating solutions whereas smaller ones require pre-enlargement coronally prior to the canal exploration. Preliminary assessment of the canal can be made with the smallest and most flexible instruments. It is unlikely that the operator will be able to determine the working length initially as files may be binding coronally.

Pre-enlargement and straight-line radicular access

Pre-enlargement is achieved by watchwinding file sizes 10–35 in series, gradually opening up narrow canal orifices to a size sufficient to take a Gates–Glidden bur. The pre-enlargement can then be developed further to produce straight-line radicular access taking care to work the drill away from furcal regions of roots. A file should stand upright in the tooth and pass undeflected deep into the canal once adequate straight-line radicular access has been achieved.

Gates–Glidden burs may be used to relocate a canal away from the danger zone; however, care should be taken to avoid overenlargement. Gates–Glidden No. 6 and 5 should only be used on the walls of the access cavity, and No. 4 no deeper than the canal orifice. The No. 3 may be used to the mid-canal region and the No. 2 to the beginning of the canal curvature, or to near full length in a straight canal. The No. 1 is quite fragile, but may be used at ultraslow speeds provided it is loose in the canal.

Advantages of pre-enlargement and establishment of straight-line access There are a number of advantages from achieving a straight-line access:

- it creates sufficient space to introduce files and irrigating needles/solutions deeper in the canal
- the bacterial count in the more coronal aspects of the canal is reduced
- a reservoir of irrigant is created that files pass through as they move apically
- the increased space allows files to fit passively in the canal, making inoculation of infected material into the periapical tissues less likely
- pressure on the coronal flutes of the file is decreased thereby increasing tactile sense and control when using files in the apical third
- precurved files remain curved, can be easily inserted and freely pass down the canal
- a greater volume of irrigant is present enhancing pulp digestion

- the bulk of pulpal and related irritants are removed reducing debris accumulation apically
- working length is more accurate because there is a more direct path to the canal terminus.
- larger files may be used for the working length radiograph.

It is important to ensure that the apical region of the canal is not blocked with dentine debris or pulp tissue when using a crown-down technique. For this reason it is important that small files +/– chelating agents are used to prevent blockage and ensure canal patency. Although apical preparation develops throughout canal enlargement, it is not completed until the end of the procedure when greater control is possible over the files in this most delicate region of the root canal.

Length determination

It is essential that care is taken over identification of the correct canal length. Clinically, the aim is to identify the apical constriction that is the narrowest point of the root canal. Apical to this the canal space widens to form the apical foramen.

The most common way of determining canal length is the working length radiograph. A file is placed in each canal at what is estimated to be the working length. This 'questimate' of length is obtained by studying the pre-operative radiograph (after adjustment for elongation or foreshortening) and using knowledge of the average lengths of teeth. Allowances obviously need to be made for fractured teeth and incisal wear. Tactile feel may also help in establishing the approximate working length provided pre-enlargement has been performed. A bisecting angle radiograph may be taken; alternatively the film may be held using a pair of Spencer Wells artery forceps or an Endo Ray film holder (the latter two techniques allow for radiographs more resembling a paralleling technique to be performed). The file position is checked on the radiograph and adjusted as necessary. It is recommended that a repeat radiograph should be exposed with the file reset if it is more than 2 mm from the desired position.

Recently, electronic apex locators have been developed that greatly assist in the placement of the first length determination file. These devices have a lip clip and a probe, which is touched against the file shaft. As the file approaches the foramen, the resistance or impedance changes and a visual display indicates when the file has touched the periapical tissues. It is usual to recheck the reading with different file sizes (08, 10, 15, 20 depending on canal size) to check for the accuracy of the reading. The file position is then checked by exposing a radiograph and adjusted as necessary. The combination of electronic apex locators and radiographs is a reliable way of determining canal length. Care must be taken to ensure that the pulp

1. In larger, straight canals the apical preparation is accomplished by preparing the apical portion using a slight rotational action of the file to an appropriate size after straight-line access has been confirmed.
2. The apical part of curved canals is generally kept small, usually a size 30 or in very curved canals a size 25. Instruments larger than size 25 rapidly lose flexibility and will attempt to cut straight ahead. Repeated use of a small file will result in a canal preparation larger than the file, in other words the canal is still being enlarged.
3. Step back preparation. Once the apical size has been determined and prepared, a greater tapering of the canal is accomplished by using successively larger instruments, each one about 0.5 to 1 mm shorter than the previous one. The distance of stepping back is determined by the degree of canal curvature.
4. Recapitulation. Canal patency must be maintained at all times. This is accomplished, after each successively larger file, by irrigating and then returning to a file smaller than the file which prepared the apical portion of the canal (No. 15 is frequently used). Irrigation is used between each file also to remove debris. Failure to recapitulate will result in canal blockage. Frequently blockage can be difficult to clear and attempts to do so may result in a ledge or even perforation (Fig. 35).
5. Further steps depend on the preparation chosen; apical stop and seat-type preparations are described in text.

chamber is dry and that there is minimal fluid in the root canals. Otherwise the fluid may short circuit the apex locator through the gingival tissues and cause a false reading. This is a particular problem in heavily restored or crowned teeth.

Apical preparation

Box 11 describes the technique used in apical preparation.

The use of excessively large files in curved canals may produce an hourglass shape termed a zip and elbow (Fig. 36).

Apical patency The concept of apical patency is considered controversial but is becoming increasingly accepted. A patency file is a small flexible instrument (08, 10) that will move passively through the terminus of a root canal without binding or enlarging the apical constricture. The aim is to prevent apical blockage, which will, in turn, reduce the incidence of ledge formation and transportation of the root canal. The use of a patency file also helps remove vital or necrotic pulpal remnants from the end of the canal. To use a patency technique, therefore, infers an intention to clean to the full canal length.

Formation of apical resistance It is important that adequate resistance form is created at the end of the root canal preparation in order to reduce the risk of overfilling. There are two ways of achieving this: an apical stop is an intentional ledge produced approximately 1 mm short of the radiographic root edge. (Fig. 37a). An apical seat is a shape that tapers back from the constriction itself blending with the rest of the canal preparation (Fig. 37b). An electronic apex locator is a useful adjunct to the working length radiograph when creating an apical seat as part of the patency technique. An apical stop is created early in the procedure and no attempt is made to gain apical patency. The seat-type preparation is usually completed as the final stage after the rest of the canal shape has been developed.

The choice of apical preparation is a personal one. Proponents of a patency technique would claim more of the canal is cleaned, whereas opponents emphasise the increased danger of extruding pulp tissue (infected or non-infected), dentine chippings or obturation material from the root canal.

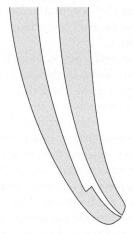

Fig. 35 Formation of a ledge in the apical third of a canal preparation. This usually occurs as a result of using files that are too large or of allowing the canal to block.

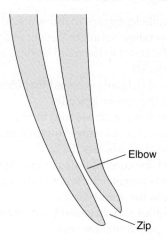

Elbow

Zip

Fig. 36 Zip and elbow formation resulting from the use of excessively large files.

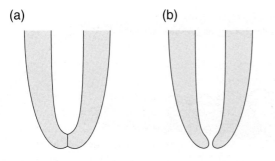

Fig. 37 Creation of apical resistance by (a) an apical stop or (b) an apical seat.

New developments in canal preparation

Considerable interest has been expressed in trying to make the mechanical aspects of canal preparation easier and quicker. The most obvious example of this is the use of rotary stainless steel Gates–Glidden drills as soon in the procedure as possible to create space coronally. File activation by means of a handpiece to speed up the creation of shape deeper in the canal system is also popular. Historically, these have used a reciprocating action or oscillatory motion (ultrasonic or sonic).

Reciprocating handpieces

Recent developments in endodontic handpieces include a refinement of the reciprocating motion to one of 60° as opposed to 90°, which provides a gentler watchwinding type motion. A variety of file designs with a latch grip attachment are available for such handpieces; however, recent innovations allow root canal files with conventional handles to be placed in the handpiece, thus negating the need for stocking files with latch attachments. Most instruments for use with the reciprocating type handpiece are manufactured from stainless steel and should be used with a light touch to prevent gouging of canal walls or instrument fracture. The watchwinding motion provided by such handpieces is particularly useful for negotiating and enlarging fine calcified canals using small files with a light touch.

Ultrasonic and sonic handpieces

Particular advantages of the vibratory systems include the use of concurrent irrigation and the associated microstreaming, which produces excellent canal debridement. The shaping ability of these instruments has proved to be disappointing, and attention has returned to the use of more conventional reciprocating or rotary handpieces.

Files

Nickel titanium alloy files

Nickel titanium (NiTi), noted for its hyperelasticity and shape memory, has radically changed endodontic file design and instrumentation techniques. Two features of NiTi have proved particularly beneficial to endodontics. First, the superior resistance to torsional failure compared with that of stainless steel has allowed the production of files that can be used in a 360° rotation. Second, the increased flexibility has allowed files of a taper greater than the standard 0.02 mm/mm used for stainless steel instruments. Such variably tapered files range from 0.02 to 0.12 mm/mm taper.

Many types are available and they can be broadly split up into those used by hand and those used in rotary handpieces.

Files of greater taper: GT files

GT files are available in a set of four, have a tip size of 20 and four different rates of taper: 0.06, 0.08, 0.10 and 0.12 mm/mm (Fig. 38). The files all have a maximum flute diameter of 1 mm to restrict overenlargement coronally. The 20/0.06 has three times the rate of taper of a standard ISO 0.02 taper file, the 20/0.08 has a taper of four times the standard etc. The flutes of the files are machined in a reverse direction and a balanced force movement is recommended for their use but in reverse in view of the flute direction. The handle on these files has been increased in size in order to make manipulation of this reverse balanced force easier. The increased taper of these files produces a predetermined shape to the canal preparation, thus reducing the need for careful stepping back of instruments to produce canal taper. Suggested criteria for use of GT files:

White	0.06 taper	fine curved canals
Yellow	0.08 taper	lower anteriors, multirooted premolars, mesial roots of lower molars and buccal roots of upper molars
Red	0.10 taper	palatal roots of upper molars and distal roots of lower molars, single canal premolars, lower canines and upper anteriors
Blue	0.12 taper	big canals, particularly those with a large apical diameter.

Variably tapered files, in view of their increased taper, are more likely to bind coronally early in the preparation procedure and thus produce a crown-down preparation. Care must be taken not to advance these files too far down the root canal at any one time as this will result in increased binding and stress along their length, greatly increasing the risk of fracture. It is important to create sufficient space in the canal before any of the variably tapered files are used.

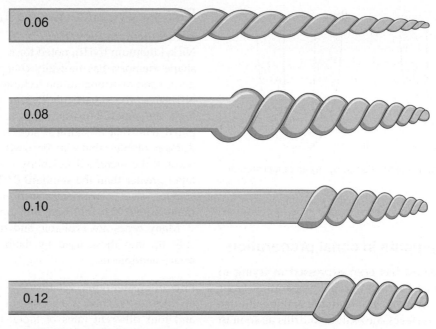

Fig. 38 GT files showing radical taper and limited flute width of 1 mm.

Rotary nickel titanium instrumentation

NiTi has allowed the production of files that can be rotated continuously in a handpiece through 360°. The advantages of the design of the present generation of rotary NiTi instruments include increased debris removal because of the continuous rotation, reduced canal transportation and smoother faster canal preparation with less operator fatigue.

Rotary instruments manufactured out of NiTi can be classified into two groups. First, those that resemble conventional files but have varying tapers (e.g. Profiles (0.04 and 0.06 taper), Rotary GTs (0.12, 0.10, 0.08, 0.06) and Quantecs) and, second, the Lightspeed, developed from the Canal Master series of instruments and resembling a Gates–Glidden drill.

Rotary nickel titanium instrumentation techniques

Profile rotary NiTi instruments are particularly effective when used in a crown-down manner. Current opinion is that the 0.06 taper Profile instruments are more appropriate for canal shaping than the 0.04. These are used in a large to small sequence (40, 35, 30, 25, 20, 15) and rotary GTs (all size 20 at the tip) are used larger taper to smaller (0.12, 0.10, 0.08, 0.06). Speed should be limited to 150 rpm in a high torque handpiece. An in and out motion is recommended (touch/retract/touch/retract) with use of each file being limited to approximately 4 seconds. The sequence is repeated as necessary until the 20/0.06 reaches full length. It is important to finish the preparation by hand as this allows gauging of the apical size of the canal and apical resistance form to be developed as necessary.

Quantec instruments are used in a sequence 1 to 10: the graduating taper technique. First, an Orifice opener size 25/0.06 taper is used in the coronal 2/3s. The apical preparation is then performed using 15/0.02, 20/0.02, 25/0.02. The apical preparation is gradually blended with the coronal preparation using the next four files, which have gradually increasing tapers (25/0.03, 25/0.04, 25/0.05, 25/0.06). Nos 9 and 10 in the series (40/0.02, 45/0.02) can then be used to increase apical size as required. Quantec Flares have now been introduced (25/0.08, 25/0.10, 25/0.12). These instruments allow a greater taper to be imparted on the canal shape if desired. Alternatively, they may be used in a crown-down manner like the rotary GTs.

Lightspeed instruments are used to create an apical stop, with canal taper being produced by using instruments in a step back manner. They have the disadvantage of not imparting a taper to the canal automatically because of their design; however, the narrow cross-sectional area of their shaft makes them very flexible. It is suggested that they are useful for apical preparation; however, there are more effective rotary instruments for imparting a taper to the root canal preparation.

Techniques for the use of rotary NiTi instruments are evolving continuously as greater understanding is gained of how best to use them safely. Pre-enlargement, coronal flaring and a crown-down approach are now recognised as being important considerations in getting best results and limiting instrument failure. Each rotary instrument should be dipped in a lubricant prior to use, with their use being preceded by irrigation and a small hand instrument. This moves irrigating solutions deeper into the canal system and maintains canal patency. Apical preparation should be completed at the end.

NiTi has good shape memory so it is difficult to see when files are fatigued. Canal curvature and calcification seem to influence fatigue more than time of use. Damaged files should always be discarded. It is important to appreciate that these instruments are for canal enlargement not canal negotiation.

It is especially important that a quality speed-reduction handpiece with high torque is used with NiTi instruments to allow appropriate speeds to be used. Instruments must be used with a light touch, similar to that which would be used with a narrow lead propelling pencil. Introduction into the canal should be gradual, using an in and out motion no more than 1 mm at a time. The instrument should be continuously introduced and removed, never being held at the same point in the canal. Any instruments that show the least sign of damage should be discarded, as should ones used in very calcified or severely curved canals.

The rotary NiTi instrumentation technique looks to be a promising development in canal preparation; however, it is important to be cautious in certain situations:

- calcified canals (ideally it should be possible to place a size 20/0.02 taper file to length prior to using rotary files in the apical third)
- canals having sharp curvature in the apical region
- two canals that join into one smaller canal at a sharp angle
- large canals that suddenly narrow.

One visit root canal treatment

Root canal therapy may be performed in one visit if time allows and the canals can be dried. However, it is important that procedures are not rushed and compromised just so that treatments can be performed in one visit. An advantage of doing a procedure in two visits is that an intracanal dressing of calcium hydroxide can be placed. This compound has a high pH and will further help to reduce the bacterial flora. Care needs to be taken to ensure that a sound coronal seal of 3–4 mm of temporary dressing material is present to prevent recontamination of the canal between visits. It is also usual to place a small pledget of cotton wool prior to placing the temporary dressing in order to prevent its inadvertant dropping into the canal between visits, or during subsequent removal.

2.5 Root canal obturation

Learning objectives

You should

- understand the reasons for obturating root canals
- appreciate that there are many different ways of achieving satisfactory canal obturation.

Obturation has three aims:

- to prevent reinfection of the cleaned canal system from the coronal end
- to prevent percolation of periradicular exudate into the root canal space
- to seal remaining bacteria within the root canal system.

The objective, therefore, is to provide a hermetic (fluid tight) seal in the canal from coronal to apical end. The apical seal is important but, recently, emphasis has also been placed on the need for coronal seal as contamination usually starts coronally, especially from saliva. If the coronal seal of the temporary or final restoration is poor, contamination of the root canal filling may occur eventually leading to failure.

Requirements before root canal filling
The tooth must be assymptomatic, chemomechanical preparation complete and the root canal dry before a root filling is inserted. Any serous exudate from the periapical tissues indicates the presence of inflammation. If there is persistent seepage, calcium hydroxide may be used as a root canal dressing until the next visit. It is advisable to recheck the canal length in situations of persistent seepage as this may frequently result from overinstrumentation and damage to the periapical tissues.

Root canal filling materials

Ideally, a root canal filling material should:

- be easily introduced into the root canal
- not irritate periradicular tissues
- not shrink after insertion
- seal the root canal laterally, apically and coronally
- be impervious to moisture
- be sterile or easily sterilised before insertion
- be bacteriostatic or at least not encourage bacterial growth
- be radio-opaque
- not stain tooth structure or gingival tissues
- be easily removed from the canal as necessary.

Ideally, a sealer should:

- satisfy the above requirements of a root filling material
- provide good adhesion to the canal wall
- have fine powder particles to allow easy mixing or be a two paste system
- set slowly.

Types of root filling material available

Solid and semisolid materials include gutta-percha and silver points. Silver points are not recommended as they do not seal the canal laterally or coronally and may cause tooth or gingival staining.

Sealers and cements include Tubliseal, AH Plus, Pulp Canal Sealer, Roths Sealer, AH 26.

Medicated pastes include N2, Endomethosone, Spad, Kri and are not recommended as they may contain paraformaldehyde, which is cytotoxic.

Gutta-percha filling techniques

Each of the techniques (except where indicated) will produce acceptable clinical results if used correctly. Proponents exist for the different techniques, although personal preference usually determines the final choice:

- single cone (not recommended as it does not seal laterally and coronally)
- lateral condensation
- thermomechanical compaction
- vertical condensation
- thermoplasticised gutta-percha
- carrier-based techniques.

Lateral condensation of gutta-percha

The objective is to fill the canal with gutta-percha points (cones) by condensing them laterally against the sides of the canal walls (Fig. 39a). The technique requires a tapered canal preparation ending in an apical stop at the working length (Box 12).

There are two main types of spreading instrument for condensing gutta-percha: long handled spreaders and finger spreaders. The main advantage of a finger spreader is that it is not possible to exert the high lateral pressure that might occur with long handled spreaders. The chance of a root fracture is reduced and it is therefore a suitable instrument for beginners.

Lateral condensation of warm gutta-percha

A modification to the cold lateral condensation technique is to perform it warm as this will soften the gutta-percha and make it easier to condense, possibly resulting in a denser root filling. The spreader may be

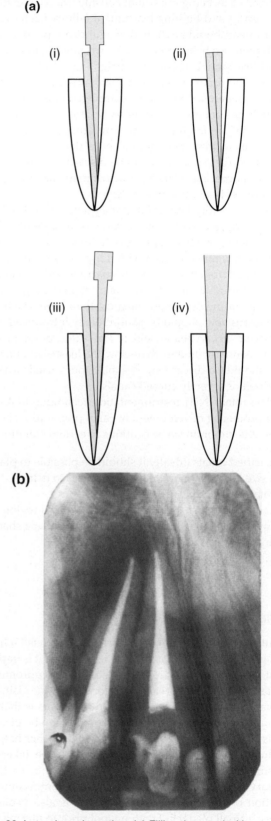

Fig. 39 Lateral condensation. (a) Filling the canal with gutta-percha condensed laterally against the sides of the canal wall (i–iv). (b) A radiograph of two canals filled using this technique.

1. A spreader is selected that reaches to within 1 mm of the working length and the length marked with a rubber stopper.
2. A master point is selected that allows a friction fit in the apical portion of the root canal. When this is marked it is called 'tug back' (like pulling a dart out of a dart board). This may be difficult to achieve with small size gutta-percha points; therefore, it is usual to accept a friction fit in narrow canals. A point one size larger than the master apical file is usually selected. If it is not possible to place the point to working length, select a point that passes to full length and trim 0.5 mm off the end using a scalpel (this has the effect of making the point slightly larger). Retry the point and adjust as necessary.
3. Mark the length of the point by nipping it with tweezers at the reference point and take a check radiograph with the cone in place.
4. Sealer placement. The sealer is mixed according to the manufacturer's instructions and introduced into the canal using a small sterile file rotated anticlockwise (omit this stage if there is a danger of sealer passing through the apical foramen, e.g. open apex). The master cone is then coated with sealer on the apical one-third and is introduced into the root canal slowly to aid coating of the canal walls and reduce the likelihood of sealer passing into the periapical tissues.
5. Once the master cone is seated, place a spreader between it and the canal wall using firm pressure in an apical direction (lateral pressure may bend or break the spreader or fracture the root). This pressure, maintained for 20 seconds, will condense the gutta-percha apically and laterally leaving a space into which an accessory point is placed.
6. An accessory cone the same size or one size smaller than the spreader is used, rotate the spreader slightly, remove it and immediately place the accessory cone. Repeat the procedure until the root canal is filled. The finger spreader condenses each cone into position. The final cone is not condensed as this would leave a spreader tract and contribute to leakage.
7. Cut off the gutta-percha 1 mm below the cementoenamel junction or gingival level (whichever is the more apical) using a hot instrument and vertically condense the gutta-percha. This is important as remaining root-filling material may stain the tooth.
8. If two or more canals are obturated with gutta-percha, undertake one at a time unless they meet in the apical third.
9. Seal the access cavity, remove the rubber dam and take a postoperative radiograph.

heated by placing it in a hot bead sterilizer before insertion into the canal. Alternatively, the friction of ultrasonic vibration may be used to introduce heat into the root filling.

Thermomechanical compaction

In this thermomechanical technique, a compactor that resembles an inverted file is placed in a slow-speed handpiece and used to help to plasticise and condense the gutta-percha. Care must be taken to use this instrument only in the straight part of the canal in order to avoid gouging of the walls. The frictional heat from the compactor plasticises the gutta-percha and the blades drive the softened material into the root canal under pressure.

Lateral condensation and thermocompaction of gutta-percha

A modification of the thermomechanical technique has been described as an adjunct to lateral condensation. Gutta-percha is first laterally condensed in the apical half of the canal, then a compactor is used to plasticise and condense the gutta-percha in the straight coronal half of the canal. The laterally condensed material in the apical half of the canal effectively prevents any apical extrusion and the softened gutta-percha is thus forced against the dentine walls.

Vertical condensation of gutta-percha

Thermal conductivity through gutta-percha occurs over a range of 2–3 mm and it only needs to be raised 3 to 8°C above body temperature (40–45°C) for it to become sufficiently mouldable. The requirements for vertical condensation of warm gutta-percha include a tapered preparation, accurate cone fit apically, suitable sealer, a heat source and a range of prefitted pluggers. Briefly, the technique of vertical condensation involves applying heat to the gutta-percha, condensing it down the root canal from coronal to apical (the downpack) and then filling the remaining space (the backfill).

The original technique of vertical condensation used two main types of instrument, a pointed heat carrier that was warmed in a Bunsen burner and a flat-ended plugger that was used cold to condense the thermoplasticised gutta-percha. The heating of the carrier took 5 to 10 seconds and posed an additional problem in that its temperature started to decrease as soon as it was removed from the flame; consequently, the carriers were heated till they were cherry red hot. Recently, the introduction of electric heat carriers has enabled more control over the length of time the heat is applied (Box 13).

The downpack procedure results in apical corkage, filling of lateral and accessory canals and an empty canal space coronally. Backfilling of the canal is achieved by using thermoplasticised gutta-percha delivered in increments and condensed (see below). Vertical condensation produces excellent results in experienced hands but has the problem of being time consuming.

1. The downpack is commenced by using the heat carrier to sear off the gutta-percha master cone at the canal orifice (Fig. 40).
2. Immediately following this, a cold plugger is introduced to condense around the periphery of the gutta-percha and seal the canal coronally.
3. A sustained push is now applied to the centre of the gutta-percha causing the sealer and warm gutta-percha to follow the path of least resistance down the main canal and along any lateral or accessory canals. This sustained push is termed a wave of condensation.
4. The heat carrier is reapplied 3–4 mm into the gutta-percha and is removed with a small bite of gutta-percha attached.
5. The filling is then condensed as described previously to form a second wave of condensation.
6. This cycle is repeated until 5 mm from the canal terminus, or to the end of the straight part of the canal, and a sustained application of apical pressure applied as the gutta-percha cools.

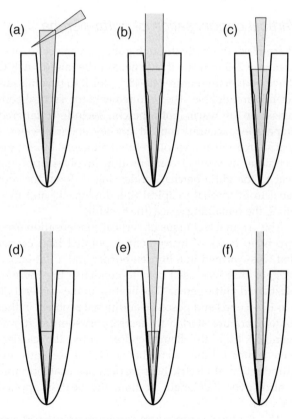

Fig. 40 The vertical condensation technique.

Continuous wave of condensation

A new technique, 'the continuous wave of obturation' has been introduced to further simplify and speed up vertical condensation. This technique uses a new device, the System B, that has four interchangeable soft steel pluggers: fine, fine/medium, medium and medium/large. The pluggers are thermostatically controlled, can be heated to preset temperatures and maintain their temperature while condensing the gutta-percha within the root canal system. The appropriate plugger is selected to match the taper of the master cone, activated and used to condense the gutta-percha to just short of its binding point 5–7 mm from the terminus of the root canal. The heat is then reactivated, the plugger drops to the binding point and is removed together with excess gutta-percha, providing an apical plug of gutta-percha. In this technique, the downpack consists of a continuous rather than several interrupted waves of condensation. Backfilling can be achieved by using the System B with a technique similar to warm lateral condensation or by increments of thermoplasticised gutta-percha.

The philosophy behind vertical condensation has not changed over three decades. The procedure aims to seal the terminus of the canal with an accurate cone fit and to obturate the coronal end once the surplus gutta-percha has been removed. The downpack then forces sealer and gutta-percha along the lines of least resistance (Fig. 41). Significant changes have been made in armamentarium, simplifying the technique and making it more operator friendly. Vertical condensation is, however, a taxing technique, which, together with the expense of the initial purchase of the equipment, probably explains the greater popularity of lateral condensation.

Thermoplasticised gutta-percha

Using the Obtura for the delivery of thermoplasticised gutta-percha is particularly useful for backfilling in

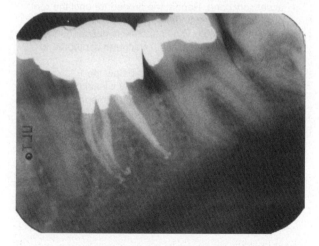

Fig. 41 Radiograph showing how vertical condensation helps obturate complex canal anatomy. Note that the mesial root has three canals with an interconnecting web running between them. The distal root has two canals and an apical bifurcation.

vertical condensation after creating the apical plug. Small increments are placed and condensed in order to keep shrinkage to a minimum. It is also useful in cases of internal resorption where the gutta-percha flows as it is condensed. Care must be taken to ensure that there is adequate apical resistance form to ensure excess gutta-percha is not pushed out of the canal system.

Carrier-based systems

These systems consist of a carrier usually made out of plastic (although originally constructed from stainless steel or titanium) that is supplied with a covering of gutta-percha. The size of the carrier required is checked using a size verification device. The carrier is placed in the oven provided and heated until the gutta-percha is soft. Sealer is placed in the canal, the carrier pushed home to the desired length and excess cut off in the pulp chamber at orifice level. Carrier-based systems produce excellent results in experienced hands but have the disadvantage of a solid central core that can complicate restoration, especially post-placement.

Coronal seal

It is important after completing canal obturation to ensure that there is an adequate coronal seal over the root filling, as coronal leakage has been shown to be an important cause of failure. This can be achieved by placing a layer of bonding resin or glass ionomer over the floor of the pulp chamber and canal orifices.

Overfills

A small amount of cement may be seen apically after obturation especially when using warm gutta-percha techniques. Cement may also be seen opposite large accessory or lateral canals (Fig. 42). It is, therefore, important that a relatively inert sealer is used. Proponents of vertical condensation argue the distinction between overfilling and vertical overextension of underfilled canal systems; that is, filling materials may be overextended or extruded beyond a canal system that has not been sealed internally. Underfilling of a canal system could also indicate that it has not been debrided satisfactorily. In such situations, necrotic pulp tissue, bacteria and their by-products would be expected to lead to failure. Overfilling infers that the whole canal system is obturated but excess material has been placed beyond the confines of the root canal and represents a quite different situation. The aim of vertical condensation is not to produce extrusion of filling material; nevertheless this can occur and histological studies have shown that these overfills do produce an inflam-

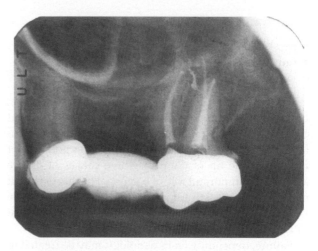

Fig. 42 Radiograph showing excess obturation material opposite a lateral canal.

matory response even though patients do not report discomfort.

2.6 Root canal retreatment

Learning objectives

You should

● appreciate the reasons why root fillings might fail

● understand how to tackle a range of retreatment problems.

Root canal treatment is not always successful, and retreatment of failed treatment is a common procedure reflecting an increasing demand to save teeth. Failure can occur for a number of reasons and it is important that the cause is diagnosed before planning treatment. There may be definite signs and symptoms of failure, such as a discharging sinus, pulpal pain or tenderness on biting. However, in the absence of symptoms, root canal retreatment decisions depend largely on radiographic findings. Retreatment may be indicated when a periradicular radiolucency is found to have appeared (or to be increasing in size) or restorative treatment is proposed that may disturb the status quo. The cause of failure may lie either inside or outside the root canal system.

Intraradicular causes of failure include:

● necrotic material being left in the root canal

● contamination of an initially sterile root canal during treatment

● persistent infection of a root canal after treatment

● loss of coronal seal and reinfection of a disinfected and sealed canal system

● bacteria left in accessory or lateral canals.

Extraradicular causes of failure include:

- persistent periradicular infection
- radicular cysts
- vertical root fractures.

Further causes of failure may be iatrogenic in nature, in particular when post space has been created without consideration being given to the intra- and extraradicular anatomy. This may result in root perforation or root fracture at the tip of the post. These causes of failure indicate the important role of bacteria. For this reason, it is essential that teeth for root canal retreatment can be isolated with rubber dam in order to prevent leakage of saliva and confine hypochlorite irrigation.

Failure, depending on its aetiology, may be treated in one of three ways: root canal retreatment, periradicular surgery or extraction. Extraction is usually indicated for root fractures in single-rooted teeth or in cases of gross caries where the tooth is non-restorable. On occasions, it may be possible to resect a fractured root in multirooted teeth or to perform crown lengthening when gross caries is present in order to make isolation and future restoration possible.

Root canal retreatment is usually considered in preference to surgical intervention despite the latter being a quicker solution, as surgery will only seal over uncleaned canal space, which will eventually leak. Additional problems with a surgical approach include the effects of compromising root length and bone support on prosthetic or periodontal grounds. If it is considered that access to the root canals cannot be gained without risk of compromising the tooth's prognosis, then surgery is indicated.

Retreatment procedures

The aim of root canal retreatment is to eliminate microorganisms that have either survived previous treatment or have re-entered the root canal system. The feasibility of root canal retreatment depends on the operator's ability to gain access to the root canal system and, in particular, the apical third. Careful assessment of the preoperative radiograph should be made with regard to whether or not a post has been used, what type it is, the type of root filling material (paste, gutta-percha, silver point) and potential problems such as curves, perforations or ledges.

In a retreatment procedure, access is usually complicated by the presence of coronal restorations, retentive devices in the root canals and root canal filling materials. The use of additional magnification and lighting is especially useful in retreatment procedures. Loupes and a headlamp will provide good visibility of the pulp chamber floor and canal orifices. Working in the middle and apical thirds of the root canal, however, requires the use of the operating microscope to see clearly.

Coronal access

The quality of the coronal restoration must be considered when gaining access. Where the coronal restoration is satisfactory, it should be retained and access made through it unless an integral post and core is present. Care needs to be taken in bur angulation as the original coronal landmarks may have been lost. Evidence of leakage coronally around the restoration margins usually indicates that it should be removed prior to performing root canal retreatment. This may involve sectioning and removal of crowns or bridges, with careful consideration being given as to the method of temporisation. At the very least any defects should be sealed internally. Removal of the restoration has the advantages of:

- ensuring removal of all caries
- allowing a thorough check to be made for cracks
- providing excellent access for identifying missed canals.

In extensive breakdown, it may be necessary to place a copper band and build up a small core prior to embarking on treatment in order to ensure a seal around the margins of the dam and avoid compromising asepsis.

Radicular access

Removal of restorative materials

It is usual to encounter a core under a coronal restoration in root canal retreatment. This can either be made out of non-tooth-coloured materials, tooth-coloured materials or cast metal. The most common non-tooth-coloured materials include amalgam and cermet cements. These can be removed using surgical length round tungsten carbide burs in the high-speed handpiece, followed by long-neck burs used at slow speed. When the floor of the pulp chamber is approached, ultrasonic tips offer a safer alternative compared with burs for dispersing material remaining over furcal areas and in the orifices of root canals. Tooth-coloured cores offer more of a challenge in removal as they may be more difficult to distinguish from dentine. Careful observation of the dried access cavity floor will usually allow differentiation between the dentine and restorative material. In addition, the texture of the restorative material is rougher than the dentine and this can be detected using an endodontic explorer. The access cavity should be thoroughly evaluated at this stage with regard to its extent and the possibility of discovering missed canals.

Removal of post and cores

Post and core build-ups may be all-in-one castings or may be a combination of preformed posts and plastic core materials. In the latter, the core should be dissected in order to expose the individual posts. In some situations it may not be necessary to remove all the posts, only the ones in the roots being retreated.

The removal of a post should not be attempted if the force to remove it could result in root fracture. Ultrasonic vibration from an appropriate insert may be used initially to try to break the cement seal, the vibrations should be directed in a coronal direction, which necessitates the cutting of a notch on the side of the core. If a specialised tip is not available, then a standard ultrasonic scaler may be used. An additional advantage of ultrasonic vibration is that heat produced from friction may also cause weakening of the lute of resin-bonded posts. It is important not to use ultrasound at high power as this may produce microcracks in the root. In some situations, ultrasonic vibrations may result in the post becoming free within the canal. If ultrasonic vibration is unsuccessful, it is necessary to use a device to pull out the post and core. This can usually be accomplished in anterior teeth using a post extractor.

The fracture of a post within a root canal can pose a major problem and care should be taken to try not to further weaken, fracture or perforate the root. Such situations should first be tackled by troughing around the post to remove the luting cement using a small long-neck bur or an ultrasonic tip. As progress is made up the root canal, then the smaller suborifice tips may be used.

Use of ultrasonic tips will remove many fractured posts without having to resort to additional means such as the Masserann kit. In this system, a suitably sized trepan is directed along the side of the post in the space created by the ultrasonic tips. A smaller trepan may then be used to grip and remove the fractured portion (additional ultrasonic vibration applied to the trepan may be useful at this point). If the post is of the screw-in type then it may be unscrewed after the use of ultrasound to weaken the cement seal, either by placing a groove in its end or grasping it with a tight fitting trepan. If this is unsuccessful, then a trepan should be selected that will cut along the threads of the post as this will minimise the amount of dentine removed while easing cutting of the metal. In exceptional cases, fractured posts may be drilled out using an end-cutting bur, this procedure is rarely necessary in view of the recent developments in ultrasonic tip design.

Access to the apical third

Access to the apical third of the root is usually restricted by the presence of materials used to obturate the canal. Those most frequently used include pastes, gutta-percha and silver points. A thorough evaluation of the access cavity should be performed, modifying it as necessary to give straight-line access to the root canals prior to attempting removal of the filling materials.

Removal of pastes

Soft pastes can usually be easily penetrated using short sharp hand files and copious irrigation. The use of an ultrasonically powered file with accompanying irrigation can be helpful in these situations, especially for removing remnants of paste from root canal walls that may remain despite careful hand instrumentation. Rotary NiTi instruments may also be used to help in removal. Hard pastes can be particularly difficult to remove and usually need to be drilled out with a small long-neck bur or chipped out using an ultrasonic insert, as described above. These procedures can only be used in the straight part of the canal and it is important to use magnification and lighting, as the risk of going off line and perforating is high. Irrigation with EDTA and sodium hypochlorite should be employed, together with frequent drying to ensure good visibility especially deep within the canal (Fig. 43).

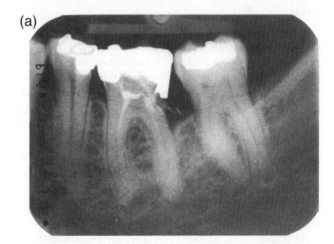

(a)

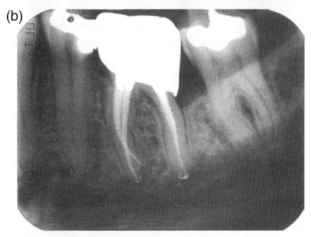

(b)

Fig. 43 Retreatment of a lower molar that had previously been root filled with a paste. (a) There is distal caries and a poor coronal seal. This needs to be rectified prior to embarking on root canal therapy. In this case a copper ring was fitted. (b) The postoperative radiograph shows that a coronal seal has been established by placing an amalcore and full coverage gold crown.

Removal of gutta-percha

Poorly condensed gutta-percha root fillings may be removed by rotating one or two small Hedstrom files around or between the root canal filling points, pulling and removing them intact. If this is unsuccessful, then removal of the root canal filling should be considered in stages, removing first the coronal, followed by the middle and apical thirds. Gates–Glidden drills may be used coronally in the straight part of the canal; these are available in a range of sizes and have a safe cutting tip that reduces the risk of perforation providing too large a size is not used. Care should be taken during their use as if too fast a speed is used then they may inadvertently screw into the canal and cause considerable damage, a suitable speed is around 1000–1500 rpm. Other rotary instruments that may be used for the removal of gutta-percha include those made from NiTi (e.g. Profiles, Quantecs). These instruments are extremely efficient at removing gutta-percha and are used at a higher speed (1000 rpm) than for canal preparation.

If gutta-percha removal is being attempted around a curvature, it is important to use a solvent such as chloroform, oil of cajaput or oil of turpentine to soften the gutta-percha, aid mechanical removal and reduce the chance of transporting the main axis of the canal. Chloroform is the most effective solvent for dissolving gutta-percha. A small drop placed in the canal is all that is required as it only softens the coronal end of the gutta-percha, which is then removed with hand files. The chloroform is replaced frequently as the softened gutta-percha is removed and progress made to the terminus of the canal. Gutta-percha softened with chloroform tends to smear the canal walls and chloroform itself has a potentially toxic effect. An alternative method of removal involves using small files dipped in Hibiscrub and working them gradually along the side of the gutta-percha to lubricate its removal. This method is more time consuming but avoids many of the problems associated with chloroform.

Removal of silver points

The seal of silver point root canal fillings is rarely as good as their radiographic appearance would suggest, and in many cases the seal relies on the cement used. If this washes out then corrosion occurs leading to failure of the root canal filling. The approach to removal depends on whether the point extends and can be seen to extrude within the pulp chamber. In such situations, many silver points can be removed easily by grasping with Steglitz forceps or pin pliers and levering. If the points cannot be removed easily, then ultrasonic vibrations can be applied to the forceps holding the point. If the silver point has been cut off at the canal orifice, then it is usually not possible to grip it. In such situations an ultrasonic tip may be used to cut a trough around the point; care needs to be taken not to touch the point as the silver is much softer than the steel used for the manufacture of the ultrasonic tip and preferential removal of the point will occur. A Masserann extractor can be used to grip the point and remove it once a trough approximately 2 mm deep has been prepared. Sometimes it may be necessary to work an ultrasonic spreader tip down the side of a point placed deep in a root canal. Removal in these situations may be facilitated by placing a Hedstrom file along the side of the point and pressing it into the soft silver in order to help to pull it coronally. Occasionally, it may help to apply ultrasonic vibrations to the Hedstrom file prior to pulling to aid removal.

Removal of separated instruments

The separation (fracture) of root canal instruments is a procedural hazard in root canal therapy. The problem may be kept to a minimum by:

- maintaining a good quality-control programme
- discarding any damaged instruments
- not forcing instruments
- using instruments in correct sequence
- not rotating stainless steel instruments more than a quarter turn clockwise.

The removal of fractured instruments has traditionally been performed using Masserann trepans and extractors together with ultrasonic vibration. New developments in ultrasonic tip designs, the use of magnification and lighting, and, in particular, the operating microscope have simplified instrument removal. Loupes and a headlamp will help in the removal of superficially placed instruments. If working deep within the canal, it is advisable to use the operating microscope, especially if using ultrasound.

It may be possible to bypass a separated instrument that cannot be removed. This becomes more difficult apically as the canal is usually rounder in cross-section in this area. If this is not possible, then the canal should be shaped, irrigated and obturated to the level of the fractured instrument, as in many situations success rate will not be affected.

Frequently, after removal of filling materials or broken instruments, a ledge will be noted in the side of the root canal. This may usually be bypassed by placing a sharp bend at the tip of a small file. The ledge may then be smoothed using a linear filing motion. Shaping and irrigation of the canal system can then be completed prior to canal obturation.

Success rate

The success of root canal retreatment is good (94–98%) when it is being undertaken to achieve a technical improvement in potential failures. When periradicular pathology is present the success rate is much lower (62–78%). Root retreatment itself can bring its own problems: perforation, separated instruments and compromised cleaning and obturation of the canal system. It is important that patients are informed of such factors prior to embarking on this procedure.

2.7 Surgical endodontics

Learning objectives

You should

• understand the indications for surgical intervention

• have an appreciation of what is involved in surgical endodontics.

Conventional orthograde root canal treatment is preferred to surgery if at all possible, even if it is considered that surgery may be necessary. Ideally, surgery should only be performed in situations that are considered hopeless. On occasions, however, retreatment of a tooth may involve the removal/destruction of expensive crown and bridgework. In such situations, a patient may opt for a surgical as opposed to orthograde approach. This should only be undertaken, however, if the patient understands that dismantling of restorations may be necessary in the future, should the surgery fail.

Incision and drainage

It is preferable in cases of acute infection to establish drainage rather than rely on antibiotics alone. Drainage may be established through the root canal. If this is not possible, then consideration should be given to incising any intraoral fluctuant swelling, the objective of the incision being to allow drainage of pus or exudate from within the tissues. Anaesthesia may be obtained by spraying ethyl chloride over the area or infiltrating local anaesthetic solution around but not into the swelling. If there is doubt as to the nature of the swelling, or a sample is required for microbiological testing, then it may be prudent to aspirate the lesion first using a wide-bore needle and syringe.

Cortical trephination

If pus or exudate is entrapped within the alveolar bone, it may be necessary to perform cortical trephination. This procedure is usually only performed if the patient is in severe pain. It involves incising first through the mucosa and mucoperiosteum and then penetrating the cortical plate with a hand or rotary instrument. Once the plate is penetrated, a root canal instrument is directed towards the apex of the tooth to allow drainage. Care needs to be exercised with this technique to ensure that roots are not damaged during the initial penetration.

Periradicular surgery

The main indication for periradicular surgery is when an endodontic treatment is failing and it is not possible to treat the root canal system by conventional means. Such situations include large posts, sclerosed canals and broken instruments. It must be remembered that the main cause of failure is inadequate debridement and bacterial contamination of the root canal system, hence the importance of root canal retreatment whenever possible. A further important indication for periradicular surgery is obtaining tissue for a biopsy.

Assessment

It is important that a thorough assessment is made prior to embarking on surgery. General factors include:

• medical history
• the patient's suitability
• access to the surgical site
• appropriate sensitivity tests on adjacent teeth.

Local factors include the strategic importance of the tooth and root end proximity to anatomical structures such as the maxillary sinus, mental foramen or inferior dental canal. These can be evaluated from angled radiographs, which will also give information on anatomical variations such as root curvatures, proximity of adjacent roots, extra canals and density/thickness of alveolar bone. Careful note should be made of the location of the pathology with regard to whether it is apical or lateral. If the pathology is lateral, it may indicate a lateral canal; these should normally be root retreated unless the resection is going to include that area of the root. Lateral lesions may also indicate a perforated post or root crack; these deserve special consideration. Note should be taken of the crown to root ratio, since periradicular surgery usually involves shortening of the root, which may lead to increased mobility. A thorough periodontal examination is essential, noting probing depth and any periodontal–endodontal communications, with consideration being given to the likely effect of root length reduction on periodontal support.

Procedure

Once appropriate assessment has been made, the procedure can be planned. This includes:

- local anaesthesia
- flap design, elevation and retraction
- bone removal
- identification of root end
- periradicular curettage
- root resection
- haemostasis
- root end preparation and filling
- debridement and closure.

Local anaesthesia

Prior to surgery, the patient should be placed on a chlorhexidine mouthrinse for 24 hours. Anaesthesia is required for patient comfort and to enhance visibility for the operator by controlled haemostasis. Regional anaesthesia is administered as appropriate, followed by multiple local infiltrations around the apex of the tooth. Xylocaine and adrenaline (epinephrine) are to be preferred in view of their superior vasoconstrictive action. Ten minutes should be allowed to elapse prior to incision to allow dispersal of the solution, as further attempts at improving anaesthesia or haemostasis during the procedure are usually only met with limited success. Muscular tissue must be avoided, as this could result in stimulation of β_2-adrenoceptors, causing vasodilatation. It is also appropriate to administer an analgesic such as paracetamol at this stage as this helps to reduce postoperative discomfort.

Flap design, elevation and retraction

A full microperiosteal flap should be considered first, with one (triangular flap) or two (rectangular flap) relieving incisions (Fig. 44a). The relieving incisions should be placed vertically in order to avoid compromising the blood supply of the non-flapped tissue and should avoid bony defects or root eminences. A distal relaxing incision may be used to relieve tension on triangular flaps. The semilunar flap (Fig. 44b) should be avoided as this provides limited access and may result in scarring. In cases where it is not considered appropriate to use a full flap, then a limited submarginal flap may be considered. In such situations 2 mm of attached gingiva must remain apical to the depth of the gingival sulcus and there must be enough tissue remaining to allow suture placement. Such submarginal designs are termed Luebke–Ochsenbein flaps (Fig. 44c).

Incisions for all flaps should be made with an appropriately designed scalpel, Nos 15 or 11 being frequently used. Flap elevation should start at the attached gingiva on the vertical relieving incision, it then progresses laterally (undermining elevation) to prevent damage to the flap margins associated with the cervical areas of the teeth. Once reflected, the flap should be retracted, taking care to keep the retractor on bone so as not to compress or damage the flap. Such damage may lead to excessive postoperative swelling or discomfort.

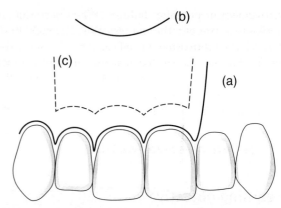

Fig. 44 Flap designs. (a) Triangular flap (a second relieving incision would convert this into a rectangular flap). (b) Semilunar flap. (c) Submarginal Luebke–Ochsenbein flap.

Bone removal

Where there is a large bony defect, loss of the cortical plate may make access to the root tip straightforward. In many instances, a round bur may need to be used to remove bone overlying the root to enable identification. Care must be taken not to damage adjacent roots.

Once access to the root end has been achieved, it is necessary to curette out soft tissue from the defect. Such tissue may be sent for histological examination. Infiltration of additional local anaesthetic may be required to improve haemostasis or anaesthesia at this stage. It is not necessary to remove every last remnant of soft tissue and care should be taken when curetting adjacent to anatomical structures such as the mental foramen or maxillary sinus.

Root end resection

The root end may be resected using a fissure bur, either by grinding it down or sectioning straight through. Care should be taken with the latter, as more may be removed than desired. In general, about 3 mm of root should be removed as this will result in removal of accessory canals forming part of the apical delta. The resection should also go right through the root but care should be taken to avoid adjacent teeth and the bevel should be minimal in order to avoid excessive exposure of dentine tubules.

Haemostasis

It is important that the region around the root be packed in order to provide haemostasis while preparing the retro cavity and placing the root end filling. Many materials may be used including bone wax, Surgiceal, adrenaline (epinephrine)-impregnated cotton wool balls, collagen-based products or calcium sulphate. The choice of material depends upon individual preference, but care must be taken to remove all remnants (except collagen-based products and calcium sulphate, which are resorbable) as, if left, they will act as a foreign body and delay healing. The material is firmly packed around the root end to ensure a dry field and good visibility.

Root end preparation

Historically, root end cavity preparation has been performed with small round or inverted cone burs, either in a straight or a miniature handpiece. It is difficult, however, even with a miniature head to place the cavity preparation in the long axis of the tooth in view of limited access. Frequently, such preparations are placed perpendicular to the resected root end and may appear to be going down the long axis of the tooth but are, in fact, directed palatally occasionally with a palatal perforation.

Recent developments involve the use of ultrasonically activated microtips, which are much smaller (Fig. 45) and allow the preparation to be placed in the long axis of the root. They need to be used at appropriate power settings in order to minimise the risk of root cracking. Several different designs are available, with different angles for easier access to posterior regions of the mouth. In addition, narrow designs are available for running out isthmus areas, which are now considered to be a previously unrecognised reason for failure in multicanaled teeth. Softened gutta-percha is packed down in the root canal and the preparation may be examined using a miniature retro-mirror. Ideally the depth should be 2–3 mm.

Root canal filling materials Amalgam has been used for many years as a first choice retro filling material although it has come under increasing criticism because of its mercury content, soft tissue staining and corrosion. Other materials that have proven success include Super EBA and IRM. Additionally, dentine bonding in the form of glassiononer or composite has been advocated. The multitude of materials used merely shows that all have weaknesses in that they show signs of leakage, hence the importance of thorough canal debridement and obturation. A new material shows great promise; this is mineral trioxide aggregate (MTA) and it is expected to become generally accepted for routine use.

Care needs to be taken when placing the retro filling that the root end is adequately isolated and dried. Materials should be mixed according to the manufacturer's instructions, and care taken to avoid excess material outwith the retro cavity. Ideally, a radiograph should be taken prior to suturing to ensure that the retro preparation and filling are adequate (Fig. 46).

(a)

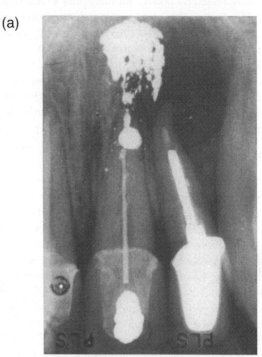

(b)

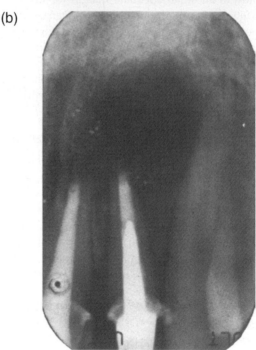

Fig. 46 Root canal filling. (a) An apicected upper central incisor. Note the periradicular area is centrally situated around the lateral incisor, the central has a fractured instrument in situ plus an incompletely debrided or sealed canal. The apex is remaining and there is a large amount of excess amalgam in the periradicular tissues. (b) The postoperative radiograph shows that the teeth have been re-root filled, a new post placed and the surgery repeated with root end super EBA fillings placed.

(a) (b)

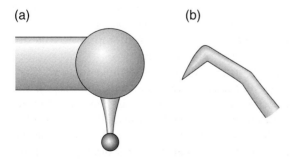

Fig. 45 The relative sizes of (a) the retrograde handpiece and (b) the ultrasonic tip.

Debridement and closure

The surgical area should be thoroughly debrided and the flap compressed for about 3 minutes prior to suturing and 10 to 15 minutes afterwards. In general, simple interrupted size 4–0 sutures will prove adequate for most situations. Suture removal is usually performed 3 to 5 days later.

It is usual for a patient to have some discomfort and swelling postoperatively. This, however, is usually minimal and can be controlled using analgesics. The area can be kept clean by continuing the chlorhexidine mouthwash until suture removal allows improved toothbrush access.

Corrective surgery

Corrective surgery may be required to seal a perforation or resect a root. The position of the perforation is of paramount importance in determining whether it is surgically accessible; parallax radiographs will help to determine the site. Perforations in the apical third of the root may be handled by removal of the apex and sealing the canal with a retro filling. Ideally, perforations resulting from post crowns should have the offending post removed and a new one placed within the root canal. Surgical correction then resembles the placement of a retro filling in the side of the root. If the post is not removed, it must be cut back sufficiently to allow an adequate margin for finishing the retro filling. Many perforations are now managed by internal perforation repair, precluding the need for surgery.

Surgical root resection may be indicated on multi-rooted teeth that have not responded to treatment or have a hopeless periodontal prognosis. Other reasons for root resection include extensive resorption, root fracture or gross caries.

Extraction with subsequent replantation

Extraction with replantation is mentioned purely for completeness. Those experienced in the technique report a high success rate. The procedure involves extracting the tooth as atraumatically as possible, performing conventional root resection and retro filling and then replanting the tooth. This procedure may be indicated when a conventional orthograde or surgical approach is not possible or advisable.

2.8 Restoration of endodontically treated teeth

Learning objectives

You should

- appreciate that posts are not always required
- understand the fundamentals of post design in the restoration of endodontically treated teeth.

Root canal treatment is performed on teeth with varying amounts of remaining tooth structure. If all or nearly all of the coronal tooth substance has been lost, then predictable long-term restoration may be problematic.

Successful restoration relies on creating adequate resistance and retention form. This involves reinforcement and replacement of remaining tooth structure. The aim is to restore the tooth with an aesthetic restoration that is both biologically and mechanically sound. Ideally, the final restoration should surround the remaining coronal tooth structure, creating a reinforcing ferrule effect.

In molar teeth, it is frequently possible to avoid the use of posts by providing an onlay or placing an amal-core. The latter involves removing the coronal 2–3 mm of root filling from the canals and using this together with the pulp chamber to provide retention for the core build up. The restoration of root-filled teeth frequently involves the use of posts.

A vast array of different post types are available. It is essential to retain as much sound tooth structure as possible as this helps in reducing leverage forces in the root and potential fracture. Screw posts are not advocated as they create additional stresses in the root. Current opinion is that posts should fit passively in the canal and only be used if absolutely necessary.

Post choice is influenced by the amount of remaining coronal dentine, root morphology and internal canal anatomy. Post length should approximate to about two-thirds of the root length, ideally with an equal amount of post below and above the alveolar crest. Care should be taken to leave an adequate amount of root canal filling material apically. Ideally this should be 5 mm; however, in short roots this may be reduced to 3.5 mm. Post length ultimately is affected by the length of the available root, the anticipated occlusal forces and the level of periodontal bone support.

The post diameter ideally should not exceed the diameter of the optimally shaped and cleaned canal. A wider post does not mean more retention, with post length being the more important factor.

Conflicting opinion exists as to post taper. Tapered posts are most sympathetic to root anatomy; however, there is considerable evidence that parallel posts are more retentive. It is advised that all cases are assessed individually giving due consideration to the root morphology and canal anatomy.

It is important that the post follows the direction of the main root canal. Failure to achieve this may result in root perforation. It is advisable to consider post hole preparation in two phases: removal of the root filling with a hot instrument or Gates–Glidden drills and then shaping of the post hole as appropriate. One should also be mindful of curvatures, especially in the apical third of the root, and the fact that roots also become narrower as one progresses apically, leaving less margin for error.

Once an adequate core (+/− post) has been placed, the coronal preparation can be finalised. This should aim to provide a minimum 2 mm ferrule effect around the coronal dentine to help to prevent fracture of tooth structure. A summary of some of the key aspects of restoration of endodontically treated teeth is provided in Figure 47.

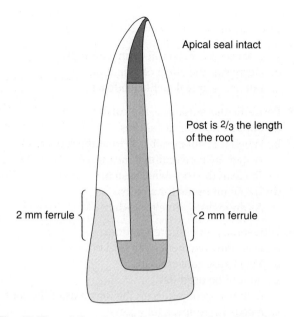

Apical seal intact

Post is 2/3 the length of the root

2 mm ferrule

2 mm ferrule

Fig. 47 The relative dimensions of post and core together with ferrule effect.

Self-assessment: questions

Multiple choice questions

1. The following are important factors in restoring an endodontically treated tooth:
   a. Preserving as much coronal tooth substance as possible
   b. Creating a ferrule effect
   c. Removing all coronal dentine
   d. Providing a wide post
   e. Producing a long post without compromising apical seal

2. Efficiency of irrigation is affected by:
   a. Depth of needle penetration
   b. Coronal pre-enlargement
   c. Frequency of use
   d. Volume and type of irrigant
   e. Temperature of irrigant

3. Major causes of failure in root canal therapy are:
   a. Placing small instruments through the foramen
   b. Presence of bacteria remaining within the root canal
   c. Presence of small amounts of filling material in the periradicular tissues
   d. Presence of necrotic material within the canal system
   e. Loss of coronal seal and reinfection of a cleaned canal system

4. Rotary nickel titanium instruments:
   a. Require a patent canal prior to use
   b. Are used for canal negotiation
   c. Can be used round any curvatures
   d. Are used for canal enlargement
   e. Should be used with a light touch

5. The following are features of irreversible pulpitis:
   a. Response lasts for minutes to hours
   b. Pain may develop spontaneously
   c. Heat may be more significant in the later stages
   d. Pain does not linger after stimulus
   e. All of the above

6. An ideal access cavity should:
   a. Provide unimpeded access to the root canal system
   b. Have convergent walls
   c. Be only large enough to allow files in to canals
   d. Provide straight-line access to each canal orifice
   e. Eliminate the pulp chamber roof in its entirety

7. Coronal pre-enlargement:
   a. Is always necessary
   b. Blocks the canal
   c. Reduces the bacterial count coronally
   d. Decreases the effect of irrigation
   e. Enhances apical tactile feedback

8. Periradicular surgery is indicated:
   a. For all endodontic failures
   b. When it is not possible to treat the root canal system by conventional means
   c. To clean the root canal system
   d. To obtain tissue for a biopsy
   e. As an investigative procedure

9. Ultrasonic root end preparation:
   a. Is an improvement over steel burs
   b. May cause root cracking
   c. Should be used dry
   d. Enables preparation up the long axis of the root
   e. Needs more space for access

10. The following are features of reversible pulpitis:
    a. Pain lingers after application of stimulus
    b. Pain is difficult to localise
    c. Tooth is tender to percussion
    d. Pain does not linger after stimulus is removed
    e. Normal appearance on a radiograph

11. A patency file:
    a. Should be small and flexible
    b. Is used to deliberately enlarge the foramen
    c. Helps to eliminate apical blockage
    d. Should be used vigorously
    e. Is a generally accepted technique

12. Root canal filling materials should:
    a. Be easy to insert into the canal
    b. Absorb moisture
    c. Expand on setting
    d. Be difficult to remove
    e. Not stain the tooth

13. The following are accepted obturation techniques:
    a. Silver points
    b. Laterally condensed gutta-percha
    c. Continuous wave
    d. Carrier devices
    e. Single point gutta-percha

14. Fractured instruments may be avoided by:
    a. Not precurving them
    b. Not sterilising them
    c. Jumping between different sizes of instruments
    d. Discarding damaged instruments
    e. Not forcing instruments

15. Root canal blockage:
    a. May be caused by dentine chips

b. May lead to perforation
c. May be reduced by use of a lubricant
d. Is increased if the coronal two-thirds is prepared first
e. Is avoidable

Picture questions

Picture 1

Figure 48 is a distal angulation view of a lower first molar. What information can you gather from this pre-operative radiograph?

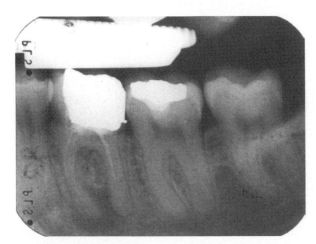

Fig. 48 Lower first molar.

Picture 2

Examine the periapical radiograph of lower left molar (Fig. 49). List four problems with how the periradicular surgery has been performed.

Picture 3

Figure 50 is a periapical radiograph of an upper incisor tooth. What is the radio-opaque object lateral to the root? How would you manage this case?

Picture 4

Figure 51 is a periapical radiograph of the upper central incisor teeth. Examine it and describe what you can see. How would you manage this case?

Short note questions

Write short notes on:

1. reactionary and reparative dentine
2. pulp sensitivity tests
3. cracked tooth syndrome
4. balanced forces
5. the accuracy of electronic apex locators.

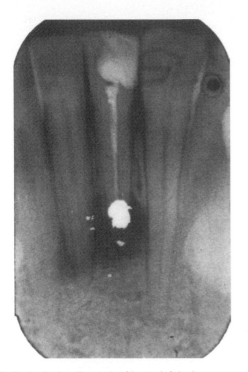

Fig. 49 Periapical radiograph of lower left incisor.

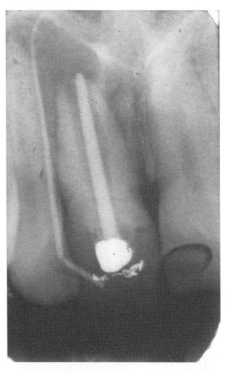

Fig. 50 Periapical radiograph of an upper incisor tooth.

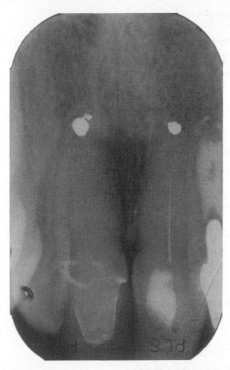

Fig. 51 Periapical radiograph of upper central incisor tooth.

Self-assessment: answers

Multiple choice answers

1. a. **True**. It is essential that sound coronal tooth tissue is retained as this enables the tooth to be restored as strongly as possible (see b, e)
   b. **True**. Retention of coronal dentine allows a collar to be placed around the remaining tooth structure. This ferrule effect strengthens the remaining tooth structure.
   c. **False**. Removing coronal dentine unnecessarily weakens the tooth, makes it more difficult to create a ferrule and produces a shorter post (see e).
   d. **False**. Wide posts weaken roots.
   e. **True**. A long post is more retentive than a short one. Leaving coronal dentine enables a longer post to be provided. It is essential however that the apical seal is not disturbed. After post preparation 3–5 mm of root filling should remain.

2. a. **True**. It is important to get deep needle penetration; this can only be achieved if the canal is large enough. Irrigant solution does not travel much further apically than the needle tip.
   b. **True**. Early radicular access increases the space available for needle penetration and irrigant exchange.
   c. **True**. It is important to refresh irrigating solutions frequently as this removes debris and ensures an active solution.
   d. **True**. A larger volume of irrigant has an increased flushing effect. Sodium hypochlorite has been shown to be more effective than water or local anaesthetic as it will kill bacteria and dissolve pulp remnants.
   e. **True**. Increasing the temperature of irrigating solutions increases their reactivity and makes them more efficient.

3. a. **False**. Small instruments placed through the foramen do not increase the likelihood of failure. It is important, however, not to overenlarge the foramen or cause damage to the periradicular tissues by using large instruments in such a manner.
   b. **True**. Successful endodontics involves removing as many bacteria as possible from the root canal system. The more bacteria that remain the greater the likelihood of failure.
   c. **False**. Small amounts of filling material outside the root cause localised inflammation, which may be detectable histologically; it is not, however, a major contributing factor to failure and does not usually cause clinical symptoms.

   d. **True**. Any necrotic tissue remaining within the canal acts as a continuing irritant.
   e. **True**. Loss of coronal seal allows reinfection of the root canal system and is a major cause of failure.

4. a. **True**. Rotary nickel titanium instruments require a patent canal as they should be used for canal enlargement, not negotiation.
   b. **False**. Using rotary nickel titanium instruments to negotiate canals increases the risk of fracture.
   c. **False**. Rotary nickel titanium instruments may be used around gradual curvatures; however, sharp curves and recurvatures put extra stress on the instruments and can lead to fracture.
   d. **True**. See (a).
   e. **True**. If too much force is used in an attempt to drive a rotary nickel titanium file down a canal there is an increased risk of binding and file fracture.

5. a. **True**. Pain from irreversible pulpitis is long lasting and may be severe.
   b. **True**. Pain may develop spontaneously, while lying down or wake the patient at night.
   c. **True**. Heat frequently becomes a more significant feature in the later stages when in fact cold may act as a relieving factor.
   d. **False**. Pain usually lingers after the stimulus is removed.
   e. **False**. See above.

6. a. **True**. It is important that the access is large enough to allow canal identification and easy placement of instruments.
   b. **False**. The walls should be divergent to enable good visualisation and support of a temporary dressing.
   c. **False**. The access should be large enough to allow unimpeded access of files into canals. This may mean offsetting it to enable straight-line coronal access.
   d. **True**. The file handle should stand upright in the canal when straight-line access has been achieved.
   e. **True**. This allows canal orifices to be identified. Commonly the roof of the pulp chamber is not completely removed over the orifice of the second mesiobuccal canal in upper molars.

7. a. **False**. Pre-enlargement is not necessary in medium to large root canals.
   b. **False**. Debris is produced during pre-enlargement; however, correct use of irrigation and a small file to disturb the dentine chips will prevent blockage.

c. **True**. Pre-enlargement removes dentine coronally that is infected with bacteria.

d. **False**. Pre-enlargement improves irrigation because there is improved access for the needle.

e. **True**. Pre-enlargement removes coronal dentine, which may restrict the passage of a file deeper into the root canal.

8. a. **False**. Root canal retreatment is the preferred option in the majority of cases.

b. **True**. It may not be possible to treat the root canal by conventional means if a very large post is present, the root canal is blocked by a fractured root canal instrument or the apical third anatomy has been destroyed by over-instrumentation.

c. **False**. Periradicular surgery aims to remove the apical 3 mm and clean a further 3 mm of canal system but is no substitute for conventional cleaning and shaping procedures.

d. **True**. The collection of biopsy material at the time of surgery is an important part of the procedure.

e. **True**. Surgery offers the opportunity to look for root fractures or perforations.

9. a. **True**. The introduction of ultrasonic techniques has been a major advancement in endodontic surgery.

b. **True**. Care needs to be taken to use ultrasonic vibration at the lowest effective power. If it is used at too high a power, for long periods or in thin roots, then fracture may occur.

c. **False**. Ultrasonic vibration produces heat. Water spray cools the tip as well as removing debris.

d. **True**. One of the major problems of instrumentation with steel burs was that it was not possible to get the retro-preparation in the long access of the root.

e. **False**. Ultrasonic tips are much smaller than conventional burs and handpieces; therefore, less space is required.

10. a. **False**. Pain from reversible pulpitis is short lasting.

b. **True**. The pulp does not contain proprioceptive receptors; consequently pain is difficult to localise until the inflammation involves the periodontium.

c. **False**. See (b).

d. **True**. See (a).

e. **True**. The inflammation is contained within the tooth; therefore, there are no changes to be seen in the periodontium.

11. a. **True**. Small flexible files help to prevent blockage without overenlarging the foramen.

b. **False**. The purpose of a patency file is to clear the foramen not enlarge it.

c. **True**. This is the main purpose of the patency file.

d. **False**. A patency file should be used with a gentle touch to avoid overenlargement of the foramen.

e. **False**. Many authorities are against passing small files through the foramen as they are concerned about damage to the periradicular tissues.

12. a. **True**. Ease of handling is an important property.

b. **False**. Root canal filling materials should not absorb moisture as this could lead to expansion or contamination.

c. **False**. Expansion on setting could predispose to root fracture.

d. **False**. It is important to be able to remove root filling materials easily for ease of retreatment and post space preparation.

e. **True**. This is important, as staining of tooth structure leads to an unaesthetic appearance for the patient.

13. a. **False**. Silver points do not seal the canal laterally or coronally and may cause staining.

b. **True**. Lateral condensation is a well-recognised technique as it seals the root canal laterally and coronally.

c. **True**. Continuous wave, a relatively new technique, is a simplified version of vertical condensation of gutta-percha and has the potential to seal lateral canals as well as the main canal system.

d. **True**. Such devices have been shown to provide an adequate canal seal. Popular examples include Thermafil and 3D GP.

e. **False**. A single gutta-percha cone will not seal the root canal laterally or coronally.

14. a. **False**. A correctly curved instrument should not have any sharp bends in it; these would increase stress in the instrument. Therefore, it will not predispose the file to fracture.

b. **False**. Sterilising instruments is an essential part of root canal therapy; it does not weaken them.

c. **False**. Jumping between different sizes of instrument is not recommended; they should be used in an ordered sequence.

d. **True**. A good quality-control programme is an essential part of endodontic therapy.

e. **True**. Root canal instruments should never be forced as they can break.

15. a. **True**. Irrigation and recapitulation with a small file will help to reduce blockage as a result of dentine chips.

b. **True**. Attempts to get past a root canal blockage may result in the file going offline and perforating the root.

c. **True**. Lubrication helps to keep debris in solution and emulsifies pulp tissue in vital cases.

d. **False**. Coronal two-thirds enlargement improves irrigation and, therefore, helps reduce the incidence of canal blockage.

e. **True**. Canal blockage is avoidable if sufficient care is take in canal preparation.

Picture answers

Picture 1

Figure 48 shows:

a. The canal system is incompletely debrided and obturated.

b. There are unistrumented mesiolingual and distolingual canals.

c. There is a subtantial periradicular radiolucency.

d. The crown is heavily restored and there is potential for coronal leakage.

Figure 52 shows the tooth postoperatively.

Picture 2

Four out of the following could be given:

a. The surgery has been performed on a tooth with an incompletely debrided and poorly obturated root canal system.

b. The bevel is steep; this resulted in failure to completely resect through the root.

c. This has not allowed for inspection for extra canals, e.g. lingual in this case.

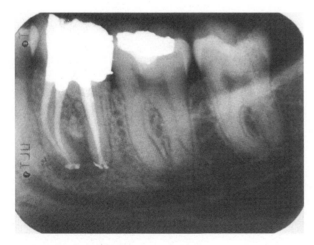

Fig. 52 Lower first molar postoperatively.

d. The root apex remains.

e. The retrograde preparation and root end filling have not been placed down the long axis of the tooth.

Picture 3

The radio-opaque object lateral to the root is a gutta-percha point that has been used to explore a sinus tract. The tooth has an open apex and requires calcium hydroxide therapy prior to obturation following barrier formation.

Picture 4

A fractured root canal instrument and two apical amalgam seals can be seen. Orthograde root canal therapy should be performed, with removal of the fractured instrument, canal cleaning and obturation up to the apical amalgam seals. Successful achievement of these goals should ensure repeat surgery is not required.

Short note answers

1. Reactionary and reparative dentine are both types of tertiary dentine, as distinct from physiological secondary dentine. Reactionary dentine is a response to a mild noxious stimulus; reparative dentine is deposited directly beneath the path of the injured dentinal tubules as a response to strong noxious stimuli.

2. Pulp sensitivity tests can be divided into thermal and electrical. Their purpose is to identify the offending tooth, although it is usual to start with a tooth expected to respond within normal limits in order to establish a baseline. Thermal tests are usually the most useful as they give an indication as to whether the pulp is alive and how healthy it is. Cold tests include ethyl chloride spray on a cotton pledget, ice or dry ice; hot tests include hot gutta-percha or hot water. Electric pulp tests are less useful as, although they provide an indication as to whether there is vital nerve tissue in the tooth, they do not give an indication of different levels of degeneration.

3. Cracked tooth syndrome is an increasingly common clinical problem and can be very difficult to diagnose in its early stages. Pain is usually short lasting but can be very sharp, especially on release of the biting pressure. A plastic bite stick (tooth sleuth) may be used over individual cusps in an effort to find the offending one. Lower second molars and upper premolars are frequently affected. Extensively cracked teeth require extraction; if the crack is less severe then extracoronal restoration may prevent further progression.

4. Balanced forces is a method instrument rotation introduced by Roane in 1985. The initial technique involved rotating the instrument 90° clockwise to set the flutes and then rotating in 180° anticlockwise while maintaining apical pressure to cut dentine. It is efficient and has been shown to maintain a central canal position even around moderate curvatures. It is usual nowadays to use a slightly less aggressive technique, which involves a 60° clockwise rotation and 120° anticlockwise rotation with the apical pressure being just sufficient to prevent the instrument backing out of the canal.

5. Electronic apex locators are used to help to determine canal length. They are accurate about 85% of the time; however, canal length should be confirmed with a radiograph. Problems can occur with the accuracy of electronic apex locators if the canal is very wet and there is fluid in the pulp chamber. These may lead to short circuiting with files in other canals or to metallic restorations. Further problems may be encountered if the file size does not closely resemble the width of the root canal.

Overview

This chapter reviews current methods for the repair and replacement of teeth using fixed restorations. These contemporary techniques have evolved more or less simultaneously with developments in dental materials. The selection, properties, advantages and disadvantages of various materials are discussed

3.1 Examination, diagnosis and treatment planning

Learning objectives

You should

- be able to record an accurate history from your patient and carry out a detailed clinical examination

- understand the basic physical and chemical properties of enamel and dentine that are relevant to the preparation of teeth for restoration

- understand the aetiology of dental caries and know how the early lesions might progress to sites of cavitation

- be able to examine a dentition to detect caries both clinically and radiographically

- be familiar with the aetiology of tooth wear and know the basic principles of management.

Examination of patients with a view to carrying out conservative procedures should follow the general principles for dental examination and history taking. (Table 4). An accurate record should be kept.

Relevant anatomy

Enamel

Enamel provides a hard durable outer coating of teeth. It is an important element in defining aesthetics of the dentition because of its opalescent/translucent qualities. Its highly crystalline structure (95–98% inorganic component by mass), while conferring important aesthetic qualities to the tooth, makes enamel particularly prone to acid demineralisation, both from caries and erosion. It is also brittle and liable to fracture, especially if unsupported by the more elastic dentine.

The inorganic component comprises 86–95% hydroxyapatite by volume. The organic component comprises 1–2%, while water contributes 4–12%. The rods and prisms are the main structural units of the material and are generally orientated at 90° to the external surface. Consequently, finishing of cavity margins and the interface with restorations should aim to provide maximum strength for the restorations and the supporting tooth structure.

Dentine

Dentine comprises 45–50% inorganic hydroxyapatite crystals, with 30% organic matrix and 25% water. Its shade varies through various hues of yellow and it is vital, elastic and permeable. As a result, it is not possible for any restorative material to provide a completely hermetic seal between itself and the cavity wall.

Dentine consists of:

intertubular dentine: the primary structural component, comprising hydroxyapatite embedded in a collagen matrix
peritubular dentine: which provides a collagen-free hypermineralised tubular wall
dentinal tubules: filled with extended processes of odontoblasts, which form the interface between the dentine and the pulp.

Table 4 Patient examination

Patient description of complaint	
Location	Site in oral cavity, referral to other sites
Type and severity (of pain)	Sharp, dull, aching types of pain
Precipitating and relieving factors	Thermal stimuli, biting
Duration	Constant/intermittent
Effect on function	Keeps awake, affects chewing
Dental history	Indication of any recent treatment
	Frequency of attendance
	Concerns about dental treatment
Medical history	All systems: noting relevant factors to planned examination, investigations and provision of treatment
Clinical examination	
Extraoral	Facial asymmetry, swellings, nodes, signs and symptoms associated with the temporomandibular joints
Intraoral	Soft tissues: white patches, ulcers, dryness, swellings, sinuses
	Periodontium: gingival appearance, plaque/calculus deposits, periodontal pocketing, recession, mobility, drifting
Dental hard tissues	
Caries assessment	Clinical diagnosis following visual, tactile, radiographic examinations
Existing restorations	Marginal integrity: evidence of creep, ditching or deterioration of the margin of the restoration indicating increased likelihood of microleakage
	Structural integrity: evidence of fracture or deterioration of the restoration
	Relationship to periodontium and periodontal health: supra-or subgingival margin, surface finish, marginal integrity/interface with tooth, e.g. overhangs, deficient margins
	Anatomy of occlusal form: correct morphology for mastication, prevention of food trapping (marginal ridges), prevention of tipping or overeruption of teeth, provision of centric contacts with opposing teeth
	Anatomy of interproximal form: prevention of food trapping, plaque accumulation, periodontal considerations
	Caries: recurrent caries related to loss of marginal integrity, leakage, failure of the restoration
	Aesthetics: satisfactory form, colour, shape
Tooth wear	Erosion: intrinsic or extrinsic causes
	Attrition: tooth-to-tooth contact, e.g. from parafunctional habits
	Abrasion: commonly caused by tooth brushing
Periodontal and prosthodontic considerations	Aesthetics, occlusion
Diagnostic tests	Radiographs, pulp vitality
Adjunctive assessments	Study models, diagnostic wax-ups, occlusal analysis

Dentinal vitality and its pathological derivative, hypersensitivity, have been hypothesised to arise from capillary action, differential thermal expansion or diffusion. No specific nerve endings lie within tubules; therefore, the ability of dentine to react to thermal stimuli is related to hydrodynamic fluid movement by which a thermal gradient results in fluid flow within the tubules (either into or out of the tooth substance) and this leads to a reaction of the tooth to this stimulus.

As a vital tissue, dentine continues to be deposited throughout life as secondary dentine, although at a slower rate than primary dentine. Deposition of secondary dentine may result from chronic low-grade trauma such as attrition, erosion, abrasion, slowly progressive caries and tooth preparation. It is then known as reparative dentine.

Dental caries

Caries can be defined as progressive dissolution of the inorganic component of dental hard tissues mediated by dental plaque. The acidic demineralisation leads to cavitation and bacterial invasion, with progressive demineralisation. A pH level of less than 5.5 is required for demineralisation to occur.

It is possible for remineralisation to occur at neutral pH. This is achieved by the buffering capacity of both saliva and plaque with calcium and phosphate ions available at the tooth surface. The equilibrium between remineralisation and demineralisation depends upon the composition and thickness of the plaque, the frequency and character of sugar intake and the composition and flow rate of saliva. Fluoride also has a modifying effect.

Aetiology and modifying factors

Bacteria
Specific bacterial species are identifiable as being involved in caries development, including *Streptococcus* spp. especially *S. mutans* (particularly implicated in root caries) and lactobacilli. This involvement has been confirmed by gnotobiotic studies, effectiveness of antibiotics and in vitro studies of enamel demineralisation by oral bacteria.

Diet
Bacteria require a source of dietary carbohydrates, the frequency of consumption being more important than the quantity. Increased frequency leads to increased periods of pH reduction (Stephen curve) and demineralisation. Adherence of plaque is also important, with sticky carbohydrate producing particularly tenacious deposits.

Saliva
Saliva has a protective effect as a result of its buffering capacity and the presence of free calcium and phosphate ions.

Development and progression

Caries can develop (Fig. 53):

- in *pits and fissures*, where it has a small site of origin with wide base (inverted 'V')
- on *smooth coronal surfaces*, where it has a wide area of origin ('V' shaped with apex towards pulp and on root surfaces)
- as a *diffuse lesion* when it originates in dentine.

Early enamel caries is subsurface: a 'white spot' with an intact surface with demineralisation occurring at a deeper level. The very early lesion progresses from *shadowing* to *white spot* to *brown spot* and surface breakdown, with resultant *cavitation*.

Dentine caries progresses more rapidly because of the decreased resistance of dentine to acid dissolution.

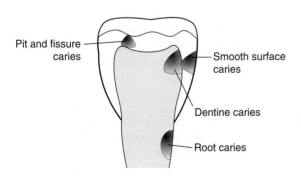

Fig. 53 Development and progression of caries.

Clinical diagnosis of caries

Diagnosis can be:

visual: transillumination with an appropriate light intensity light source can be particularly helpful, showing shadowing of the carious lesion; the tooth should be dry and clean with good illumination
tactile: sticky to sharp probe
radiographic: best for interproximal caries, but the accuracy of bitewings in diagnosis is only 40–60%.

Caries management

Management varies with the stage of progression. A preventive approach is indicated for early white spot, with fluoride application and dietary analysis. A cavitated lesion will require restoration.

Tooth wear
Aetiology

The terminology used for the various types of tooth wear is specific to the aetiology.

Erosion
Tooth wear resulting from the effect of acids is known as erosion. Erosion may be exaggerated by reduction/cessation of salivary flow. This can be idiopathic, age-related, associated with medications or following local radiotherapy.

Intrinsic acids include gastric acid reflux from gastric/peptic ulceration, hiatus hernia, chronic dyspepsia, recurrent vomiting, anorexia/bulimia nervosa.

Extrinsic acids are dietary mainly from carbonated drinks, citrus fruit, fruit juices, pickles. They are also an occupational hazard, for example for those working with manufacture of batteries.

Attrition
Attrition is tooth wear from tooth–tooth or tooth–restoration contact. It can commonly result from parafunctional habits such as bruxism or clenching.

Tooth substance opposing porcelain (particularly unglazed) may exhibit significant rates of wear.

Reduction of posterior support through tooth loss may lead to a rapid degree of wear of the remaining teeth.

Abrasion
Abrasion is tooth wear from extrinsic sources, for example tooth brushing (especially cervically in areas of gingival recession) and 'occupational' for those working in a dusty environment with inadequate protection.

Diagnosis

Diagnosis is achieved by clinical observation and history.

Management

The first stage in management of tooth wear is to identify the aetiology and, where possible, modify or preferably eliminate the causative factor(s). This may involve education of the patient and provision of:

- dietary counselling
- oral hygiene advice
- general medical and occasionally psychiatric advice and treatment (eating disorders).

Thereafter, intervention is governed by the extent of the damage sustained by the dentition. Simple maintenance and monitoring are often the best policy where limited damage has occurred and may include:

- provision of protective appliances (soft vinyl or hard acrylic mouth guards)
- adhesive restorations applied to the worn surfaces
- topical fluoride application and oral hygiene instruction
- use of accurate study models for regular comparison of tooth wear.

Active treatment requires careful planning, looking at all aspects of the dentition and its prognosis. It may involve:

- conventional or adhesive intracoronal restorations
- extracoronal restorations, ranging from veneers/shims to full coverage crown and bridgework (see relevant sections below).

3.2 Conventional intracoronal restorations

Learning objectives

You should

- be familiar with the historical classification of carious lesions
- understand the basic strategies behind the preparation of cavities.

The destruction of tooth substance by caries or other factors requires restoration of lost tooth substance. This usually necessitates preparation of a cavity within that tooth to support and retain the chosen restorative material.

Cavity preparation requires the instrumentation of a tooth to remove caries or any other congenital or acquired defects to allow placement of an appropriate restorative material that will re-establish form, function and/or aesthetics.

Black's classification

G. V. Black classified carious lesions by location. As restorations essentially conform to caries location, the cavities that require to be prepared are similarly classified.

Class I	pit and fissure caries: mainly occlusal of molars or premolars, although may be buccal or palatal fissures
Class II	proximal surfaces of molars or premolars
Class III	proximal surfaces of incisors or canines
Class IV	proximal surfaces of incisors or canines extending to incisal edge
Class V	cervical cavity
Class VI	an addition to the original classification: occlusal or incisal cusp tip wear.

Indications for restoration

- treatment of caries
- replacement/repair of an existing restoration
- repair of a fractured tooth
- restoration of form/function/aesthetics (e.g. of a congenitally affected tooth)
- as part of other restorative needs (e.g. in preparation for removable prosthodontics).

Objectives and stages of cavity preparation

Access

Access should be sufficient to allow adequate visualisation of caries and to allow complete removal. It should also aim to retain as much sound tooth substance as is compatible with this objective. The old concept of 'extension for prevention' is now regarded as undesirable, as restoration margins are not 'self-cleansing'.

Caries removal

All stained and softened tooth substance should be regarded as carious. Stained and firm tooth substance requires careful evaluation before removal. Staining at the amelodentinal junction should be removed wherever possible. The pulp should be protected when the caries is deep.

Removal of unsupported enamel

As previously suggested, enamel is brittle and if unsupported by dentine will have a high risk of fracture under functional loading, with probable failure of the associated restoration.

Outline form

Margins should be placed in areas accessible for cleaning and maintenance and at a position on the tooth where functional loading will not adversely affect the restoration/tooth interface. Outline form should be compatible with the chosen restorative materials' properties.

To provide adequate resistance/retention form

Resistance form is defined as an aspect of cavity design whereby both the restoration and tooth should, upon completion of the restoration, be able to withstand functional forces.

Retention form results from opposing cavity walls being parallel or slightly convergent to 'resist' any forces that will tend to dislodge the restoration from the cavity.

Dentine pins Where adequate mechanical retention cannot be achieved by cavity design, particularly where a cusp has been lost, auxiliary retentive elements are required. The most common type is the dentine pin. This may be friction grip (manually placed), cemented or self-threading. The last is the most common in present day usage and utilises a slightly undersized predrilled hole in the dentine, prepared to a depth of approximately 2 mm. Care in placement is required to avoid encroachment on the pulp, periodontal ligament and the enamel–dentine junction. A preliminary depression should be prepared in the dentine using a medium round latch grip bur, just within the enamel–dentine junction. This prevents travel of the twist drill across the dentine surface during preparation. The smallest size of pin should be used whenever possible.

Care should also be taken to place the pin where it will not encroach upon the occlusion. Although it is possible to bend most pins (commonly made in stainless steel and occasionally now in titanium) or to reduce them in height following placement, this should be avoided where possible to prevent stress distribution. It is acknowledged that dentine pins reduce amalgam's tensile and compressive strengths and they should only be used to augment retention of a restoration that might not survive without such auxiliary retention. A minimum number of pins should be used to achieve this objective. A rule of thumb is to use one pin to replace each missing cusp.

Preventive resin restorations

Recent developments in dental materials (particularly adhesive techniques) have led cavity design away from the very prescriptive form originally described by Black, which often led to removal of excessive amounts of sound tooth substance.

Techniques have been developed whereby cavity preparation is employed only for caries removal. Replacement of the lost, diseased tooth substance is with a resin-based restorative material (often bonded to the tooth tissue) together with sealing of any sites deemed to be more caries-prone (such as pits and fissures) with a related resin-based material.

While the theory behind placing such restorations is sound, 'tunnel preparations', advocated for treatment of interproximal caries with preservation of the marginal ridge, are technically very demanding. They do not allow good visualisation for adequate caries removal and the subsequent sealing of the interface between tooth and restoration. They should, therefore, be used with caution.

3.3 Adhesive dentistry

Learning objectives

You should

- know the biological principles behind bonding materials to tooth tissue

- know the limitations of adhesive dentistry

- know the technical stages for bonding to enamel and dentine.

Adhesion or bonding of materials to enamel and/or dentine requires an intimate link between the restorative material and the tooth substance, with adequate 'surface wetting' to decrease surface tension. Bonding may occur by:

- weak physical electrostatic attraction (van der Waal forces)
- chemical bonding, with interatomic bonds developing across the tooth/restoration interface
- mechanical bonding, with development of irregularities allowing undercuts to be filled with a suitable bonding agent providing 'micromechanical retention'; this is the most common mechanism, with perhaps a small contribution from the weak electrostatic forces.

The quality of bonding may depend upon:

- the materials being bonded and their properties
- the functional loads applied to the tooth and the restoration
- moisture or other contaminants
- the effects of repeated thermocycling.

Other factors affecting bonding include salivary pellicle and the 'smear layer' formed following instrumentation. The smear layer is defined as any debris, calcific in nature, that is produced by reduction or instrumentation of dentine, enamel or cementum.

Indications

Adhesive restorative techniques may be used for:

- restoration of carious cavities
- aesthetic correction of dental anomalies (e.g. shape, position, dimension, shade)
- bonding of ceramic or metal to tooth substance
- cementation of crowns or bridges
- splinting
- repair of fractured restorations.

Advantages

Use of adhesives has a number of advantages:

- less-invasive tooth preparation because of the reduced need for mechanical retention or stabilisation of the restoration
- reduction in microleakage
- possible better stress transmission to tooth substance
- improved aesthetic treatment options.

Biology of bonding

Enamel bonding

Bonding to enamel is principally micromechanical. Use of mild acids such as phosphoric acid (30–40%) results in dissolution and removal of approximately 10 μm of the surface organic component of enamel and leaves a microporous layer of 5–50 μm. The pitted surface enables an unfilled resin bonding agent (usually a low viscosity bis-GMA acrylic (bisphenol-α-glycidyl methacrylate) resin) to flow into the pits and form resin tags, which then provide micromechanical retention. The tags are either 'macro-tags' between the prism peripheries or 'micro-tags' formed at the core of prisms in the individual crypts of dissolved hydroxyapatite crystals. The latter contribute most of the bond strength. The bonding resin is then chemically bonded to a filled acrylic resin restorative material.

The etching effect of the acid is dependent upon:

- the acid used and its concentration
- the vehicle for the application (liquid, gel); gel is preferred
- the times allowed for etching and rinsing: etch for 15–60 seconds (time depends on the acid used)
- the method of activation (rubbing, agitation): agitation preferred
- the enamel structure, anatomy and previous instrumentation.

Dentine bonding or conditioning

The higher organic component of the smear layer means that it must be removed and hydrophilic monomers (such as 2-hydroxyethylmethacrylate (HEMA)) are required.

Dentine remains 'wet' as a result of a persistent fluid exudate from the dentinal tubules that have been cut during instrumentation. Also, dentine tends to vary in its composition, with areas of sclerosis and hypermineralisation.

The aim of dentine conditioning is to demineralise the surface dentine gently and dissolve or modify the smear layer to expose a microporous scaffold of collagen fibrils. These tend to collapse without the support of the inorganic component.

The depth of demineralisation depends on several factors:

- the acid used
- concentration and application time
- other components of the etchant.

Techniques for enamel and dentine bonding

Acid etching of enamel should be carried out using a 30–40% solution of phosphoric acid in a gel form, which is applied for no less than 15 seconds. The enamel is then washed for 10–20 seconds. Excessive exposure to more concentrated solutions for increased periods of time results in poorer bond strengths as the critical 'tag' structure is lost and a precipitate of monocalcium phosphate monohydrate forms.

The use of a drying agent is sometimes suggested to remove more water from the etched pattern to improve resin penetration. Most primers tend to consist of a hydrophilic monomer dissolved in an organic solvent such as acetone or ethanol. This leads to displacement of water from the dentine surface, allowing improved infiltration of the monomer into the collagen network.

Dentine conditioning may be carried out using a range of acids for varying periods of time, but it always should avoid extreme demineralisation of the dentine. The acids used include 10–40% phosphoric acid, 2.5% nitric acid, 10% citric or maleic acids and 1.6–3.5% oxalic acid.

Total etch technique

The total etch technique involves using one of the above acids to achieve etching of enamel simultaneously with conditioning of dentine. Desiccation of the dentine surface is undesirable, with slight dampness allowing hydrophilic materials to bond more successfully.

Self-etching acidic monomer primers or 'condiprimers' have been developed that form a continuum between the tooth surface and the adhesive material by simultaneous demineralisation and resin penetration with monomers. These can be 'air dispersed' (but not rinsed) and polymerised by light activation in situ.

Bonding resins are used to link the resin primer to the restorative material. They are usually hydrophobic

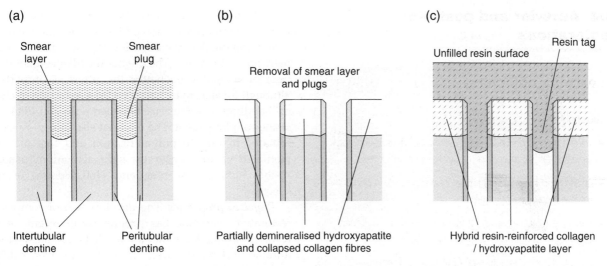

Fig. 54 Dentine conditioning and adhesion. (a) Freshly cut dentine surface. (b) Conditioned dentine. (c) With bonding agent applied.

monomers based on the bis-GMA molecule or more hydrophilic monomers such as TEG, DMA and HEMA. The resins act to stabilise the hybrid layer and form resin extension tags into tubules, providing retention (Fig. 54). They may be light or chemically cured. The light-cured types require the bonding agent to be applied before the restorative resin to avoid its displacement or inadequate curing through insufficient light intensity reaching the material. As a result of oxygen inhibition of curing, the most superficial 15 μm will remain uncured, but it still offers sufficient double MMA bonds for co-polymerisation of the adhesive resin to the restorative resin. Brush thinning of the material is preferred to air thinning to maintain sufficient film thickness to prevent the air-inhibited layer permeating the resin.

Bonding to ceramics

Bonding to ceramics is achieved by use of both micromechanical and chemical bonding. Porcelain requires to be etched with hydrofluoric acid, while glass-ceramics require ammonium bifluoride. Both these chemicals result in expansion of the ceramic surface area by creation of microporosity. This allows a flow of resin into the ceramic surface to provide tags, forming micromechanical retention similar to that with tooth substance.

Additionally, chemical 'silane' bonding acts by use of a bifunctional coupling agent that chemically links to both the ceramic and to the adhesive resin. Bonding agents have undergone significant development since their introduction and are often viewed as having evolved through several 'generations' (Table 5).

Table 5 Generations of bonding agents used in restorative dentistry

	Suggested mode of action	Product examples	Reasons for failure
1st generation	Bifunctional organic monomer with reactive groups reacting with calcium, hydroxyapatite or collagen	Cervident	Poor bond strength; hydrolytic breakdown
2nd generation	Phosphorus esters of methacrylate derivatives	Clearfil Bond	Poor hydrolytic stability
		Scotchbond	The primary bond was to the smear layer, preventing formation of strong resin–dentine bonds
3rd generation	Used total etch concept: removal/modification of the smear layer. Used a separate conditioner acid. Most used a 4-META molecule with hydrophobic/hydrophilic groups	C&B Metabond, Superbond Gluma	Questionable long-term hydrolytic stability
4th generation	Acidic primers with no separate conditioner, thereby reducing the number of steps. Applied by 'rubbing in' and air drying, curing and then applying bond and cure	Scotchbond 2, Optibond	

3.4 Anterior and posterior restorations

Learning objectives

You should

- understand how the developments in adhesive technology have influenced the design of cavities in anterior teeth

- understand the principles of cavity design and, in particular, the finishing of cavity margins

- know the advantages and disadvantages of the materials used to restore anterior and posterior teeth

- be able to make an informed choice of the most appropriate material for each clinical situation

- understand the principles behind the construction of indirect posterior restorations

- know the clinical indications and materials for indirect posterior restorations.

Cavity design in anterior teeth

The design of cavities for anterior tooth restoration should be governed by the extent of caries, as adhesive technology has, in most cases, superseded the need for incorporation of retentive elements such as grooves or slots. This allows retention of the maximum amount of tooth substance and, therefore, retains strength and aesthetics of the restored tooth.

Caries removal remains a priority especially at the amelo-dentinal junction. The use of a lining material that is compatible with the final restorative material (i.e. not a liner based on zinc oxide/eugenol with composite materials) is necessary in deeper cavities. Calcium hydroxide bases (Life, Dycal) are useful, although recent innovations in light-cured glass ionomer and *compomer* (combined glass ionomer and composite resin materials) also provide a satsifactory lining and often a better seal with the tooth substance because of their adhesive nature.

Materials for anterior teeth

Composite

Composite remains the most common material used for tooth-coloured, anterior, directly placed restorations. The material is based on a polymer resin matrix with filler particles. Most are based on the bis-GMA resin developed by Bowen in 1962. Filler particles are usually a type of glass (barium glass) or silicon dioxide. They provide improved translucency, alter (reduce) the coefficient of thermal expansion and make the material more wear resistant, dense and harder. They also reduce polymerisation shrinkage. The greater the filler content (volume or weight), the better the physical properties, although this has to be balanced by a reduction in clinical handling. The interface between resin and filler is a silane coupling agent. The material also incorporates an initiator to initiate polymerisation and this may be mediated chemically or by light activation (usually visible light at the blue end (460–480 nm) of the spectrum).

Physical properties The development of composite restorative materials has progressed in recent years, resulting in materials that are aesthetically satisfactory, durable and handle well. They do, however, exhibit a number of properties that are undesirable. Polymerisation shrinkage can lead to a reduction in volume of up to 7% and cause contraction forces of 4–7 MPa. This can cause cracking or flexure of tooth substance. It can also lead to gap formation between the tooth and the restoration, causing microleakage, recurrent caries and sensitivity. Incremental placement and curing of the restoration has been recommended to minimise this problem.

The coefficient of thermal expansion of composites is two to six times higher than that of the tooth; as a result, thermocycling, as occurs during normal consumption of hot and cold foods and drinks, results in microleakage and loss of adhesion between the tooth and restoration.

The ratio of filler particles in composites varies with the materials, being defined as microfilled or hybrid resins.

Microfilled resin composites incorporate submicron inorganic filler particles, usually averaging 0.04 μm, and increase the viscosity of the material. The incorporation of greater amounts of filler particles in this way reduces polymerisation shrinkage and improves the surface finish. This allows high polishability, allowing the restorations to be used for maximum aesthetics. Microfilled resins are not as strong as other composites.

Hybrid resin composites contain a mixture of submicron (0.04 μm) and small particle (1–4 μm) fillers. These allow the maximum filler loading and, therefore, improved physical properties.

Glass ionomer

Glass ionomer materials tend to be used anteriorly in cervical (class V) restorations because of their caries-inhibiting properties. They were first developed in the 1970s and have since undergone significant modifications. They have traditionally contained fluoroaluminosilicate glass (previously found in the silicate cements) but are less soluble than the cements as a result of incorporation of carboxylic and phosphoric acids. The glass has high levels of fluoride, aluminium and also calcium, sodium and silica. The liquid component is a polyacrylic acid. The setting occurs by the acid attacking the surface of the glass, forming a gel layer, with resultant cross-linking as the material sets. The leaching of fluoride is suggested to contribute to their caries-inhibitory property. Glass ionomers are mildly adhesive to tooth substance. They have a similar coefficient of thermal expansion to tooth and minimal setting contraction; they are therefore, reported to give good marginal seal and reduced microleakage.

Handling of glass ionomers is difficult as they have short working and long setting times, and they are particularly susceptible to moisture contamination or drying early in the setting process. Moisture contamination leads to surface disruption, while desiccation causes shrinkage and crazing. It is, therefore, essential to cover the material immediately after insertion with a varnish or resin to protect the material during early setting.

More recent innovations have seen glass ionomers being combined with acrylic resin materials, sometimes known as compomers. These allow the materials to be light cured although they tend in fact to be dual cured. They are generally easier to handle than conventional glass ionomers and have a longer and more controllable working time as a result of the light curing, which also contributes to a more rapid hardening with increased compressive, flexural and tensile strengths, fracture toughness and wear resistance. The incorporation of composites also has improved the aesthetics of the materials. They, therefore, have the benefits of both composite and glass ionomers. Some examples of recently available materials are included in Table 6.

Direct posterior restorations

Cavity design in posterior teeth

Cavities in posterior teeth conform to Black's classification I, II, V and VI. As with anterior direct restorations, cavity form should now be governed by the extent of the caries and the material to be used. Cavity preparation should, therefore, be as conservative as possible. Where direct posterior composite materials are used, the question of bevel placement remains controversial. Where enamel is available, the bevel will provide more area for acid etching and

bonding. Additionally, the bevelling will result in exposure of transversely cut enamel rods. This results in a significantly stronger bond being created. However, the bevelling results also in formation of very thin sections of composite that are vulnerable to occlusal stress.

The placement of bevels is more appropriate at some sites of a cavity than others. A bevel of less than 1 mm on the buccal or lingual cavo–surface margin of a box improves retention and bonding and allows margins to be more accessible for finishing. Placement of a bevel at the gingival margin of the box is more technically demanding and there may also be limited enamel remaining. The gingival margin, therefore, should only be bevelled when it is well above the amelocemental junction. Occlusally, placement of bevels should be avoided at points on the surface where occlusal stops may be present.

Materials for posterior teeth

Materials for direct restoration of posterior teeth need to be strong and durable because of the forces applied to them during normal masticatory function.

Amalgam
Amalgam has been used for over 150 years. The continued use of amalgam has become a controversial topic in recent years with concerns being raised about its safety, particularly in relation to the release of mercury during removal, placement, carving and, in the longer term, during chewing. There remains however, considerable evidence to support its safety as a dental material, with no apparent firm scientific evidence to indicate an association with any systemic disease. Some countries have taken steps to ban its use, but at present, no direct restorative material exists that has the same ease of handling, relative cost effectiveness and clinical serviceability.

Amalgam is an alloy of mercury with other metals. High copper alloys are most commonly used nowadays with 12–30% copper (by weight) in addition to silver, tin and zinc. The increased copper levels results in elimination of the weak gamma 2 phase, which was very corrodible. The exclusion of moisture during packing of the restoration is highly desirable as moisture reduces the clinical effectiveness of the material.

Advantages
Amalgam has many advantages:

Table 6 Compomer resins

Material	Manufacturer	Setting mechanism		
		Acid–base	Visible light	Chemical
Dyract	DeTrey Dentsply	+	+	
Fuji II LC	GC	+	+	+
Photac-Fil	ESPE	+	+	
Vitremer	3M	+	+	+

- strength
- ease of handling
- wear resistance
- reduced microleakage, resulting from slow corrosion
- longevity
- cost-effectiveness.

Disadvantages

The disadvantages of amalgam are:

- poor aesthetics
- lack of bonding to tooth substance
- mercury hazard to operator, associated staff and possibly to patients.

Posterior composites

Recent developments in composite technology have seen improvements in the compressive and tensile strengths of these materials for use in posterior teeth. Sufficient concerns remain about their wear resistance, setting characteristics and thermal properties to suggest that they should be used for posterior restorations with caution.

The demand of patients for increasingly aesthetic restorations has seen a significant rise in the use of composite materials for posterior restorations in recent years. However, as with most dental materials, they have both advantages and disadvantages.

Advantages

Aesthetics. Composite resins have been developed that give a wide range of shades, tints and opaqueness, allowing production of very aesthetically satisfactory restorations matching almost any natural tooth shade and appearance. Stability of this colour appears good, although extrinsic staining may result with time as a result of surface deterioration. Microfilled composites suffer less from this problem.

Reduced destruction of sound tooth substance. Adhesive technology allows limited removal of tooth substance beyond that required to eliminate caries and undermined enamel (preventive resin restorations). Tooth preparation differs from that for conventional amalgam cavities by being shallower and narrower (both of which reduce material volume and, therefore, polymerisation contraction). There is reduced undercutting of the cavity walls with rounding of internal line angles, thus reducing the development of stress and improving adaptation of the material during placement.

Adhesion. Composite resins are compatible with bonding agents, which allow a chemical bond to be developed between the tooth and the bonding agent and then between the bonding agent and the composite resin (see Enamel and dentine bonding).

Low thermal conductivity. Less ability to conduct heat providing insulation.

Elimination of galvanism. Lack of electrical conductivity.

Disadvantages

Polymerisation contraction. Modern composites tend to shrink by between 2 and 7% as they set. This may result in a number of changes that may lead to the ultimate failure of the restoration:

- sufficient force may be applied to the cusps of the tooth that they are 'pulled' inwards and microcracks develop, leading to weakening of the cusps and later failure under functional loading
- the forces generated may pull the restoration away from the walls or margin of the cavity leading to microleakage
- force vectors resulting from the contraction are very specific, with visible light-cured (VLC) resins polymerising towards the light source and chemically cured resins towards the centre of the material mass.

Various techniques are advocated to reduce the effects of polymerisation shrinkage:

- incremental placement allows curing of small amounts of material at a time, reducing the overall contraction and ensuring that the curing light penetrates to the full depth of the resin
- beta-quartz inserts (made of the same quartz glass material that acts as a filler particle for most composite resins) are placed in the body of a composite resin restoration to reduce the volume of composite and thereby the contraction (while these have been available for some time, they are difficult to use clinically and they are yet to be accepted as a realistic means of reducing polymerisation shrinkage on a routine basis).

Postoperative sensitivity. This occasionally arises from placement of composite restorations in posterior teeth. Its incidence has, however, reduced since dentine-bonding agents have improved. The reasons suggested for this symptom include polymerisation shrinkage, which results in microleakage, and plaque and fluid ingress.

Susceptibility to occlusal wear. Developments in materials have resulted in a reduction in this problem, but composites continue to wear as a result of both chemical breakdown and mechanical forces. The higher the volume of filler particles, the lower the rate of wear, although resins with large filler particles tend to show some susceptibility to abrasion wear as a result of three-body wear.

Factors of clinical significance in wear rates include:

- the size of the restoration in relation to the tooth
- the position of the tooth in the arch
- the type of tooth or restoration opposing it
- the ability of the patient to exert heavy occlusal loads.

Effectively, a restoration will be most susceptible to wear if it is placed in posterior teeth, is large in proportion to the surface area of the tooth and is in a patient with a bruxist habit.

Water absorption. The resin component of the material can absorb water, which tends to allow hydrolytic breakdown.

Degree of polymerisation. The effectiveness of cure is dependent upon several factors:

- material selection: different materials show variable degrees of polymerisation, with a better result arising with those cured by visible light
- lighter shades cure better and there is better light transmission through those materials with larger filler particles
- positioning of the light source is also critical as is the quality and regular maintenance of the light unit.

Guidelines for directly placed posterior composites As a result of the disadvantages, careful consideration should be given before using directly placed posterior composites. The following are useful guidelines for their use:

- where aesthetics is the prime consideration
- where cavity width is no greater than one-third the intercuspal width of the tooth
- when the gingival margin of the restoration is placed on intact enamel
- when centric stops allow occlusal support on tooth substance rather than on the restoration
- when occlusal parafunction is absent
- when there is good access to allow careful placement technique (preferably under rubber dam).

Finishing and polishing

Finishing/polishing involves the contouring and smoothing of the restoration to anatomical form with all marginal discrepancies eliminated. Polishing provides a smooth or shiny surface finish. Many products are available for finishing and polishing, including diamond burs, impregnated rubber points and various flexible discs. The smoothest surface is created by using an acetate strip. Care is required in finishing to avoid adversely affecting the wear characteristics of the materials. Overheating or an excessively traumatic technique will tend to damage the surface, resulting in more rapid wear. Increasingly finer grades of abrasives should be used to finish these materials.

Indirect posterior restorations

Indirect posterior restorations are constructed by first preparing a cavity in the tooth and then taking an impression or other record (e.g. CAD–CAM) before the restoration is fabricated in the laboratory (indirectly) for subsequent placement in the mouth. Such restorations can be fabricated as either a metal casting (e.g. gold

inlays) or as a tooth-coloured restoration in either composite or ceramic. They involve multiple stage techniques, with transfer of the clinical information from the mouth to the laboratory. This increases the possibility of errors and, therefore, great care is required to ensure maximum accuracy at each stage of the procedure.

Indications

Cast metal inlays/onlays

Cast metal inlays are preferred to amalgam restorations when the higher strength is desirable or when significant recontouring of the restoration is required and this cannot be achieved by a direct restoration.

Onlays are indicated where there has been a significant loss of occlusal tooth substance or where caries or breakdown of a pre-existing large restoration has grossly weakened the remaining tooth substance. The improved strength of the alloy under occlusal forces is the important property.

Bonding of occlusal shim restorations in tooth wear has become increasingly popular since the advent of more reliable dentine-bonding materials. Aesthetics of the direct metal inlays/onlays, while better than amalgam, are less satisfactory than a tooth-coloured material and considerable development has occurred in recent years.

Tooth-coloured inlays/onlays

Aesthetic considerations are often paramount in the choice of tooth-coloured resin or porcelain materials to restore posterior teeth. The use of inlays or onlays reduces the need for tooth preparation by utilisation of bonding technology.

Wear is an important consideration with the use of these materials, as porcelain is abrasive against natural tooth tissue while composites are prone to wear by the opposing dentition. The use of laboratory-cured composite resin materials for inlays has addressed, to some extent, the problems encountered in relation to their strength in function. Polymerisation is by secondary application of intense light, heat or pressure, in addition to the initial light cure as with direct materials. This 'extra' processing may include the use of temperatures of 250°C for periods of up to 7 minutes or of a specially designed light box. This results in an improvement in physical properties of the material while conferring no significant advantages in terms of reducing wear.

Indirect laboratory construction of these restorations allows improved accuracy of contact points, proximal contours and of the gingival margin of the restoration, sites where direct composite restorations can frequently be inadequate.

Polymerisation shrinkage, a major consideration with direct restorations, is less important with indirect restorations as the latter are polymerised prior to cementation and, therefore, the only shrinkage to occur at placement is within the very thin layer of luting agent. With porcelain onlays, an adequate thickness of coverage at vulnerable occlusal surfaces, such as over cusps, is required because porcelain is brittle and prone to fracture under occlusal stress if used in thin section. Porcelain, however, provides better long-term occlusal stability compared with composite. Patients should not exhibit any parafunctional habits and the occlusal scheme should allow centric contact but minimal eccentric contact.

Indirect tooth-coloured onlays are particularly useful for premolar restorations and also when the tooth has a short occluso-gingival height, where a full veneer crown may be an inadequate form of restoration.

Ceramic restorations can also be fabricated using CAD–CAM technology. Instead of taking a conventional impression, the preparation is scanned using an intraoral camera. The image created is processed by a computer and the milling machine manufactures the restoration from a solid ceramic block. The process, while being very expensive, has the benefit of being able to provide the ceramic restoration in a single visit.

CAD–CAM, however, is unable to recreate occlusal anatomy or full veneer crowns. There is also some concern about the marginal fit of CAD–CAM restorations, with some reports of gaps of 125 to 175 μm prior to cementation. This deficit appears, however, to be resolved at the time of cementation by filling the potential space with the luting cement.

Tooth-coloured restoration technique

The different materials available for indirect inlays and onlays require minor differences in preparation and, as most are technique sensitive, the protocol identified by the manufacturer of the chosen restorative material should be adhered to as rigorously as possible. Basic principles in preparation of the cavity include caries removal and development of an 8 to 10° divergence of the cavity walls. All internal line angles should be rounded.

For onlays, 2 mm occlusal reduction is desirable to give adequate strength of the finished restoration. The impression should be taken using an accurate material such as a silicone-based material. Temporisation can be with any material that is non-irritant and will not inhibit a composite resin material.

The restoration is constructed in the laboratory by pouring the impression to form a master cast. Porcelain restorations are constructed on a duplicate refractory die. Placement of the restorations requires care, particularly with isolation, as bonding is severely compromised if oral fluids contaminate the preparation. Isolation using rubber dam is usually required.

3.5 Extracoronal restorations

Learning objectives

You should

- know the principles of tooth preparation for veneers and full veneer crowns

- be aware of the different types of margin preparation

- know the principles of soft tissue management to maximise the opportunity for recording a satisfactory impression and working model.

Veneers

The porcelain veneer has become an increasingly popular aesthetic restoration used to modify the appearance of anterior teeth. This restoration is a thin shell of porcelain that is applied directly to tooth structure. Initially, composite materials were used as facings for teeth that required changes to their colour, shape, spacing or orientation. These materials, however, were unsatisfactory as long-term aesthetic restorations as they were subject to wear and discoloration. Porcelain veneers have become more predictable as bonding materials have continued to be developed.

The patient must be aware of the uncertain long-term prognosis for veneers, with the possibility of fracture, marginal discoloration and occasionally postoperative sensitivity. It is particularly important to assess the patient's expectations of treatment fully in order to avoid unwanted disputes at a later date.

Prior to preparing teeth, it is useful to use some form of aid such as a diagnostic wax-up. This is carried out by modification of a stone cast of the patient's dentition by making simple wax additions to tooth morphology or alignment. This gives both the practitioner and the patient a preview of the aesthetics of the finished restoration(s). An alternative chairside option is direct placement of composite to simulate the change in tooth morphology but without the use of a bonding agent. This allows removal of the restorative material at the end of the session. Clinical photographs are a useful adjunct to any form of cosmetic treatment, protecting the dentist from potential medicolegal problems and reminding the patients of their preoperative situation. They can also be useful for the technician in helping with shade matching and tooth morphology.

Early composite resin and acrylic (Mastique) veneers did not usually utilise tooth preparation. In addition, they required a thick bulk of material for adequate aesthetics. This almost inevitably led to overcontouring of the restorations, with resultant gingival problems and less satisfactory aesthetics. Glazed porcelain has now superseded composites for anything other than for short-term restorations, as it is much more resistant to abrasion and stains, it is aesthetic and it is well tolerated in the oral environment. The ability to bond porcelain to acid-etched enamel was developed in the early 1980s, with porcelain being etched using a hydrofluoric acid. A composite resin luting agent is used to bond the veneer to acid-etched enamel. Silane coupling agents have also been used to improve bond strength, by providing a weak chemical bond between the silicon dioxide in the porcelain and the bis-GMA polymer of the composite resin. Where insufficient enamel exists, it is necessary to use dentine-bonding agents. As these have improved, the range of situations in which the veneers can be utilised is continuing to increase.

Tooth preparation

It is now recognised that tooth preparation is required to provide the best cosmetic and functional result with porcelain veneers. The preparation should be minimal and kept within enamel, although adequate thickness of enamel must be removed to allow space for a correctly contoured restoration. Reduction should be approximately 0.5 mm. The gingival finishing line should be a fine chamfer, preferably at the gingival crest or just within the gingival sulcus. Where possible, the finishing line should be on enamel to provide reduced marginal leakage. As enamel thickness at the gingival margin is less than elsewhere on the crown of the tooth, reduction should be kept to 0.3 mm in this area.

In order to minimise loss of sound tooth substance, it is preferable to use some form of depth cutting technique, whereby grooves of the appropriate depth are cut at various points across the tooth surface. Specifically designed burs such as three-wheeled diamond depth cutters may be used (Fig. 55). Interproximally, care should be taken to reduce the tooth adequately. It is important to extend fully the reduced area into the embrasure space, particularly cervically, and in situations where the tooth has darkened.

There are two views on the most appropriate point at which to finish the incisal reduction:

* finish the prepared labial surface at the incisal edge with no reduction of the incisal tooth substance or continuation of the preparation onto the lingual surface (Fig. 56a).
* slight reduction of the incisal edge with overlap of the porcelain onto the lingual tooth surface (Fig. 56b).

Some authorities feel that overlapping of the incisal edge allows the porcelain to function in compression, where it tends to be stronger. This may also improve the stability of the veneers during seating. The margins of

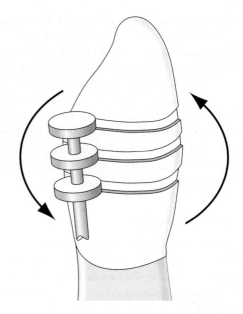

Fig. 55 Depth cutting for a veneer preparation.

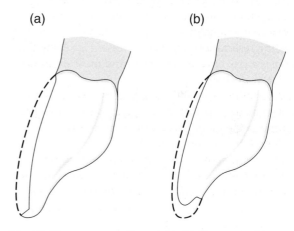

Fig. 56 Veneer preparations. (a) Labial face only. (b) Incorporating the incisal edge.

the preparation should be carefully blended and finished to remove any sharp angles, as these tend to lead to stress concentration and increase the risk of fracture propagation.

Both techniques appear to provide equally acceptable results in clinical service. The decision as to which technique to use will tend to be governed by any occlusal considerations in addition to the aesthetic needs such as a requirement to lengthen the tooth.

Impression taking is with any material used for conventional fixed restorations. Gingival retraction should be used where the gingival margin lies within the gingival sulcus. In most cases where the preparation remains within the enamel, patients are unlikely to require provisional restoration. Where it is required, a layer of directly applied light-activated composite resin can be retained by using a small dot of acid etchant and bonding agent in the centre of the labial surface.

The porcelain veneer is constructed in the laboratory using conventional porcelain techniques on a refractory die. It is important to incorporate adequate opaque porcelain in order to mask any discolouration of the tooth. The fitting surface of the veneer has to be etched with hydrofluoric acid so it can bond to conventional bonding resins. As with posterior tooth-coloured inlays, it is important to isolate the teeth at the time of the veneer placement to minimise any contamination with moisture.

Full veneer crowns

Where tooth destruction by dental disease is extensive, restoration may only be possible with full coverage restorations or crowns. Full evaluation of teeth to be restored in this way is required prior to commencement of treatment:

- All caries should be eliminated, with construction of an appropriate core of material (reinforcement of existing tooth substance or provision of a suitable replacement: amalgam, composite, cast post/core). If existing restorations have been present for some time there is a risk of recurrent caries and most should be replaced electively.
- Radiographic assessment and vitality testing of non-root-treated teeth should be carried out to allow for appropriate endodontic treatment prior to a definitive crown being placed.
- Occlusion in both centric and eccentric positions should be fully assessed, particularly in cases where restoration is required because of tooth wear. This may require the use of a semi-adjustable articulator and diagnostic casts in addition to a clinical assessment.
- Periodontal health should be achieved prior to provision of coronal restorations as gingival inflammation will prevent good quality preparation of margins and their accurate reproduction during impression taking, especially anteriorly where margin placement just within the gingival sulcus may be desirable for aesthetic reasons.

Similar criteria to those for intracoronal restorations apply to design of the preparation, namely maintenance of maximum sound tooth structure and provision of satisfactory resistance and retention form. The last are governed to a great extent by the preparation of the walls of the tooth. Absolute parallelism of opposing walls gives a theoretical maximum resistance and retention but will not allow seating of the restoration fully, leading to marginal leakage and occlusal interference. The actual angle of taper will vary with the tooth being prepared, and the skill of the clinician. An ideal taper of 12 to 16° has been recommended, but studies have shown that tapers of up to 24° may be required on posterior teeth. It is, therefore, advisable to aim for the minimum taper consistent with elimination of undercuts and satisfactory cementation of the final restoration. Extra taper may be required for cementation of bridges where abutment teeth have differing alignment. Reliance on the adhesive potential of more modern cements should never take the place of careful tooth preparation.

Provision of satisfactory resistance form to counteract rotational displacement forces requires the operator to:

- maximise the length of the preparation while avoiding disruption of the periodontal tissues
- allow for an adequate occlusal thickness of restorative material while creating a preparation that maximises the surface area for increased retention.

On occasions, the occluso-gingival height may be insufficient to provide adequate resistance and retention and additional features such as pinholes, grooves, slots or boxes (Fig. 57) may have to be incorporated into the preparation to provide auxiliary retention. It is imperative that these are parallel to the long axis of the tooth preparation.

A common error in preparation of teeth for full coronal restorations is inadequate tooth reduction. Failure to remove adequate tooth substance in all dimensions will result in overbulking of the crown or provision of a crown with insufficient thickness for strength or wear resistance. All-ceramic restorations should have at least 2 mm of clearance both on buccolingual or proximal aspects. Metal ceramic restorations should have 1.5 to 2 mm thickness on functional cusps where metal *and* porcelain coverage is provided, or 1 to 1.5 mm on all other aspects of the tooth. For gold alloys, 1.5 mm is required for functional cusps but 1 mm is adequate on most other surfaces. The functional cusps are the palatal of upper molars and premolars and the buccal of mandibular molars and premolars in a class I occlusion. The extra space is achieved by the use of a 'functional cusp bevel' in the tooth preparation. Similarly, over-preparation of teeth is undesirable, particularly where the pulp remains vital, as even if the pulp chamber is not

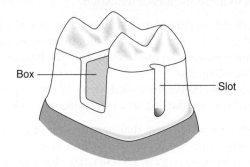

Box

Slot

Fig. 57 Methods for gaining auxiliary retention.

breached, the physical trauma and thermal changes created by tooth preparation can lead to irreversible pulp damage and necrosis and abscess formation.

The interface between the natural tooth and the restoration is obviously critical to the success of the restoration. A number of finishing lines may be used, the chosen design being governed to a great extent by the type of restoration being placed.

Ceramic restorations benefit from having a shoulder (Fig. 58). This improves the strength of the potentially weak porcelain and gives a good resistance to occlusal forces. It is, however, more destructive of tooth substance. The alternative is a heavy chamfer (Fig. 59a).

A chamfer finish is the preferred option for metal finishing margins both for full veneer gold crowns and in metal ceramic crowns with a metal margin (Fig. 59b).

One other margin, which is occasionally used, is the shoulder bevel (Fig. 59c). It is more commonly used with inlay or onlay preparations but can be also be used for metal ceramic restorations when the aesthetics at the gingival margin are not important (such as with restorations on posterior teeth).

As with veneers, tooth preparation is assisted by the use of depth grooves, which should be cut into the tooth surface at the initial stage of preparation. This allows an accurate estimate of the amount of tooth reduction. An optional technique is to use a putty index, made before the tooth is prepared. Replacement of this index against

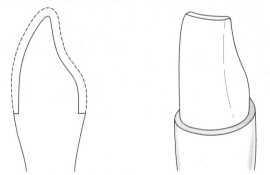

Fig. 58 The shoulder preparation.

(a)   (b)   (c)

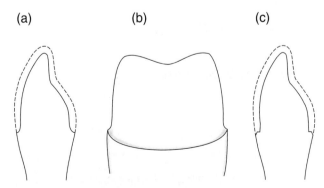

Fig. 59 Chamfer preparations. (a) Deep chamfer.
(b) Chamfer for metal finishing margins. (c) Shoulder-bevel chamfer.

the adjacent teeth allows one to assess the amount of tooth reduction that has been carried out. For more detail on individual crown preparations, you should refer to a more comprehensive text on crown and bridgework.

Crown and bridge impression technique

As most crown and bridge impression materials are now based on rubber polymers, they tend to be somewhat hydrophobic. As a result, it is vital that careful moisture control is achieved prior to impression taking.

Most crown preparations result in crown margins that are at the gingival crest or just within the gingival sulcus. The gingival margin, therefore, should be both healthy and not traumatised during tooth preparation. The presence of gingivitis and traumatised gingiva increase the risk of gingival haemorrhage during impression taking, leading to a loss of accuracy.

There are a number of ways to manipulate the gingival tissues to optimise the chance of achieving a workable impression, the most common being the use of retraction cord. Such cords tend to be either braided or woven cotton, often impregnated with some form of astringent material.

Astringent materials include aluminium sulphate, ferric sulphate and aluminium chloride. Ferric sulphate is incorporated in the Tissue Management System marketed by Ultradent. This system also allows the astringent to be presented in a syringe that has a brush end and can be used to massage the material into the gingival sulcus to inhibit bleeding. The appropriate gauge of cord should be chosen for each individual gingival sulcus.

The cord should be placed carefully into the gingival sulcus with the aim being to displace the gingival tissues laterally away from the tooth rather than attempting to force the cord into the depth of the sulcus (Fig. 60). The cord should be placed with slight pressure towards the last placed part to reduce the tendency for it to spring out of the sulcus again.

Electrosurgery may also be used on occasions when use of retraction cord alone is insufficient. There may be occasions where the tissues have overgrown slightly, for example where a temporary crown has been slightly undercontoured. The main concern with the use of electrosurgery is the potential for damage to the adjacent bone if local heat production is excessive, as the bone can be readily damaged. However, careful use of the electrocautery tip will allow removal of excess tissue, or creation of a new or deepened gingival sulcus. The machine should produce a fully rectified, filtered current that allows only minimal transfer of heat away from the operative site. It is important that the patients are fully informed of the nature of the procedure, as it can be quite disconcerting for them to suddenly become aware of the unpleasant odour which this procedure

(a) (b)

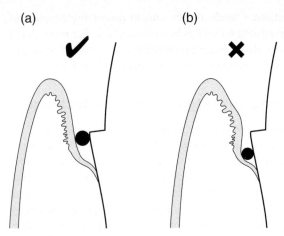

Fig. 60 Retraction cord technique. (a) Correct placement. (b) Incorrect placement.

generates. The instrument should be passed along the gingival sulcus with light pressure and quick continuous strokes. It is important that the electrode is not allowed to remain in one place for any length of time, as this is when damage may occur. High-volume suction should be used to remove the unpleasant odour of cauterisation. Care should be taken to avoid contact of the electrode with metal restorations as this can lead to excessive heat transmission to the pulp of the tooth.

On occasions, the crown length may be insufficient and conventional crown lengthening surgery may also be required.

The impression should provide an accurate model of the prepared tooth and surrounding tissues for the technician to produce a functionally and cosmetically satisfactory restoration. This requires accurate duplication of all dimensions of the preparation and particularly the finishing line, usually at, or just within, the gingival sulcus. Potential contact points with adjacent teeth must be accurately represented.

The material chosen to record the impression usually depends upon clinical preference, but it should have a number of desirable properties:

- ease of mixing and presentation
- long setting time
- strength and tear resistance
- moisture tolerance
- patient acceptability
- readability
- dimensional stability
- compatibility with disinfection solutions and cast materials
- reasonable cost.

Materials commonly used for crown and bridge impressions are:

- polyvinyl siloxane rubber-based materials, e.g. Extrude, President, Express, Permagum, Reprosil

- polyether rubber-based materials, e.g. Impregum, Permadyne
- polysulphide rubber-based materials, e.g. Permalastic
- reversible hydrocolloid.

Each type of material has its own particular handling characteristics, of which the operator requires to be aware, and may suit one operator more than another.

Many systems now are manufactured in a 'gun' dispensing system. This allows for ease of mixing, with almost complete elimination of air bubbles in the mixed material and a regular consistency of mix with predictable setting characteristics.

Most materials come with a range of viscosity for use in *putty and wash* or *heavy and light* body impression techniques. These techniques essentially allow use of the less viscous materials, which have improved flow properties, for accurate representation of the preparation. They are usually applied using a syringe to allow injection of the material into the gingival sulcus and around the preparation without inclusion of air pockets. These pockets can result in air blows on the impression surface and blebs, pimples or other irregularities on the surface of the cast. The heavy body or putty materials are used as a matrix for the lighter body material to minimise distortion during clinical and technical handling of the impression.

When a putty and wash technique is used, commonly in a stock tray, a two-stage impression technique is usually recommended, with a first-stage impression being taken in the putty material and using a polythene spacer. The second stage involves use of a free-flowing light body material applied directly to the preparations with a syringe to minimise air-blows and to which the putty matrix is applied. This reduces distortion, which may occur as a result of the use of some stock trays. More rigid stock trays, including metal 'rim-lock' trays, are available that reduce this problem and allow use of the single-stage technique using heavy and light body materials, although a special tray is recommended for this purpose.

3.6 Bridgework

Learning objectives

You should

- be able to give a classification for bridge design
- understand the indications for the provision of fixed bridges
- be able to advise patients on the advantages and disadvantages of replacing teeth with a fixed conventional bridge.

Where natural teeth are missing, the options for replacing them include removable partial dentures, fixed bridges and dental implants. A fixed bridge can be a so-called *conventional bridge* based on metal ceramic retainers with a porcelain and metal pontic (artificial tooth or teeth restoring the edentulous space). Alternatively, an *adhesive bridge* can be bonded to abutment teeth by use of composite adhesive technology.

Fixed bridges vary in the level of support provided by adjacent natural teeth. For a single-span edentulous area, a cantilever or fixed–fixed design would be appropriate:

- a cantilever design utilises support from only one side of the saddle area, although support may be from more than one tooth (Fig. 61).
- a fixed–fixed bridge design utilises support from both sides of the edentulous span (Fig. 62).

For multiple spans with a pier abutment (a single tooth lying between the two edentulous areas) more complex designs are required:

- a fixed–movable bridge utilises a custom-made or proprietary precision attachment to provide a degree of flexibility between the two component parts of the bridge (Fig. 63)
- a compound bridge uses a combination of fixed–fixed and cantilever elements in a single casting bridge (Fig. 64)
- hybrid bridges incorporate conventional and adhesive components but should be avoided unless no other option is feasible; placement of the bridge using conventional cements and adhesive resins at the same time is complicated and may lead to

(a)

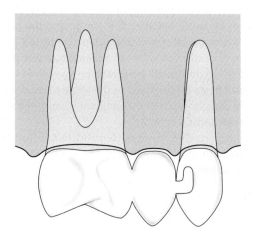

(b)

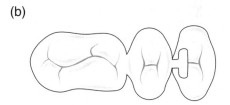

Fig. 63 Fixed–movable bridge replacing the second premolar has a fixed retainer on the first molar with a flexible dovetail attachment to distal of the retainer on the first premolar. (a) Side view. (b) Cross-section.

(a)   (b)

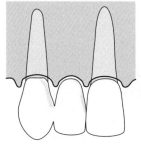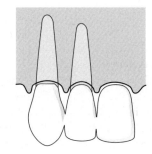

Fig. 61 Cantilever design for bridgework. (a) A single abutment (canine) cantilever replacing the lateral incisor (pontic). (b) A double abutment (canine and lateral incisor) cantilever replacing the central incisor (pontic).

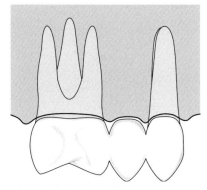

Fig. 62 Fixed–fixed bridge design replacing the second premolar (pontic) using the first premolar and first molar as the abutments.

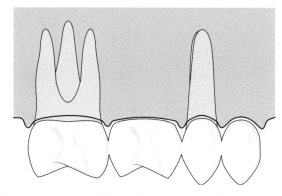

Fig. 64 Compound bridge with retainers placed on the second molar and the second premolar; the fixed pontic is the first molar and the cantilevered pontic is the first premolar.

inadequate seating unless a very experienced operator carries out treatment.

Pontic design is important in allowing the patient to maintain satisfactory oral hygiene to prevent recurrent caries or periodontal disease, while providing a cosmetic replacement for the missing tooth where that is appropriate. Designs include (Fig. 65):

- sanitary pontic
- bullet-nose pontic
- ridge-lap pontic
- modified ridge-lap pontic.

Of these, a ridge-lap design is undesirable as it does not allow for cleaning between the pontic and the mucosa. Sanitary and bullet-nosed pontics are preferred posteriorly where aesthetics is less of a concern, while a modified ridge lap design allows cleansibility with maximum aesthetics by overlying part of the ridge to mimic emergence of the pontic from the gingival tissues in a similar way to the natural tooth.

For any bridge design, appropriate planning is required with a full assessment of the periodontal and occlusal status.

A healthy periodontium is essential prior to provision of bridgework. Teeth that have previously suffered periodontal bone loss remain satisfactory bridge abutments provided the disease has been treated and stabilised. There should be enough remaining bone for teeth to contribute satisfactorily to support of the bridge without detriment to themselves or to the function and longevity of the restoration. The suitability of individual teeth will vary between different teeth in different areas of the mouth as well as between different patients. Assessment is, therefore, required on an individual basis.

Tooth contacts. Opposing and adjacent tooth contacts are important. Overeruption of an opposing tooth into an edentulous saddle may mitigate against bridgework for that saddle, unless treatment to address the overeruption is carried out. Similarly, tipped and tilted teeth adjacent to a saddle area will, if their long axes are not parallel, prevent construction of any form of fixed–fixed bridge. Orthodontic uprighting can be used to overcome this problem.

Previous restoration. The extent to which an individual tooth has been previously restored will likewise govern suitability as a supporting element in bridgework. Non-vital teeth are no longer regarded as being more

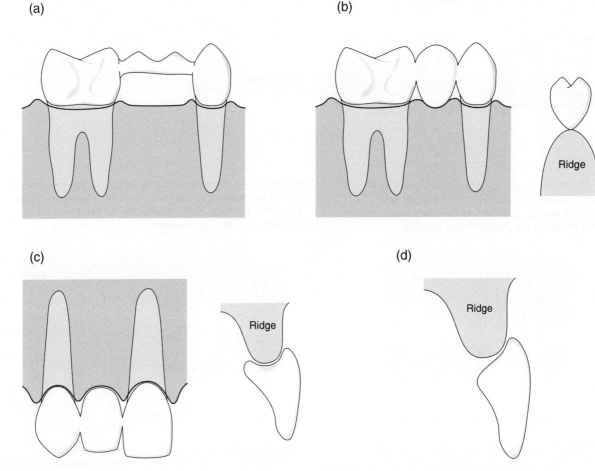

(a)

(b)

(c)

(d)

Fig. 65 Pontic designs. (a) Sanitary pontic. (b) Bullet-nose pontic. (c) Ridge-lap pontic. (d) Modified ridge-lap pontic.

brittle than vital teeth. Where a post has been required to augment the support of the core for the crown or bridge abutment, there is a potential inherent mechanical weakness in that tooth. Root-filled teeth with posts should be viewed with some caution as potential bridge abutments.

Occlusal factors. When doubt exists about occlusal factors in the design of the bridge, or where extensive restoration of the arch has the potential to alter guidance or occluso–vertical dimension, the use of a face-bow registration and a semi-adjustable articulator is mandatory. This will allow use of a diagnostic wax-up as part of the planning procedure.

Self-assessment: questions

Multiple choice questions

1. The following factors are important in remineralisation and demineralisation of early carious lesions:
   a. Plaque composition
   b. Frequency of sugar intake
   c. Fluoride content of dentifrices
   d. Gingival inflammation
   e. Salivary flow rate

2. The following factors are contraindications to provision of a metal ceramic crown:
   a. Bruxism
   b. Persistent apical pathology
   c. Acute gingivitis
   d. Temporomandibular joint dysfunction (TMD)
   e. Xerostomia

3. A hybrid composite:
   a. Has a single size of aluminosilicate particles
   b. Requires acid etching to allow retention in the cavity
   c. Is only suitable for posterior restorations
   d. Is used for bonding veneers
   e. Has the same coefficient of thermal expansion as tooth

4. Which of the following may be used in a cavity to be restored with composite:
   a. Non-setting calcium hydroxide
   b. Dentine bonding agent
   c. Glass ionomer
   d. Unmodified zinc oxide eugenol
   e. Zinc polycarboxylate

5. The following definitions in occlusion are correct:
   a. Group function is the bilateral tooth contacts in lateral excursion
   b. RCP (retruded contact position) is CO (centric occlusion)
   c. Freeway space is a positive interocclusal space arising as the difference between test free height (RFH) and occlusal free height (OFH)
   d. Deflective contact is a tooth contact deflecting the mandible from natural path of closure
   e. Approximately 80% of the dentate population will have a CR (centric relation) to CO slide

6. The following are methods of recording the relationship of mandibular teeth to maxillary teeth:
   a. Occlusal wax registration
   b. Transfer copings
   c. Gothic arch tracing
   d. Face bow transfer
   e. Diagnostic wax-up

7. Methods of recreating adequate crown height when restoring teeth with severe erosion include:
   a. Orthodontic extrusion
   b. Dahl therapy
   c. Crown lengthening surgery
   d. Electrosurgery
   e. Devitalisation with post and core provision

8. Bleaching:
   a. Always requires rubber dam isolation
   b. Can only be carried out on non-vital teeth
   c. A 'walking bleach' uses carbamide peroxide
   d. Is always effective in severe tetracycline staining
   e. External bleaching is more effective if heat is applied

9. Indications for resin bonded fixed–fixed bridgework are:
   a. Mobile abutments
   b. Abutments with proximal restorations
   c. Evidence of attritive tooth wear
   d. Short span
   e. Translucent incisal enamel on abutments

10. With respect to auxiliary pin retention of directly placed restorations:
   a. These should be placed at the enamel dentine junction
   b. Two pins should replace each missing cusp
   c. Self-threading pins are less retentive than friction lock or cemented
   d. The ideal depth within tooth substance is 1 mm
   e. Pins decrease the compressive and tensile strength of amalgam

Case history questions

Case history 1

A 35-year-old female patient attends complaining of gradual discoloration of an upper right central incisor tooth over the last 2 years. It is presently symptom free, but she is unhappy about its appearance and wishes this to be improved.

1. What questions would you ask in relation to the history?
2. What investigations would you carry out?
3. What treatment options exist?

Case history 2

A 50-year-old male patient attends complaining of intermittent discomfort from a lower molar tooth, mainly on chewing or biting on the tooth in one position. The tooth has been restored a few years previously with a large MOD amalgam. The pain is sharp in nature, related to the one tooth, and each episode lasts only a few minutes at most.

1. What investigations might you carry out?
2. What is the differential diagnosis?
3. How would you treat it?

Case history 3

A 20-year-old female patient attends with a complaint of severe sensitivity of many teeth, especially to thermal stimulus (hot and cold). She looks frail and underweight.

1. What might you expect to see intraorally?
2. What might be its aetiology?
3. How would you deal with the patient?
4. How would you deal with her dentition?

Short note questions

Write short notes on the following:

1. Enamel caries
2. Aetiology of tooth wear
3. Cavity preparation for a class II plastic restoration
4. Methods of tissue management in crown impressions
5. Pontic design in crown and bridgework

Essay question

Discuss treatment planning for a three unit metal–ceramic bridge.

Self-assessment: answers

Multiple choice answers

1. a. **True**. The thickness and viscosity of plaque, in addition to the types of bacteria incorporated in it, will have an effect on the transfer of ions into and out of a carious lesion.
   b. **True**. The plaque ecology will be altered by regular consumption of refined sugar allowing the pH level to reduce (Stephan curve) and increasing demineralisation.
   c. **True**. Any form of topical fluoride will provide free fluoride ions, which will be incorporated in the remineralisation process.
   d. **False**. Gingival inflammation, while being an effect of plaque accumulation and toxin production, does not in itself affect the remineralisation/demineralisation process.
   e. **True**. Salivary flow rate, if reduced, will reduce the available ions for remineralisation. Saliva generally has an important function in modifying caries development.

2. a. **False**. Bruxism is a common habit and while its aetiology may not be identifiable, some patients brux because of an occlusal discrepancy; it is important to identify and eliminate this if the crown is to be placed in proximity to the problem. Where bruxism is present and no obvious aetiology can be identified, recognition of the condition in preparing the supporting tooth, designing the restoration and possibly protecting by use of an occlusal splint after placement should all be considered.
   b. **True**. Any apical pathology should be addressed before a crown is placed on the affected tooth. If there is any suspicion of loss of vitality of an abutment tooth, it should be fully evaluated and, if necessary, definitive restoration deferred until the prognosis is more certain.
   c. **True**. Gingival health should be maximised before crown preparation and placement – this will improve the accuracy of margins and, therefore, the prognosis for the restoration.
   d. **True**. As with bruxism, TMD should be addressed first to avoid any potential occlusal conflicts and also to allow satisfactory access during treatment without exacerbating symptoms.
   e. **False**. Xerostomia has a wide range of causes and provided the patient is aware of the potential for a higher caries rate as a result of their condition, xerostomia cannot be regarded as a contraindication to crown placement.

3. a. **False**. Hybrid composites contain a variety of particle sizes to allow a greater filler load within the material. This improves physical characteristics of the material.
   b. **False**. While acid etching is now recommended for all composite restorations, cavity preparation with appropriate undercuts will cause the material to be retained. However, shrinkage of the material will increase the risk of microleakage if no etching/bonding is carried out.
   c. **False**. While hybrid materials are stronger and are, therefore, more applicable to posterior sites, they may be used anteriorly, although their aesthetics are slightly poorer.
   d. **False**. Composites with low filler content are more appropriate for bonding.
   e. **False**. Virtually no restorative material has the same coefficient of thermal expansion as natural tooth, leading to concerns about the detrimental effect of thermocycling over time.

4. a. **False**. Non-setting calcium hydroxide is used as an interim root filling material. It is not suitable for lining a cavity.
   b. **True**.
   c. **True**.
   d. **False**. Unmodified zinc oxide eugenol is too slow setting and may also interfere with setting if composites are used.
   e. **True**.

5. a. **False**. Group function is defined as multiple tooth contacts on the working side during lateral excursion but with no non-working side contact.
   b. **False**. RCP is CR (centric relation) i.e. the jaw position with the condyles in the most retruded position in the glenoid fossa. CO is ICP (intercuspal position), which is the jaw position with maximum interdigitation of teeth.
   c. **True**.
   d. **True**.
   e. **True**. Only 20% of the population have coincidence of the most retruded mandibular position with maximum interdigitation of the teeth.

6. a. **True**.
   b. **True**.
   c. **True**. Occlusal wax registrations, transfer copings and the gothic arch tracing devices are all means of recording the intermaxillary relationship.

d. **False**. A face bow only records the relative position of the maxilla to the hinge axis.

e. **False**. A diagnostic wax-up is used as a tool to assess changes in occlusion or tooth shape prior to an advanced restorative procedure.

7. a. **True**.

b. **False**. Dahl therapy, while often used as an adjunct to treatment of tooth wear, does not result in increased crown height but rather alters the interincisal space to allow space for subsequent restoration.

c. **True**.

d. **False**. Electrosurgery is not advocated for increasing crown height in most erosion cases as it cannot be used for tissue removal where bone is in close proximity and it is positively contraindicated for bone removal.

e. **True**.

8. a. **False**. A 'walking bleach', where the active agent is sealed within the tooth, by its nature does not require rubber dam isolation, although dam should be used during placement. (Bleaching techniques are discussed in detail in Chapter 6.)

b. **False**. Vital and non-vital bleaching can be carried out.

c. **False**. The agents commonly used for a 'walking bleach' are usually hydrogen peroxide (30%) and/or sodium perborate (Bocosan). Carbamide peroxide is the active agent in recent vital bleaching agents (e.g. Opalescence)

d. **False**. Severe tetracycline staining, while it may be improved by bleaching in many cases, does not always improve with bleaching.

e. **True**. Heat can improve the effectiveness of hydrogen peroxide bleaching techniques.

9. a. **False**.

b. **False**.

c. **False**.

d. **True**. All except a short span are potential contraindications to resin-bonded bridgework.

e. **False**.

10. a. **False**. Pins should avoid the enamel dentine junction.

b. **True**. Only one pin per cusp is recommended.

c. **False**. Retention of self threading > friction lock > cemented.

d. **False**. The ideal depth in dentine is 2 mm.

e. **True**. Pins actively weaken the strength of amalgam restorations and are used simply to aid retention.

Case history answers

Case history 1

1. You should ask for the
   - history of trauma: its nature, severity, timing.
   - incidence and timing of previous symptoms: sensitivity, pain, gingival swelling/discharge, mobility
   - history of previous treatment: restorations, endodontic treatment
   - patient's views on appearance and on improving appearance.

2. Investigations would include
   - clinical examination: careful examination in good light, assessment of degree and nature of discolouration (including comparison with shade guide as necessary), quality of existing restorations, periodontal status, mobility, presence of gingival sinus
   - pulp vitality tests: electric, hot (heated gutta-percha), cold (ice, ethyl chloride)
   - radiographs: to identify the morphology of the root canal system and the presence of any apical pathology.
   - assess the nature and quality of previous dental treatment (root fillings, restorations).

3. Treatment could include bleaching, internal/external, a veneer or a crown. Alternatively the tooth could be extracted and replaced with fixed or removable prosthesis. All options, with their indications and contraindications, should be presented to the patient to ensure that she is fully informed.

Case history 2

1. Examination would include:
   - clinical examination: assessment of existing restoration (presence of fracture, recurrent caries, occlusal contacts), assessment of remaining tooth structure (caries, fracture lines – careful use of transillumination often required), removal of restoration if required to fully visualise fracture
   - vitality testing: thermal and electric
   - Radiographs to identify recurrent caries, deficient restoration, possible fracture (although fractures are rarely identifiable in these circumstances on radiograph)
   - occlusal tests: using either a rubber burlew wheel or a 'Tooth Sleuth' placed over individual cusps and with patient occluding on the instrument with the opposing tooth; a positive response for a

cracked cusp/tooth is for the patient to experience a sharp pain on release of the occlusal pressure, which arises from flexure of the two parts of the tooth.

2. Differential diagnosis includes cracked cusp/tooth syndrome, recurrent caries, reversible pulpitis, possibly dentine hypersensitivity and, less commonly, trigeminal neuralgia or atypical facial pain or odontalgia.

3. Treatment will vary with the diagnosis, but from the information given, the most likely cause will be a cracked cusp. Treatment will depend upon the extent and position of the fracture. Where it simply involves a cusp and the fracture is supragingival, the best way of treating it is to remove the cusp and the fracture line and restore the tooth, with a cuspal coverage restoration in amalgam or gold, composite or porcelain. Where the fracture is not immediately evident, but the tooth has a large restoration, the restoration should be removed and the cavity floor and walls carefully examined to identify any fracture line. If the fracture runs longitudinally through the root or significantly subgingivally, the only option may be extraction.

Case history 3

1. In such cases, extensive erosive tooth wear may be seen affecting almost all natural tooth surfaces and resulting most commonly from frequent vomiting. The tooth surfaces may be eroded through to dentine and if the condition is severe enough and progressing rapidly, sensitivity will result from thermal stimuli because the rate of wear is more rapid than the ability of the pulp to generate secondary dentine. Cusps will be rounded and the tooth surface will tend to be smooth and glossy. Any restorations previously present in teeth may lie proud of the tooth surface. The patient may be dehydrated and have a dry appearance to the skin and oral tissues.

2. A patient of this age who appears very underweight may well suffer from an eating disorder such as anorexia or bulimia. If this is the case, sensitivity is required in eliciting a history, as the patient may be reluctant to admit to this.

3. It is important, where possible, to identify the aetiology of the symptoms. If the patient can acknowledge the nature of their problem, liason with their medical practitioner for further investigation and treatment of the condition is desirable. Failure to do so will make dental treatment more difficult and lead to more rapid failure.

4. Treatment depends on the extent of the erosion and

the level of patient co-operation. Full or partial veneer restorations, with minimal preparation (to avoid loss of further tooth tissue) and utilising dentine and enamel bonding technology where necessary, is likely to be required. Fluoride supplements and oral hygiene advice (particularly prior to active treatment) are also beneficial.

Short note answers

1. Enamel caries arises in pits, fissures and on smooth coronal (e.g. proximal) surfaces as a result of progressive dissolution of the inorganic component mediated by dental plaque. Plaque metabolism of dietary sugars leads to acid production and this leads to demineralisation at a pH level of less than 5.5. The carious lesion is clinically visible, dependent on the site, by shadowing of the tooth substance particularly with transillumination. Early enamel caries occurs below the enamel surface, developing as a 'white spot'. The surface remains intact with demineralisation occurring deeper. It then progresses to a brown spot and to surface breakdown with resultant cavitation. These can be diagnosed by radiographs or, if cavitation is occurring, with a sharp dental probe. The pattern of progress depends on the site: in pits and fissures it has a small site of origin at the surface with a wide base towards the pulp, while on smooth coronal surfaces it has a wide area of origin with a narrow apex towards pulp. Remineralisation occurs at neutral pH. This is achieved by the buffering capacity of both saliva and plaque with calcium and phosphate ions available at the tooth surface. Fluoride modifies enamel's crystalline structure, conferring increased resistance to acid demineralisation.

2. Tooth wear can be categorised as three types. These are attrition, erosion and abrasion, each with a different aetiology. Attrition arises from the movement of tooth surfaces against each other. It mainly results from bruxism (grinding habits) although it is an age-related phenomenon in non-bruxists. It mainly affects the occlusal surfaces of the teeth, commonly across the whole dentition. Erosion arises from acidic demineralisation of the surface of the tooth. The origin of the acid may be extrinsic (dietary, including carbonated drinks, fresh fruit juices, citrus fruits, vinegar and pickles, or environmental/occupational, although health and safety issues have reduced this) or intrinsic (arising from gastric reflux/vomiting – these may arise from conditions including hiatus hernia, gastric or peptic ulceration, anorexia, bulimia, alcoholism). The pattern of wear will vary greatly dependent on the

source of the acid, with localised wear to the palatal surfaces of the upper anterior teeth in dietary erosion resulting from excessive consumption of carbonated drinks (increasingly seen in teenagers), while anorexic or bulimic patients may show much more widespread erosion, including buccal and lingual erosion of posterior teeth. Abrasion is commonly a result of incorrect tooth brushing, often affecting the cervical area of the tooth, where gingival recession may have exposed root surface dentine, which is readily abraded by a scrubbing technique. Cervical enamel can also be damaged in this way. Again rarely seen nowadays as a result of health and safety regulations, in the past abrasion was sometimes seen in those working in a very dusty environment.

3. Cavity preparation for a class II plastic restoration will vary slightly with the type of plastic restorative material used, options usually being either amlagam or composite. Given that a class II cavity is by definition a cavity in a premolar or molar tooth, the material should be chosen with care to ensure longevity and functionality of the restoration. It is undesirable to use a directly placed composite material in a tooth with extensive carious destruction, as the material may be too weak to withstand normal functional loads. Principles for cavity preparation include:

   a. *Access*. This should be sufficient to allow adequate visualisation of caries to allow its complete removal, while aiming to retain a maximum amount of sound tooth substance compatible with this objective.

   b. *Caries removal*. Removal of stained and softened tooth substance regarded as carious. Tooth substance that is stained and *firm* requires careful evaluation. Staining at the amelo-dentinal junction should be removed wherever possible. The pulp should be protected if the caries is deep.

   c. *Removal of unsupported enamel*. Enamel is brittle and if left unsupported will have a high risk of fracture under functional loading, with resultant failure of the associated restoration.

   d. *Outline form*. The cavity margin should remain accessible for cleaning and maintenance whenever possible. It should be placed where functional loading will not impinge on the restoration/tooth interface.

   e. *Resistance/retention form*. Resistance form is that aspect of cavity design whereby both the restoration and tooth should, upon completion of the restoration, be able to withstand functional forces. Retention form results from opposing cavity walls being parallel or slightly convergent to 'resist' any forces that will tend to dislodge the

restoration from the cavity. In amalgam cavities, this remains an important aspect of cavity design, although again minimal preparation is desirable. In composite restorations, dentine bonding technology is applicable and retention may be augmented in this way.

4. Tissue management in crown and bridgework involves moisture control and appropriate soft tissue handling in order to achieve an accurate impression, which is essential for maximum accuracy in the fit of the final restoration. Careful moisture control should be achieved prior to impression taking as most crown and bridge impression materials are hydrophobic. This can be achieved by use of cotton rolls, saliva ejector and dry-guards, with close support assistance by a dental nurse. The gingival margin should be both untraumatised and healthy, with no gingivitis as this is more likely to increase the risk of gingival haemorrhage and therefore result in inaccuracies. The close proximity of crown, bridge or veneer margins to the gingival tissues does, however, necessitate careful handling of even healthy gingiva. Methods include the use of retraction cord (with or without astringent), or electrosurgery. Occasionally, crown-lengthening surgery may be required. Retraction cords are either braided or woven cotton cords. The appropriate gauge of cord should be chosen for each individual gingival sulcus. A variety of astringent materials have been used and include aluminium sulphate, ferric sulphate and aluminium chloride. The cord should be placed carefully into the gingival sulcus with the aim being to displace the gingival tissues laterally away from the tooth rather than attempting to force the cord into the depth of the sulcus (Fig. 60). Placement of the cord should be with pressure applied slightly towards the area into which it has already been placed as this reduces the tendency for it to spring out of the sulcus again. Electrosurgery may also be used on occasions where use of retraction cord alone is insufficient. There may be occasions where the tissues have overgrown slightly, e.g. where a temporary crown has been slightly under-contoured. The main concern with the use of electrosurgery is the potential for damage to the adjacent bone if local heat production is excessive, as bone can be readily damaged. However, careful use of appropriate equipment will allow removal of any excess tissue or creation of a new or deepened gingival sulcus. The machine should produce a fully rectified, filtered current, which allows only minimal transfer of heat away from the operative site. It is important that the patient is fully informed of the nature of the procedure, as it can be quite disconcerting for them to become aware suddenly of the unpleasant odour

that this procedure generates. The instrument should be passed along the gingival sulcus with light pressure and quick continuous strokes. It is important that the electrode is not allowed to remain in one place for any length of time as this is when damage may occur. High-volume suction should be used to remove as much of the smell of the procedure as possible. Care should be taken to avoid contact of the electrode with metal restorations, as this can lead to excessive heat transmission to the pulp of the tooth. On occasions, the crown length may be insufficient and crown-lengthening surgery may be required.

5. Pontics in bridgework should be carefully designed and an appropriate prescription provided for the technician. Ideally, they require to be functional, aesthetic, cleansable and maintainable. There are several types of pontic used in conventional bridgework; however, certain designs do not satisfy the requirements of an ideal pontic, for example, ridge lap pontics are not to be recommended. The other types of pontic commonly used are modified ridge lap, bullet-nose and sanitary. The modified ridge lap is perhaps the most commonly used, particularly anteriorly where the overlap of the cervical portion onto the ridge allows for maximum aesthetics, while the palatal or lingual portion is contoured to allow maximum cleansability. Bullet-nose and sanitary pontics are used posteriorly, where aesthetics are less critical but access for cleaning and maintenance is important. A bullet-nose pontic has a single point of contact against the alveolar ridge and is designed to have wide embrasure spaces. The sanitary pontic is usually constructed in gold and should have at least 3 mm clearance from the crest of the alveolar ridge. This minimises the tendency for food accumulation and maximises the ability to clean the area. Embrasure spaces in bridgework should be designed not only to mimic normal anatomy but also to allow the patient to use appropriate interproximal clean aids such as Super floss, interproximal brushes or wood sticks. Both the clinician and the technician should, therefore, carefully design the junction between the abutments and the pontics. Care is required to reproduce the appropriate occlusal contact between the pontic and the opposing tooth. This requires careful occlusal registration in an appropriate medium, correct mounting of the working and opposing casts and provision of a fully functional occlusal scheme.

Essay answer

Your answer should consider:

- Position of bridge in the mouth
- Occlusion, including
  — the completeness of the dentition and the need for other restoration
  — occlusal support
  — classification of the occlusion
  — local occlusal factors: rotation, overeruption, tipping
  — eccentric occlusal guidance: lateral and protrusive
  — parafunction.
- Diagnostic aids: radiographs, photographs and study models, the last potentially mounted on an appropriate articulator and with diagnostic wax-up.
- General dental health
  — caries incidence/activity
  — tooth vitality
  — apical pathology
  — periodontal health and maintenance, and, therefore, the suitability of the potential abutment teeth to support the proposed bridge.
- Bridge design: given that a three unit conventional metal ceramic restoration has been specified, the main considerations are pontic design and abutment margin placement and design.
- Aesthetic/phonetic/functional requirements: i.e. what the patient is expecting from the bridge cosmetically and in speech and eating.
- Other treatment options.

4 Prosthodontics

Overview

The discipline of prosthetics has evolved in the 1990s from being a discipline heavily weighted to complete denture construction to a speciality concerned more and more with the reconstruction of the partially dentate patient. As people are living longer and retaining their dentitions into later life, the demands on the prosthetist have changed to match the increasing demands of a changing population. This chapter will address the clinical stages involved with complete and partial denture construction and highlight other areas of interest to the prosthetist. Detailed information on material science, preprosthetic surgery and prosthetic laboratory techniques has not been included and indeed this text should be seen as an introduction and summary of the areas covered.

4.1 Complete dentures

Learning objectives

You should

- appreciate the importance of correct patient assessment
- understand the clinical and laboratory stages in complete denture construction
- have some understanding of solving complete denture problems.

Patient assessment

The evaluation of a patient who requires any form of dental treatment should begin at the earliest stage of meeting that patient. On an initial meeting with the patient, the points that should be subconsciously noted, even before any dialogue occurs, are the sex and age of the patient, their physical stature, the appearance they wish to present to the public and, finally, their present dental status. These brief thoughts about a new patient can often provide reliable predictions of the expectations of the patient and, based on that, the possible outcomes. As a generalisation, an edentulous smartly dressed, physically healthy, middle-aged female is more likely to have higher expectations from her prosthesis than an edentulous, elderly physically impaired male. It is vitally important, nevertheless, not to categorise definitively patients as a result of initial impressions. A patient's appearance and demure can be deceptive; therefore, a detailed history is required to give a broader, more structured assessment of the patient's oral status, dental demands and psychological attitude towards treatment. A short but concise evaluation of the presenting complaint or reason for attendance is required, and in this respect it is important that words are not placed into the patient's mouth. Such interference will severely compromise treatment outcomes. Structured questioning should only begin after the patient has clearly indicated their reasons for attendance, complaints and any wishes they may have. A detailed dental history should then be built up gradually. Important features that must be gained from such a history are:

- When did you become edentulous?
- Why did you lose your teeth?
- Did you wear partial dentures prior to this?
- Did you have immediate dentures fitted?
- How many sets of dentures have you had?
- How long did each set last?
- Did you attend the dentist for any denture maintenance visits?
- How old is your present set of dentures?
- Which set of dentures was the most successful in your opinion?

- Do your dentures cause you discomfort?
- Do you wear both dentures at night?
- Do you like the appearance of your present dentures?
- Can you eat with your present dentures?

A clear and concise medical history is also required with certain features being of particular note for denture wearers (Table 7).

An extraoral assessment for any temporomandibular joint problems, facial asymmetry, lymph node enlargement, lower face height and soft tissue support are all clinical requirements. Following this, the patient should be asked to remove their dentures and an intraoral assessment should be carried out. All soft tissues should be inspected, including the floor of mouth and tonsillar region and the health of the tissues evaluated. The elderly edentulous patient is more likely to present with oral lesions, and a dentist may often be the first person to detect such problems. In this respect, it is important to appreciate the possible oral manifestations of systemic disorders. The ridges should then be palpated and a note made as to the remaining hard tissue support. A classification system of the type shown in Figure 66 is of great benefit.

Once the health of the extraoral and intraoral hard and soft tissues has been examined, *detailed* examination of the dentures themselves should be carried out away from the mouth to assess their cleanliness and condition. Each denture in turn should then be placed intraorally to assess:

- retention: it is often beneficial to classify retention as being good, adequate or poor; reasons for lack of retention should be listed such as under- or overextension of the periphery, position of post dam, adaptation of the fitting surface
- stability; a scale of good, adequate or poor should be used and the reasons for lack of stability listed such as flabby ridge, unsupported ridge, extensive resorption or inadequate muscle control
- occlusion: a classification should be used to describe the occlusal relationship of the dentures and a general assessment of occlusal contact and support should be made; a measure of the interocclusal clearance provided by the dentures is also essential.

Once the history has been completed, it is important that a treatment plan should be developed for every patient, which will be dependent upon the presenting complaints together with the findings from the clinical examination. The proposed treatment should include any preliminary requirements followed by the intended technique of denture construction including any special considerations. It is not satisfactory for the treatment plan to be simply the construction of complete dentures. It should also clearly indicate the impression materials, freeway space present, balanced occlusion, tooth selection and selection of acrylic matrix. Specific indication should be given of the indications for copy dentures, functional impression, neutral zone technique or flat cusped teeth.

Clinical techniques

Preliminary impressions

Preliminary impressions are taken in stock trays using impression compound. These trays may need modification (usually reduction) to improve their suitability for the patient. In some cases the detail of such impressions can be improved using an alginate wash.

Laboratory prescription
As the next appointment will be for recording master impressions, it is essential at this and subsequent stages to indicate precisely your technical requirements. The prescription on the laboratory card should be clear and comprehensive. If there is any possibility of confusion, it is most valuable to discuss the patient personally with the technician involved. If a laboratory card is not completed and dated properly, the work may not be available at the next appointment.

Requirements for trays
Lower trays. Close-fitting light-cured trays for use with zinc oxide/eugenol paste should be requested. If extensive undercuts are present, a spaced tray for alginate is required.

Upper trays. Spaced (two thickness of modelling wax) light-cured trays should be prescribed for use with impression plaster, or alginate if undercuts are present.

Borders. The peripheral border of all trays should finish 2 mm short of the depth of the sulcus when the

Table 7 Important medical factors for denture wearers

Area	Significant factors
Physical disabilities	Disability (mental or physical), arthritis
Neuromuscular disorders	Parkinsons' disease, epilepsy, stroke
Airway/breathing disorders	Asthma, bronchitis
Skin/mucosal disease	Pemphigus, pemphigoid, lupus erythematosus
Medication	Any medication that may cause dry mouth

Anterior mandible

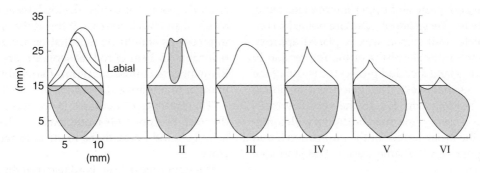

Posterior mandible

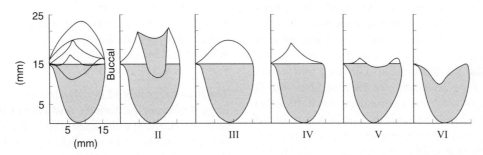

Anterior maxilla

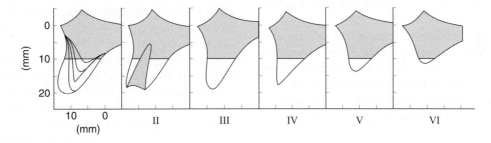

Posterior maxilla

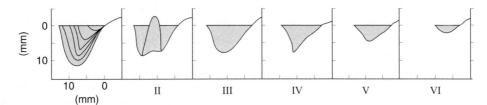

Fig. 66 A classification system for edentulous jaws (from Cawood, Howell 1991 Reconstructive preprosthetic surgery I. Anatomical considerations. Int J Oral Maxillofac Surg 20: 75–82).

spacer is in place. This is approximately the position of the mucogingival line.

Master impressions

The master impression should record detail of the denture-bearing area together with the depth *and* width of the functional sulcus so that the finished denture maintains an effective facial seal. In some cases, the tray will require modification to its peripheral border and this should be carried out using autopolymerising acrylic resin or greenstick compound prior to the impression being recorded.

Normally lower impressions will be recorded using zinc oxide/eugenol paste and upper impressions using impression plaster. These impressions are not to be considered complete until ribbon wax is placed approximately 2 mm from the periphery of the impression in order to provide a land area and protect the width of the sulcus on the resultant cast. This placement of ribbon wax is called beading (Fig. 67). In the very few cases where alginate is used, a line must be drawn with indelible pencil on the facial surface of the impression 2 mm from the periphery for the same reason. This land area must not be removed!

Laboratory prescription

Casts should be poured in dental stone and a prescription provided regarding the construction of occlusal rims. The material to be used for the occlusal rim bases must be specified. This may be polystyrene (a vacuum formed base) or shellac for the maxilla with wax and a wire strengthener being acceptable for the mandible. Acrylic resin may also be used and if permanent acrylic bases are requested these should be made in clear, heat-cured resin. In this event you must prepare a post dam on the upper cast and indicate the position of a palatal relief if required. Wax bases are *never* suitable for upper rims.

It is always advisable after pouring the master casts to retain the individual trays until all treatment has been completed.

Recording jaw relations. It is important to remember that previous dentures may provide useful information on the appropriate jaw relationship, occlusal plane, incisal level and the relationship of teeth to soft tissues. Any alterations to these factors that may be required should have been noted at the treatment-planning stage.

Clinical procedure

If the occlusal rims are constructed on acrylic bases, the fitting surfaces should be examined for sharp edges, acrylic 'pearls' and excessive undercuts. These must be corrected before proceeding. If the acrylic resin has been extended into bony undercuts, disclosing wax or pressure relief cream may be used to locate any area requiring adjustment. The stability, retention and peripheral extension of upper and lower occlusal rims should be

assessed and modified if necessary. If retention is persistently poor it must be decided whether this is the result of an inaccurate cast. If this is the case, the master impressions should be repeated or a wash impression recorded if heat-cured baseplates are being used. Remember to chill occlusal rims frequently in cold water in order to minimise distortion.

The presence of dentures in the mouth will modify the rest position. Measurements of the resting face height should normally be made with the lower rim in place.

The upper record rim is adjusted so that:

- lip support is correct
- incisal height is correct
- occlusal plane is correct (parallel to the alar-tragus and interpupillary lines)
- labial and buccal contour is correct
- the centre line is marked.

The lower rim should be adjusted to correct the buccolingual contour posteriorly and correct the labial contour anteriorly. The rim should sit in the neutral zone. It should be trimmed to establish even bilateral contact at the retruded contact position. In this respect, the patient should be asked to close until the rims first contact. Excessive pressure may cause them to tilt or be displaced into the alveolar mucosa, giving the appearance of even contact when, in fact, it does not exist. In some cases, the patient may be helped to find the retruded position by asking them to curl the tongue back to contact the posterior border of the upper occlusal rim.

An assessment should be made of the rest vertical dimension and vertical dimension of occlusion both from facial appearance and from measurement using the Willis gauge or the two dots technique. This should ensure that there is an adequate intraocclusal clearance.

When satisfied that the patient is consistently occluding in the retruded jaw relation at the correct vertical dimension of occlusion, make locating marks in the midline and buccally. Remove the rims and place them together outside the mouth using the locating marks. The jaw relation is now ready to be recorded but prior to this cut 'V'-shaped notches in upper rim and the buccal locating mark and remove 2 mm of occlusal rim height from the mesial aspect of the locating mark to the distal end of the rim on the lower.

Place modelling wax on the trimmed posterior surface of the lower rim and soften it thoroughly. Stabilise the rims with fingers and encourage the patient to close into retruded jaw relation (check locating marks are coincident) and wait until the wax has hardened. After removing rims from the mouth, check that casts can be placed into the rims without any premature contacts distally. Also ensure that the rims can be separated and re-located accurately.

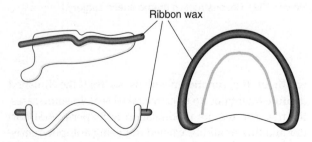

Fig. 67 Positioning of red ribbon wax for beading to create a land area on a master model.

Select teeth that are appropriate for the age, sex and racial characteristics of the patient. Reference may be made to previous dentures if the patient was happy with their appearance.

Cut the post dam on the master cast and outline any areas of the cast requiring relief (this will have been done at an earlier stage if heat-cured bases are used).

Final laboratory prescription

Record the shade, mould, and material to be used for the artificial teeth on the Laboratory Card. Indicate the type of articulator (average movement or semi-adjustable) on which the dentures are to be set up and indicate any aspects of the occlusal rims that are to be copied in the trial dentures. Indicate the type of bases required for the trial dentures. All casts should be mounted using a split cast technique.

Trial dentures

An examination of the completed set up on the articulator should be carried out before trying in the mouth, and any discrepancies noted. The occlusion is then assessed, checking balance in excursive movements. If the trial dentures are not correct on the articulator, this must be rectified before proceeding.

In the mouth, carry out a complete assessment of the trial dentures including:

- stability and retention
- peripheral extension and shape of polished surfaces
- positioning of teeth in relation to neutral zone
- occlusion should be assessed visually (articulating paper is *not* necessary at this stage, but care must be taken to stabilise the bases on their respective supporting tissues)
- interocclusal clearance to give a satisfactory interocclusal clearance is assessed using the Willis bite gauge
- appearance including the shade, mould and position of the anterior teeth and the contour of the labial flanges; check that the appearance is natural (a completely even arrangement of teeth usually looks *unnatural*), and modify if necessary
- re-check occlusion if the positions of the anterior teeth have been modified as this may result in occlusal interference.

After carrying out any corrections that are necessary, obtain patient's comments. *Do not proceed to finish unless the patient is satisfied, especially with the appearance* (record this in the notes).

If the occlusion and vertical dimension of occlusion is incorrect it means that the previous jaw registration was also incorrect. Accordingly, a new jaw registration will require to be recorded using the trial denture as an occlusal rim. In this case, it is usually necessary to remove all posterior teeth from the lower denture and replace them with a miniature occlusal rim. This can then be modified until the correct occlusion is obtained, and the dentures sealed together at the new registration.

Where the occlusion of trial dentures is subject to such modifications, the casts must be remounted on the articulator to the new registration as the jaw relationship has been changed. The dentures would then proceed to being re-set and tried in again at the next visit.

Laboratory prescription

The prescription should state definitely whether dentures can be finished or if a further trial is required. If the jaw relationship has been re-recorded, the casts are re-mounted on the articulator and a second trial stage is carried out.

If the dentures are to be processed, use of the split-cast technique will avoid occlusal errors during processing. Instructions should be given for any special colouring of the acrylic matrix.

One of the possible faults that can occur in the laboratory is porosity within the acrylic resin.

Porosity

Contraction porosity results when insufficient acrylic dough has been placed to create an excess or flash. Alternatively, the application of insufficient pressure during curing can lead to porosity voids dispersed throughout the whole mass of the denture base.

Gaseous porosity results if the temperature of the dough is raised significantly above the boiling point of the monomer (100°C), producing spherical voids in the hottest part of the curing dough. This occurs most commonly in the lingual flanges of a lower denture.

Granular porosity results from evaporation of the monomer during preparation. Proportioning of the powder to liquid ratio is dependent on allowing each powder particle to become wetted by monomer. The mixture is left to stand until it reaches the right consistency suitable for packing into the gypsum mould. During this standing period a lid should be placed on the mixing vessel to prevent evaporation of the monomer. Loss of monomer during this stage can produce granular porosity in the set material, which is characterised by a blotchy opaque surface.

Final dentures

The processed dentures should be checked for any sharp edges, acrylic 'pearls' or excessive undercuts on the fitting surface. Insert each denture separately and check on fit and comfort to patient. An examination of the occlusion in the mouth can be done either visually or using articulating paper.

Visual assessment is made by observing and by asking the patient if the teeth are meeting with equal pressure on both sides of the mouth when the mouth is closed gently.

Articulating paper is used to confirm these findings and to locate precisely any premature contacts. A heavy mark made by the paper may indicate where the initial contact is being made. Fossa rather than cusp tips should be ground at this stage only. Beware of artefacts, such as those produced by tilting of the dentures. This would produce marks from the articulating paper on both sides of the mouth, whereas initial observations may have indicated that the first occlusal contact is only on one side.

Remember if any occlusal faults are diagnosed, it is a clinical and not a laboratory error providing the split-cast technique has been used. Relatively minor occlusal discrepancies may be adjusted at the chairside until:

- the occlusal pressure on both sides of the mouth is the same
- the occlusal *contacts* indicated by articulating paper are primarily on 654/456; heavy contacts distally or anteriorly should be avoided as these may cause tipping of the dentures
- lateral and protrusive movement is possible without cuspal interference causing displacement of the dentures.

Chairside occlusal adjustments are particularly difficult; where there is any doubt, a check record should be obtained.

Check record

A check record is advisable for the correction of occlusal errors that are too large to adjust easily at the chairside. This technique is also more reliable and accurate than major adjustment made at the chairside using articulating paper. Narrowed wax wafers, constructed from one thickness of pink modelling wax, are sealed to the occlusal surfaces of the lower posterior teeth and adjusted so that the patient occludes evenly on the wafers in retruded jaw relation with the teeth separated by a distance less than the freeway space. The teeth should not penetrate through the wax, otherwise tooth contact may cause displacement of the dentures and/or the mandible. This occlusal registration may be refined using registration paste. The dentures are then re-mounted on an average movement, or semi-adjustable, articulator.

The articulator is closed with the incisal pin removed, and the occlusal contacts are checked visually and with articulating paper. Adjustments are carried out until an even occlusion is obtained. The dentures are re-inserted and the occlusion checked in the mouth. This is often a major saving in time if an occlusal error is found at the initial insertion stage. A face bow is unnecessary for check record adjustments.

The time taken for re-mounting can be reduced significantly if the need for a check record is anticipated at the trial stage. The laboratory should be asked to return the processed dentures for the fit stage with the upper denture and cast located by the split cast mounting. It is then only necessary for the occlusal record to be obtained and the lower denture to be re-mounted before the adjustments can be carried out.

Advice to patients

Preferably a printed leaflet giving instructions in respect of new dentures should be discussed with your patient after the final dentures have been inserted. In particular, the importance of good denture hygiene should be emphasised. If an immersion cleaner is recommended, a hypochlorite type is the most suitable. Any mechanical cleaning should be done with a brush that allows access and has good adaptability to all surfaces of the denture. A small multitufted toothbrush is very suitable.

If the patient has to leave the new dentures out because of pain or soreness, request that the dentures be worn for 24 hours before the review appointment, in order that the cause of the discomfort may be more readily detected. Under no circumstances should the patient attempt adjustment of the dentures.

Cleaning routine
- A twice daily routine of brushing, soaking and then brushing again should be adopted. This will help keep the denture clean, fresh and free from plaque.
- Brushing the denture helps to get rid of food and other difficult debris. Using a small-headed toothbrush helps to gain access to awkward corners and a soft brush avoids damaging the denture. Toothpaste should never be used as it is too abrasive and will leave small scratches on the acrylic surface.
- After brushing, the denture should be soaked in a specialist cleaner to help to remove stubborn stains, calculus and plaque.

Common complaints of the edentulous patient

Most prosthetic complaints can be prevented or minimised by adequate diagnosis, treatment planning and treatment plus attention to F/F. Preprosthetic radiographic investigation can prevent the finding of retained roots, unerupted teeth and bone pathology after the new dentures have been constructed; however, this should not be done as a matter of course. Pretreatment case history and clinical investigation with a detailed assessment of any existing dentures should aid the solution of such problems as correct face height, tooth position and polished contour.

Table 8 Common complaints of patients with dentures

Complaint	Probable cause	Treatment
Generalised discomfort over the denture-bearing areas	Increased occlusal face height	Occlusal adjustment or, more commonly, remake
	Occlusal interference in lateral and protrusive movements	Occlusal adjustment
	Movement of denture bases over basal tissues	Soft reline; balanced articulation with free sliding contact
	Incorrect anteroposterior relationship of dentures, i.e. non-coincidence of tooth and muscular positions	Occlusal adjustment
	Increased free monomer	Remake with correct curing cycle
Lack of chewing pressure, 'collapsed face', generalised facial discomforts	Decreased occlusal face height	Use cold-cure acrylic (occlusal pivots) or splint to build up occlusal face height then remake one or both dentures
Angular cheilitis	Lack of facial support (rarely occlusal face height)	Build up canine prominence or move anterior teeth forward; use antifungal cream; increase denture hygiene
Pain over crest of ridge (especially lower anterior region)	Irregular bony contour following abnormal healing pattern	X-ray, surgery
	Irregular soft tissue following socketed immediate dentures	Resilient lining for patients, for whom surgery is contraindicated
Localised pain	Irregularities on fitting surface	Adjustment
	Premature contact	Occlusal adjustment
	Buried roots, unerupted teeth, cysts, etc.	X-ray, surgery
	Excess undercut utilised	Relieve
Pain in sulcus		
Ulcer	Overextension	Relieve
Denture-induced hyperplasia	Overextension	Severe relief; may not resolve, then surgery
Localised pain in lower premolar region	Pressure on superficial mental nerve	Relieve denture, surgery: repositioning only to be used in exceptional cases Resilient lining
Pain on one side	Premature contact, poor articulation	Analyse occlusion (check record) and articulation, then adjust
Pain from cheek and tongue	Teeth not set in neutral zone; especially if no horizontal overlap	Reduce width of teeth and provide horizontal overlap
Denture displaces on opening or in speech	Overextension of border	Reduce border, develop new border and replace in acrylic resin
	Underextension of border	Develop new border and replace in acrylic resin
	Anterior teeth too far forward of ridge	Reposition anterior teeth, F/F will probably have to be remade
Upper denture	Inadequate post dam	Trace and reprocess or cold-cure
	Excessively deep post dam	Remove excess and polish post dam area
	Interference of coronoid process on opening	Reduce thickness of flange
	Bulky flange	Reduce thickness of flange
Lower denture	Incorrect shape of polished surfaces	Recontour
	Excessive thickness of flange in region of modiolus	Reduce
	Posterior teeth outside neutral zone	Reduce width of teeth or remake
	Insufficient room for tongue	Increase/remake
Speech defect	New F/F	Encouragement and perseverance Reduce thickness of denture to provide more tongue space Speech analysis and adjustment

(Continued overleaf)

Table 8 (*contd.*)

Poor mastication	Cuspless teeth Acrylic teeth replacing porcelain	Provide grooves in teeth (inverted cusps) Replace with porcelain
Dry mouth	Systemic factors and medication	Salivary substitute
General inability to accommodate	Menopausal Age changes High oral awareness Change in denture shape	Meticulous attention to detail and encouragement
Nausea	Denture extended onto soft palate Lack of retention Reduced tongue space Inability to accept such a large amount of acrylic	Reduce Correct Recontour polished surface Horseshoe design for upper
'Teeth meet too soon', 'can't open mouth far enough for food'	Increased occlusal face height	Reduce or remake F/F
Appearance	Insufficient attention at try-in Unwillingness of patient to put function before aesthetics	Correct Attempt to reach understanding
Denture stomatitis	Ill-fitting denture Fungal infection Increased free monomer	Reline/remake Denture hygiene; antifungal cream Remake: correct curing cycle
Midline fracture	Ill-fitting dentures Teeth set excessively off the ridge F/– against lower standing teeth Fatigue	Reline/remake Remake Metal palate/sufficient overjet Rebase

However, complaints will still occur with both new and old dentures. Table 8 lists some of the more common complaints, their probable causes and suggested treatment.

Relines or rebases

A reline involves the addition of a material to the fitting surface of a denture base. A rebase involves the removal and replacement of virtually all the denture base, namely the fitting and polished surface of the denture.

Advantages of a reline

- can be done at the chairside or in the laboratory
- can be permanent or temporary
- will improve the retention of an ill-fitting denture
- a resilient lining can be added to a previous denture base.

Advantages of a rebase

- will not increase the thickness of the palate
- will remove the majority of the previous denture base if, for example, bleaching has occurred.

There are few indications these days for a full rebase as it is often more satisfactory to consider a copy technique of the denture that would have been rebased; this will not necessitate the removal of the denture from the patient.

4.2 Copy dentures

Learning objectives

You should

- understand the indications and advantages of a copy denture technique over a more conventional approach to complete denture construction

- appreciate the clinical and technical stages involved in such a technique.

Tradition in dentistry dies hard as it does in other fields, and many dentists still persist in starting from the assumption that a patient presents no valuable information from the existing prosthesis and a conventional technique of denture construction can always produce a better result. This, of course, is not always the case, as patients who have worn dentures satisfactorily over a long period of time have developed a neuromuscular feedback with relation to the spatial relationship of the denture to the surrounding tissues. It is for such patients that the concept of the copy denture can yield satisfactory results.

In this respect, however, it is important to realise that the copy denture does not simply replicate the current dentures worn by the patient. It is designed specifically to reproduce the favourable aspects of the current prosthesis such as tooth position and polished surfaces, while improving the adaptation and occlusion. Copy dentures are particularly useful for elderly patients with good denture-wearing experience.

Indications

There are a number of situations where copy dentures are advisable:

- correct position of teeth in the neutral zone or correct zone of adaptation and the polished surfaces are satisfactory
- loss of retention in otherwise favourable dentures requiring replacement
- wear of the occlusal surfaces
- replacement of immediate dentures
- spare set of dentures.

Typical dental history that would suggest an indication for copy dentures:

- elderly patients presenting with satisfactory complete dentures
- worn occlusal surfaces, indicating long-term acceptability
- deterioration of denture base materials
- patient requests 'spare set' of dentures
- patient with a history of denture problems, make controlled modifications to copy previously most successful dentures.

Clinical advantages include:
- no alteration or mutilation of existing dentures
- no period for the patient without their dentures
- three clinical stages
- simple duplication procedure, less time than conventional impressions.

Technical advantages include:
- no individual trays or record blocks required
- infrequent re-articulation of teeth for try-in necessary
- elimination of repolishing after border adjustments
- no thickening of palate in the finished denture, as occurs in some reline procedures
- only two laboratory stages.

Alginate copy box technique

First clinical stage

Any modifications are made at the first clinical stage (Box 14).

Laboratory stage

Wax-acrylic replicas are poured by adding wax into the mould to 1 mm past the gingival margins of the

---

Box 14 Technique for copying existing denture

1. Correct any under- or overextension using greenstick or acrylic border moulding material.
2. Add labial flange (if required) to open face denture using impression compound.
3. Use a wax wafer to provide desired occlusal face height and decide whether increase to be on F/ alone or /F alone or shared between the two. It may be necessary to use occlusal pivots if the occlusal vertical dimension needs increased significantly.
4. Choose shade.
5. Copy denture utilising alginate and copy boxes (Fig. 68).
6. Send copy boxes to laboratory with prescription.

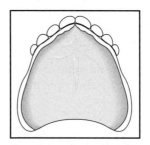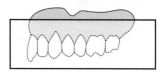

Fig. 68 Denture copied by insertion in a copy box.

teeth and allowed to set. The base of the wax is then scored and self-cured acrylic is poured into the closed mould through previously cut sprue holes and allowed to polymerise. A stone duplicate is cast into the mould once the wax and acrylic copy has been removed. This stone mould can be used for comparison of the copy try-in. The denture templates are then removed from the moulds and articulated using the wax wafer provided. The wax teeth are then removed and replaced by acrylic denture teeth of appropriate shade and mould. This will provide trial dentures for the second clinical stage. Grooves are cut in the palate and filled in with wax (Fig. 69) to allow removal of palate at a later stage.

Second clinical stage

At the second clinical stage the trial dentures are assessed by clinician and patient and any errors in occlusion or tooth position corrected, necessitating a retry. When the trial dentures are satisfactory they should be prepared for impression taking. This involves removing any undercuts, reduction of the peripheral border and modification using greenstick or a border moulding self-cured acrylic resin. The surfaces of the replica are polished with vaseline and wash impressions are recorded using zinc oxide/eugenol or low-viscosity elastomer (if hard tissue undercuts are

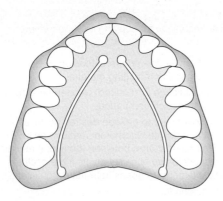

Fig. 69 Grooves cut in the palate to allow its removal later.

present in the mouth) using the closed mouth technique. Occlusal relationships should be maintained. The position, width and depth of required post dam are determined.

Final laboratory stage

The functional borders are preserved and stone casts are poured. The acrylic palate is removed and an even thickness palate is waxed-up.

Third clinical stage

The new dentures are checked for fit, extension and occlusion. A later review is arranged.

Common problems

The dentist may have several problems:

- the copy technique itself (some dentists have never been taught this technique as undergraduates)
- attempting the impossible, by using the copy denture technique in a patient for whom it is clearly not indicated
- copy flasks; some flasks are very expensive
- forgetting to take the shade
- finding a laboratory that is comfortable with the technique
- inadequate information on the prescription.

Similarly, certain problems are encountered by technicians:

- duplicating the dentures; many laboratories duplicate the denture completely in wax or self-cured acrylic
- articulating the copy
- setting up, copying the previous arrangement
- waxing up
- finishing, removing the palate and replacing a wax palate
- grinding of denture teeth to fit acrylic base
- registration problems
- the NHS fee.

4.3 Immediate replacement dentures

Learning objectives

You should

- understand the concept of immediate replacement dentures

- comprehend the clinical stages involved in immediate denture construction.

An immediate denture is defined as a denture that is made prior to the extraction of the natural teeth and which is inserted into the mouth immediately after the extraction of those teeth. It may involve total or partial replacement. In our society, it is important that people are seen with teeth, and generally it is unacceptable that patients should be rendered edentulous without any replacement prosthesis. As overall dental health has improved, the total removal of teeth followed by the provision of complete dentures has become uncommon. It is now more usual to provide simple immediate additions to existing dentures or to provide an immediate partial denture.

Advantages of immediate dentures

There are several advantages for the patient:

- maintenance of the soft tissue contour of the face
  — dentures will support the soft tissues around the face in their correct position once teeth are lost
  — prevent collapse of tissues together with the occurrence of infection, such as angular cheilitis
- maintenance of mental and physical well-being
  — the patient is not seen to be edentulous; this is important for business, domestic and social purposes
  — aesthetics are maintained by placing the artificial teeth in a position similar to natural teeth or improved by changing the position
- adaptation to dentures is aided
  — maintain tooth position
  — maintain muscle balance
  — prevent the formation of abnormal mandibular movements
  — aids chewing and mastication
- patients adapt to immediate dentures provided at time of extraction; consequently, the copy denture technique may be utilised to reproduce successful design features.

There are also advantages for the dentist:

- the use of existing occlusion for jaw registration procedures: teeth may act as occlusal stops, which

will provide the intercuspal position and the correct occlusal vertical dimension
- Aesthetic consideration: shape and size of the teeth are known, which will assist selection (this may prove to be a problem rather than an advantage if teeth have drifted owing to periodontal disease)
- haemorrhage control.

Disadvantages of immediate dentures

Immediate dentures do have a number of disadvantages:

- good co-operation is required, with the need for close supervision
- alveolar bone resorption occurs rapidly, leading to loss of adaptation
- after care may require many visits including relines/rebases/new dentures
- increased cost: the provision of relines and further denture provision makes the treatment costly
- no trial denture stage possible: this is a big disadvantage as it is not possible to show the patient what the teeth will eventually look like
- gross irregularities of teeth make processing difficult, e.g. class II division II, bulbous tuberosities/tori
- surgical and anaesthetic difficulties
  — cysts/osteosclerosis may present difficulties in planning shape of ridge
  — special care for infective endocarditis/diabetes/coronary heart disease
  — dilaceration
  — multirooted teeth.

Types of immediate denture

Immediate dentures can be flanged or socket fit.
Flanged dentures are:

- retentive
- easier to reline and rebase
- may be difficult to place where there is an undercut – use of partial flange.

Socket-fit dentures are:

- made so the teeth sit into sockets of the extracted teeth
- aesthetically good initially
- contraindicated in mandible as have uneven ridge
- prone to loss of aesthetics as resorption continues
- difficult to reline/rebase or to add flange
- have poor retention
- used in practice because of poor technical understanding of biological problems.

Wherever possible, a flange denture should always be designed.

Diagnosis

The difficulties involved with immediate denture provision *must* be explained to patients. The patient needs:

- clear explanation of the technique
- visits to be planned
- to know which teeth are to be removed beforehand
- motivation.

The health of the oral and facial tissues must be assessed:

- soft tissues: basic periodontal evaluation, probing depths give an indication of the initial collapse/retraction of soft tissues; pre-extraction scaling and polishing
- hard tissues: edentulous areas, charting of teeth, use of an orthopantomograph and periapical radiographs of the teeth to be removed.

Treatment planning

For a one tooth immediate denture when no denture is present:

1. Preliminary and/or master impressions, usually in alginate
2. Select shape and shade of tooth
3. Extraction of tooth/teeth and delivery of dentures.

For a one tooth addition to an existing denture:

1. Impression of mouth with denture in situ
2. Addition of denture tooth/teeth as soon as possible
3. Extraction of tooth/teeth and delivery of denture (preferably within 1 to 2 days).

For multiple teeth immediate denture, one of three options is possible:

1. Extract all the teeth at one time and insert immediate dentures

or

2. Extract posterior teeth prior to making immediate dentures to replace anterior teeth (disadvantage is that it may lead to tongue spread)

or

3. Post immediate dentures.

In general, options 1 or 2 are undertaken. If option 3 is selected, difficulties can arise because of resorption of ridges during denture construction.

Clinical stages

The clinical stages are:

1. Preliminary impressions in alginate with or without impression compound

2. Master impressions in alginate
3. Occlusal record rims for existing edentulous areas
4. Trial stage
5. Delivery of dentures and extraction of teeth
6. Review appointments.

Laboratory stage

Trimming of casts occurs between try-in and before processing of dentures. The cast must be prepared by the dental surgeon as he/she alone has seen the patient and undertaken the clinical examination. The cast is marked with a pencil to show the gingival margin, the long axis of the teeth and the length of the teeth. The teeth are removed from the cast. The stone is removed to a depth that is predetermined by the probing depth around the teeth and information from any radiographs. In a flanged denture, the stone is trimmed to simulate the ridge following tooth extraction.

Surgery

In extreme cases, surgery (alveolectomy; very rare nowadays) of the ridges is undertaken at the same time as tooth extraction. This may be indicated if there is a large undercut or if marked repositioning of the teeth is to be undertaken. It is undesirable to remove the cortical plate of bone as the rate and amount of bone resorption is unpredictable.

Review appointments

It is important to review a patient with an immediate denture at regular intervals especially in the first few weeks and months. The initial days are primarily concerned with the postoperative care of the healing tooth sockets, while the later reviews are directed at the management of the resorption.

A simple timetable for reviewing a patient is as follows:

at 24 hours, a general check is made of the overall comfort of the dentures and to ensure no major ulceration has occurred and that the sockets are healing well

at 1 week, a more detailed check and adjustment of dentures can be made

at 1 month, the socket has healed and a chairside temporary reline may be required

at 3 to 6 months, the management of loss of fit of the dentures owing to bone resorption is undertaken; this may involve relines and/or rebases, which are undertaken at either the chairside or with the aid of the production laboratory

at 12 months, a replacement denture is made using the copy denture technique.

4.4 Overdentures

Learning objectives

You should

- comprehend the advantages of overdentures over more conventional dentures

- acknowledge the different overdenture preparations that can be prepared and the advantages and disadvantages of each.

An overdenture is a prosthesis that gains additional support by covering one or more teeth, prepared roots or implants beneath its impression surface.

Indications
- converting a partially dentate individual to complete dentures
- elderly patient with a few remaining teeth and a mucosal borne partial denture
- attrition/erosion/abrasion
- cleft plate and surgical defects
- hypodontia
- potentially difficult complete denture requirements.

Contraindications
- poor oral hygiene
- rampant uncontrolled caries in the remaining dentition
- uncontrolled periodontal disease
- inadequate interarch space.

Advantages of overdentures
- maintenance of alveolar bone
- sensory feedback
  — assistance in control of masticatory force
  — recognising size and texture of objects
  — position of mandible during function
- minimal load thresholds
- tactile sensitivity discrimination
  — complete denture wearers are six times less efficient at detecting small objects
  — patient with an overdenture is able to exert high forces during mastication with more precision
- reduction of psychological trauma.

The ideal overdenture scenario would be the retention of four root-filled teeth in the lower arch, the canines and the first molars. This situation, however, is highly improbable as the first molars are commonly amongst the first teeth to be lost and, therefore, are unlikely to be one of four remaining teeth. The canines are important teeth as they have long roots and are highly proprioceptive but also command an important position in the line of the arch.

Abutment

Abutment selection depends upon:

- periodontal status
- number and location in arch
- canines and molars where possible
- conservation status
- need for root canal therapy
- presence of bony undercuts
- extra retention from teeth
- economics.

Periodontal disease

With respect to periodontal disease in patients wearing overdentures, it has been shown that:

- 35% show a significant loss of attachment within the first 3 years
- Only 50% of dentures are plaque free, and the majority of patients wear their dentures at night
- Disease is related to both poor denture and poor oral hygiene.

Caries prevalence within 5 years of placement in studies of overdenture abutments varies from 13 to 35%. The use of topical fluorides (0.4% stannous fluoride) is indicated on a daily basis for these patients.

Preparation of coronal root surface

Table 9 describes various preparations of the coronal root surface for overdenture placement.

The presence of overdenture abutments allows the loads from occlusal forces to be dissipated over a large area as the support of the periodontal ligament is brought into function. This along with the increase in tactile discrimination and the maintenance of alveolar bone levels make the benefits of this technique invaluable in dealing with certain clinical denture problems.

4.5 Removable partial dentures

Learning objectives

You should

- understand the basic concepts of partial denture construction

- appreciate the importance of design for the prevention of further dental disease

- be able to classify and describe a partial denture using terminology that will be understood by colleagues.

Treatment planning for partial dentures is commonly misunderstood. This can only be undertaken following a careful examination for caries, periodontal disease and any surgical requirements, and then by recording casts of the mouth and mounting them on an articulator. This will indicate where restorations or periodontal treatment are appropriate and also where tooth modification might be required prior to design. In all patients requiring removable partial dentures, this should be undertaken before embarking upon any other form of restorative treatment. This is because the type of denture required may influence the overall treatment plan, for example rest seats incorporated into class II restorations, full veneer crowns contoured to provide undercut areas for retention or tooth extraction as a result of overeruption. Partial denture design intends to:

- preserve what remains
- restore what is missing
- prevent future disease.

When making a partial denture the following questions need to be addressed:

- Is the prosthesis necessary?
- Is the patient healthy?
- Is the patient suitable for the prosthesis?
- How large a space is to be restored?
- By what structures is the prosthesis to be supported?
- How is the prosthesis to be made?

Partial denture classification

A simple and effective classification is one that describes partial dentures in terms of the nature of the support utilised by the partial denture:

- teeth
- mucosa
- teeth and mucosa.

Further information can be gained by a classification of the partially edentulous arches which relates the edentulous spaces to the remaining teeth (Fig. 70; Kennedy 1928).

The following points should be noted when using this classification:

- the most posterior edentulous area determines the class
- additional edentulous areas are called modifications
- the size of the modification is not important
- if a third molar is missing and not to be replaced, it is not considered in the classification.

Preliminary impressions

A stock tray is selected and modified with impression compound or autopolymerising acrylic as appropriate. Normally a high-viscosity alginate should be used as this will compensate for the lack of fit of the stock tray. A thin layer of adhesive should be applied to the tray prior to mixing the alginate.

Table 9 Preparation of the coronal root surface for overdenture placement

Preparation	Advantages	Disadvantages
Flat facing	Plenty of occlusal clearance; no lateral forces applied; easy to place attachments	Risk of gingival overgrowth; difficult to keep clean; no real additional stability
Dome-shaped facing	Favourable crown:root ratio; efficient plaque control; sufficient occlusal clearance	RCT normally required; may provide less retention and stability than thimble shape
Thimble-shaped facing	Provides maximum retention and stability; RCT may not be required; patient is aware that a tooth still remains	May be insufficient occlusal clearance; unfavourable crown:root ratio; minimal room for attachment placement; protection of tooth surface may be required

The presence of overdenture abutments allows the loads from occlusal forces to be dissipated over a large area as the support of the periodontal ligament is brought into function. This along with the increase in tactile discrimination and the maintenance of alveolar bone levels make the benefits of this technique invaluable in dealing with certain clinical denture problems.

Laboratory prescription

It is essential at this and at subsequent stages to indicate precisely what is required for the next appointment. The prescription on the laboratory card must be clear and comprehensive. If there is any possibility of confusion, it is essential to discuss the case personally with the technician involved. Indicate the type and material of individual trays required. If the laboratory card is not completed and dated, work may not be available for the next appointment.

Design

The design of a partial denture should always be determined before the master impressions are recorded. In this respect, the preliminary casts should be mounted on an articulator and surveyed to produce the desired design. In many cases where there are sufficient teeth, casts can be placed in occlusion by hand prior to mounting. In other situations, it will be unnecessary to construct occlusal rims to register the jaw relationship

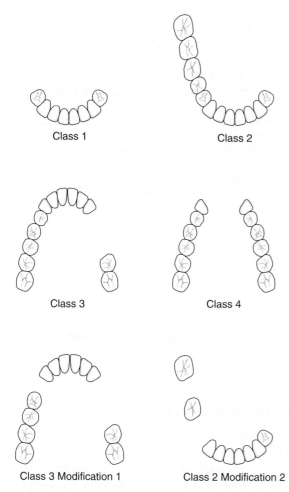

Fig. 70 Classification of the partially edentulous arches. Class 1 = bilateral free end saddles; Class 2 = Unilateral free end saddle; Class 3 = unilateral bounded saddle; Class 4 = single bounded saddle anterior to abutment teeth (from Kennedy 1928 Partial denture construction. In: Dental Items of Interest, pp. 3–8. New York).

of the patient. A provisional design should then be produced and at this stage a decision should be made on the need for possible tooth preparation or modification. This may indicate that the following may be necessary:

- rest seat preparation to provide sufficient space and horizontal surface for any support component
- modification of tooth contour by grinding or the addition of light-cured composite resin to improve the action of clasp arms or the occlusal relationship.

The proposed design should then be transferred to the study cast, which should be retained for reference until the trial stage has been completed. The design prescription must be clear and comprehensive. The design will describe:

- saddles
- support
- retention

- bracing and reciprocation
- connector
- indirect retention.

Second clinical visit

Normally the second visit will be for master impressions where the casts have already been mounted and a design determined. When the casts cannot be mounted however, the second visit will be devoted to recording the jaw relationship of the patient prior to mounting casts on the articulator and developing a design.

Recording jaw relationships

If an occlusal stop is present in the mouth, it may be that the associated intercuspal position is acceptable. If there is horizontal (antero-posterior or lateral) deviation of the mandible after the initial occlusal contact, it may be necessary to correct the deflective occlusal contact by tooth modification or, in extreme situations, extraction. If there is loss of vertical dimension of occlusion (OVD), the appropriate increase will have to be determined by adjusting occlusal rims in relation to the rest vertical dimension (RVD).

For the purpose of jaw relationships and their registration, partially dentate patients can be divided into two categories:

- patients without an occlusal stop to indicate the correct intercuspal position or vertical dimension of occlusion
- patients with occlusal contact in the intercuspal position.

No occlusal stop to indicate intercuspal position
The OVD is determined by establishing the RVD and modifying the occlusal rims until the OVD is some 2–4 mm short of the RVD, this distance indicating the amount of interocclusal clearance. The horizontal jaw relationship recorded should be the retruded position. Box 15 outlines the procedure.

Occlusal contact in intercuspal position
If there is occlusal contact, the rims should be adapted until the natural occlusal contact is observed (Box 16).

Laboratory prescription
The prescription will cover a number of points:

- shade, material and mould of artificial teeth
- if the next stage is the try-in of a metal framework, the design should be drawn on the laboratory card and full instructions given, including the path of insertion decided by the clinician
- the study casts should be retained as a guide for the technician

Box 15 Technique to establish jaw relationships in patients without an occlusal stop

1. Occlusal rims (and wax trial dentures) should only be placed in the mouth long enough to carry out a particular clinical procedure. On removal, they should be chilled in a bowl of cold water to avoid distortion.
2. In the mouth, the fit and extension of the rim should be checked and modified if necessary to produce acceptable stability.
3. The upper occlusal rim should be adjusted so that the occlusal plane is correct in relation to the remaining upper natural teeth. If there is an anterior saddle, the rim must indicate the correct incisal level and degree of lip support. Removal of wax from the palatal aspect of this rim might be necessary in order to allow closure of the mandible into the tooth position while retaining the incisal level.
4. The occlusal stop should be checked when the patient closes with the upper rim in place. If the occlusion shows a premature contact between a tooth and the opposing occlusal rim, the offending part of the rim should be adjusted until the occlusal stop is re-established.
5. The lower rim should then be adjusted until the occlusal stop has again been established.
6. Wax should be removed or added from the buccal and lingual surfaces of the rims until they lie in the neutral zone and blend with the natural teeth.
7. The lower rim should be modified so that there is a small gap (about 1 mm) between the occlusal surface of the rim and the opposing teeth or rim when the natural teeth are in contact.
8. The intercuspal or retruded contact position should be recorded using wax or an occlusal registration material such as Bite Registration Paste. Petroleum jelly should be spread thinly over the opposing wax rim to act as a separating medium.
9. The casts should be placed in occlusion using the occlusal rims and checked to determine that the tooth relationship on the casts is the same as that in the mouth. If there is a premature contact between the heels of a cast and the opposing block or cast, this should be eliminated.

- if the metal denture is restoring lower free-end saddles, consider the need for the altered cast technique (see below): if the technique is to be employed, request the addition of acrylic trays to the framework in the saddle areas
- if the anterior teeth require metal backings, request a wax trial denture for the next stage so that the appearance and position of the teeth can be checked before the framework is made.

Box 16 Technique to establish jaw relationships in patients with occlusal contact

1. The occlusal stop should be checked with the natural teeth when the patient occludes with the upper rim in place. If the vertical dimension of occlusion has been increased as a result of a premature contact between a lower tooth and the occlusal rim, the offending part of the rim should be reduced until the occlusal stop is re-established.
2. The lower rim should be adjusted until there is an even occlusion at the OVD determined by the intercuspal position.
3. Locating notches should be cut in the upper rim, petroleum jelly applied as a separating medium and the intercuspal position recorded with the rims in place, using wax or registration paste.
4. The casts are placed in occlusion using the occlusal rims and checked to ensure that there is no premature contact between the heels of a cast and the opposing block or cast. Correct if necessary.

Master impressions

Master impressions are obtained at the second or third clinical visit.

Wax stops should be placed on the fitting surface of the individual trays before modifying the peripheral extension and any overextension should be corrected. Any underextension should be corrected with the addition of autopolymerising acrylic resin. When mandibular free-end saddle areas are present, border moulding of the tray in the retro-mylohyoid areas should be undertaken routinely.

The impression is recorded as described in Box 17.

Box 17 Recording the impression

1. The tray is dried and a thin layer of adhesive is applied to the whole of the inner surfaces of the tray and to an area extending 3 mm beyond the periphery of the tray. The adhesive is allowed to dry before loading the tray.
2. A low-viscosity alginate is used to record the impression. In some cases, it may be beneficial to use silicone-based or rubber-based materials.
3. If the impression is satisfactory, a cast should be poured in improved hardened dental stone as soon as possible.
4. All individual trays should be retained until treatment is completed.

Laboratory prescription

The laboratory prescription should indicate that casts are to be poured in hardened dental stone. Bearing in mind that the occlusion has already been determined naturally or by occlusal rims prior to establishing a design, the subsequent stage should be either trial dentures or the production of a metal casting. In the former situation a shade and mould of teeth must be selected.

The metal framework

- The framework must conform to the original design
- The framework must fit the cast. If the fit is unsatisfactory on the cast it will also be unsatisfactory in the mouth
- The casting should be free from porosity or other imperfections.

Note: if any of the above points are not met the casting should be returned to the laboratory.

- The position of the retentive and bracing arms should be checked relative to the survey lines
- All components that are designed to be clear of the gingival margin area should be checked to ensure that the clearance is adequate
- In the mouth, these aspects should be checked again, remembering that the likelihood of some instability in free-end saddle designs may be caused by spacing beneath the mesh retention
- The occlusion is examined to ensure that there are no premature contacts; this should be done by visual examination, from comments by the patient and with the use of articulating paper or disclosing wax. Any premature contact must be removed at this stage.

If the metal framework is satisfactory, request the setting of the teeth on the framework after choosing an appropriate shade and mould of tooth.

Altered cast technique

The altered cast technique is an impression method designed to compensate for the differential support provided to a lower partial Kennedy I or II denture base by the abutment teeth and the mucosa of the edentulous part of the alveolar ridge (Box 18).

The trial denture

The trial denture is the last stage at which modifications can be made before the wax is replaced by acrylic. A careful routine must be followed to prevent any mistakes continuing through to the finished dentures. The dentures should be examined first on the mounted casts for:

- fit of dentures on the casts
- occlusion

> **Box 18** The altered cast technique
>
> 1. The Cobalt–chromium (CoCr) casting is tried in the mouth.
> 2. A closely fitting tray is added to the framework of the free-end saddle of the CoCr skeleton with border moulding using self-cured acrylic resin or greenstick.
> 3. The recording of an impression uses zinc oxide/eugenol, with pressure only applied to the rest seat areas of the framework. No direct pressure is applied to the edentulous saddle area. The original technique used impression waxes.
> 4. The original master cast is sectioned, removing the posterior part of the model that had recorded the free-end edentulous ridge area.
> 5. The framework is seated back on the sectioned model and a new posterior section cast into the tray area.

- position of artificial teeth with regard to adjacent natural ones
- the arrangement of anterior teeth
- extension and contouring of wax flanges.

The trial dentures are then examined in the mouth for:

- fit of the dentures
- occlusion and OVD
- contouring of wax flanges with regard to peripheral extension, shaping of polished surface, coverage of gingival margins
- appearance: modify positions of teeth and incisal edges of anterior teeth to achieve a pleasing result that is acceptable to the patient
- patient's comments on appearance: as seen in the mirror and ensure that they are satisfied.

If, at this stage, the occlusion is incorrect, modifications must be carried out before continuing with the next stages. An increase in occlusal height may be achieved by adding pink modelling wax to the occlusal surfaces of posterior teeth on one of the dentures. A reduction in occlusal height is achieved by replacing the posterior teeth on one denture with wax rims and adjusting these to occlude evenly at the correct vertical dimension. Wax or bite registration paste may be used for the final recording. If the occulusion has been re-recorded it will be necessary to have a re-try to check that the occlusion is satisfactory.

Laboratory prescription

Carefully list and describe any modifications you wish the technician to carry out before finishing the dentures. Modifications at this stage should always be minor.

To ensure that interference with insertion of the finished denture will not occur as a result of inadequately blocked out tooth undercuts, request the following instructions and procedure:

- undercuts should be blocked out in wax on master cast, in respect of vertical path of insertion
- the master cast should be duplicated
- denture should be processed on duplicate cast
- the processed denture should be fitted back onto the master cast.

Final denture insertion

The denture should be checked to see that there are no sharp edges or acrylic 'pearls' on the fitting surface of the saddle areas. Insert denture into the mouth. Occasionally, the denture cannot be seated because acrylic has been processed into an undercut area on the cast; this results from inadequate blocking out of the undercuts. If the area of acrylic to be removed is not immediately apparent, use pressure relief cream. Always remove the acrylic by approaching with the bur from the fitting surface. The seal between denture and tooth in the non-undercut area should *never* be touched. In the mouth, check:

- fit of components
- retention and stability
- occlusion.

Occlusal contact is checked by asking for the patient's comments, by visual inspection and by the use of articulating paper. Articulating paper should be inserted bilateral and not unilaterally. In the latter, the patient may be encouraged to deviate the mandible to the side on which the paper is placed.

Occlusal adjustment should be continued until both the patient's comments and visual inspection confirm that even contact has been achieved in intercuspal position. Attention should be given to occlusal contacts in lateral and protrusive positions. In many patients, the dentures will be adjusted so that they conform to the occlusal guidance provided by the remaining natural teeth.

Advice to the patient

The patient must be taught the correct way to handle the denture for insertion and removal and vulnerable components must be pointed out. A printed sheet of instructions should be provided for the patient. This will mention, in particular, aspects such as cleaning/eating/wearing at night/pain/need for regular recall, including recall with the hygienist.

It is important to discuss these points verbally with the patient first of all. The purpose of such a sheet is simply to act as an aide-memoir. Finally you should ensure that the patient knows whom to contact in the event of problems arising with the denture.

The responsibility for the prosthetic care of the patient does not end with the insertion of a denture.

Review appointment

The patient should be asked for comments on the first week of wearing the dentures. A history must be taken of any complaint. Subsequent examination must be directed to diagnosing the cause of the complaint before making any adjustments. Whether or not there are any problems reported by the patient, the denture-bearing tissues must be examined and the occlusion must be checked. At times, a patient may claim to be perfectly comfortable even though extensive ulceration is present.

Any inflammation of the denture-bearing tissues that is not related to the peripheral area is most likely from occlusal causes. Therefore, a careful inspection must be made of occlusal contact in tooth position and excursive movements, and the necessary adjustments made. The impression surface of the denture must not be 'eased' empirically. Should attention of the impression surface be required, a disclosing material such as pressure indicator paste should be used.

A check must be made on the patient's oral and denture hygiene. This can be done with the use of disclosing solution. Steps to reinforce plaque control must be taken if appropriate.

Self-assessment: questions

Multiple choice questions

1. Complete denture assessment should include:
   a. A history of tooth loss
   b. A denture history
   c. A medical history
   d. A social history
   e. A summary of the patient's expectations

2. Impression compound contains:
   a. Stearic acid
   b. Borax
   c. Talc
   d. Paraffin wax
   e. Copper

3. An immediate denture is advisable for:
   a. A single tooth replacement in the anterior region of the mouth
   b. A patient who will require the surgical removal of the broken down tooth
   c. A patient who is at risk of tooth movement if a replacement unit is not placed soon after extraction
   d. A patient losing an upper second molar tooth
   e. A case where haemorrhage control may be required

4. A partial denture clasp made of cast cobalt chromium:
   a. Should not be used as an occlusally approaching clasp arm on a premolar
   b. Is more flexible than a wrought gold clasp of similar length
   c. Engages 0.5 mm undercut
   d. Is a potential food trap
   e. Can be circumferential, occlusally approaching or ginigivally approaching in design

5. The altered cast technique is used to:
   a. Account for the differential compression between hard and soft tissues
   b. Remount flasked dentures to perfect the occlusion
   c. Destroy unwanted models
   d. Construct a master cast that is altered by partial replacement with a cast of an additional impression
   e. Modify a cast to allow for rest seat preparation intra-orally

6. The indications for the 'copy denture' technique include:

   a. Recurrent fracture of a previous upper denture base
   b. A spare set of satisfactory dentures
   c. An elderly patient who has worn a satisfactory set of dentures for many years
   d. Incorrect positioning of the anterior teeth
   e. Replacement of immediate dentures

7. The choice of denture teeth:
   a. Is dependent on the age of the patient
   b. The patient's complexion
   c. Should be determined by the patient
   d. Should conform to the patient's facial contour
   e. Is related to the upper lip length

8. The neutral zone technique:
   a. Can be used in the maxilla
   b. Should have the upper denture in place while it is being recorded
   c. Is used to record the zone of minimal conflict
   d. Helps to determine the pre-extraction position of the natural dentition
   e. Requires the use of laboratory stents to locate the teeth

9. Elastic impression materials include:
   a. Plaster
   b. Alginate
   c. Zinc oxide/eugenol
   d. Agar
   e. Silicone

10. At the jaw registration stage in complete dentures:
    a. The freeway space of the dentures should be determined
    b. The horizontal relationship of the jaws is recorded
    c. The tooth shade is chosen
    d. The tooth mould is selected
    e. Heat-cured base plates may provide increased stability

11. Surveying for partial denture construction:
    a. Is only carried out on the preliminary model
    b. Is always carried out at 90° to the occlusal plane
    c. Should use an analysing rod prior to deciding the angle of survey
    d. Determines naturally occurring guideplanes
    e. Is not necessary in acrylic partial denture construction

12. Various techniques used in the management of the free-end saddle situation include:

a. Split cast technique
b. RPI (rest, plate, I bar) design
c. Altered cast technique
d. Balance of forces
e. Flexible connectors

Case history questions

Case history 1

A 60-year-old male presents complaining of a loose upper denture. He has been edentulous for over 20 years and has had two sets of complete dentures in this time. On examination, his palate presents as seen in Figure 71.

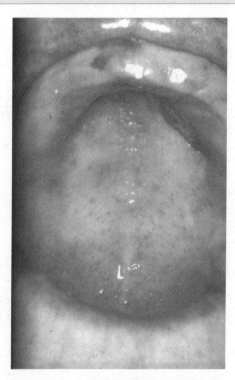

Fig. 71 Male with loose upper denture.

1. What questions in the history of this patient are important in this problem?
2. What are the priorities in the management of this patient?
3. What are the differential diagnoses?

Case history 2

A 50-year-old lady presents with an unretentive upper denture and a lower denture that causes recurrent ulceration (Fig. 72).

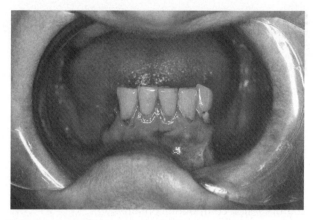

Fig. 72 Ulcerated lower arch of a 50-year-old lady.

1. What are the likely causes for the symptoms that this patient presents with?
2. How could you resolve the problem of the unretentive upper denture?
3. What treatment would be suggested to resolve the problems of her lower arch?

Essay question

List the basic principles of removable partial denture design and describe their importance in relation to the maintenance of oral health.

Short note questions

Write short notes on:

1. Disinfection of impression materials
2. Special trays
3. Heat-cured base plates
4. The important features in complete denture construction that contribute to the retention of a denture, naming three anatomical features that may affect the retention of complete dentures
5. Every denture design
6. Gingival stripping caused by partial dentures
7. Spoon dentures
8. The properties that a clasp should exhibit and list three commonly utilised materials used to construct denture clasps
9. Denture stomatatis
10. Angular cheilitis
11. Denture hygiene.

Self-assessment: answers

Multiple choice answers

1. a. **True**. A history of tooth loss will provide an approximate time-scale for the resorptive processes of that individual patient.
    b. **True**. A denture history will give some indication as to the tolerance of the patient to a prosthesis.
    c. **True**. A medical history may provide information regarding current medication that could result in a dry mouth and, therefore, affect the possible retention of a prosthesis. Several other factors in a medical history may also affect complete denture construction.
    d. **True**. A history of smoking and/or drinking will increase the prevalence of oral malignancy and may necessitate more frequent reviews to monitor the oral mucosa.
    e. **True**. It is important to assess the patient's expectations as these can often be unrealistic and may affect the patient's acceptance of a prosthesis.

2. a. **True**. Because stearic acid improves flow properties of material.
    b. **False**. Borax is used as a retarder in gypsum products.
    c. **True**. Talc increases the viscosity of the material, reducing its thermal contraction.
    d. **True**. Determines the softening temperature.
    e. **False**. Copper is metallic and is not in impression compound.

3. a. **True**. An immediate denture can provide an aesthetic replacement of an anterior tooth.
    b. **False**. An immediate denture would not be indicated as the bone contour of the area after surgical intervention is uncertain.
    c. **True**. An immediate denture can be used as a space maintainer.
    d. **False**. It is rarely necessary unless an addition to an existing partial denture can be carried out to replace a posterior unit in this manner.
    e. **True**. Although this point is often one of debate, it is generally accepted that an immediate denture can assist in haemorrhage control if constructed carefully.

4. a. **True**. A cast cobalt chromium clasp of this length will not be flexible enough to engage an undercut.
    b. **False**. A gold clasp is more flexible.

c. **False**. Engages a 0.25 mm undercut.
d. **True** Partial dentures themselves could be considered as food traps but the clasp component particularly causes a problem.
e. **True**. These are the three traditional designs of clasp arm.

5. a. **True**. This is the concept of the altered cast technique.
    b. **False**. That is the split cast technque.
    c. **False**. This is not the purpose of the technique.
    d. **True**. This is how an altered cast is carried out.
    e. **False**. This is not the purpose of the technique.

6. a. **False**. The reason for the recurrent fracture of the denture base would need to be addressed prior to remaking the denture.
    b. **True**. This is a method of duplicating dentures.
    c. **True**. If a patient has become accustomed to the polished surfaces of an existing denture then it is often advantageous to copy this.
    d. **False**. There would be no advantage of a copy technique if the tooth position had to be changed.
    e. **True**. This would mean that the original tooth position was copied.

7. a. **True**. The age of the patient will dictate tooth colour and length.
    b. **True**. This will determine tooth colour.
    c. **False**. Often patients will choose tooth colour to be too white; therefore, their approval should be sought after the dentist's selection.
    d. **True**. This will help to determine the tooth mould.
    e. **True**. The length of the upper incisors will be partly determined by the upper lip length.

8. a. **False**. The neutral zone can only be used in the mandible.
    b. **True**. Upper lip support is essential to record the neutral zone.
    c. **True**. The neutral zone is often called the zone of minimal conflict.
    d. **True**. The technique helps to determine the likely position of the original dentition.
    e. **True**. This is how the technician positions the teeth from the neutral zone impression.

9. a. **False**. Plaster is a non-elastic impression material.
    b. **True**. Alginate is an elastic impression material.

c. **False**. Zinc oxide/eugenol is a non-elastic impression material.

d. **True**. Agar is an elastic impression material.

e. **True**. Silicone is an elastic impression material.

10. a. **True**. The occlusal face height of the denture should be recorded at the jaw registration stage.

b. **True**. The relationship of the mandible to the maxilla in the retruded contact position is recorded.

c. **True**. The technician needs this information for the try-in stage.

d. **True**. The technician needs this information for the try-in stage.

e. **True**. The use of heat-cured bases does provide a more stable record rim for the registration stage.

11. a. **False**. The master model has to be surveyed also.

b. **False**. Although this is often the first choice of survey it is often the case that the path of insertion should follow a different path.

c. **True**. The use of an analysing rod helps to assess the path of insertion prior to the initial survey.

d. **True**. The use of naturally occurring guideplanes will aid greatly in the retention of a denture.

e. **False**. Undercut areas must be blocked out prior to processing an acrylic partial denture.

12. a. **False**. This technique is used to remount casts after processing.

b. **True**. The use of a mesial rest, distal plate and I bar design is commonly applied in this situation.

c. **True**. The altered cast can be used to address this clinical situation.

d. **True**. This design concept has been used in the free-end saddle situation.

e. **True**. The use of stress breaking or flexible connectors can be used in this clinical situation.

Case history answers

Case history 1

1. History taken would reveal:
   - *Social history*: this patient was a heavy smoker who smoked around 60 cigarettes a day. He was also a heavy drinker.
   - *Dental history*: the patient had experienced surgery to his front teeth prior to their extraction 10 years ago. The lesion in his palate was first noticed 6 months ago and has progressively got larger since then resulting in his denture no longer fitting.
   - *Medical history*: this may have some relevance to the problem but did not in this case.

2. Resulting from this patient's presentation and history it is unlikely that the lesion in the palate is a simple traumatic ulcer and, therefore, an urgent referral to a oral maxillofacial surgeon or an incisional biopsy must be carried out. The suggestion that the denture should be left out for a week and the situation reviewed given the history and presentation of the lesion would be ill-advised.

3. Differential diagnosis. The main palatal lesion was an adenoid cystic carcinoma, but it could have been a squamous cell carcinoma, a pleomorphic adenoma or an mucoepidermoid carcinoma. The histological appearance would have confirmed the diagnosis. The lesion on the ridge was an amalgam tattoo.

Case history 2

1. The upper denture problem is likely to be related to a flabby ridge that has developed as result of the retention of the lower natural dentition. This often results in the patient having a problem of support or stability of the denture, although there can also be a problem of retention. The recurrent oral ulceration of the lower ridge is likely to be a result of an unretentive and unstable lower denture caused by the lack of denture-bearing area and also the height discrepancy between the occlusal plane and the residual ridge.

2. The management of a unsupported or flabby ridge is by use of a selective compression impression technique or the use of a mucostatic impression technique. A brief summary of these two techniques should be included.

3. The problem of the lower arch is complex; however, the extraction of the remaining lower dentition may just transfer the problem from that of a partial denture problem to one of a complete lower denture problem. This particular case was managed by root filling the lower canines and using stud attachments to retain an acrylic partial lower denture. This solved the presenting complaints because the stud retainers stopped the movement of the lower denture, thus eliminating the traumatic ulceration.

Short note answers

1. Answer should include a summary of the guidelines on the disinfection of dental impressions (Control of Substances Hazardous to Health Regulations, 1999). An impression should be rinsed under running

water on removal from the mouth to remove any saliva, blood or debris. The impression should then be disinfected. Possible disinfectant solutions should be listed and the duration of soak stated (e.g. sodium hypochlorite 10 000 ppm for 5 minutes minimum). The effects of such disinfectants on the stability of the impression material should also be commented on.

2. Special trays are constructed of a variety of materials including shellac, acrylics and light-cured composite materials. The use of adhesives can be complemented by the addition of perforations within the tray design. Trays should be extended ideally to 2 mm short of the functional sulcus depth. The spacing of a tray is dependent on the impression material being used and varies from 3 mm spacing for impression plaster to 0.5 mm for zinc oxide/eugenol.

3. Heat-cured base plates can be used at the jaw registration stage of complete denture construction. They provide increased stability to the denture for use at this stage and give a good guide to the likely retention and stability of the completed denture. They potentially can have disadvantages in that if there is minimal inter-arch space then premature contact of the baseplates between the maxillary tuberosity region of the upper plate and the retromolar pad region of the lower can occur. The processing of the final denture can potentially cause distortion of the baseplate if it is not carried out carefully.

4. Features that contribute to retention include:
   - peripheral (border) seal
   - area of impression surface
   - accuracy of fit
   - adhesion between the saliva, denture and oral mucosa
   - cohesion within saliva film
   - orientation of the denture-supporting structures: the shape of the palate for example will influence the retention, a flatter palate providing better retention but less stability
   - correct positioning of the denture base in relation to displacing forces, namely soft tissue forces of the lips, cheeks and tongue
   - anatomical features: for example, maxillary and mandibular tori, fraenal attachments, muscle attachments, genial tubercles, hard/soft palate junction, maxillary tuberosity.

5. An Every denture conforms to a specific design to ensure gingival health. It is restricted to use in the upper arch. The denture design requires the presence of bounded saddles. The design should incorporate the following features: point contact between natural teeth and artificial teeth, wide embrasures, uncovered gingivae, distal stabilisers and a 'free occlusion'. The general principles of partial denture design should be followed.

6. An acrylic or cobalt chromium connector of a denture can cover the gingival margins of teeth. If insufficient support for the partial denture exists, then gingival stripping can occur of the dentition under load. This can be avoided by providing adequate tooth support for the denture, using dental connectors that do not cover the gingival margins of teeth and by the maintenance of good oral hygiene.

7. Spoon dentures are simple acrylic dentures made to replace one or more anterior maxillary teeth. They derive their support from the ridge and palate. They are used commonly as they are cheap, easy to construct and modify. However, such a denture is weak and non-rigid and it is commonly unretentive and poses a possible airway risk.

8. Properties should include the following.
   Strength. Should be strong enough in thin cross-section to withstand oral forces. Adding molybdenum in small amounts to cobalt chromium alloy increases its strength; however, the addition of nickel decreases its strength while increasing its ductility.
   Ductility. In cobalt chromium the grains tend to be large and, therefore, there are only two to three grains across the thickness of a clasp. This reduces its ductility and it is easily broken or distorted.
   Malleability. A malleable material can be worked into thinner sections; this property is of importance in wrought clasps.
   Proportional limit. The limit beyond which a clasp will permanently deform or fracture.
   Torsional elasticity. The rigid position of a clasp arm should be above the survey line. The torsional elasticity of the metal in the more rigid upright part provides flexibility to the horizontal arm and a more effective distribution of stress throughout the structure.
   Modulus of elasticity (resilience). The higher the modulus the shallower the undercuts that can be engaged.
   Appearance. A tooth-coloured clasp may be more aesthetically pleasing but may not provide other optimal properties. Often gold alloys are more aesthetically acceptable intra-orally than 'silver' coloured alloys.
   Three commonly used materials could be chosen from cast cobalt chromium, wrought stainless steel, cast gold, wrought gold, tooth-coloured resin clasps.

9. Denture stomatitis is a multifactorial condition, the aetiological factors include poor denture hygiene, trauma, *Candida albicans* infection, endocrine imbalance, iron deficiency anaemia, reduced salivary

flow, folate deficiency and diabetes mellitus. The clinical picture is normally a diffuse erythematous area associated with denture support. Treatment includes the establishment and control of the relevant aetiological factors.

10. Angular cheilitis is usually as a result of an infection with *Candida albicans*, *Staphylococcus aureus* and/or streptococci. It is commonly related to denture stomatitis, but other causes include iron deficiency, hypo-vitaminoses, malabsorption conditions, HIV infection and other immune defects. Investigations can include blood pictures, smears for fungal hyphae and bacteriological cultures. The treatment should involve the resolution of any systemic predisposing factors where possible and the use of topical antifungals and antibacterial agents.

11. Denture hygiene should involve a regimen of brush, soak, brush. The adherance of plaque to both acrylic and cobalt chromium requires that hygiene measures are carried out at least twice daily. The initial brushing will remove any food debris and then the use of a proprietary soaking solution will loosen and remove stains, plaque and calculus deposits. The final brushing stage will remove any residual debris. It is essential that a brush or cleanser that is not too abrasive is used as otherwise this will scratch the acrylic and potentially provide a rougher surface for plaque attachment.

Essay answer

This essay plan is to be seen as a template to the structure of the essay. The content is not exhaustive but gives an example in each area of the content that could be included.

Introduction

All removable prostheseses will by their nature attract or retain more plaque in the mouth than if an appliance were not present. However, various features of design can influence this, as well as factors of patient motivation and instruction on cleaning techniques and materials. The maintenance of oral health is also not purely dependent on oral hygiene but also relies on the design of the prosthesis, which should aim to preserve what remains and prevent future disease.

Important features to discuss include:

Saddles. Number of saddles and the need to replace all missing units to prevent overeruption or drifting has important implications.

Support. The choice between tooth support or mucosal support of the denture will influence the load distribution to the oral structures and could, therefore, affect the health of the oral tissues.

Retention. All forms of clasps will cause plaque retention; therefore, the correct number and positioning of clasps is essential to maintain oral health.

Bracing/reciprocation. The prevention of movement of a denture base during function will aid in the protection of the dental tissues.

Connector. If a connector is designed to cover as little gingival margins as possible, this will minimise gingival damage and limit plaque and debris accumulation.

Indirect retention. The provision of indirect retention will help to prevent rotational forces being applied to abutment teeth and will, therefore, be important in the maintenance of oral health.

5 Conscious sedation in dentistry

Overview

The use of drugs to help in the management of patients' anxieties regarding dental care is not new. The use of alcohol predates the invention of local analgesia, and a perusal of many art galleries will show travelling tooth pullers where patients sedate themselves prior to treatment.

The use of sedative techniques in dentistry tends to fluctuate in popularity. The administration of centrally acting drugs by dentists is also an area that has attracted some concern over safety.

The techniques described in this chapter are safe and amenable to use by suitably trained dentists working in general dental practice, community dental clinics or hospitals.

5.1 Sedation

Learning objectives

You should

- understand what sedation means

- know the indications for sedation

- know when not to use sedation

- be able to assess a patient with regard to sedation use.

There have been many definitions of sedation put forward over the years. The current definition that must be accepted in the UK is the General Dental Council's definition:

A technique in which a drug, or drugs, produces a state of depression of the central nervous system enabling treatment to be carried out, but in which verbal contact is maintained throughout the period of sedation. The drugs and techniques used should carry a margin of safety wide enough to render unintended loss of consciousness unlikely.

Although the definition allows for the use of more than one sedative agent, it must be emphasised that the vast majority of patients can be adequately and safely sedated with a single drug technique as described in this chapter. Details of more advanced techniques can be found in specialist texts.

Indications for sedation

The indications for sedation can be considered under three main headings: psychosocial, medical and dental.

Psychosocial indications

Indications relating to anxieties regarding dental treatment include:
- phobias
  — specific: drills, needles, extractions
  — general: things in mouth, all dental procedures
- gagging: inability to tolerate objects intraorally without retching
- persistent fainting during procedures, often associated with the administration of local analgesics
- idiosyncrasy to local analgesics: patients who have a problem where local analgesics appear not to work; the cause of the failure is psychological rather than physical.

Medical indications

Some conditions may be aggravated by the stress of undergoing dental treatment:

- ischaemic heart disease
- hypertension
- asthma
- epilepsy
- psychosomatic illnesses.

Many patients with these conditions can be treated quite 'normally' with local analgesic injections and tender loving care (TLC) on the part of a sympathetic dentist. There are, however, a group of patients who, in addition to having a medical condition, also become quite anxious about dental treatment. A history of aggravation of the pre-existing condition in the dental environment may be the only clue as to the patient's concerns.

Some conditions affect the patient's ability to co-operate with dental treatment:

- mild-to-moderate mental and physical handicap
- spasticity disorders
- Parkinson's disease.

The use of sedation aids the management of these patients. The most important requirement is that the patient is able to understand what is being done. Lack of understanding will lead to failure of the technique. The assessment of a patient's understanding is extremely difficult.

Dental indications

Sedation may be required for difficult or unpleasant procedures (e.g. extraction of wisdom teeth) or for orthodontic extractions, particularly in patients with limited previous dental care experience. The proper prescribing of sedation for these indications can help to prevent many patients having to suffer unpleasant experiences. It is well recognised that patients who have had a wisdom tooth surgically removed are more likely to fail than attend the appointment for the second surgical removal.

Contraindications to sedation

Contraindications can be grouped in a similar manner as indications.

Psychosocial contraindications

Patients must be willing and co-operative. A failure to consent for treatment is an absolute contraindication to the provision of care under sedation. Similarly, patients must co-operate to allow the administration of the sedative agents by a given route. Failure to do so will prevent the dentist being able to treat the patient.

Unaccompanied patients
A responsible adult, who will remain with them until their recovery is complete, must accompany patients who are receiving sedation. The only exception to this rule is for adult patients who are receiving inhalation sedation with nitrous oxide and oxygen. Such patients may be allowed to attend without an escort provided that the dentist feels it is appropriate. A responsible adult must accompany children receiving inhalation sedation.

Medical contraindications

Severe or uncontrolled systemic disease
Patients who are to receive sedation should have any general medical problems controlled prior to the commencement of their dental treatment. The administration of sedative drugs masks the patient's ability to detect if they are becoming unwell. It is recommended that patients who would be considered as grade III or worse in the American Society of Anesthesiologists' (ASA) classification of anaesthetic risk (Table 10) should not receive sedation outside an environment where the staff are trained to deal with the potential problems. This generally will mean these patients should not be treated outside a hospital setting.

Severe learning or movement difficulties
The key to success in sedation is that the patient understands the procedure. If this understanding is lacking, then sedation is prone to failure.

Chronic obstructive pulmonary disease
Chronic bronchitis causes an severe upset in respiratory physiology. It results in the respiratory drive being dictated by hypoxia rather than by changes in carbon dioxide levels. The clinical importance of this is, first, that the patient is significantly more sensitive to respiratory depressant drugs (including the benzodiazepines used in intravenous sedation) and, second, that high levels of oxygen, as used in inhalation sedation, may also cause the patient to stop breathing as hypoxic drive is reduced.

Table 10 American Society of Anesthesiologists' classification of anaesthetic risk

Grade	Description
I	Fit and well patient, no intercurrent disease
II	Patient with mild intercurrent disease that is well controlled and does not affect lifestyle
III	Patient with moderate intercurrent disease that does affect lifestyle
IV	Patient with severe intercurrent disease that is a constant threat to life
V	Patient who is unlikely to survive 24 hours with or without medical intervention
VI	A clinically brain dead patient awaiting organ harvest

Severe psychological/psychiatric problems

Patients suffering from delusional states such as psychoses or schizophrenia are notoriously difficult and unpredictable in their response to sedation. This relates to the frequently unpredictable reaction of the patient to the feelings of being sedated. Most of these patients are also taking heavy-duty antipsychotic drugs, which may interact with the sedatives that they are being given as part of their dental treatment. Consequently, only experienced sedationists should treat these patients.

Thyroid dysfunction

Individuals who suffer from hypothyroidism are significantly more susceptible to the effects of central nervous system depressant drugs. Sedation should be avoided in this group.

Hyperthyroid patients may be difficult to sedate and care has to be taken with the use of vasoconstrictors in local analgesic solutions.

Pregnancy and lactation

It is wise to carry out as little treatment as possible for pregnant patients. Almost any drug that is given to the mother will cross the placenta and enter the fetal circulation. While the effects on the mother are easily observed, the effects on the fetus are masked from direct observation. The use of sedation during pregnancy should be restricted to the absolute minimum. It is, however, permissible to use sedation to provide emergency dental care, perhaps in the situation where the fetus would be at greater risk from the repeated administration of antibiotics than from a single visit for treatment under sedation.

Inhalation sedation should be avoided during the first 3 months of pregnancy when there is the greatest risk of damage to the fetus. After this point, there is no evidence of any problem in the use of inhalation sedation with nitrous oxide. Common sense indicates that this will be the case, given the regular use of nitrous oxide as an obstetric analgesic.

There is no evidence that intravenous midazolam causes any fetal abnormalities. It can be used during the first 6 months of pregnancy if required. There is evidence that intravenous midazolam can cause hypotonia in the older fetus and, therefore, it should not be used during the last 3 months of pregnancy.

Contraindications to inhalation sedation with nitrous oxide

In addition to the general contraindications above, blocked nasal airways is a specific contraindication for the use of nitrous oxide sedation. Inhalation sedation will not work when a patient cannot breathe through the nose. Some blockages are temporary, such as hay fever or the common cold, and treatment may merely have to be postponed. Other blockages of the nasal airway are permanent. These could include enlarged adenoids or a deviated nasal septum. Alternative means of anxiety control may have to be used unless surgical correction is planned.

Contraindications to intravenous sedation with midazolam

The following conditions are contraindications to the use of benzodiazepine sedation (in addition to those described in the general section above.)

Hepatic insufficiency. Midazolam is detoxified in the liver. If hepatic function is greatly reduced then its metabolism is also reduced. Because there is considerable extrahepatic metabolism of midazolam, it is generally accepted that a clinically significant decrease in the metabolism of midazolam would only occur when other hepatic functions, such as the production of blood clotting factors, are also significantly reduced.

Porphyria. In this condition the use of certain drugs sensitises the sufferer to the effects of sunlight. The most notable drugs that cause these effects are barbiturates, although the benzodiazepines have also been implicated.

Myasthenia gravis. This autoimmune condition causes impairment of transmission at the neuromuscular junction. The resultant decrease in impulse transmission makes the sufferer very susceptible to the effects of other muscle relaxant drugs, including the benzodiazepines. Administration of benzodiazepine can lead to the patient being paralysed but awake.

Allergy to the benzodiazepine group of drugs. Although very rare, this must be considered as an absolute contraindication to the use of intravenous midazolam.

Dental contraindications

The dental contraindications to sedation fall into two groups:

- those procedures considered too long or too difficult to be carried out under local analgesia
- where the presence of spreading infection in the floor of the mouth threatens the airway, in such cases the airway must be secured under general anaesthesia.

All forms of dental treatment may be carried out under sedation. The judgement as to whether it is appropriate to carry out any particular treatment must be made on a patient-to-patient basis.

Patient assessment

The aims of patient assessment are to discover what sedation is required and suitable.

Patient's psychological ability to tolerate dental treatment. There are many patients who find dentistry difficult to cope with. Some of those are so phobic of dental treatment that they avoid attending at all costs, unless driven by intractable pain. It is important to find out what the patient's specific fears are, and what their previous experiences of dental treatment have been. This also ensures that basic mistakes, such as suggesting that claustrophobic patients have inhalational sedation, are avoided.

Patient's physiological ability to tolerate dental treatment. If a patient suffers from any of the medical conditions highlighted above, it is important to establish how well they have tolerated receiving dental treatment previously. A history of aggravation of the medical condition in the dental setting should be taken as an indication for sedation.

The type and amount of dental treatment required. It is important to establish that the patient actually requires dental treatment prior to the administration of sedation. It is also impossible for the patient to give informed consent (see below) if the dental treatment has not been explained.

Is the treatment practical under sedation? It must be established that the treatment needed can be carried out under sedation

Does the patient need sedation? Information in the above areas will allow an informed decision as to whether or not the patient requires sedation. As in all areas, the provision of treatment should not be complicated unnecessarily. Sedation should only be used where there is a definite indication.

Are there any contraindications to sedation? It is important to ensure that there are no reasons to avoid sedation prior to offering it to a patient.

The assessment process

The assessment process follows similar lines to the history taking and examination of all dental patients.

Dental history
In addition to the current dental history, it is important to establish the patient's pattern of attendance, and any specific fears. This will aid in treatment planning and will also give an indication of the potential co-operation once sedated. Those who are phobic of anything in their mouths tend to co-operate less well than those with a specific fear (e.g. needles or drills). There are specially designed questionnaires available for this purpose, but many tend to pose their questions in a threatening way. It is often better to ask the patient to say in their own words what they find difficult to cope with.

Medical history
In addition to the standard questions, it is important to establish if there has been a previous history of sedation,

and how the patient coped. Other factors that are of importance in sedation terms are:

- current drug history
- past drug history
- allergies (including to sticking plaster).

Dental examination
It is frequently not possible to carry out a full dental examination. Anxious patients do not tolerate the use of probes (even periodontal) well. The reaction to the examination helps in the assessment of the level of anxiety. It also allows appropriate radiographs to be prescribed.

Physical examination
All adult patients should have their blood pressure recorded as part of the assessment for sedation. Patients who are found to be hypertensive (systolic pressure more than 160 mmHg or diastolic more than 100 mmHg) should be referred for investigation.

If inhalational sedation is proposed, then the patency of the nasal airway should be confirmed. If intravenous sedation is proposed, it is important to establish if there are visible veins, along with ascertaining if there have been previous problems with having cannulae sited.

Establish rapport with the patient and deal with misconceptions
The importance of this process cannot be overstated. Most patients needing sedation will relate tales of a previous bad experience at the dentist. The most important part of building a rapport is to try (difficult as it is) to persuade the patient that you are different from the previous dentists. It is also important to deal with any misconceptions such as the difference between amnesia, as induced by sedation, and unconsciousness.

The patient should also give written informed consent form at the assessment appointment.

5.2 Pharmacology of sedative agents

Learning objectives

You should

- understand the clinical effects of the major sedatives used in dentistry

- understand their side-effects

- appreciate the hazards of occupational exposure to nitrous oxide.

The two groups of drug to be considered are the benzodiazepines for oral and intravenous sedation and nitrous oxide for inhalation sedation. Many other agents have been used for sedation but are either now obsolete or are not recommended for routine general practice use.

The benzodiazepines

The benzodiazepines form a large group of drugs comprising over 50 marketed preparations. All of the group have basically the same effects on the body system (they are pharmacodynamically the same). Differences between the drugs primarily relate to the potency of the drug, which is a measure of affinity the drug has for its receptor, the strength of effect that it has on the receptor and also the length of time required to eliminate the drug from the body (pharmacokinetic properties). The pharmacokinetic differences relate to two areas:

- the length of time it takes to eliminate the parent drug (the elimination half-life)
- whether the elimination process produces metabolites that are themselves pharmacologically active.

The principal pharmacological effects of the benzodiazepines, listed as seen with increasing dose (with anxiolysis occurring with the lowest dose), are as follows:

- anxiolysis
- anticonvulsive
- mild sedation
- decreased attention
- amnesia
- more profound sedation
- muscle relaxation
- anaesthesia or hypnosis.

Mechanism of action

Benzodiazepines have two distinct mechanisms of action. In higher centres of the brain, benzodiazepines bind to a receptor that controls sodium ion movement. The receptor is closely associated with a receptor for the endogeneous, inhibitory neurotransmitter gamma-aminobutyric acid (GABA). The action of GABA allows chloride ions from the extracellular fluid to enter the cell. This makes the cell more negatively charged and, therefore, less likely to fire. The benzodiazepines increase the affinity of the GABA receptor for its transmitter and, thus, increases the inhibitory action of GABA. This action of the benzodiazepines is responsible for the sedative and anticonvulsant properties of this group of drugs.

The second mechanism of action is seen at lower centres in the brain stem and spinal cord. Here the benzodiazepines mimic the action of another inhibitory neurotransmitter, glycine. This action of the benzodiazepines is responsible for the anxiolytic and muscle relaxant actions.

Repeated administration of benzodiazepines, (for example when used as oral anxiolytic agents) produces tolerance to the effects that are mediated via GABA. The effects produced by mimicking glycine are, however, largely unaltered.

The amnesic actions of benzodiazepines are poorly understood. The administration causes anterograde amnesia (i.e. from the point of administration forwards in time). Long-term memory is affected more than short term and, therefore, patients remember less the week after the appointment than at the point of discharge.

Side-effects of intravenous benzodiazepines

The principal side-effect of intravenous benzodiazepine administration is respiratory depression. This is produced by two mechanisms. First, the muscle relaxant actions of the drugs affect the respiratory muscles, namely the intercostal muscles and the diaphragm. This reduces the efficiency of the contractions. Second, as with all drugs that depress the CNS, the carbon dioxide receptors in the brain are affected, resulting in a lesser response to changes in blood carbon dioxide. Consequently, although the patient can breathe and will take deep breaths with suitable encouragement, they do not feel the need to breathe.

The second notable side-effect is that of sexual fantasy production. Such fantasies have been described in the literature, although again the mechanism is unclear. It is also unclear why patients may remember the fantasy but yet have no memory of any treatment that has been carried out. The incidence is unknown, but it appears to be dose related with a threshold for midazolam of 0.1 mg/kg body weight. No member of the dental team must ever be left alone with a sedated patient, in case this should result in an allegation being made.

Available benzodiazepines for sedation

Diazepam

Diazepam is a non-water-soluble benzodiazepine. It is available as either a solution in propylene glycol or as a soya-based emulsion. The solution is irritant to inject and is associated with pain and thrombophlebitis. Both the solution and the emulsion contain 5 mg/ml.

Pharmacokinetic properties Diazepam is a long-acting drug. Its elimination half-life is 48 hours. It is metabolised to active metabolites with an elimination half-life in excess of 3 days.

Its use as an intravenous sedative is associated with rebound sedation, occurring 4–6 hours after administration. This occurs after the patient has been discharged and, consequently, is not under professional supervision.

Midazolam

Midazolam is a water-soluble imadazobenzodiazepine, which is painless on intravenous injection. It is available in two concentrations: 10 mg in 5 ml or 10 mg in 2 ml. The more dilute solution is used for intravenous sedation.

Pharmacokinetic properties Midazolam is a short-acting drug with an elimination half-life of about 90 minutes. Its metabolites are largely inactive.

The metabolism of midazolam occurs both in the liver and extrahepatically. The half-life of midazolam is less affected by liver disease than any of the other benzodiazepines.

The effects of a single titrated dose are not prolonged by renal disease.

Midazolam is between two and five times as potent as diazepam.

Midazolam is currently becoming more popular as an oral sedative, despite the lack of a product licence for this use in the UK and the availability of an oral preparation. Midazolam tablets are available in other countries.

Other benzodiazepines

Although there are in excess of 50 benzodiazepines currently available, no others are commonly used for dental sedation.

Benzodiazepine antagonist drugs

Flumazenil

Flumazenil was the first benzodiazepine antagonist drug to be marketed commercially. It is an imadazobenzodiazepine that has a structure very similar to that of midazolam.

Flumazenil acts competitively to displace the active benzodiazepine molecule from the receptor site, thus blocking any potential action.

Pharmacokinetics Flumazenil is a very short-acting drug. Its elimination half-life is 53 minutes, which is significantly shorter than that of any of the sedatives it may be used to reverse.

Contraindications to the administration of flumazenil Flumazenil is a non-selective antagonist that will block the effects of all benzodiazepines. It should not be given to patients who are taking protracted courses of oral benzodiazepines as it may produce an acute withdrawal reaction. Where oral benzodiazepines are used to control epilepsy, the administration of the antagonist will antagonise the anticonvulsant action of the benzodiazepine, potentially leading to fitting.

Flumazenil is a benzodiazepine and must not be administered if an allergic reaction to the sedative is suspected.

Propofol

Propofol (2,6-diisopropylenol) is a synthetic sedative hypnotic, which was introduced for the induction and maintenance of general anaesthesia. In common with other anaesthetic agents it will produce sedation when given in lower doses.

Propofol is lipid soluble and thus is presented in a 1% (10 mg/ml) emulsion.

Clinical effects of propofol

The action of propofol is to enhance the effect of GABA. This is accomplished via a different mechanism from the benzodiazepines, allowing its use in regular benzodiazepine users.

Sedative doses of propofol produce a different quality of sedation from benzodiazepines. The effect is closer to a pure anxiolysis. This can be associated with patients becoming more talkative.

The amnesic actions of propofol are less predictable than those of benzodiazepines.

Side-effects of propofol

Propofol causes depressant effects on the cardiovascular system. It will cause a fall in arterial blood pressure and heart rate. Falls of 25–35% in systolic blood pressure have been recorded, but are of little clinical significance to young, fit and healthy patients treated in the supine position.

Although propofol does produce profound respiratory depression in anaesthetic doses, it would appear that in sedative doses less respiratory depression is seen with propofol than with midazolam.

Pain on injection (especially when small veins are used) is the most common cause of complaint from patients. Mixing a small amount of plain lignocaine with the solution can prevent this.

As with the other sedatives described, sexual fantasies have been described by patients receiving propofol sedation.

The distribution and elimination of propofol

Propofol has an extremely short redistribution half-life. This accounts for the rapid patient recovery from sedation. The elimination from the body takes longer, and thus patients may have residual effects that they fail to appreciate.

Nitrous oxide

Nitrous oxide is the oldest sedative currently in use in clinical dentistry. It is the only drug that is in general use for inhalational sedation in dentistry.

Physical properties of nitrous oxide

Nitrous oxide is a gas at room temperature and pressure. It is colourless and is sometimes described as having a sweet odour. It is 1.5 times as heavy as air and tends to collect at floor level. Pressurised nitrous oxide will liquefy, as its critical temperature (the temperature above which it cannot exist as a liquid) is 36.5°C. Nitrous oxide cylinders contain a mixture of gaseous and liquid nitrous oxide at a pressure of approximately 640 psi.

Anaesthetic and analgesic properties

Nitrous oxide is a weak anaesthetic agent. The MAC_{50} value (the theoretical value that would provide surgical anaesthesia for 50% of the population) is 110%. This can be contrasted with isoflurane at 1.15%. Nitrous oxide is very insoluble in blood (blood:gas partition 0.47), which means that there is a rapid equilibration between the concentration of nitrous oxide in the alveoli and that in the blood, and induction of and recovery from sedation is extremely rapid.

The main effects of nitrous oxide are mood alteration, particularly euphoria, and analgesia. An inspired concentration of 50% nitrous oxide equates to approximately 15 mg morphine, particularly when considering ischaemic muscle pain.

Effects of chronic exposure to nitrous oxide

It should be emphasised that there are virtually no problems of acute exposure for patients, provided that physiological concentrations of oxygen are administered with the nitrous oxide. There are, however, a number of potential problems with chronic exposure:

- decreased fertility in female staff
- increased rate of miscarriage in staff and partners of staff
- combination with cobalt-containing vitamins
  — oxidation of vitamin B_{12}
  — impairment of DNA synthesis
- depression of haematopoiesis
- neurological effects: CNS degeneration
- liver disease
- malignancy, especially cervical carcinoma.

All of these effects tend only to be seen when there is not active scavenging of waste gases.

5.3 Current sedation techniques

Learning objectives

You should

- know the advantages and disadvantages of each type of sedation

- be aware of the techniques involved

- appreciate the need for post graduate training prior to independent practise of sedation

- understand the principles of monitoring patients under sedation

- understand clinical and electromechanical monitoring.

Oral sedation

The administration of oral drugs is an attractive way of producing sedation. This is largely because of the simplicity of the technique as far as the dentist is concerned and the acceptability for patients, particularly in the UK.

Disadvantages

There are significant disadvantages to this type of sedation.

Prolonged latent period. Drugs taken orally will take a long time to act. It will usually be at least 30 minutes to 1 hour until there is a significant degree of sedation. The main problem is that patients who require sedation do not enjoy being in the dental environment, and waiting for the sedation to act can be traumatic.

Unpredictable dose. The other techniques that are recommended for sedation involve titrating the dose of sedative drug to the patient's response. The long latent period involved with oral sedation means that once the dose has been administered it cannot be altered. Recommended doses range between 10 and 40 mg temazepam. This wide variation in the amount of drug means that success is unpredictable.

Unpredictable absorption. There are many factors that affect the absorption of drugs from the gastrointestinal tract. Elixirs and gelatin filled capsules tend to be absorbed more rapidly than tablet formulations. Other factors include the amount, timing and constituents of any food in the stomach. Consequently it cannot be predicted exactly when the drug that has been administered will have its effect.

First-pass metabolism. All drugs that are administered orally and are absorbed from the upper part of the gastrointestinal tract pass to the liver via the portal circulation.

A significant proportion of the dose is metabolised as it passes through the liver prior to reaching the systemic circulation (first-pass metabolism). As a result, a higher dose must be used for oral drugs to achieve the desired effect.

Technique for oral sedation

Midazolam is administered mixed in a drink. The dose for children is 0.5 mg/kg body weight up to a maximum of 20 mg. The adult dose is 20 mg.

The onset of sedation is more rapid than with other benzodiazepines, with the patient being adequately sedated 20–30 minutes after administration. A suitably trained member of the dental team must supervise the patient once the sedative has been administered.

Once sedation is achieved careful consideration should be given to siting an intravenous cannula to give i.v. access as when intravenous sedation is undertaken. The patient should be either sedated in the dental surgery or, if this is not possible, moved to the surgery as soon as sufficiently relaxed to allow this. Electromechanical monitoring should ideally be commenced before administration of the sedative.

Discharge after sedation depends on the patient being sufficiently recovered to walk unaided and being sufficiently co-ordinated to be discharged into the care of a responsible adult.

Monitoring of sedated patients is discussed below.

Inhalational sedation

Techniques of inhalational sedation tend to fluctuate in popularity. It has also been described by a number of names such as relative analgesia, inhalation sedation, or inhalation psychosedation. All the widely available techniques involve the use of mixtures of nitrous oxide and oxygen.

Advantages of inhalational sedation

Rapid onset of sedation. The relative insolubility of nitrous oxide in blood results in the peak levels of nitrous oxide being attained within 3–5 minutes of inhalation.

Rapid recovery. There is effectively no metabolism of nitrous oxide, recovery being effected by exhalation of the gas via the lungs. The same factors that produce rapid induction of sedation lead to rapid recovery.

Recovery is independent of treatment time. Once a stable level of sedation is achieved, the continued administration of nitrous oxide merely maintains the equilibrium of blood:alveolar concentration. Consequently, patients recover as rapidly whether they have been treated for 10 minutes or 2 hours.

Absence of metabolism. Only 0.0004% of the inspired nitrous oxide is absorbed. The almost total absence of metabolism accounts for the safety of nitrous oxide and its ability to be used in a wide range of patients.

The technique does not involve an injection. Many patients are frightened of needles and the fact that nitrous oxide administration does not require an invasive technique is an advantage.

A degree of analgesia is produced. Although the use of inhalation sedation will not provide sufficient analgesia to allow dental treatment to be carried out, it will make the administration of local anaesthetic injections easier.

Inhalation sedation can be used on virtually all patients. Inhalation sedation has very few contraindications and is the only technique currently recommended for patients of all ages.

Disadvantages of inhalational sedation

Bulk of equipment. The equipment required for the administration of inhalational sedation is bulky and can cause problems in a small surgery.

Expense of equipment. The equipment that is to be used must be a dedicated inhalational sedation machine. It is not acceptable to have a general anaesthetic machine that is used for both types of treatment. This is because (GA) machines do not have the same safety features as relative analgesia machines. In addition to the equipment for drug administration, a scavenging system to remove expired gases is required. Finally, once in use, the costs of the gases must be taken into account.

Intrusion of nosepiece into the operating field. This can be a problem when treating upper anterior teeth (see Fig. 73). Disruption of the seal in this area will result in both a decrease in the effectiveness of sedation and an increase in chronic exposure of staff.

Patient's perception of equipment. Patients who have had a previous bad experience associated with general anaesthesia may find that the nosepiece reminds them of the GA mask.

Chronic exposure of staff. The major health problems that may be associated with the use of nitrous oxide will affect staff, not patients. Measures must be taken to ensure that occupational exposure is kept to a minimum.

Potential addiction. Nitrous oxide is an addictive drug; dentists should be aware of the risks to both their staff and themselves.

Technique for inhalational sedation

The technique described (Box 19) is based on the use of the Quantiflex MDM Relative Analgesia Machine, which is the most widely used equipment for this type of sedation (Fig. 74).

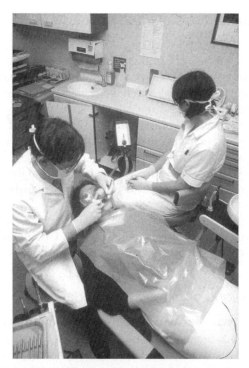

Fig. 73 The nosepiece of the Quantiflex MDM Relative Analgesia Machine adapts against the upper lip, impairing access to the upper anterior teeth.

Signs and symptoms of adequate sedation with nitrous oxide

Signs The signs are what the operator sees:

- the patient is awake
- the patient is relaxed and comfortable

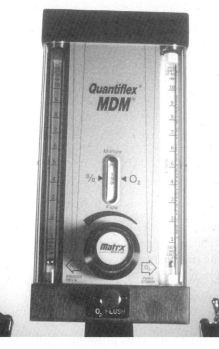

Fig. 74 The Quantiflex MDM Relative Analgesia Machine.

> **Box 19** Technique for inhalational sedation
>
> 1. Preprocedural machine checks. It is vital for the patients well-being that all equipment is in working order and that there is a sufficient supply of nitrous oxide and, more importantly, oxygen for the session. The manufacturer's instructions for checking and servicing equipment should be followed.
> 2. The correct size of nosepiece for the patient should be selected. This is often best done at an assessment appointment as part of introducing the patient to the process of sedation.
> 3. The patient is brought into the surgery, and pretreatment discussions completed.
> 4. The relative analgesia machine is turned on, with 100% oxygen at a flow rate of 6 l/min.
> 5. The nosepiece is fitted to the patient, and the flow rate titrated until the reservoir bag on the machine can be seen to move with each breath but does not fully collapse when the patient breathes in.
> 6. Nitrous oxide is introduced. The initial introduction is 10% increments at 1 minute intervals. After an inspired concentration of 20% has been reached, the increments are reduced to 5%. Throughout the process, the patient must be reassured and encouraged. The most important part of sedation is the patient management. Inhalational sedation will not work without the hypnotic suggestions of the operator.
> 7. Once adequate sedation has been achieved, dental treatment can commence.

- vital signs are within normal limits: heart rate, respiration rate and blood pressure (if measured) will all be normal
- blink rate is reduced
- mouth remains open on request: in this respect inhalational sedation is very different from intravenous sedation
- protective reflexes are normal
- hyperactive gag reflexes are reduced, allowing dental treatment
- decreased response to painful stimuli.

Symptoms The symptoms are what the patient feels:

- relaxed and comfortable
- lessened awareness of pain
- paraesthesia/tingling
- mild intoxication
- euphoria
- detachment
- warmth
- indifference to the passage of time
- dreaming.

Patients will not necessarily show all the signs, or experience all the symptoms of sedation that are listed above. It is a matter of judgement as to when adequate sedation has been achieved. The majority of patients will require between 25 and 40% nitrous oxide to achieve sedation. It is very important to avoid oversedation, as patients find overdoses of nitrous oxide unpleasant.

Signs and symptoms of oversedation Oversedation can cause:

- persistent mouth closing
- spontaneous mouth-breathing
- patient complains of unpleasant feelings
- lack of co-operation
- nausea and vomiting.

The treatment of a patient who is oversedated involves reducing the concentration of inspired nitrous oxide by 5–10%, and reassuring the patient that things will improve.

Recovery from sedation

Once dental treatment has been completed, the patient is allowed to breathe 100% oxygen for 2 minutes. This allows the nitrous oxide to be exhaled via the scavenging system rather than into the surgery. It can also prevent a phenomenon called diffusion hypoxia, which may arise owing to the rapid release of nitrous oxide from blood when it is removed from the inspired air.

After recovery, a child patient must be discharged into the care of a responsible adult. Adults may be discharged alone and it is the dentist's responsibility to decide if the patient needs to be accompanied or not.

Intravenous sedation

Intravenous sedation is normally used for anxious adult patients. It is particularly useful for the extremely anxious or for those who feel claustrophobic when undergoing dental treatment.

Advantages of intravenous sedation

Speed of onset of sedation. The hand-to-brain circulation time is of the order of 20 seconds; as a result, the onset of sedation is very rapid. This prevents an increase in anxiety while waiting in the dental environment.

The dose of sedative can be titrated against the patient's response. The patient receives the correct dose of sedative for their needs.

Administration is comfortable. Once venous access is achieved, the patient is not troubled (unlike intramuscular or subcutaneous injections).

Intravenous access is preserved. This allows the administration of other agents if required (as in the case of a medical incident).

Recovery. This is shorter than for drugs administered via the oral or intramuscular route.

Disadvantages of intravenous sedation

The establishment of intravenous access. Many patients find the process of having an intravenous cannula sited unpleasant. It is, however, amazing how many patients find that it is acceptable to have an injection in the hand but will not tolerate intraoral injections.

Rapid onset. The rapid onset of the effects of intravenous drugs means that care must be taken to ensure that patients are not oversedated.

Adverse reactions. Any adverse reactions to the drugs tend to be more severe if the drugs are administered by injection rather than orally.

No easy reversal is possible. There is no way to recover the drug once it has been administered. The only way to reverse sedation is by the use of antagonist drugs.

Technique of intravenous sedation

The primary prerequisite for the use of intravenous sedation is that all those involved in the patient's treatment have received the appropriate training and the surgery is equipped with the appropriate scale of equipment for administering the sedation, monitoring the patient and dealing with any emergencies. Both dentist and dental nurse should have attended relevant postgraduate/postcertification courses.

Equipment required for intravenous sedation
Administration

- surgical wipe to disinfect skin
- gauge intravenous cannula
- surgical tape to fix cannula
- syringes (5 ml) to administer sedative and saline flush
- gauge needle to draw up drug
- labels to distinguish syringes
- tourniquet
- disposable tray.

Monitoring equipment

- stop watch
- non-invasive blood pressure recording facility
- pulse oximeter.

Emergency equipment As for all dental surgeries and

- flumazenil
- facility to give supplemental oxygen at a flow of 2 l/min (most emergency cylinders are set to a minimum of 5 l/min).

Special dental equipment

- mouth props
- dental chair with a fast prone facility that will work in the event of power failure.

Preparation of the drugs

All drugs to be used for sedation (including normal saline) must be drawn up by the dentist administering the sedation. This task must not be delegated to a dental nurse.

As with all agents to be administered to patients (including local anaesthetics), agents must be checked to ensure that they have not passed their expiry date and that there are no signs of damage to the containers in which they are supplied. Once drawn up, drugs must be clearly labelled as there are many clear solutions, which can easily be confused.

Preparation of the patient

It is important to ensure that all the formalities have been completed before the patient is sedated. This will include checking that the patient has signed a consent form and that their blood pressure has been recorded. It is also good practice to ensure that the patient has visited the toilet before embarking on a procedure that will keep the patient in the dental chair for about an hour or so. The patient's medical and dental histories should also be checked to ensure that nothing has happened since the previous appointment either to change the dental treatment plan or to modify the choice of sedation technique.

Intravenous cannulation

Cannulation is a prerequisite for carrying out intravenous sedation. It is important to select a site that is accessible to the dentist, acceptable to the patient, away from structures that might be damaged in the process but where there are adequately sized superficial veins present. The dorsum of the hand is the usual choice in this situation. The process of cannulation is shown in Figure 75.

Once the cannula has been sited, its correct location is confirmed using a dose of saline. The sedative agent can then be administered. The usual choice is midazolam (10 mg in 5 ml formulation). The dose should be titrated according to the patient's response. A small dose is administered, allowed to have its effect and then a decision made as to whether or not sufficient has been administered. If not, the cycle is repeated. The usually recommended regimen is:

1. Slow bolus of 2 mg (1 ml)
2. Wait for 90 seconds
3. Administration of 1 mg increments at 1-minute intervals until the patient is adequately sedated.

Signs of adequate sedation

A depth of sedation that will allow the patient to have treatment is often referred to as the 'endpoint', implying that it is discrete, and apparent. This is not the case. There is a plane of sedation within which the patient needs to be to allow treatment to be undertaken. Different patients will require to be at different levels within this plane of sedation; indeed, the same patient may require to be at different levels of sedation depending on the type of treatment proposed, and how they are feeling in general.

The judgement of the correct depth of sedation largely comes down to clinical experience. An adjunct to assessing the adequacy of sedation is to ask the patient if they are ready to have dental treatment. A slow, ponderous answer is usually indicative of the correct level of sedation. Tests of co-ordination, such as asking the patient to touch their nose (and watching them miss), tend to embarrass patients and have the added disadvantage of being of little clinical use.

In general, once an adequate level of sedation has been achieved, the duration of the dental treatment should be tailored to the duration of the sedation, and no further increments of sedative given.

The dosage of midazolam required to produce sedation is extremely variable. Given that the ethos of sedation is that the dose of sedative is judged according to the patient's response, it is difficult to justify setting maximum doses. However, well over 95% of patients will be adequately sedated on a dose of 10 mg of midazolam or less. Doses in excess of this should only be given after careful assessment and consideration.

Dental treatment under intravenous sedation

Patients recover from the effects of intravenous sedation while they are being treated. Consequently, the longer the appointment progresses, the less sedated the patient will become. The pattern of dental treatment must be tailored to suit. The most invasive treatment (the administration of local anaesthetic and use of rotary cutting instruments) should be confined to the first 25 minutes of treatment. The remaining treatment (placement of restorations) can take place during the next 20 minutes or so. It should, however, be emphasised that all patients are different, and each patient should be treated for the amount of time that they are happy to receive treatment.

Recovery from intravenous sedation

Patients recover much more slowly from intravenous sedation than from inhalational sedation. It is impossible to set strict time limits on when patients should be discharged. It is more important to assess the patient's state of mind and ability to leave the surgery premises. A useful test is to ask the patient to walk across the room, turn and walk back. If they can negotiate that test without undue loss of balance, they are probably fit to be discharged. It is also worth checking that the patient is happy to leave, and that the escort is happy to take them.

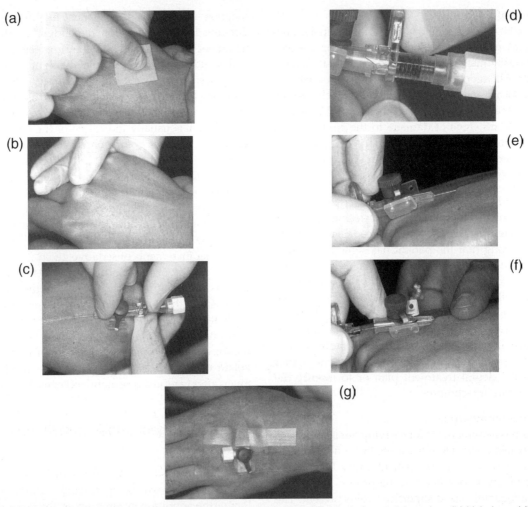

Fig. 75 The cannulation sequence. (a) Site for venepuncture disinfected with alcohol-containing wipe. (b) Vein immobilised with skin traction from operator's left hand. (c) Cannula inserted into vein. (d) Correct position confirmed by seeing flashback of blood. (e) Cannula slid down needle to site completely. (f) Vein occluded by assistant while needle removed. (g) Cap placed on end of cannula and wings secured with tape.

All patients receiving intravenous sedation *must* be charged into the care of a responsible adult.

Complications of intravenous sedation

Complications associated with intravenous cannulation
All of the following responses are difficult to cope with, and patients in these categories should be treated by those who are experienced in using sedation.

Venospasm. This is a condition, probably anxiety related, where the veins collapse at attempted cannulation. It is difficult to prevent even for those skilled at cannulation.

Extravascular injection. This results from an incorrectly sited cannula. The main thing is to prevent the extravascular injection of any pharmacologically active agent by testing that the cannula is correctly sited.

Intra-arterial injection. Injection of drugs into an artery is a potentially serious event. Once again it should be prevented by careful technique, particularly by checking that any vessel that is selected as a potential cannulation site does not pulsate.

Haematoma formation. Haematomata form as a result of blood leaking from a blood vessel into the subcutaneous tissues. Formation may occur at cannulation, as a result of multiple vein wall punctures or when the cannula is removed as a result of insufficient pressure being applied to the site.

Pain on cannulation. Venous cannulation is uncomfortable, but for most patients it can be overcome with the use of distraction techniques.

Problems associated with sedation
Oversedation. The most likely sign of a patient being oversedated is respiratory depression. In the majority of patients, this can be managed by encouraging the patient to breathe and by support until the overdose wears off. In more severe cases, supplemental oxygen

may be required; should that fail, the sedation should be reversed with the benzodiazepine antagonist.

Hyporesponse. The patient fails to sedate despite the use of large doses of sedative.

Paradoxical reaction. The patient appears to have sedated normally but reacts in an uncontrolled fashion when treatment is attempted.

Hyper-response. The patient sedates very deeply on a very small dose of sedative.

Sexual fantasy. It appears that some patients who are sedated feel that they have been interfered with in a sexual way. Such allegations are potentially distressing to the dentist, not to mention legally difficult as they may result in imprisonment. Consequently, no member of the dental team should be left alone with a sedated patient. Dentist and dental nurse act as each other's chaperone.

Reversal of intravenous sedation

The advent of flumazenil raised the possibility of being able to reverse a patient's sedation. This is, however, not recommended as a routine practice.

Indications for reversal

- oversedation
- patients with a difficult journey home
- patients who will be difficult to manage either because of a learning difficulty or who are much larger than their escorts.

Contraindications to reversal

- patients taken concurrent oral benzodiazepines (especially if used to control epilepsy)
- patients who have had a suspected allergic reaction to the sedative.

Intravenous sedation with propofol

There are a number of techniques described using propofol for intravenous sedation. All involve using a syringe pump to deliver the solution to the patient. The techniques fall into two groups.

In the first group the sedationist controls the level of sedation by altering the rate of infusion. The second group of techniques allows the patient to control the depth of sedation with the use of sophisticated technology.

Currently these techniques are used predominantly in hospital settings and are unsuitable for the operator–sedationist.

Monitoring of sedated patients

All patients who are having any form of dental treatment should be monitored by those who are providing that treatment. The importance of monitoring is greater when patients have been sedated, as they are less aware of their surroundings, and any changes that are occurring within their own bodies.

Clinical monitoring

The cornerstone of all monitoring is the clinical observation of the patient.

Is the patient conscious? In this context consciousness is defined as the ability to respond to verbal command.

Does the patient look relaxed and comfortable? This will show that they are tolerating treatment without undue distress. The patient's facial expression and general demeanour in the dental chair are good indications of their level of comfort.

Skin colour. Any changes in skin colour should be noted, as they may be indicative of an impending medical incident, for example a bluish tinge may result from hypoxia secondary to respiratory depression. Reddening, particularly in an area where there has been contact with surgical gloves or rubber dam, may indicate an allergy.

Pattern and depth of respiration. Given that respiratory depression can occur with benzodiazepine sedation, patients should have the rate and depth of breathing monitored. Patients who are receiving inhalational sedation should also be monitored, as mouth-breathing is an early sign of overdose.

Electromechanical monitoring

The clinical monitoring is complemented by the use of electromechanical devices.

Pulse oximetry

The use of a pulse oximeter, which will pick up falls in arterial oxygen saturation before they are clinically evident, provides an early warning of respiratory depression. Falls of 4–5% must be corrected, and any fall below 90% saturated must be treated as potentially serious. The reasons for this will become apparent when the oxygen–haemoglobin dissociation curve is studied (Fig. 76). The oximeter should be attached to the patient and be switched on prior to the administration of any sedative so that the normal saturation can be noted. The pulse oximeter also displays a reading of the patient's pulse. Changes (particularly increases) may indicate distress or pain during treatment.

Pulse oximetry is not routinely used with inhalational sedation, as high concentrations of oxygen are always administered; the minimum is 30%.

Non-invasive blood pressure recording

Adult patients should have their blood pressure recorded both as part of the assessment process and immediately prior to sedation. This allows the establishment of a

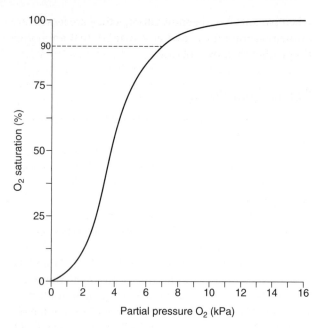

Fig. 76 The oxygen–haemoglobin dissociation curve; 90% saturation is at the top of the steep portion of the curve. Further respiratory depression will result in rapid falls in saturation.

baseline reading. There is no requirement to monitor a patient's blood pressure continuously, unless there are medical reasons for so doing. Any patient in this category should be treated by an experienced sedationist. It is not normal to measure blood pressure for fit and well children prior to sedation.

Reservoir bag on a relative analgesia machine
In addition to the above, when inhalational sedation is used, observation of the movements of the reservoir bag allow an assessment of the patient's pattern of breathing. Increases in rate or depth may indicate anxiety, while a decrease in the amount of movement of the bag while the chest movements remain the same may indicate that the patient is mouth-breathing.

As most sedation is carried out by an operator sedationist, the main burden of monitoring tends to fall on the dental nurse. The issue of training for the dental team is covered below

5.4 Dental treatment planning

Learning objectives

You should

- appreciate which procedures benefit from the use of sedation

- understand how to encourage patients to complete treatment.

All dental procedures that might be carried out under local anaesthesia can be carried out under sedation and local anaesthesia. Some procedures are more easily carried out under one form of sedation than another, for example apicectomies on upper incisors are difficult under inhalational sedation as the nosepiece tends to interfere with the operating field.

The main decision rests on what treatment is advisable to carry out for patients. As in all other areas of dentistry, these decisions depend much on the patient's co-operation.

Patients requiring sedation often have very poor attendance records, largely because they are terrified of being in the dental environment. Previous non-attendance means that they have not been exposed to oral health education, such as diet advice and oral hygiene instruction. In these patients, poor oral hygiene at first attendance should not be taken as an indication of lack of will to co-operate.

The ideal for dental treatment planning is to deal with any periodontal problems, manage the routine conservative work, provide advanced conservation (fixed prosthodontics and endodontics) with removable prosthodontics as the final stage. Berating an anxious patient on the merits of good oral hygiene and forcing them to have all hard and soft deposits removed from their teeth as a first stage will result in the patient failing to return for treatment. It is important to engage the patient in treatment first to show them that they can attend and cope with receiving treatment.

The decision of what treatment to provide will then depend on the patient's ability to cope with treatment under sedation, as well as their response to the health education message. It is inappropriate to promise patients advanced treatment prior to the initial sedation appointment, as it may well be that even with sedation co-operation may be limited.

Treatment such as molar endodontics, multiple crowns and bridges and technique-sensitive procedures should be reserved for only the very co-operative and compliant patients.

5.5 Medicolegal aspects

Learning objectives

You should

- appreciate the obligations on the dental profession using sedation

- know the importance of compliance with GDC requirements.

Sadly, all aspects of medical and dental practice are being affected by the need to consider the possibility of legal action for negligence.

There have been many reports written on the practice of sedation, and although those who wish to practise in this field must be aware of the contents of such reports, it is the edicts of the General Dental Council (GDC) that are the legal framework under which we operate.

The gist of the principal requirements from the GDC's guidance in its 1997 publication *Maintaining Standards* are reproduced below.

- The definition of sedation is as given at the beginning of this chapter. Although it allows latitude in the techniques that may be used for sedation, it does go on to say that usually single-drug techniques (such as described in this chapter) are the most appropriate. There are other more complicated techniques, which are inappropriate for the undergraduate and thus are not discussed here.
- Dentists are entitled to act as operator/sedationist, with the proviso that they must have undertaken the relevant postgraduate training. This will mean attendance at a suitable course that provides the theoretical background and, ideally, supervised clinical practice.
- If a dentist is to exercise this right, then the appropriate assistance must be available. This may be from a suitably trained dental nurse. Such a dental nurse should hold the National Certificate from the National Examining Board for Dental Nurses (NEBDN) and, as a minimum, should have attended an appropriate postcertification course. The ideal is that dental nurses who are assisting with sedation also hold the Certificate in Dental Anaesthetic Nursing from the NEBDN. The training allows the dental nurse to monitor the patient's clinical condition, which is particularly important as the dentist may become distracted by the dental treatment.
- All patients should be carefully monitored during sedation (Section 5.3).
- All patients who are to have sedation must have their medical history checked. This practice should be routine for all who are attending for even the most basic procedure, whether or not sedation is used.
- All patients having any treatment under sedation of any sort must give consent in writing. This consent should be informed; that is that the dentist who is to administer the sedation explains the procedure to the patient and any alternative treatments that may be possible. This allows the patient to give their consent based on knowledge of the treatment options.
- Patients who are recovering from sedation must be protected and monitored in adequate facilities. They should only be discharged when the person administering the sedation is satisfied that they have recovered sufficiently. Patients receiving intravenous or oral sedation must be discharged into the care of a responsible adult, as must children receiving inhalational sedation. Adults receiving inhalational sedation with nitrous oxide and oxygen may be discharged alone at the dentist's discretion. This will largely depend on the patient's response to sedation and, therefore, can only really be suggested once the dentist has assessed the patient's reaction to having dental treatment in this manner.
- All of those who practise dentistry must be capable of dealing with a patient collapse. The GDC believe that sedation increases the risk of a collapse, although there is no evidence to support this view. There are, however, no additional requirements on those practising sedation in terms of resuscitation skills from those required of all dentists. All who provide dental treatment should practise their emergency skills regularly in simulated emergency situations.
- The possibility of sexual fantasies must be taken seriously. The GDC recommends that dentists should always be accompanied by a dental nurse, but that this is mandatory when sedation is being used.

Although any discussion of medicolegal issues tends to cause panic, it should be remembered that those who practise ethically in accordance with guidelines have little to fear.

Self-assessment: questions

Multiple choice questions

1. Assessment for sedation involves:
   a. Dental examination
   b. A trial attempt at dental treatment
   c. Recording the patient's blood pressure
   d. Taking a full medical history
   e. Obtaining verbal consent for treatment

2. Nitrous oxide is:
   a. A colourless gas with a pungent odour
   b. Is lighter than air
   c. Is highly soluble in blood
   d. Is a weak anaesthetic with a MAC_{50} value of about 110%
   e. Can only be used to sedate children

3. Flumazenil:
   a. Is recommended for routine use in order to hasten recovery
   b. Is not a benzodiazepine
   c. Antagonises the action of all benzodiazepines
   d. Is useful for managing allergic reactions to benzodiazepines
   e. Has a shorter half-life than midazolam

4. The following are contraindications to intravenous sedation:
   a. Myasthenia gravis
   b. Chronic bronchitis
   c. Liver failure
   d. Well-controlled angina
   e. Mild learning difficulty

5. The pharmacodynamic properties of the benzodiazepine group of drugs include:
   a. Anxiolysis
   b. Analgesia
   c. Antiemetic effect
   d. Sedation
   e. Anaesthesia

6. Nitrous oxide cylinders:
   a. Contain gaseous nitrous oxide at high pressure
   b. The pressure of the cylinder contents is directly proportional to the volume of gas remaining
   c. Are light blue with a white quartered top
   d. Must be stored vertically
   e. Can be connected to the same mounts as Entonox cylinders

7. Nitrous oxide sedation:
   a. Can only be used for children
   b. Produces such deep sedation that a mouth prop is required to maintain intraoral access
   c. Produces sufficient analgesia for soft tissue surgery
   d. Relies heavily on the operator's ability to use suggestion
   e. Is useful in patients with gagging problems

8. Oral sedation:
   a. Is less predictable than intravenous sedation
   b. Drugs may be subject to first-pass metabolism
   c. May be achieved with midazolam
   d. Means that the patient can attend without an escort
   e. Should be titrated against the patient's response

9. An overdose of intravenous benzodiazepine:
   a. Will most often present as respiratory depression
   b. May result in lack of consciousness
   c. May produce severe systemic effects including liver damage
   d. Always requires treatment with flumazenil
   e. Will result in the dental treatment having to be postponed until a future occasion

10. An overdose of nitrous oxide:
    a. Can lead to the patient laughing uncontrollably
    b. Reduces patient co-operation
    c. Occurs at the start of treatment but is unlikely later
    d. Can lead to vomiting
    e. Results in the patient's mouth becoming fixed in an open position

11. Midazolam:
    a. Is water soluble at all pH values
    b. Is half as potent as diazepam
    c. Has an elimination half-life of about 2 hours
    d. Metabolism is reduced by erythromycin
    e. Causes thrombophlebitis on injection

12. Scavenging must be used with relative analgesia sedation because nitrous oxide:
    a. Reacts with cobalt-containing enzymes
    b. Reduces the sperm count of male dentists
    c. Can cause vitamin B_{12} deficiency
    d. Makes female staff less fertile
    e. May increase incidence of cervical carcinoma in female staff.

Case history question

A 14-year-old female is referred for the extraction of four first premolars for orthodontic reasons. She is a pleasant but anxious child who attends a local boarding school.

Medical history. The patient says she faints easily but has not been investigated. She has an allergy to elastoplast.

Dental history. Although a regular attender for as long as she can remember, the patient has previously only had one small filling that did not require local analgesia.

Intraoral examination. The patient has good oral hygiene, with all teeth bar the third molars fully erupted. There is crowding evident in both arches.

1. What are the treatment options?
2. Which is the best option and why?
3. What is the major problem with providing treatment for this girl?

Picture questions

Picture 1

1. What is the piece of equipment shown in Figure 77?
2. What are the features labelled A–G?

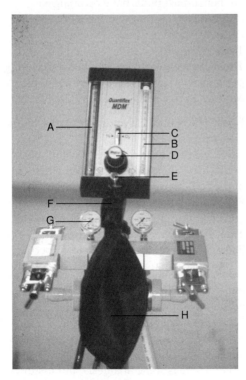

Fig. 77 Equipment used in sedation.

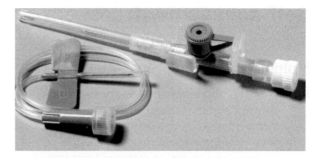

Fig. 78 Equipment for venous access.

Picture 2

1. What are the pieces of equipment in Figure 78?
2. Given the choice, which would be used for dental sedation and why?

Short note questions

Write short notes on:

1. the advantages of midazolam over diazepam as an intravenous sedative
2. the disadvantages of oral sedation
3. the signs and symptoms of oversedation with nitrous oxide
4. factors that could cause the arterial saturation reading on a pulse oximeter to fall to 85% during sedation with intravenous midazolam
5. the principal clinical effects of the benzodiazepine group of drugs
6. factors observed during the clinical monitoring of a sedated patient.

Viva questions

1. How would you assess a patient who attends asking to be referred for intravenous sedation?
2. Describe how you would explain inhalational sedation to a 10-year-old child who is referred for treatment.

Self-assessment: answers

Multiple choice answers

1. a. **True.** It is important to at least have a look in the patient's mouth to establish that there is a treatment need and give the patient an idea of the amount of time required. If the patient is very anxious, then probing cavities and restoration margins or doing a periodontal assessment will tend to distress the patient.
    b. **False.** It is cruel and heartless to imply that patients must be shown to be unable to tolerate treatment before offering sedation.
    c. **True.** The only exception to this rule is that fit children who are to receive relative analgesia do not normally have their blood pressure recorded. It may also be that with some patients with moderate learning difficulties there may be insufficient co-operation for what is an uncomfortable procedure.
    d. **True.** All patients undergoing any dental intervention should have a full medical history recorded.
    e. **False.** Written informed consent is required for all treatment under any form of sedation.

2. a. **False.** Although colourless, nitrous oxide has a sweet odour.
    b. **False.** Nitrous oxide is about 1.5 times as dense as air.
    c. **False.** Nitrous oxide is very insoluble in blood, a fact in the rapid onset of and recovery from sedation.
    d. **True.**
    e. **False.** Nitrous oxide is suitable for just about all ages of patient. It is vastly underused in adult patients.

3. a. **False.** It is currently recommended that flumazenil is only used in an emergency.
    b. **False.** Flumazenil is a benzodiazepine. In fact it is very closely related to midazolam in chemical structure.
    c. **True.**
    d. **False.** If a patient is allergic to any other benzodiazepine, they will almost certainly be allergic to flumazenil. Giving it in this situation will make things worse, not better.
    e. **True.** The shorter half-life has been used as an argument against its routine use.

4. a. **True.** The muscle-relaxant properties of the benzodiazepines coupled with the poor

transmission of motor impulses to muscles can lead to paralysis.
    b. **True.** The altered respiratory drive associated with chronic hypoxia in severe chronic bronchitis makes patients extremely sensitive to the respiratory depressant effects of the sedative agents.
    c. **True.** Midazolam is principally broken down in the liver. There is, however, significant extrahepatic breakdown. Consequently liver failure will only be a problem when the function is sufficiently severe to cause problems with breakdown of local anaesthetics and a failure of clotting.
    d. **False.** If the angina is well controlled, sedation may be used. It may also be of great value if the patient normally has few problems but gives a history of exacerbation of the problem during dental treatment.
    e. **False.** Sedation may help such patients to cope with treatment.

5. a. **True.**
    b. **False.** Relief of anxiety may influence the patients perception of stimuli or reaction to chronic pain, but benzodiazepines have no analgesic properties.
    c. **False.**
    d. **True.**
    e. **True.** Large enough doses of benzodiazepines, particularly if given rapidly intravenously, will produce loss of consciousness.

6. a. **False.** The cylinders contain both gas and liquid under pressure.
    b. **False.** The pressure remains constant until all the liquid has vaporised. This occurs when only 1/8 of the contents are left.
    c. **False.** The cylinders are light blue. The white quartered top denotes an Entonox cylinder.
    d. **True.** This prevents liquid entering the gas outlet.
    e. **False.** The pin index system is gas specific.

7. a. **False.** This technique is useful for a wide range of patients. Adults can be managed extremely well with inhalational sedation.
    b. **False.** Spontaneous mouth closing is a sign of overdose; consequently, mouth props should not be used with this type of sedation.
    c. **False.** There is some analgesia, but insufficient for surgical procedures.
    d. **True.**
    e. **True.**

8. a. **True.** The pattern of drug absorption is unpredictable and, therefore, the effects of the dose and the time to onset of sedation are unpredictable.
   b. **True.** The drug once absorbed from the gastrointestinal tract passes via the portal circulation to the liver. Here a significant proportion is metabolised.
   c. **True.**
   d. **False.** The effects may persist longer than intravenous agents. Temazepam has a significantly longer half-life than midazolam.
   e. **False.** The long latent period for the absorption of oral drugs means that the dose has to be given on a best guess basis.

9. a. **True.**
   b. **True.**
   c. **False.** There are no toxic effects to systems. The effects are of respiratory depression and anaesthesia. If the patient is supported until the drugs are eliminated they will make an uneventful recovery.
   d. **False.** Minor overdose can be managed by encouraging the patient to breathe and supporting them until they recover to a normal level of sedation.
   e. **False.** Once the patient has returned to a normal level of sedation (if managed as in (d)), treatment can be carried out.

10. a. **True.** Hence the name laughing gas.
   b. **True.** It feels unpleasant to the patient, and they often become disorientated.
   c. **False.** Overdose often occurs later in treatment, when the part of the procedure that the patient dislikes most is past and their requirement for anxiolysis reduces.
   d. **True.** This is a relatively late sign of overdose, and one would hope that remedial action would be taken before this stage was reached.
   e. **False.** Spontaneous mouth closing is an early sign of overdose.

11. a. **False.** It is lipid soluble at physiological pH and can cross the blood–brain barrier.
   b. **False.** It is about two to five times as potent as diazepam.
   c. **True.**
   d. **True.**
   e. **False.** This is one of midazolam's great advantages over diazepam.

12. a. **True.**
   b. **False.**
   c. **True.**

   d. **True.**
   e. **True.**

Case history answer

1. The treatment options are:
   • local anaesthesia
   • inhalational sedation
   • intravenous sedation if child appears mature for her years
   • oral sedation
   • general anaesthesia.
2. Inhalational sedation is the best option, although all are potentially possible. Local anaesthesia alone is asking a child with little experience of dental treatment to tolerate a total of eight local anaesthetic injections (including two palatal) and cope with four extractions. In an attempt to avoid gas, many dentists tried to persuade children in this category to have treatment under local, and the result was an increase in the number of children referred to have three first premolars out under general anaesthesia.

   Intravenous and oral sedation are less predictable although possible for children; inhalational sedation remains the method of choice.

   General anaesthesia should be avoided if at all possible. Its use for a minor cosmetic procedure cannot be justified, particularly in the light of recent publicity.
3. The major problem in this case is medicolegal, not clinical. Obtaining consent for treatment for this patient is a problem, as the parents presumably live a long way from the school. The Head Teacher will have the power to act as guardian and give medical consent in an emergency situation, but this would not be the case for orthodontic treatment. The parents must at least be spoken to on the telephone and be sent a consent form to sign if they cannot be seen face to face.

Picture answers

Picture 1

1. This is the head of a Quantiflex MDM Relative Analgesia Machine.
2. Features are:
   A nitrous oxide flow rotameter
   B oxygen flow rotameter
   C gas mixture control
   D gas flow rate control
   E oxygen flush button
   F air entrainment value
   G common gas outlet.

Picture 2

1. These are (a) an intravenous cannula and (b) a butterfly needle.
2. The cannula is used in preference to the butterfly. The use of the butterfly leaves a needle in the patient's vein. This can cut out of the vein if the site is subject to movement. The cannula is soft, blunt ended and flexible and so once sited will not tend to cut out. The cannula is teflon coated and does not encourage the clotting of blood, whereas cells can coagulate around the steel of the butterfly. The cannula is more likely to give intravenous access for the duration of the appointment.

Short note answers

1. Midazolam is water soluble and, therefore, does not cause pain on intravascular injection. It has a shorter half-life than diazepam; consequently, patients will recover more rapidly. The absence of active metabolites from midazolam mean that there is no rebound sedation, also hastening recovery.
2. The disadvantages of oral sedation are:
   - prolonged latent period
   - unpredictable dose
   - unpredictable absorption
   - first-pass metabolism.
3. The signs of oversedation with nitrous oxide are:
   - persistent mouth closing
   - spontaneous mouth-breathing
   - disorientation
   - irrational or sluggish response to command
   - poor co-operation
   - unconsciousness.

   The 5 symptoms of oversedation with nitrous oxide are:
   - loss of control
   - unpleasant sensations
   - anxiety
   - headache
   - nausea.
4. Technical causes of fall of in arterial oxygen saturation recorded by the pulse oximeter are:
   - probe loose or misplaced
   - cuff partially inflated on same limb.

   Patient causes of fall in arterial oxygen saturation are:
   - obstruction owing to oversedation
   - obstruction by foreign body
   - obstruction because of treating dentist's activity
   - respiratory depression caused by sedative agent

   - pre-existing respiratory or cardiovascular disease
   - collapse, e.g. faint.
5. The clinical effects of the benzodiazepines are:
   - anxiolysis
   - anticonvulsion
   - sedation
   - reduced attention
   - amnesia
   - muscle relaxation
   - anaesthesia
   - respiratory depression
   - fall in blood pressure (minimal)
   - increase in heart rate (slight)
   - potential sexual fantasy.
6. Factors monitored clinically during sedation:
   - level of consciousness (response to verbal command)
   - level of relaxation
   - response to treatment (effectiveness of sedation)
   - respiration
     — rate
     — depth
     — signs of obstruction
   - pulse
     — heart rate
     — rhythm
   - colour: skin and mucosa.

Viva answers

1. You should describe assessment in terms of:
   - medical history: any problems or contraindications to a particular type of sedation
   - dental history: current pain, previous care, particular fears, particular wishes regarding current treatment
   - social history: alcohol or drug abuse; availability of an escort
   - physical evaluation: blood pressure measurement
   - dental examination
   - radiographic examination
   - explanation of the likely treatment options.
2. It is important in answering this type of question to use words that a 10-year-old child would understand. Thus terms like 'tingly' should be used not paraesthesia. In all events, it is important to emphasise that it will feel pleasant, warm, etc., but always use phrases like 'you may feel' as not everyone has all of the symptoms described in the section on inhalational sedation. It is also wise to talk about a nosepiece rather than a mask in case the child has had a previous bad experience with general anaesthesia.

6 Paediatric dentistry

Overview

The successful practice of paediatric dentistry requires an intimate knowledge of normal child development and behaviour as well as the technical and clinical skills that are necessary to work in a small mouth. The aim of every clinician who treats children should be to deliver that child into adolescence and young adulthood without fear and with tolerance for dental treatment. If that is achieved and, in addition, the young adult has an appreciation of the importance of oral health to overall general health then the hours spent in behaviour management and practical prevention will have been worthwhile.

6.1 Tooth development and eruption

Learning objectives

You should

- know at what age primary teeth begin to mineralise, at what age their root formation is complete, and at what age they erupt
- know at what age permanent teeth begin to mineralise, at what age their root formation is complete, and at what age they erupt.

Tooth development

Tooth germs develop from the dental lamina, which itself develops from the primary epithelial band. The dental lamina forms a series of epithelial buds that grow into surrounding connective tissue. The buds become associated with a condensation of mesenchyme and together they represent a tooth germ at its early 'cap' stage of development. The epithelial bud becomes the enamel organ and the mesenchymal cells the dental papilla and follicle. The cells at the margin of the enamel organ grow to enclose some mesenchymal cells, the 'bell' stage of development. Histodifferentiation of the enamel organ now occurs into external and internal enamel epithelia, stratum intermedium and stellate reticulum.

On the lingual aspect of each primary tooth germ, the dental lamina proliferates to produce the permanent successor tooth germ. Permanent tooth germs with no primary precursors are produced by distal extension of the dental lamina.

Dentine formation occurs after differentiation of dental papilla cells into odontoblasts, which is induced by the internal enamel epithelium. Once dentine formation has begun, the adjacent cells of the internal enamel epithelium differentiate into ameloblasts and produce enamel. The dentine of the roots of teeth is produced in a similar fashion by differentiation of odontoblasts induced by the internal enamel epithelium, and root growth is controlled by the epithelial cells at the margins of the enamel organ – the root sheath of Hertwig. Root growth is not complete until 1–2 years in the primary dentition and 3–5 years in the permanent dentition after eruption of the crowns of the teeth. The beginning of mineralisation for both dentitions is given in Tables 11 and 12.

Eruption

The exact controlling mechanism of eruption has not yet been identified. It is likely that the dental follicle has a major part to play as the connective tissue of the follicle is a rich source of factors responsible for the local mediation of bone deposition and resorption. Typical eruption times are given in Tables 11 and 12.

Table 11 Typical times for calcification and eruption of deciduous teeth

	Calcification begins (weeks in utero)	Eruption (months)
Upper		
Central incisor (a)	12–16	6–7
Lateral incisor (b)	13–16	7–8
Canine (c)	15–18	18–20
First molar (d)	14–17	12–15
Second molar (e)	16–23	24–36
Lower		
Central incisor (a)	12–16	6–7
Lateral incisor (b)	13–16	7–8
Canine (c)	15–18	18–20
First molar (d)	14–17	12–15
Second molar (e)	16–23	24–36

Root calcification is complete 1–1.5 years after eruption.
Typical eruption sequence is a, b, d, c, e.

Table 12 Typical times for calcification and eruption of permanent teeth

	Calcification begins (months)	Eruption (years)
Upper		
Central incisor	3–4	7–8
Lateral incisor	10–12	8–9
Canine	4–5	11–12
First premolar	18–21	10–11
Second premolar	24–27	10–12
First molar	At birth	6–7
Second molar	30–36	12–13
Third molar	84–108	17–21
Lower		
Central incisor	3–4	6–7
Lateral incisor	3–4	7–8
Canine	4–5	9–10
First premolar	21–24	10–12
Second premolar	27–30	11–12
First molar	At birth	5–6
Second molar	30–36	12–13
Third molar	96–120	17–21

Root calcification is complete 2–3 years after eruption.
Typical eruption sequence: upper 6 1 2 4 5 3 7 8; lower 6 1 2 3 4 5 7 8.

6.2 Management of the child patient

Learning objectives

You should

- know the milestones of child development
- be able to relate the milestones to what an individual child can be expected to cope with in the dental surgery
- know the strategies that a dentist could employ to help children to cope
- appreciate the importance of an accurate and comprehensive history and examination.

Psychological aspects

Child development

Development should be regarded as a continuum as it may differ from child to child. It is an uneven process and is influenced by periods of rapid bodily change. There are certain 'psychological signposts' that are important for the dentists and his staff to recognise.

Motor development
Motor development occurs in a predictable order and failure to attain 'motor milestones' enables remedial intervention that will aim to improve motor skills. The environment can influence motor development, and

generalised motor development is completed in early life. Skills or changes that follow walking are refinements rather than new skills. Dominance of one hand emerges early. Motor retardation in a child may be manifested by no specific handed dominance. At 6–7 years of age, a child will have sufficient co-ordination to brush their teeth reasonably well. Below 6–7 years, many areas of the mouth will be inaccessible without parental help.

Cognitive development
Sensorimotor at 0–2 years. Infant can think of things as permanent without having to see them directly.

Pre-operational at 2–7 years. Thought patterns are not well developed; the child is egocentric and inflexible.

Concrete operations at 7–11 years. The child can apply logical reasoning and consider another person's point of view.

Formal operations at 11 years or older. Transition to adult thinking results in the development of logical abstract thinking and different possibilities for action can be considered.

Perceptual development
By age 7 years, children do develop selective attention and can determine which advice merits attention and which can be ignored. Concentration skills also improve. By age 9, children achieve adult proficiency.

Language development
Language and thought are inter-related and lack of stimulation will retard both. Keep dental jargon to a minimum and always assess patients before offering advice.

Social development
Separation anxiety is high until age 5 years and then declines rapidly so do not expect a child younger than this to enter the surgery on their own.

Adolescence
Increasing independency and self-sufficiency develops in adolescence. Young people do tend to be moody, are oversensitive to criticism and often feel miserable for no apparent reason. Therefore, do not criticise adolescents excessively and try to give them support and reassurance.

Parental influence and dental treatment

Parents are vital for positive reinforcement over any treatment objective. Programmes of treatment must be designed to reduce any chances of making parents or their children feel guilty. Design of treatment programmes should also allow goals to be achieved one by one, never overloading parent or child.

Dentist–patient relationship

Each patient is a unique individual and should be treated as such. Overall, it is fair to conclude that while the technical skill of a dentist is of concern, the most important factors for a patient are gentle friendly manner, explanation of treatment procedures and the ability to keep pain to a minimum.

The structure of the dental consultation
1. Greeting – by name
2. Preliminary chat: non-dental topics first, then dental; *listen* to the answers!
3. Preliminary explanation: clinical and preventive objectives in language that can be understood
4. Business: during treatment, constantly check the patient is not in pain and explain and discuss what you are doing; summarise what you have done to patient and parent and offer aftercare advice
5. Health education: constantly reinforce advice about maintaining a healthy mouth and give advice as though you mean it; always set realistic objectives
6. Dismissal: a clear signpost that the appointment is over, using the child's name and a definite farewell.

Anxious and unco-operative children

The extent of anxiety does not relate to dental knowledge but is an amalgam of personal experiences, family concerns, disease levels and general personality traits. It is, therefore, not easy to pinpoint aetiological agents and measure anxiety. In addition, there is no standard measure of anxiety.

Helping anxious patients cope
Several approaches can help to reduce coping problems:
- reducing uncertainty
  — tell, show, do
  — send letter home explaining details of proposed visit
  — acclimatisation programmes
- modelling: videos or a live model
- cognitive approaches
  — identification of beliefs: try to get individuals to identify and alter their dysfunctional beliefs, useful for all focused types of anxiety
  — distraction attempts to shift attention from dental setting towards another kind of situation, e.g. videos, headphones with music or stories
- relaxation: useful for high levels of tension; aims to bring about deep muscular relaxation; trained therapist is required
- systematic desensitisation: working through various levels of feared situations from 'mildest' to 'most anxiety'
- inhalation sedation: usually for ages 5 and over.

Care programme

History involves social, medical and dental information

Social. Name, address, age, school, siblings, parental occupations. This allows clinician to establish rapport. Try and assess social background, knowledge of dentistry and the family's expectations.

Medical. Apart from allowing safe delivery of dental care, two additional factors can be gleaned: children with medical conditions may have a negative attitude to treatment because of the time they have spent in hospitals; they may also be more likely to fail dental appointments owing to the disruption in education that the medical problem has already caused.

Dental. Past dental experiences may give an indication of how the child will cope with proposed treatment. Parental attitude to treatment is important. A treatment plan must be modified to accommodate this. Establish exactly why they have come. The answers from child and parent may be different!

Examination

Clinical examination

The clinical examination need not involve sitting in the dental chair at the first visit. Examine the child as a person not just a mouth.

Extraoral. General appearance is noted; percentile charts are useful way of monitoring height and weight. The head and neck is examined making a sketch of any lesions/marks.

Intraoral. Soft tissues may be indicator of systemic disease. The relationship between periodontal condition and oral hygiene may indicate an underlying condition. Occlusion factors include crowding, malalignments, mandibular deviations and habits. The condition of the teeth is noted; are they clean and dry?

Radiographic examination

Guidelines for prescription of radiographs in children are shown in Table 13.

There are 3 general indications for taking radiographs in children.

Caries diagnosis. At least 50% more approximal lesions can be diagnosed by bitewing radiographs than with clinical examination. New orthopantogram (OPT) films may be very efficient at diagnosing occlusal caries, but bitewings remain essential in diagnosis of 'occult' occlusal caries.

Abnormalities in dental development. All children at age 8 or 9 years should have an OPT to identify disturbances in development of the dentition in terms of the number, position and form of the teeth. Precise location of maxillary canines can then be achieved by intraoral parallex technique.

Detection of bony or dental pathology. Periapicals examined for individual teeth; panoramic views for larger pathology or trauma.

Special investigations

There a number of special tests that are sometimes relevant:

- vitality testing: not suitable for primary dentition; in permanent dentition, no tests are reliable but the electric pulp tester is probably the best
- culture and sensitivity: bacterial, fungal and viral infections
- blood tests: haematological, biochemical, bacteriological and virological examination.

Treatment planning

Planning should incorporate:

- management of pain: consider all teeth of poor prognosis
- long-term treatment planning: to include attitudes and motivation

Table 13 Guidelines for prescription of radiographs in children

| | Child | | |
	Primary dentition	Mixed dentition	Adolescent (permanent dentition)
New patient	Bitewings (lateral obliques)	Bitewings, orthopantogram, occlusals/periapicals	Bitewings, orthopantogram

Recall patient
   Clinical caries: high caries risk
   No clinical caries: low caries risk
   For growth and development
	6–12 monthly bitewings
	 12–24 monthly bitewings
	 Not usually indicated unless specific problem
		6–12 monthly bitewings
		 12–24 monthly bitewings
		 Orthopantogram if considering extractions owing to caries (i.e. whether to balance or) if compensate planning active orthodontic treatment; if monitoring a developmental anomaly
			12 monthly bitewings
			 24–36 monthly bitewings
			 An orthopantogram at about 18 years of age to assess the position of unerupted third molars

- preventive care: tailored to each individual
- restorative care: realistic aims are important.
- aesthetic considerations: children can be under considerable peer pressure over their appearance.

6.3 Caries

Learning objectives

You should

- be able to explain the development of caries to any patient/parent

- know the current clinical methods and possible future methods to detect caries

- know the four practical 'pillars of prevention'

- know the current materials in use for the restoration of primary and permanent teeth, and their respective advantages and disadvantages.

Development of caries

Fermentation of dietary sugars by microorganisms in plaque on the tooth surface produces organic acids. This rapid acid formation lowers the pH at the enamel surface below the level (critical pH $\simeq$ 5.5) at which enamel will dissolve. When sugar is no longer available to the plaque microorganisms, the pH within plaque will rise through the outward diffusion of acids and their metabolism and neutralisation in plaque. As a result, remineralisation of enamel can occur.

Dental caries progresses only when demineralisation is greater then remineralisation. The early caries lesion is subsurface with a surface white demineralisation (precavitation). This may be because a layer of dental plaque on the tooth acts as a partial barrier to diffusion. Plaque forms on tooth surfaces that are not cleaned and it is visually obvious within 2–3 days if there is no toothbrushing. Plaque does not consist of food debris but is 70% microorganisms. Diet influences plaque flora composition; in diets rich in carbohydrate, *Streptococcus mutans* predominate and is very efficient at metabolising sugars to acids. Precavitation carious lesions are reversible by remineralisation if the plaque pH is high (alkaline). This can occur during the periods where there is no sugar intake. The concentrations of calcium, phosphate and fluoride in plaque are very important in the remineralisation process.

Once cavition has occurred and the thin white surface layer has collapsed, it is necessary to restore the tooth surface with a restoration. Cavitation lesions are not reversible.

Epidemiology of caries

The size of the problem of caries in the population has changed over time. Prevalence and extent have fallen markedly since the late 1970s in many countries and this fall can largely be attributed to fluoridated toothpaste. However, caries is becoming more of a problem in preschool children in many countries.

Diagnosis of caries

- visual (eye alone)
- visual tactile (eye plus probe)
- radiography (usually bitewing radiographs)
- fibre-optic transillumination (FOTI)
- electrical resistance methods (ERM).

Visual tactile supported by bitewing radiographs remain the most satisfactory combination for the diagnosis of occlusal and approximal caries. ERM shows great promise and is worthy of further development. However, overall systematic and random errors in diagnosis are great.

Prevention

The four practical 'pillars of prevention' are: diet, fluoride, fissure sealants and plaque control.

Dietary factors

Fluoride is the only dietary nutrient that has any preeruptive influence on a tooth's future susceptibility to caries (major effect is posteruptive).

Non-milk extrinsic sugars (NME) are the dietary threat: sucrose, glucose, fructose, maltose. Intrinsic sugars (lactose in milk and sugars in fruit and vegetables) are not generally a threat to dental health. However, even lactose in milk in a bottle at night or in on-demand breast feeding can be cariogenic. Starchy staple foods (potatoes, bread, rice, pasta) are not a cause of dental caries, but mixtures of finely ground heat-treated starch and sugars (biscuits) are likely to be cariogenic. The frequency of sugar intake and the total quantity of sugar intake are important. In British schoolchildren two-thirds of NME intake is from confectionery, soft drinks and table sugar. Unnecessary addition of extra sugars to milk and other feeds is the cause of caries in young children, especially in immigrant minorities.

Non-sugar sweeteners allowed for use in food and drinks can be considered for practical purposes as noncariogenic. A very slow metabolism for some bulk sweeteners in plaque is not important. There are two groups of non-sugar sweeteners:

- bulk: sorbitol, mannitol, isomalt, xylitol, lactitol and hydrogenated glucose syrup
- intense: saccharin, acesulphame K, aspartame, thaumatin.

Bulk sweeteners have a laxative effect and should not be given to children under the age of 3 years.

Dietary advice

Dietary advice should be positive, practical and personal to the patient and parent, and take into account cooking skills and financial considerations. It can only be achieved with a written 3- or 4-day diary history. Advise against drinks with a high sugar content and titratable acidity.

NMEs should be kept to main meals and acceptable alternatives should be suggested for between meal snacks. No food or drink should be taken within 1 hour of bed and no drink should be available (apart from water) during night.

Fluoride

Fluoride has the ability to increase enamel resistance to demineralisation as well as decreasing acid production in plaque and increasing remineralisation. Although it has a preeruptive effect its major role is posteruptive.

Fluoride can be delivered systemically (swallowed) or topically (applied to the teeth). Water, salt and milk have and are being used throughout the world as systemic vehicles for fluoride. In the USA, 56% of the population receive fluoridated water, in Ireland 60% and in the UK 10%. Fluoride drops/tablets, which have a topical and a systemic effect, are an established and proven method of fluoridation. However, there has been a recommended daily reduction in dosage during the 1990s because it is recognised that the original dose was probably too high and that fluoride is now more likely to be ingested from other sources (toothpaste and water). Toothpastes have been responsible worldwide for the large fall in caries. In 1970, virtually no toothpaste contained fluoride; by 1978, 97% contained fluoride. Most adult pastes contain 1000–1500 ppm fluoride ions (used by those over age 5 years). Children's pastes containing up to 500 ppm are available for those under 5. Only a smear of paste should be used and supervision of brushing is needed to prevent swallowing as this is a risk for fluorosis. Fluoride mouthrinses for age 6 years and over are a valuable daily adjunct. The 0.05% NaF ($\simeq$ 225 ppm F^-) mouthrinse probably has better compliance than weekly 0.2% NaF ($\simeq$ 900 ppm NaF) application. Finally, professionally applied fluoride solutions, gels and varnishes complete the fluoride armamentarium. Varnishes are easier to apply than the solutions and gels and can be applied effectively to all ages.

Although each individual method of fluoride application is effective, a combination of methods may achieve greater benefit (Table 14).

Fissure sealing

The most effective sealant is bis-GMA. At least 50% of sealants are retained for 5 years and their effectiveness in reducing and delaying the onset of caries is not in doubt. Both unfilled and filled resins and clear and opaque resins have been used to equal effect. Isolation after etching and drying is essential to success.

Indications for patient selection and tooth selection are:

- special needs: medical, physical, intellectual, social disability
- caries in primary dentition
- occlusal surfaces of permanent molars, cingulum pits of upper incisors

Table 14 Fluoride preparations

Risk groups	Under 6 years	6–15 years	Adults
Fluoridated community			
Low caries risk	Toothpaste	Toothpaste	Toothpaste
Average caries risk	Toothpaste	Toothpaste	Toothpaste
High caries risk	Toothpaste, topical varnish	Toothpaste, topical gel/varnish, mouthrinse	Toothpaste, topical gel/varnish, mouthrinse
Low-fluoride community (less than 0.3 ppm)			
Low caries risk	Toothpaste	Toothpaste	Toothpaste
Average caries risk	Toothpaste, drops/tablets	Toothpaste, tablets	Toothpaste, mouthrinse
High caries risk	Toothpaste, drops/tablets, topical varnish	Toothpaste, tablets, topical gel/varnish, mouthrinse	Toothpaste topical gel/varnish, mouthrinse

- seal as soon as moisture control permits
- continue to monitor sealed teeth clinically and radiographically.

Plaque control

Caries reduction cannot be achieved by tooth brushing alone. However, toothbrushing will control gingivitis and periodontal disease and is an important way of conveying fluoride to the tooth surface.

Chemical control of plaque with chlorhexidine is effective, but because of its side-effects (staining of teeth, altered taste sensation) it should only be used as a short term adjunct to periodontal care.

The effects of all the practical 'pillars of prevention' are additive and all treatment plans should take into account age, caries risk, water fluoride level and co-operation.

Treatment

The treatment of carious teeth should be based on the needs of the child; the long-term objective should be to help the child to reach adulthood with an intact permanent dentition, no active caries, as few teeth restored as possible and a positive attitude toward their future dental health.

Restorative materials

Amalgam. Its main advantage is that it is economical and simple to use. However, there is current concern over its safety. In Scandinavia, its use is banned in children, with concern over environmental issues rather than amalgam toxicity itself. It does seem prudent to avoid its use whenever possible, especially in the paediatric population where other materials may give sufficient longevity.

Glass ionomer cements (GIC). These consist of basic glass and acidic water-soluble powder; they set by an acid–base reaction between the two components. The cement bonds to enamel and dentine and releases fluoride to the surrounding tissues.

Resin-modified GIC. A hybrid of GIC/resin that retains significant acid–base reaction in its overall curing process to set in the dark. There are two setting reactions: the acid–base reaction between glass and polyacid and a light-activated, free radical polymerisation of methacrylate groups of the polymer. This material has some physical advantages over conventional GIC, together with its ability to 'command set'.

Polyacid-modified composite resin (compomer). This contains either or both essential components of a resin-modified GIC but it is not water based and, therefore, no acid–base reaction can occur. They will not set in the dark and cannot strictly be described as GICs.

Composite resins. Their introduction revolutionised clinical dentistry and their aesthetic benefits are unquestioned. Problems of resistance to wear, water absorption and polymerisation contraction have restricted their use in the permanent posterior teeth and almost ruled them out of a role in caries management in posterior primary teeth. Nevertheless they do have clearly defined roles in the anterior teeth of both dentitions.

Preformed crowns. These preformed extracoronal restorations are essential in the restoration of grossly broken down teeth, primary molars that have undergone pulp therapy, hypoplastic primary and permanent teeth and teeth in those children at high risk of caries, particularly those having treatment under general anaesthesia.

Isolation

Adequate isolation is necessary for any restorative material to have a chance of success. Rubber dam isolation is the optimum and may necessitate local anaesthesia for the gingival tissues. Clamps should be secured individually with floss ligatures. Additional advantages of the rubber dam include airway protection, soft tissue protection and reduced risk of caries infection from saliva aerosol. In the absence of rubber dam, good moisture control can be achieved with cotton wool rolls, dry tips and saliva ejector.

Primary teeth

Pit and fissure caries

The primary fissures are shallower than their permanent counterparts and the presence of caries is a sign of high caries activity. The material of choice is an adhesive material either a GIC, resin-modified GIC, or compomer. Manufacturers' instructions for these materials should be followed assiduously utilising tooth conditioners and bonding resins where stated.

Approximal caries

Minimal approximal cavity A minimal approximal cavity with no occlusal dovetail is repaired using the 'retentive box preparation'. The material of choice is a compomer, which has greater mechanical strength than GIC or resin-modified GIC and which still releases fluoride. The approximal box is prepared as in Box 20 but without an occlusal dovetail. Additional retention grooves may be achieved by placing grooves into dentine using half-round burs along the gingival floor and lingual wall. The buccal wall is avoided because of the large buccal pulp horn in primary molars (Fig. 79).

Approximal caries with occlusal extension The success rate of amalgam in approximal caries with occlusal extension has been reported as being 70–80%. (Box 20).

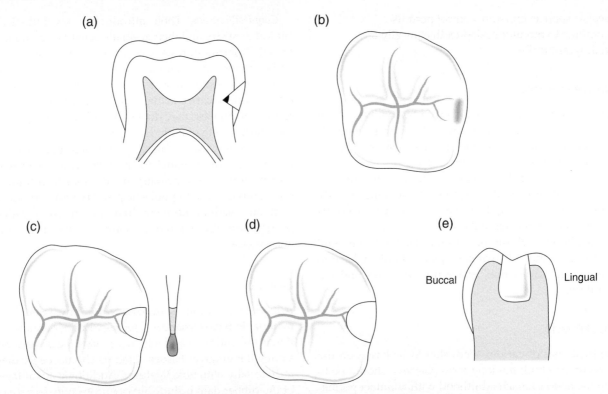

(a)

(b)

(c)

(d)

(e)

Buccal   Lingual

Fig. 79 Approximal posterior caries without pit and fissure caries: the 'retentive box preparation'. (a) Position of the caries. (b) Occlusal view showing cavity or shadow. (c) Access leaving sliver of enamel. (d) Extension of walls and removal of caries from the amelodentine junction. (e) Grooves placed on lingual wall and gingival floor, not on buccal wall.

The failure rate of GICs is higher than amalgam: 33% over 5 years compared with 20% for amalgam.

Box 20 Technique for two-surface restorations

Figure 80 outlines the steps for two-surface restoration.

1. Local anaesthesia and isolation.
2. Complete occlusal part of restoration incorporating a small isthmus and a dovetail for retention. Usually a small pear-shaped diamond in a high-speed handpiece is ideal. The dovetail does not need to extend into all fissures to produce an adequate form.
3. Extend cavity proximally and proceed gingivally creating a box and remove remaining enamel at the contact point. Buccolingually, the cavity should just clear contact points so that an explorer can reach the restoration margins.
4. Remove deep caries with a slow-speed bur.
5. Bevel axio-pulpal line angle to increase the strength of the restoration.
6. Place a calcium hydroxide liner in deep restorations.
7. Place matrix band and wedges.
8. Inset amalgam incrementally starting in the box.
9. Slightly overfill and curve occlusal form with a small ball-ended burnisher and then carver.
10. Remove matrix and pass floss between contact point to remove debris.
11. Check occlusion.

Consequently, amalgam is still the material of choice. However, recent clinical trials of 3 years' duration show that compomers can be as durable as amalgam.

Restorations on more than two surfaces Restorations extending onto more than two surfaces include cusp replacement and endodontically treated teeth. The stainless steel crown is the material of choice, with survival times in excess of 40 months. Their replacement rate is low at 3% compared with 15% for amalgams. Although initially they are more expensive, in the long term they are cost-effective. Problems of colour are gradually being overcome by the introduction of tooth-coloured veneer crowns. Once learnt, their placement technique (Box 21) is less technically demanding than intracoronal restorations in primary teeth and they should certainly be considered for any tooth for which the dentist cannot be sure that an alternative restoration would survive until the tooth is exfoliated.

Anterior teeth

Treatment options for anterior teeth depend on the severity of the decay and the age and co-operation of the patient. In the pre-school child, caries of the upper primary incisors is usually a result of 'nursing caries syndrome': frequent or prolonged consumption of fluids containing NME sugars from a bottle or feeder cup. Progression of decay is rapid, commencing on the labial

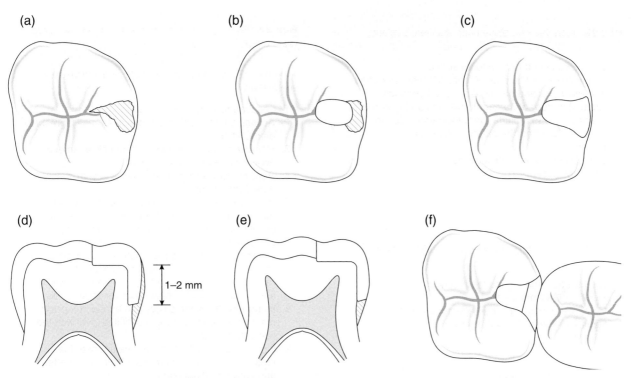

(a) (b) (c)

(d) 1–2 mm (e) (f)

Fig. 80 Posterior caries with pit and fissure caries. (a) Position of the caries. (b) Removal of the occlusal caries. (c) Access to the approximal caries (sliver of enamel left). (d) Establish gingival floor of box and remove remaining enamel at the contact point. (e) Deepen the axio-pulpal line angle centrally as shown (f) in the cavity profile. The buccal and lingual walls of the cavity should be just clear of the broad contact areas.

Box 21 Technique for preformed crowns

1. Local anaesthesia and isolation.
2. Restore tooth with GIC prior to preparation.
3. Reduce occlusal surface by 1.5 mm using flame-shaped or tapered diamond bur.
4. Cut interproximal slices with 10 to 15° taper ensuring the contact point is clear and there are no stops.
5. Buccolingual reduction is not usually necessary unless there is a prominent accessory cusp. These walls are essential for retention.
6. Choose size of crown by measuring mesiodistal width.
7. Trial fit. No more than 1 mm of crown should be subgingival, so trimming with scissors and smoothing with a stone may be required.
8. Cement with GIC or polycarboxylate cement. Seat the lingual side first to bring most of the excess cement to the buccal aspect.
9. Allow to set. Remove excess cement from margins.
10. Small occlusal interferences will adjust by movement of nearby teeth.

---

surface and quickly encircling the teeth. The most suitable form of restoration is the 'strip crown technique', which uses a celluloid crown former with light-cured composite resin to restore crown morphology. In older children over 3 or 4 years of age, new lesions of primary incisors indicate high caries activity. These lesions usually occur approximally and do not progress as quickly as nursing caries. They can be restored with GIC, compomer or composite resin.

Permanent teeth

Bitewing radiographs should be taken prior to any instrumentation of a tooth surface. For a clean fissure with no radiographic evidence of caries, a fissure sealant is the treatment of choice in molar teeth. If the fissure is stained with no radiographic evidence of caries, it will require clinical exploration. If clinical exploration reveals dentinal caries, then a restoration will be required. If dentinal caries is detected radiographically, a restoration is obviously necessary.

Fissure sealants

Consideration needs to be given whether to use a clear, coloured or opaque resin sealant or whether to use a non-filled or filled resin (Box 22). Early sealants were clear in order to check that caries was not developing under the sealant. However, the margins were difficult to see and coloured and opaque materials were introduced in order to see areas of sealant fracture and loss. The final choice is with the individual clinician.

Box 22 Technique for placement of a resin sealant

1. Clean, wash and dry the tooth surface.
2. Etch with gel or liquid for 30 seconds then wash and dry with water and air irrigation for 20 seconds.
3. Apply thin coat of sealant to the pits and fissures, making sure to include the buccal extension in lower molars and the palatal groove in upper molars.
4. Light polymerise for 20 seconds.
5. Check occlusion.

Box 23 Technique for placement of a GIC sealant

1. Clean, wash and dry the tooth surface.
2. Run/flow GIC into the fissures.
3. Compress using a gloved finger for 3 minutes.
4. Remove excess GIC with excavator.
5. Varnish.

Box 24 Technique for placement of a preventive resin restoration

Figure 81 shows the placement of a preventive resin restoration.

1. Local anaesthesia and isolation.
2. Access questionable fissure with a small high-speed diamond bur.
3. Remove carious dentine and enough enamel to allow complete caries removal.
4. Remove caries from deeper dentine with a slow-speed round bur.
5. Place GIC liner over dentine, extending it up to amelodentinal junction, light-curing if necessary.
6. Gel/liquid etchant is placed on enamel margins for 20 seconds, followed by wash and dry. It is not necessary to etch the liner, sufficient roughening of the surface of GIC will result from washing.
7. Place a thin layer of bonding resin into the cavity and onto enamel margins. Cure for 20 seconds.
8. Incrementally fill the cavity with hybrid composite resin. Polymerise the resin until it is level with the occlusal surface.
9. Flow opaque unfilled fissure sealant over the restoration and the entire occlusal fissure pattern and cure for 20 seconds.
10. Check the occlusion.

Bitewing radiographs are an important part of sealant review as it only needs failure of one small part of the sealant–enamel bond for leakage to occur.

GIC may be useful as temporary sealants in individuals with highly active caries until teeth have erupted sufficiently to allow conventional sealants (Box 23). Indeed they are similarly applicable for patients in whom isolation for placement of conventional sealants is impossible. They may require more frequent replacement because of their brittleness in thin section but they will provide occlusal protection and a reservoir of fluoride for release to surrounding enamel.

Stained fissure with no radiographic caries
The fissure should be explored with a small round bur. If the lesion stays within enamel, a fissure sealant is placed. If the lesion extends into dentine the treatment is as for pit and fissure caries.

Pit and fissure caries
If occlusal contacts are retained on enamel in a pit and fissure caries, a composite restoration is applicable, taking the opportunity to fissure seal non-carious fissures; this is known as a 'preventive resin restoration' (Box 24). The durability of preventive resin restorations is proven to be as good as occlusal amalgam restorations and is achieved with removal of significantly less enamel.

If the occlusal contacts are not retained on enamel, then amalgam is the material of choice as it will not wear significantly, nor will it wear opposing teeth.

Approximal caries
Amalgam remains the material of choice even in modern conservative cavity designs that do not sacrifice as much sound tissue as Black's original designs. Non-metallic restorative materials in these situations show significant wear after 4–5 years, which may be a manifestation of fatigue within the resin matrix.

Anterior teeth
Composite resin or the newer reinforced compomers should be the materials of choice. Incisal edge restorations require careful design to utilise more surface area of normal enamel rather than resorting to dentine pins.

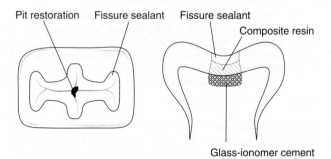

Fig. 81 Preventive resin restoration.

6.4 Tooth discoloration

Learning objectives

You should

- know the causes of extrinsic and intrinsic tooth discoloration

- know which treatments are appropriate for each type of discoloration.

The colour of a young persons teeth is of great importance. Peer group pressure can be significant, and teasing about size, position and colour of teeth can be very harmful. The most useful method of classification for the clinical management of discoloration is one that identifies the main site of discoloration (Table 15).

Once the aetiology has been identified, the most appropriate method of treatment can be chosen. Treatment emphasis should be on minimal tooth preparation. As a general rule, microabrasion should be the first-line treatment for all cases of enamel opacities and mottling; composite resin in the form of localised or full veneers is used in preference to porcelain.

Treatments

Treatments for discoloured teeth can be used in children and adults, although some are not suitable for children younger than teenage. Techniques use abrasion, bleaching and restorations. The exact mechanism by which bleaching occurs remains unknown. Theories of oxidation, photo-oxidation and ion exchange have been suggested.

The hydrochloric acid pumice microabrasion technique

The microabrasion method is a controlled removal of surface enamel in order to improve discolorations that are *limited* to the outer enamel layer (Box 25). It is achieved by a combination of abrasion and erosion and the term 'abrosion' is sometimes used. No more than 100 μm of enamel are removed. Once completed, the procedure should not be repeated. Too much enamel removal is potentially damaging to the pulp and cosmetically the underlying dentine colour will become more evident.

Indications
- fluorosis
- idiopathic speckling
- postorthodontic demineralisation
- prior to veneer placement for well-demarcated stains
- white/brown surface staining, e.g. secondary to primary predecessor infection or trauma (Turner teeth).

Effectiveness
Critical analysis of the effectiveness of the technique should not be made immediately but delayed for at least

Table 15 The aetiology of tooth discoloration

Staining type	Cause
Extrinsic staining	Beverages/food
	Smoking
	Poor oral hygiene (chromogenic bacteria give a green/orange stain)
	Drugs: iron supplements (black stain), minocycline (black stain), chlorhexidine (brown/black stain)
Intrinsic discoloration of enamel	
Local causes	Caries
	Idiopathic
	Injury/infection of primary prececessor
	Internal resorption
Systemic causes	Amelogenesis imperfecta
	Drugs, e.g. tetracyclines
	Fluorosis
	Idiopathic
	Systemic illness during tooth formation
Intrinsic discoloration of dentine	
Local causes	Caries
	Internal resorption
	Metallic restorative materials
	Necrotic pulp tissue
	Root canal filling materials
Systemic causes	Bilirubin (haemolytic disease of newborn)
	Congenital porphyria
	Dentinogenesis imperfecta
	Drugs, e.g. tetracyclines

Box 25 The hydrochloric acid pumice microabrasion technique.

Armamentarium

- Bicarbonate of soda/water
- Copalite varnish
- Fluoridated toothpaste
- Non-acidulated fluoride (0–2 years: drops)
- Pumice
- Rubber dam
- Rubber prophylaxis cup
- Soflex discs
- Hydrochloric acid 18%.

A complete kit for the acid–pumice microabrasion can be purchased commercially as PREMA (Premier Dental Products).

Technique

1. Take preoperative vitality tests, radiographs and photographs.
2. Isolate teeth to be treated with rubber dam and paint Copalite varnish around necks of the dam.
3. Place a mixture of sodium bicarbonate and water on the dam behind the teeth to protect in case of spillage.
4. Mix 18% hydrochloric acid with pumice into a slurry and apply a small amount to the labial surface on either a rubber cup rotating slowly for 5 seconds or a wooden stick rubbed over the surface for 5 seconds before washing for 5 seconds directly into an aspirator tip. Repeat until the stain has reduced, up to a maximum of 10, 5-second applications per tooth. Any improvement that is going to occur will have done so by this time.
5. Apply the fluoride drops to the teeth for 3 minutes.
6. Remove the rubber dam.
7. Polish the teeth with the finest Soflex discs.
8. Polish the teeth with fluoridated toothpaste for 1 minute.
9. Review in 1 month for vitality tests and clinical photographs.
10. Review biannually, checking pulpal status.

1 month as the appearance of the teeth will continue to improve over this time. Experience has shown that although white mottling is often incompletely removed it does become less perceptible. This phenomenon has been attributed to the relatively prismless layer of compacted surface enamel produced by the 'abrosion' technique, which alters the optical properties of the tooth surface.

Long-term studies of the technique have found no association with pulpal damage, increased caries susceptibility or significant prolonged thermal sensitivity. Patient compliance and satisfaction is good and any dissatisfaction is usually a result of inadequate preoperative explanation. The technique is easy to perform for operator and patient and is not time consuming. Removal of any mottled area is permanent and is

achieved with an insignificant loss of surface enamel. Failure to improve the appearance by the microabrasion technique does not have any harmful effects and may make it easier to mask some lesions with veneers.

Non-vital bleaching

Non-vital bleaching is used for teeth that have become discoloured by the diffusion into the dentinal tubules of haemoglobin breakdown products from necrotic pulp tissue (Box 26).

Box 26 Non-vital bleaching

Armamentarium

- Rubber dam
- Zinc phosphate cement/GIC
- Phosphoric acid 37%
- Sodium perborate powder (Bocasan)
- Cotton wool
- Glass ionomer cement
- White gutta-percha
- Composite resin.

Technique

1. Preoperative periapical radiographs are essential to check for an adequate root filling.
2. Clean teeth with pumice and make a note of the shade of the discoloured tooth.
3. Place rubber dam isolating the single tooth. Ensure adequate eye and clothing protection for the patient, operator and dental nurse.
4. Remove palatal restoration and pulp chamber restoration.
5. Remove root filling to the level of the dentogingival junction; it may be necessary to use adult burs in a mini-head.
6. Place 1 mm zinc phosphate cement or GIC over the gutta-percha.
7. Freshen dentine with a round bur. Do not remove excessively.
8. Etch the pulp chamber with 37% phosphoric acid for 30–60 seconds. Wash, and dry. This will facilitate the ingress of the perborate mixture.
9. Mix distilled water and the sodium perborate into a thick paste. This should be done immediately before placement. Place into the tooth either alone with a flat plastic instrument or on a cotton wool pledget.
10. Place a dry piece of cotton wool over the perborate mixture.
11. Seal the cavity with glass ionomer cement.
12. Repeat process at weekly intervals until the tooth is slightly overbleached.
13. Place non-setting calcium hydroxide into the pulp chamber for 2 weeks. Seal with glass ionomer cement.
14. Finally, restore the tooth with white gutta-percha (to facilitate reopening pulp chamber again if necessary at a later date) and composite resin.

Indication
- discoloured non-vital teeth with a well-condensed gutta-percha root filling and no clinical or radiographical signs of periapical disease.

Contraindications
- heavily restored teeth
- staining from amalgam.

Effectiveness
If the colour of a tooth has not significantly improved after three changes of bleach, it is unlikely to do so and further bleaching should be abandoned. The maximum number of bleach applications is usually accepted as 10. Failure of a tooth to bleach could be caused by inadequate removal of filling materials from the pulp chamber. This should be checked before abandoning a procedure.

Slight overbleaching is desirable, but the patient should be instructed to attend the surgery before the next appointment if marked overbleaching has occurred.

Non-vital bleaching has a reputation for causing brittleness. This may be the result of previous injudicious removal of dentine (which only needs to be 'freshened' with a round bur) rather than a direct effect of the bleaching procedure itself.

This method of bleaching has been associated with the later occurrence of external cervical resorption. The exact mechanism is unclear, but it is thought that the previously used hydrogen peroxide diffused through the dentinal tubules to set up an inflammatory reaction in the periodontal ligament around the cervical region of the tooth. In a small number of teeth there is a gap between the enamel and the cementum, and in these the above explanation is tenable. The purpose of the 1 mm layer of zinc phosphate cement is to cover the openings of the dentinal tubules at the level where there may be a communication to the periodontal ligament. In the same way, non-setting calcium hydroxide is placed in the pulp chamber for 2 weeks prior to final restoration in order to eradicate any inflammation in the periodontal ligament. It is unknown whether the perborate mixture is associated with external cervical resorption.

Clinical studies have demonstrated that regression can be expected with this technique. The longest study after 8 years gave a 21% failure rate. However, if white gutta-percha has been placed within the pulp chamber, it can be readily removed and the tooth easily rebleached.

The advantages of the technique are:

- easy for operator and patient
- conserving of tooth tissue
- maintenance of the original crown morphology
- no irritation to gingival tissues
- no problems with changing gingival level in young patients compared with veneers or crowns
- no technical assistance required.

Chairside vital bleaching

Vital bleaching in the surgery involves the external application of hydrogen peroxide to the surface of the tooth followed by its activation with a heat source (Box 27). The technique is lengthy and time consuming and

---

Box 27 Technique of vital bleaching

Armamentarium
- Rubber dam with clamps and floss ligatures
- Orabase gel
- Topical anaesthetic
- Gauze
- Phosphoric acid 37%
- Heating light with rheostat
- Hydrogen peroxide 30 volume
- Polishing stones
- Fluoride drops (0–2 years).

Technique

1. Take preoperative periapical radiographs and vitality tests. Any leaking restorations should be replaced.
2. Clean teeth with pumice and water to remove extrinsic staining. Preoperative photographs should be taken with a tooth form, a 'Vita' shade guide registering the shade, adjacent to the patient's teeth.
3. Apply topical anaesthetic to gingival margins.
4. Coat the buccal and palatal gingivae with Orabase gel as extra protection from bleaching solution.
5. Isolate each tooth to be bleached using individual ligatures. The end teeth should be clamped (usually from second premolar to second premolar).
6. Cover the metal rubber dam clamps with damp strips of gauze in order to prevent them from getting hot under the the heat source.
7. Etch the labial and a third of the palatal surfaces of the teeth with the phosphoric acid for 60 seconds, wash and dry. Thoroughly soak a strip of gauze in the 35% hydrogen peroxide and cover the teeth to be bleached.
8. Position the heat lamp 13–15 inches from the patient's teeth. Set the rheostat to a mid-temperature range, increase it until the patient can just feel the warmth in their teeth and then reduce it slightly until no sensation is felt.
9. Keep the gauze damp by reapplying the hydrogen peroxide every 3–5 minutes using a cotton bud. The bottle should be closed between applications as the hydrogen peroxide deactivates on exposure to air.
10. After 30 minutes, remove the rubber dam, clean off the Orabase gel and polish the teeth using the shofu stones. Apply the fluoride drops for 2–3 minutes.
11. Postoperative sensitivity may occur and should be relieved with paracetamol.
12. Assess the change; it may be necessary to repeat the process 3 to 10 times per arch. Treat one arch at a time. Keep the patient under review, as rebleaching may be required after 1 or more years.
13. Take postoperative photographs with the original 'Vita' shade tooth included.

---

demands a high degree of patient compliance and motivation. Within paediatric dentistry, it is appropriate only for the teenager. Its main remit is in the older patient to treat the yellowing of teeth that occurs with ageing.

Indications
- very mild tetracycline staining without obvious banding
- mild fluorosis
- single teeth with sclerosed pulp chambers and canals.

Nightguard vital bleaching

The nightgaurd vital bleaching technique involves the daily replacement of carbamide peroxide gel into a custom-fitted tray of either the upper or lower arch (Box 28). Like the previous technique, it demands a high degree of patient compliance and motivation and is appropriate in paediatric dentistry only for the teenager. Its main remit is in the older patient to treat the yellowing of teeth.

Indications in paediatric dentistry
- mild fluorosis
- moderate fluorosis as an adjunct to microabrasion.

Carbamide peroxide gel (10%) breaks down in the mouth into 3% hydrogen peroxide and 7% urea. Both urea and hydrogen peroxide have low molecular weights, which allow them to diffuse rapidly through enamel and dentine. This explains the transient pulpal sensitivity occasionally experienced with bleaching systems for use at home.

Localised composite resin restorations

Defective enamel can be replaced with a tooth-coloured restoration that bonds to, and blends with, enamel (Box 29). It is indicated for well-demarcated white, yellow or brown patches.

The localised restoration is quick and easy to complete. Despite the removal of defective enamel down to the amelodentine junction, there is often no significant sensitivity and, therefore, no need for local anaesthesia. If the hypoplastic enamel has become carious and extends into dentine, a liner of glass ionomer cement (correct shade) prior to placement of composite resin will be necessary. In these cases, local anaesthesia will probably be required. Advances in bonding and resin technology make these restorations simple and obviate the need for a full labial veneer. Disadvantages are marginal staining, difficulty in achieving an accurate colour match and reduced composite translucency when lined by a glass ionomer cement.

Box 28 Nightguard vital bleaching technique

Armamentarium

- Upper impression and working model
- Soft mouthguard, avoiding the gingivae
- Carbamide peroxide gel 10%.

Technique

1. Take an alginate impression of the arch to be treated and cast a working model in stone.
2. Relieve the labial surfaces of the teeth by about 0.5 mm and make a soft pulldown vacuum-formed splint as a mouthguard. The splint should be no more than 2 mm in thickness and should not cover the gingivae. It is only a vehicle for the bleaching gel and is not to protect the gingivae.
3. Instruct the patient on how to floss their teeth thoroughly. Perform a full mouth prophylaxis and instruct the patient how to apply the gel into the mouthguard.
4. The length of time the guard should be worn depends on the product used.
5. Review the patient about 2 weeks later to check that they are not experiencing any sensitivity, and then at 6 weeks, by which time 80% of any colour change should have occurred.

Box 29 Localised composite resin restorations for defective enamel

Armamentarium

- Rubber dam/contoured matrix strips (Vivadent)
- Round and fissure diamond burs
- Enamel/dentine bonding kit
- New generation highly polishable hybrid composite resin
- Soflex discs and interproximal polishing strips.

Technique

1. Take preoperative photographs and make shade selection.
2. Apply rubber dam or contoured matrix strips.
3. Remove demarcated lesion with round diamond fissure bur.
4. Etch enamel margins, wash and dry.
5. Apply dentine primer to dentine and dry.
6. Apply enamel and dentine bonding agent and light-cure.
7. Apply chosen shade of composite using a brush lubricated with the bonding agent to smooth and shape. Light-cure for the recommended time.
8. Remove matrix strip/rubber dam.
9. Polish with graded Soflex discs (3M), finishing burs and interproximal strips if required. Add characterisation to surface of composite.
10. Take postoperative photographs.

Composite resin veneers

Although the porcelain jacket crown (PJC) may be the most satisfactory long-term restoration for a severely hypoplastic or discoloured tooth, it is not an appropriate solution for children for two reasons: the large size of the young pulp horns and chamber, and the immature gingival contour.

Composite veneers may be direct (placed at initial appointment; Box 30) or indirect (placed at a subsequent appointment having been fabricated in the laboratory). The conservative veneering methods may not just offer a temporary solution but may also offer a satisfactory long-term alternative to the PJC. Most composite veneers placed in children and adolescents are of the 'direct' type as the durability of the indirect composite veneers is as yet unknown. Composite veneers are durable enough to last through adolescence.

Before proceeding with any veneering technique, the decision must be made whether to reduce the thickness of labial enamel before placing the veneer. Certain factors should be considered:

- increased labiopalatal bulk makes it harder to maintain good oral hygiene; this may be courting disaster in the adolescent with dubious oral hygiene
- composite resin has a better bond strength to enamel when the surface layer of 200–300 μm is removed
- if a tooth is very discoloured, some sort of reduction will be desirable as a thicker layer of composite will be required to mask the intense stain
- if a tooth is already instanding or rotated, its appearance can be enhanced by a thicker labial veneer.

New-generation, highly polishable hybrid composite resins can replace relatively large amounts of missing tooth tissue as well as being used in thin sections as a veneer. Combinations of shades can be used to stimulate natural colour gradations and hues. The exact design of the composite veneer will vary with each patient. Usually it will be one of four types: intraenamel or window preparation, incisal bevel, overlapped incisal edge or feathered incisal edge (Fig. 82).

Indications
- discoloration
- enamal defects
- diastemata
- malpositioned teeth
- large restorations.

Box 30 Technique for placement of composite resin veneers

Armamentarium
- Rubber dam/contoured matrix strips (Vivadent)
- Preparation and finishing burs
- New-generation, highly polishable hybrid composite resin
- Soflex discs (3M) and interproximal polishing strips.

Technique
1. Clean teeth with a slurry of pumice in water. Wash and dry and select shade.
2. Use a tapered diamond bur to reduce labial enamel by 0.3–0.5 mm. Identify finish line at the gingival margin and also mesially and distally just labial to contact points.
3. Isolate the tooth either with rubber dam or a contoured matrix strip. Hold this in place by applying unfilled resin to its gingival side against the gingiva and curing for 10 seconds.
4. Etch the enamel for 60 seconds, wash and dry.
5. Where dentine is exposed, apply dentine primer.
6. Apply a thin layer of bonding resin to the labial surface with a brush and cure for 15 seconds. It may be necessary to use an opaquer at this stage if the discoloration is intense.
7. Apply composite resin of the desired shade to the labial surface and roughly shape it into all areas with a plastic instrument before using a brush lubricated with unfilled resin to 'paddle' and smooth it into the desired shape. Cure 60 seconds gingivally, 60 seconds mesio-incisally, 60 seconds disto-incisally and 60 seconds from the palatal aspect if incisal coverage has been used. Different shades of composite can be combined to achieve good matches with adjacent teeth and a transition from a relatively dark gingival area to a lighter more translucent incisal region.
8. Flick away the unfilled resin and remove the contoured strip.
9. Finish the margins with diamond finishing burs and interproximal strips and the labial surface with graded sandpaper discs. Characterisation should be added to improve light reflection properties.

Contraindications
- insufficient available enamel for bonding
- beware patients who play woodwind instruments!

Porcelain veneers

Normally, porcelain veneers are considered at around 18 years of age when the gingival margin is at an adult level and the standard of oral hygiene is acceptable. However, a non-standard application which may be applicable at an earlier age is the restoration of the peg lateral with a three-quarter wrap-around veneer finished to a knife edge at the gingival margin.

Table 16 Treatment technique for tooth surface loss

Technique	Advantages	Disadvantages
Cast metal (nickel/chrome or gold)	Fabrication in thin section: requires only 0.5 mm space Very accurate fit possible Very durable Suitable for posterior restorations in parafunction Does not abrade opposing dentition	May be cosmetically unacceptable because of 'shine through' of metallic grey Cannot be simply repaired or added to intraorally
Composite Direct	Adequately durable for labial veneers only Least expensive May be used as a diagnostic tool	Technically difficult for palatal veneers Limited control over occlusal and interproximal contour Inadequate as a posterior restoration
Indirect	Can be added to and repaired relatively simply Aesthetically superior to cast metal Control over occlusal contour and vertical dimension	Requires more space: minimum of 1.0 mm Unproven durability
Porcelain	Best aesthetics Good abrasion resistance Well tolerated by gingival tissues	Potentially abrasive to opposing dentition Inferior marginal fit Very brittle: has to be used in bulk section Hard to repair

(a) (b)

(c) (d)

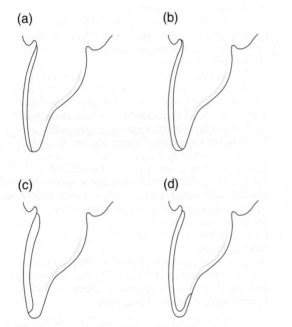

Fig. 82 Types of veneer preparation. (a) Feathered incisal edge. (b) Incisal bevel preparation. (c) Intra-enamel or window preparation. (d) Overlapped incisal edge preparation.

6.5 Tooth surface loss (wear)

Dentists have been aware of the problem of tooth wear or non-carious loss of tooth tissue for a long time. However, it is only more recently that it has been associated increasingly with our younger population. There are three processes that make up the phenomenon of tooth wear:

attrition: wear of tooth as a result of tooth contact
erosion: irreversible loss of tooth substance brought about by a chemical process that does not involve bacterial action
abrasion: physical wear of tooth substance produced by something other than tooth-to-tooth contact.

In children, abrasion is relatively uncommon. The most frequent cause of abrasion is overzealous tooth brushing, which tends to develop with increasing age. Attrition during mastication is common, particularly in the primary dentition where almost all upper incisors show some signs of attrition by the time they exfoliate. However, in the 1990s, the contribution of erosion to the overall process of tooth wear in the younger population has been highlighted.

While erosion may be the predominant process, attrition and abrasion may be compounding factors, e.g. toothbrush abrasion may be increased if brushing is carried out immediately after the consumption of erosive foodstuffs or drinks. It is often difficult to identify a single causative agent in a case of tooth wear so the general term *tooth surface loss* may be more appropriate.

Prevalence

There is very little published evidence on the prevalence or severity of tooth wear in children. In 1993, the National Child Dental Health Survey included assessment of the prevalence of erosion of both primary and permanent incisor teeth for the first time. The survey reported that 52% of 5-year-old children had erosion of the palatal surfaces of their primary incisors with 24% showing progression into the pulp. The prevalence of erosion of the palatal surfaces of permanent incisors was also alarmingly high: 27% in 15 year olds. However, only 2% in this age group showed progression into the pulp. What is unclear is whether the problem of tooth surface loss is actually increasing or whether these figures reflect an increased awareness.

Aetiology

In young patients there are three main causes of tooth surface loss:

- dietary
- gastric regurgitation
- parafunctional activity.

In addition to these, certain environmental factors have been linked to tooth wear. With the exception of frequent use of chlorinated swimming pools, most environmental and occupational hazards do not apply to children.

Dietary causes of tooth surface loss

The most common cause of erosive surface loss is excessive intake of acidic food or drink. Food and drink implicated in erosive tooth surface loss in young patients include:

- citrus fruits, e.g. lemons, oranges, grapefruits
- tart apples
- vinegar and pickles
- yoghurt
- fruit juices
- carbonated drinks, including low-calorie varieties, sparkling mineral water and 'sports' drinks
- vitamin C tablets.

Acidic drinks, in particular, are available to all age groups of children. Pure 'baby' fruit juices are marketed for consumption by infants and these have been shown to have pH values below the critical pH for the dissolution of enamel (pH 5.5). Many of these drinks are given to infants in a feeding bottle, and the combination of the highly acidic nature of the drink and the prolonged exposure of the teeth to the acidic substrate may result in excessive tooth surface loss as well as dental caries. While a wide range of foods and drinks is implicated in the aetiology of tooth surface loss, soft drinks make up the bulk of the problem. Soft-drink consumption has increased dramatically since the 1960s, to a staggering 151 litres per capita of the population in the UK in 1991. Adolescents account for up to 65% of these purchases. Pure fruit juices do contribute to this figure but, increasingly, carbonated drinks make up a large part of the younger population's intake. These are now widely available in vending machines located in schools, sports centres and other public areas. Both normal and so-called 'diet' carbonated drinks have very low pH values and are associated with tooth surface loss. While there is no *direct* relationship between the pH of a substrate and the degree of tooth surface loss, pH does give a useful indication as to the potential to cause damage. Other factors such as titrateable acidity, the effect on plaque pH and the buffering capacity of saliva will all influence the erosive potential of a given substrate. In addition, it has been shown that erosive tooth surface loss tends to be more severe if the volume of drink consumed is high or if the intake occurs at bedtime.

The pattern of dietary erosive tooth surface loss depends on the manner in which the substrate is consumed. Carbonated drinks are commonly held in the mouth for some time as the child 'enjoys' the sensation of the bubbles. This habit may result in a generalised loss of surface enamel. Generalised loss of surface enamel of posterior teeth is often evident, particularly on the first permanent molars. Characteristic saucer-shaped lesions develop on the cusps of the molars. This phenomenon is known as *perimolysis*.

Gastric regurgitation and tooth surface loss

The acidity of the stomach contents is below pH 1.0; therefore, any regurgitation or vomiting is potentially damaging to the teeth. As many as 50% of adults with signs of tooth surface loss have a history of gastric reflux. The aetiology of gastric regurgitation may be divided into those with upper gastrointestinal disorders and those with eating disorders.

In young patients long-term regurgitation is associated with a variety of underlying problems:

- gastro-oesophageal reflux
- oesophageal strictures
- chronic respiratory disease
- disease of the liver/pancreas/biliary tree
- overfeeding
- feeding problems/failure to thrive conditions
- children with mental handicap
- Reye's syndrome
- rumination.

In addition, there are a group of patients that suffer from gastro-oesophageal reflux disease (GORD). This may be either symptomatic, in which case the individual knows what provokes the reflux, or the more insidiously asymptomatic GORD, in which the patient is unaware of the problem and continues to ingest reflux-provoking foods.

Parafunctional activity

Localised tooth surface loss frequently occurs in patients who exhibit abnormal parafunctional habits. The excessive grinding that is a feature of this problem is not always apparent to the patient. However, apart from the marked tooth tissue loss, other signs of bruxism may be evident including hypertrophy of the muscles of mastication, cheek biting and tongue faceting. An example of erosion and parafunction having a disastrous effect on the dentition may be seen (and heard) in children who have cerebral palsy. These children often have chronic gastric regurgitation and also severe bruxism, resulting in excessive tooth surface loss.

Management

Immediate management

The most important part of management is early recognition. It is important to establish the aetiology and where possible eliminate the cause prior to treating any sensitivity. Dietary counselling should be personal, practical and positive. Suitable alternatives should be suggested with the most appropriate times for their intake:

- inform patients of types of foods and drinks that have greatest erosive potential
- suggest still/non-carbonated drinks as an alternative
- limit the intake of acidic foods/drinks to meal times
- advocate use of neutral fluoride mouthwash or gel for daily use to try and minimise the effect of the acids
- encourage use of bicarbonate of soda mouthrinse in those with recurrent gastric reflux
- where attrition is marked, neutral fluoride gel can be placed into an occlusal guard during the night or during episodes of vomiting.

Immediate temporary coverage of sensitive teeth with GIC or composite resin can relieve symptoms and act as a diagnostic acid.

Definitive management

The main treatment objectives are:

- resolve sensitivity
- restore missing tooth structure
- prevent further tooth tissue loss
- maintain a balanced occlusion.

Study models must be taken at initial diagnosis and at periodic intervals to monitor progress. Table 16 outlines the merits of the restorative materials available.

Adhesive metal castings

Box 31 describes fitting of adhesive metal casts.
  Indications

- amelogenesis imperfecta
- dentinogenesis imperfecta
- dental erosion, attrition, abrasion
- enamel hypoplasia.

Long-term review
Long-term review is necessary to:

- monitor future tooth surface loss
- maintain the existing restorations
- provide support for the patient.

Box 31 Technique for production of adhesive metal casts

Armamentarium
- Gingival retraction cord
- Elastomeric impression material
- Face bow system and semi-adjustable articulator
- Rubber dam
- Panavia-Ex (Kuraray).

Technique
1. Study models are essential, with photographs if possible.
2. Institute full mouth prophylaxis.
3. Ensure good moisture isolation.
4. Place retraction cord into the gingival crevices of the teeth to be treated and remove immediately prior to taking the impression.
5. Take an impression using an elastomeric material: a putty/wash system is the best and check the margins are easily distinguishable.
6. Take a face bow transfer and interocclusal record in the retruded axis position.
7. Mount the casts on a semi-adjustable articulator.
8. Construct cast onlays, a maximum of 1.5 mm thick occlusally, in either nickel/chrome or gold.
9. Grit blast the fitting surfaces of the occlusal onlays.
10. Return to the mouth and check the fit of the onlays.
11. Polish teeth with a pumice and isolate under rubber dam where possible.
12. Cement onlays using Panavia-Ex.
13. Check occlusion.
14. Review in 1 week for problems and regularly thereafter.

6.6 Endodontics

Learning objectives

You should

- know the indications and contraindications for primary molar pulp treatment

- know the medicaments used in primary molar pulp treatment

- know the treatment for vital and non-vital immature permanent incisors

- know the initiating factors in the different types of resorption.

Primary teeth

The question of whether to retain primary teeth should be based on three factors: medical, behavioural and dental.

Medical contraindications to extraction

- bleeding disorders and coagulopathies
- hypodontia associated with syndrome (e.g. ectodermal dysplasia).

Medical indications for extraction
- congenital cardiac disease
- immunosuppression
- poor healing potential (unstable diabetes).

Behavioural reason for retention Poor co-operation makes extraction difficult.

Dental contraindications to extraction

- well-maintained arch
- orthodontic considerations
- hypodontia: lack of permanent successor.

Dental indications for extraction

- extensive caries with gross coronal breakdown and caries penetrating pulpal floor
- acute infection with large collection of pus
- excessive tooth mobility
- natural exfoliation
- poorly maintained mouth.

Pulpal treatment options

Indirect and direct pulp capping

Pulp capping can be applied successfully to the primary dentition provided strict selection criteria are applied.

Indirect capping. Gentle excavation of the majority of softened dentine is achieved without exposing the pulp.

The remaining softened dentine is covered with setting calcium hydroxide to destroy any remaining micro-organisms and to promote the deposition of reparative secondary dentine. The tooth is then restored at the same visit.

Direct capping. The small mechanical exposure on a vital symptom-free tooth that is well isolated is the only situation where direct capping should be applied. If direct capping is applied in other situations, pulp inflammation usually persists and results in total pulp necrosis. In the majority of children, pulpotomy is the preferred treatment, with a high rate of success.

Pulpotomy

Pulpotomy involves the extirpation of vital inflamed pulp from the coronal chamber as a means of preserving the vitality and function of the remaining portion of radicular pulp (Box 32).

There is a controversy over the most appropriate medicament for vital pulpotomies. It is currently widely held that formocresol in 1:5 dilution is an acceptably safe medicament with a success rate of 90–98%. However, calcium hydroxide has been used and is the only medicament that promotes biological healing and the formation of a hard tissue barrier over amputated radicular pulp. Success rate with calcium hydroxide is 60%. Unfortunately it has been associated with internal resorption and further research is necessary.

If successful, the treated tooth should be asymptomatic. Failure will result in pain, swelling, increased

---

Box 32 Technique for pulpotomy

1. A preoperative radiograph is taken of the affected tooth.
2. Use local anaesthesia and isolation.
3. Removal of caries and formation of an endodontic access cavity (slow speed Batt bur).
4. Excavation of coronal pulp with slow speed 6 or 8 bur or a spoon excavator (Fig. 83b).
5. Haemorrhage control. Place several pellets of cotton wool firmly into the excavated coronal pulp chamber to apply pressure to the radicular pulp stumps. Pellets may be soaked in LA solution. Remove the pellets after 5 minutes. Repeat until haemorrhage has ceased. If haemorrhage is profuse, it indicates a more serious inflammation and a pulpectomy is indicated.
6. Place pledget moistened in formocresol solution into chamber for 4 minutes (Fig. 83c). On removal, the pulp stumps will appear dark brown or black.
7. Restore pulp chamber with reinforced zinc oxide/eugenol cement and reinforced glass ionomel cement (Fig. 83d).
8. Restore the tooth with a preformed crown (Fig. 83e).

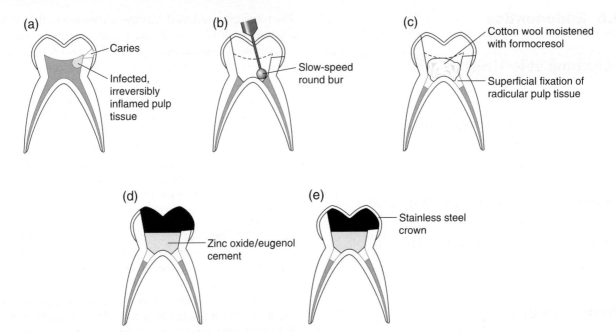

Fig. 83 Primary molar pulp amputation (vital pulpotomy) (with permission from Whitworth, Nunn 2001. In: Welbury RR (ed) Paediatric Dentistry, 2nd edition, p. 171. Oxford: Oxford University Press).

mobility, fistulae and radiographic signs of either radio-lucency at the furcation or apex or internal/external resorption of the root.

Radiographic assessment every 12 months is necessary to check the above and the developing underlying permanent successor.

Pulpectomy

Pulpectomy involves the chemomechanical preparation of primary root canals with endodontic hand instruments and irrigants (Box 33). Because of the anatomy of the root canals and the presence of the permanent successor, greater emphasis is often placed on the use of antimicrobial and tissue-fixative medicaments, especially in primary posterior teeth. The success rate is 60–80%.

Pulpectomy for anterior primary teeth If the pulpal tissue is vital, the procedure can be completed in one visit otherwise the two-stage procedure (Box 33) should be followed.

Pulp treatments under general anaesthesia It is usual to extract all teeth of dubious prognosis in a child who is not co-operative or cannot co-operate and requires treatment under general anaesthesia. However, one-stage procedures are possible and the operator will have to assess pulpal status and radiographic signs accordingly.

Clinical problems with pulpally involved primary teeth There are situations where it is clinically impossible or inappropriate to complete ideal pulp therapy and these are usually associated with the behaviour of the child:

- when an unexpected exposure is encountered and no local anaesthetic has been given
- when local anaesthesia is inadequate
- when the child is in acute pain.

Box 33 Technique for pulpectomy

1. Take a preoperative radiograph of the affected tooth.
2. Use local anaesthesia and isolation (may be remnants of vital tissue).
3. Caries removal and endodontic access. As described in the text Batt burs that are non-end-cutting will allow pulp chamber roof removal without fear of furcal or lateral perforation.
4. Debridge pulp chamber with normal saline or 0.5–1.0 hypochlorite solution and file canals to within 2–3 mm of radiographic apex (Fig. 84b). Dry canals with paper points.
5. Seal a pledget of cotton wool barely moistened with formocresol into the pulp chamber with a hard setting cement for 7–10 days (Fig. 84c). The intention is to fix any remaining pulpal remnants and kill any microorganisms remaining after canal preparation.
6. At review, if the signs and symptoms of periapical or furcal pathosis have resolved, the canals can be filled with non-reinforced slow-setting zinc oxide/eugenol cement. Fluid mixture may be introduced with spiral fillers or stiffer mixes packed with cotton wool pledgets or pluggers (Fig. 84d). Care should be taken not to extrude material beyond the root apices.
7. Restore the tooth with preformed crown (posterior) or strip crown (anterior) placed over quick-setting zinc oxide/eugenol cement (Fig. 84e).

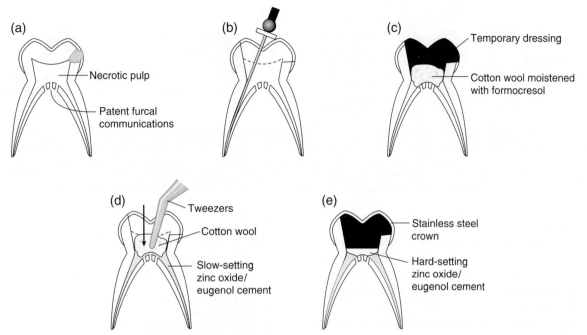

Fig. 84 Primary molar non-vital pulp therapy (with permission from Whitworth, Nunn 2001. In: Welbury RR (ed) Paediatric Dentistry, 2nd edition, p. 175. Oxford: Oxford University Press).

> **Box 34** Treatment when pulp therapy cannot be completed
>
> 1. Place Ledermix paste into pulp chamber, canals, or over site of exposure.
> 2. Place dry cotton wool pellet over Ledermix and restore with a temporary cement.
> 3. Review within 7 days and re-assess. If inflammation or infection persists, proceed to pulpectomy or extraction. Otherwise the decision regarding pulpotomy or pulpectomy will depend on pulp status.

The aim of treatment is to control pain and to prevent further pain (Box 34).

Young permanent molar teeth with immature apices

The treatment of choice for the cariously exposed young permanent tooth is dependent on:

- stage of root development
- status of the crown
- orthodontic considerations for the tooth and the arch
- psychological and behavioural factors.

The final decision has to balance the long-term advisability of retaining the tooth and the practicality of restoring the crown. Coronal destruction in an immature molar tooth is associated with pulpal exposure, which will mean that this tooth will require maintenance throughout life.

Vital teeth with immature roots

For vital teeth with immature roots the aim of therapy is to preserve vitality to ensure completion of root development.

Indirect pulp cap
An indirect pulp cap is indicated in teeth with minimal symptoms (Fig. 85). A thin layer of carious dentine is left over the pulp because its removal would create an exposure. Caries control is a variation of indirect pulp capping. Calcium hydroxide cement is usually placed over the softened dentine but GIC or Ledermix have also been advocated.

Direct pulp cap
Permanent teeth respond well to direct pulp capping procedures, unlike primary teeth. Selection of appropriate cases is important.
  Indications

- small carious exposures
- teeth with no history of swelling or spontaneous pain
- no radiographic changes
- controllable bleeding at exposure site.

Calcium hydroxide or Ledermix cement is placed directly onto the exposed pulp, covered with a GIC base and then the final restorative material is placed over the GIC.

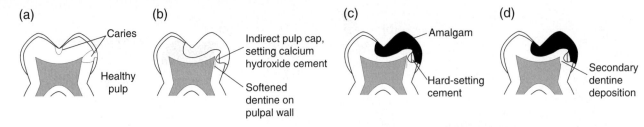

Fig. 85 Indirect pulp capping. (a) Symptom-free molar tooth with deep proximal caries. (b) The caries is excavated to the brink of pulpal exposure leaving a small amount of softened dentine. A thin layer of setting calcium hydroxide cement is applied to the softened dentine as an indirect pulp cap. (c) The indirect pulp cap is covered with hard cement and the tooth restored with amalgam. (d) Some months later, the pulp has remained vital and secondary dentine deposition is evident (with permission from Whitworth, Nunn 2001. In: Welbury RR (ed) Paediatric Dentistry, 2nd edition, p. 168. Oxford: Oxford University Press).

Pulpotomy

Calcium hydroxide results in rapid bridge formation over the radicular pulp stumps. It can be used to great effect to delay extraction for orthodontic purposes but may preclude root canal therapy at a later stage if the tooth is retained.

Formocresol has no place in the treatment of permanent teeth.

Ledermix cement may have a place as a pulpotomy medicament as it not only has the advantages of the obtundent effect of corticosteroid and antibiotic but also contains both calcium hydroxide and zinc oxide/eugenol.

Non-vital teeth with immature roots

Non-vital teeth with immature roots should be removed, although short-term retention for orthodontic reasons may be desirable. After root canal instrumentation and cleaning, a medicament such as Ledermix or non-setting calcium hydroxide should be placed and the crown restored.

Young permanent incisor teeth with immature apices

Vital

Permanent vital incisors can be treated with calcium hydroxide pulpotomy or Cvek pulpotomy (apexogenesis). The aim is removal of contaminated pulp tissue with a clean round high-speed diamond bur in order to allow radicular growth with vital radicular pulp (Box 35).

Success rate is 80–96%. Prognosis is best if the procedure is completed within 24 hours of the injury.

Non-vital incisors

Non-vital incisors are treated with calcium hydroxide pulpectomy (apexification) to create an apical head–tissue barrier against which a root filling can be placed (Box 36).

Box 35 Pulpotomy of vital permanent incisors

1. Clinical examination (Fig. 86a) shows a complicated fracture with microbial invasion of the coronal pulp. The pulp has been exposed to the mouth for longer than 24 hours.
2. Use local anaesthesia.
3. Place rubber dam.
4. The coronal pulp is accessed with a diamond bur running at high speed with constant water cooling (Fig. 86b).
5. Wash pulp with saline until haemorrhage stops. Remove any clots with gentle saline washing.
6. Non-setting calcium hydroxide is placed over pulp remnant. Cover with setting calcium hydroxide and semi-permanent restorative material (Fig. 86c).
7. Review at 6 weeks. If there is no evidence of pulp pathosis, review at a further 6 weeks and then 6 monthly for evaluation of pulp vitality and assessment of calcific bridge formation clinically and radiographically. Direct visual assessment of a calcific bridge is sometimes possible. Figure 86d shows a calcific barrier with healthy pulp at 12 months.
8. If vitality is lost, non-vital pulp therapy should be undertaken through the calcific bridge.
9. Pulpectomy when root development is complete may be required if the root canal is required for restorative purposes. A modified Cvek pulpotomy, where the surface 1–2 mm of exposed pulp tissue is removed by a slow bur, is also used with equal success.

Endodontic complications in young permanent incisor teeth

Root fractures

Root canal therapy can often be confined to the non-vital coronal portion of the canal. Instrumentation by rotation of hand files and placement of non-setting calcium hydroxide to the fracture line aims to produce a stop at the coronal side of the fracture line. The coronal portion can then be obturated with gutta-percha and sealer.

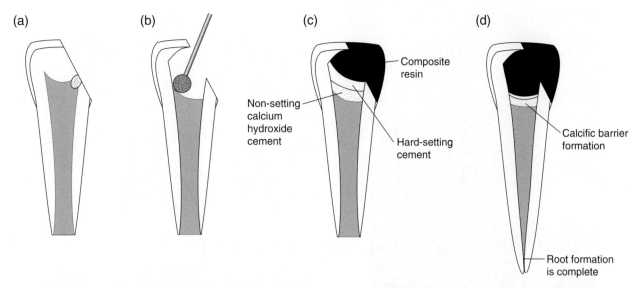

(a)   (b)   (c)   (d)

Composite resin

Non-setting calcium hydroxide cement

Hard-setting cement

Calcific barrier formation

Root formation is complete

Fig. 86 Permanent incisor pulpotomy (apexogenesis) (with permission from Whitworth, Nunn 2001. In: Welbury RR (ed) Paediatric Dentistry, 2nd edition, p. 173. Oxford: Oxford University Press).

Box 36 Permanent root end closure for non-vital incisors

1. Use local anaesthesia.
2. Place rubber dam.
3. Access cavity (Fig. 87a).
4. Extirpate nectrotic pulp tissue.
5. Prepare canal 1 mm short of radiographic apex.
6. Gentle instrumentation and irrigation with 1% sodium hypochlorite solution to remove and dissolve organic debris and kill microorganisms. Use gentle debridement in a crown–apex direction and determine working length (Fig. 87b).
7. Press canal with calcium hydroxide.
8. Re-dress with non-setting calcium hydroxide after 1–2 weeks, then 3-monthly (Fig. 87c).
9. Compression of non-setting calcium hydroxide with a cotton wool pellet or plugger to ensure good condensation in the canal.
10. Dry cotton wool and then GIC or IRM temporary dressing is added.
11. Average time for apical stop formation is 1 year.
12. Obturation with gutta-percha using a warm vertical condensation technique or thermoplastic gun (Fig. 87d).

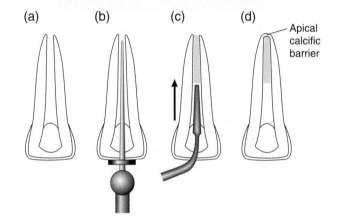

(a)   (b)   (c)   (d)

Apical calcific barrier

Fig. 87 Permanent incisor root-end closure (apexification) (with permission from Whitworth, Nunn 2001. In: Welbury RR (ed) Paediatric Dentistry, 2nd edition, p. 178. Oxford: Oxford University Press).

Root resorption

Inflammatory

External. Resorption is initiated by damage to the periodontal ligament but propagated by necrotic pulp tissue via dentinal tubules. Diagnosis is by asymmetrical radiolucent shape of surface of root with intact root canal walls (Fig. 88).

Internal. Resorption is initiated by cells of the pulp within the root canal. Diagnosis is as a ballooning of the root canal with intact root surface (Fig. 89).

Treatment of both types is by thorough mechanical and chemical debridement followed by non-setting calcium hydroxide paste in a bid to halt the process. Obturation with thermoplastic gutta-percha is used if cessation of resorption occurs.

If the apical portion is non-vital it may be possible to instrument across the fracture line, although it can be very difficult to prevent bleeding into the canal. When the canal is eventually dry after changes of non-setting calcium hydroxide, obturation is with gutta-percha and sealer. Failure to instrument a non-vital apical fragment necessitates surgical removal of the fragment. Splinting across fracture lines with a post is a radical temporary solution with a poor long-term prognosis.

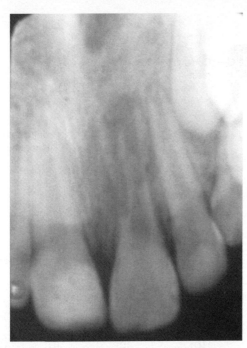

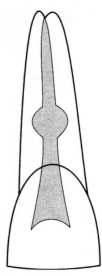

Fig. 89 Ballooning of the root canal caused by internal resorption. (With permission from Whitworth, Nunn 1997. In Welbury RR (ed) Paediatric Dentistry. Oxford University Press, Oxford)

Fig. 88 Radiograph showing the radiolucent shape of external root resorption.

Cervical. This is an unusual form of external inflammatory resorption initiated by damage to the root surface in the cervical region and propagated either by infected root canal contents or by periodontal microflora. Treatment is usually by obturation of the root canal followed by surgical external repair and restoration.

Replacement

Replacement is progressive resorption of tooth structure and its replacement with bone as part of contin-ued bone remodelling. It occurs after trauma in which there is significant periodontal ligament injury, i.e. luxation, intrusion and avulsion. It cannot be treated. The tooth should be maintained in the mouth for as long as possible with intracanal non-setting calcium hydroxide dressings while plans are made for permanent prosthetic replacement.

Self-assessment: questions

Multiple choice questions

1. The mineralisation of these teeth may be affected by maternal illness during pregnancy:
   a. Primary molars
   b. Primary incisors
   c. Permanent incisors
   d. Primary canines
   e. Permanent first molars

2. With regard to childhood development and dental treatment:
   a. Separation from parents is possible after age 5 years
   b. Adequate manual dexterity for good oral hygiene is possible at age 5 years
   c. Parental influence is important
   d. By age 5, children have developed selective attention
   e. Teenagers respond well to criticism

3. Bitewing radiographs should be taken every 6–12 months for:
   a. Primary dentition with high caries risk
   b. Primary dentition with low caries risk
   c. Mixed dentition with low caries risk
   d. Mixed dentition with high caries risk
   e. Permanent dentition with low caries risk

4. Orthopantograms:
   a. Diagnose occlusal caries accurately
   b. Diagnose interproximal caries accurately
   c. Identify abnormalities in dental development of number, position or form
   d. Can precisely localise teeth
   e. Identify larger areas of pathology

5. In caries development:
   a. Plaque consists mainly of food debris
   b. Precavitation lesions are reversible
   c. Pre-school caries prevalence is falling
   d. In the UK, 56% of water is fluoridated
   e. Dietary advice is easy to give

6. In caries diagnosis:
   a. Diagnosis of interproximal caries in the primary dentition is easy
   b. Marginal ridge breakdown in primary molars suggests pulpal involvement
   c. Stained fissures in first permanent molars should be explored
   d. Occlusal caries is reliably diagnosed clinically
   e. Electrical resistance methods aid caries diagnosis

7. In caries epidemiology:
   a. The fall in caries prevalence since the 1970s is largely a consequence of toothbrushing
   b. Pre-school caries is related to maternal *Strep. mutans* levels
   c. Nursing caries is associated with frequent use of sugared drinks
   d. Nursing caries can be prevented by correct advice
   e. Caries levels in school-age children in the UK have fallen since 1973

8. Fluoride supplementation should be given:
   a. Systemically to all patients with special needs
   b. As a mouthwash to a 5 year old
   c. From birth
   d. In only one systemic form of delivery
   e. In topical form to all patients with orthodontic appliances

9. With regard to restorative materials in the primary dentition:
   a. Amalgam is the material choice for pit and fissure caries
   b. Nursing caries is best treated with glass ionomer cement
   c. Approximal cavities without occlusal extension should be restored with amalgam
   d. Preformed metal crowns are the most durable restorations for large cavities and endodontically treated teeth
   e. Glass ionomer cement is suitable for two-surface cavities

10. With regard to the restoration of permanent teeth:
    a. Composite can be placed in pit and fissure location as long as occlusal contacts are retained on enamel
    b. Composite can be placed in approximal cavities
    c. Regular bitewing radiographs are required for fissure-sealed teeth
    d. Stained fissures should be investigated early to conserve tooth tissue
    e. 'Occult' caries is easy to diagnose clinically

11. In extrinisc tooth discoloration:
    a. Stains can be removed by polishing
    b. Bleaching is an accepted treatment
    c. Mouthwashes can be an important factor
    d. Liquid oral medicines are never involved
    e. Food and beverages are a common cause

12. Intrinsic discoloration:
    a. May be caused by internal resorption

b. Is caused by some drugs
c. If caused by fluorosis, it can be treated by microabrasion
d. May be caused by previous trauma to primary teeth
e. In non-vital teeth can be treated by bleaching

13. In primary molar endodontics:
    a. Vital pulpotomy has a low success rate
    b. Calcium hydroxide is the medicament of choice for vital pulpotomy
    c. Teeth with furcation caries should be extracted
    d. Treatment is indicated in children with cardiac defects
    e. Treatment is indicated in children with bleeding coagulopathies

14. In permanent incisors with open apices:
    a. Pulpotomy is preferred to pulp cap for pulpal exposures
    b. Pulpotomy medicament of choice is formocresol
    c. Pulpotomy enables radicular development with vital pulp tissue
    d. Non-vital pulpectomy with non-setting calcium hydroxide stimulates root end closure
    e. Non-vital pulpectomy root end closure occurs in 6 months

Case history question

> An 8-year-old child who was previously caries free suddenly develops interproximal lesions.

1. What investigations would you do?
2. What treatment would you advise?

Picture questions

Picture 1

Figure 90 shows teeth that erupted 12 days after birth.

1. What is the name given to these teeth?
2. Are these teeth usually part of the normal dentition?
3. What problems can arise with these teeth?
4. How should they be treated?

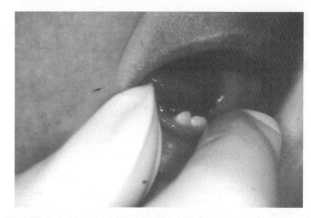

Fig. 90 Teeth that erupted 12 days after birth.

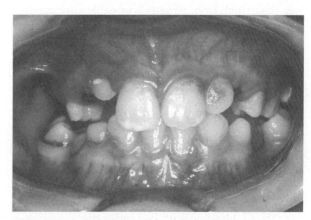

Fig. 91 Staining of teeth.

Picture 2

Figure 91 shows stained teeth.

1. What type of staining is shown?
2. What is the likely cause of the staining?

Short note questions

Write short notes on:

1. drinks to avoid for a patient with tooth surface loss of dietary origin
2. the main clinical features and risk factors for 'nursing' caries
3. indications and contraindications for inhalation sedation.

Self-assessment: answers

Multiple choice answers

1. a. **True**. Primary molars begin mineralising at 3.5–6 months of pregnancy.
   b. **True**. Primary incisors begin mineralising at 3–4 months of pregnancy.
   c. **False**. Permanent incisors do not begin mineralising until 3–4 months after birth.
   d. **True**. Primary canines begin mineralising at 3.5–4.5 months of pregnancy.
   e. **True**. Permanent molars begin mineralising at 7–8 months of pregnancy. They are the only permanent teeth for which mineralisation can be affected by events during pregnancy.

2. a. **True**. Separation anxiety is high until the age of 5.
   b. **False**. Co-ordination is normally sufficiently developed at age 6–7.
   c. **True**. Absolutely vital for positive reinforcement.
   d. **False**. By age 7 years, children have developed selective attention and can determine which advice is important.
   e. **False**. Teenagers require support and reassurance.

3. a. **True**. This is the correct frequency.
   b. **False**. Bitewings should only be taken every 12–24 months.
   c. **False**. Bitewings should only be taken every 12–24 months.
   d. **True**. This is the correct frequency.
   e. **False**. Bitewings should be taken every 12 months.

4. a. **False**. They may suggest that caries is present, but bitewings give a more accurate diagnosis.
   b. **False**. They may suggest that caries is present, but bitewings give an accurate diagnosis.
   c. **True**. They are invaluable in this regard.
   d. **False**. Only in conjunction with intraoral radiographs can they be used to localise teeth.
   e. **True**. They are excellent for the diagnosis of larger pathological lesions.

5. a. **False**. Plaque is 70% microorganisms.
   b. **True**. Once the surface layer is broken and cavitated they need to be restored.
   c. **False**. It is rising, which is extremely worrying.
   d. **False**. Only 10% of UK water is fluoridated.
   e. **False**. It requires time and thought. It must be personal, practical and positive.

6. a. **False**. The wide contact area makes diagnosis of interproximal caries difficult. Bitewing radiographs increase diagnosis of caries by 50%.
   b. **True**. In over 50% of teeth this is the case.
   c. **True**. Fissure biopsy should be performed prior to restoration with either a fissure sealant if the lesion stays within enamel or a preventive resin restoration if it involves dentine.
   d. **False**. It remains one of the most difficult diagnoses to make.
   e. **True**. These recent developments will make caries diagnosis easier in the future.

7. a. **False**. It is linked to fluoridated toothpaste.
   b. **True**. Levels of maternal *Strep. mutans* have been shown to correlate with caries levels in pre-school children.
   c. **True**. Especially if the sugared drinks are taken on demand throughout the night.
   d. **True**. Advice at birth to the new mother by the health visitor is probably the most important factor in establishing correct habits.
   e. **True**. Fortunately this is the case.

8. a. **False**. Water fluoride levels must be obtained prior to advising on systemic supplementation.
   b. **False**. Mouthwashes cannot reliably be handled under the age of 6 years.
   c. **False**. Current guidelines in the USA and UK recommend that 6 months is the earliest to consider supplementation.
   d. **True**. Giving fluoride tablets to someone who lives in an optimally water fluoridated area will produce fluorosis.
   e. **True**. Prescription of a daily 0.05% sodium fluoride mouthwash is recommended in these circumstances.

9. a. **False**. Glass ionomer cement or compomer are better.
   b. **False**. Strip crowns with composite resin.
   c. **False**. Compomer is preferred to amalgam.
   d. **True**. Less than 5% of metal crowns will require replacement.
   e. **False**. Compomer or amalgam is used.

10. a. **True**. It is currently accepted that wear of the composite could be excessive in occlusal loading situations.
    b. **False**. Amalgam is the material of choice.
    c. **True**. A macroscopically intact sealant is not necessarily microscopically intact.
    d. **True**. A fissure biopsy is the treatment of choice.

e. **False**. By definition, it is difficult and requires bitewing radiography.

11. a. **True**. Polishing should be completed on all discoloured teeth to allow accurate assessment, diagnosis and treatment planning.
    b. **False**. Bleaching is a treatment for intrinsic discoloration.
    c. **True**. Chlorhexidine mouthwash binds tannin to produce black staining around the gingival margin.
    d. **False**. Iron supplements will produce a black stain and some antituberculosis drugs a red-brown stain.
    e. **True**. Especially in the presence of poor oral hygiene.

12. a. **True**. This gives a characteristic 'pink spot' appearance to the overlying enamel.
    b. **True**. Tetracyclines are the most notorious offenders, producing a yellow-grey discoloration with intensification of the colour and banding in the cervical third of the crown.
    c. **True**. The majority of fluorotic stains involve the outer 100–300 μm enamel. Controlled microabrasion removes approximately 100 μm enamel and changes the optical properties of enamel to render residual stains less perceptible.
    d. **True**. Previous trauma to primary teeth can produce localised hypoplasia of permanent crowns: so-called Turner teeth.
    e. **True**. Historically, peroxide has been the medicament of choice. However, a sodium perborate and distilled water mixture may produce similar results, possibly without the risk of external cervical resorption.

13. a. **False**. Formocresol pulpotomy has 90–98% success rate.
    b. **False**. It only has a 60% success compared with 90–98% for formocresol.
    c. **True**. These cannot be restored.
    d. **False**. Absolutely contraindicated. Extract.
    e. **True**. This avoids extraction, which would have bleeding complications.

14. a. **True**. Its chance of success and hence its ability to retain vital radicular pulp is superior to pulp capping.
    b. **False**. Formocresol should not be used in permanent teeth.
    c. **True**. This is the important factor in choosing pulpotomy as opposed to pulp capping.
    d. **True**. As long as the cells of Hertwig's root sheath are not damaged.
    e. **False**. Commonly in about 12 months.

Case history answer

1. It is essential to establish the cause of the caries. A 3-day diet analysis is very important. The family circumstances may have recently changed and there may have been an increased exposure to sugared sweets and snacks.
2. Dietary advice, suggesting that sugars are kept to main meal times with savoury snacks between meals. Drinks should not contain sugar and no food or drink should be taken within an hour of going to bed. Addition therapy could include topical fluoride toothbrush instruction and fissure sealant placement on first permanent molars.

Picture answers

Picture 1

1. Neonatal teeth. If these teeth are present at birth they are called natal teeth.
2. Yes. Lower incisors are the commonest teeth involved.
3. Ulceration of the infant's tongue or the mother's breast and a danger to the airway if they are excessively mobile.
4. If they fulfil any of the above or if they are supernumaries, then they should be extracted. If they are part of the normal dentition then retention is beneficial.

Picture 2

1. Extrinsic staining.
2. Foods and beverages, chlorhexidine mouthwash, oral drug suspensions e.g. iron preparations.

Short note answers

1. The acidogenic potential is a term that takes into account a liquid's resistance to changes in its pH, i.e. its inherent buffering capacity. Natural juices have a very high acidogenic potential, followed by fruit-flavoured carbonated waters and drinks, and then carbonated cola drinks. Patients should be advised to try and eradicate all carbonated beverages except on special occasions and at these times to try to take them at a main meal with a straw. Natural fruit juices should be advised only at meal times.
2. The main clinical features are rapidity of onset, surfaces and teeth affected, characteristically the smooth labial and/or palatal surfaces of upper incisors; pattern of attack characteristically (with exception of lower incisors) is teeth as they erupt.

The risk factors include use of a pacifier dipped in a sugar solution, prolonged on-demand sugary drink feeding, lower social class and certain ethnic groups.

3. Indications for inhalation sedation include:
   - dentally anxious
   - marked gag reflex
   - traumatic procedures
   - sickle cell trait/anaemia
   - bleeding disorders
   - cardiac disorders
   - physical handicap
   - asthma
   - epilepsy.

Contraindications include:
   - common cold
   - tonsillar and adenoidal enlargement
   - severe pulmonary conditions
   - undergoing psychiatric treatment
   - learning difficulties
   - myasthenia gravis
   - first trimester of pregnancy.

Special situations

Overview

This chapter covers dental trauma, dental anomalies and the special needs of medical, physical and intellectual disability.

Increased knowledge of the pathophysiology of dental trauma has resulted in an improvement in the standard of care for traumatised teeth and an increase in the prognosis for such teeth. Teeth that would have been extracted in the recent past can now often be maintained in function during adolescence and early adulthood. The category of special needs has increased with successful scientific advances in paediatric medicine and surgery. More children now survive previously fatal illnesses. However, they often do so with either direct oral and dental side-effects of the original illness or its treatment or with significant risk of morbidity or mortality from oral or dental infection.

7.1 Traumatic injuries

Learning objectives

You should

- know the most common injuries in the primary and the permanent dentitions

- be able to classify crown/root fractures and periodontal ligament (displacement) injuries

- know the appropriate treatments for each classification of injury

- appreciate the importance of a high index of suspicion in child physical abuse and know what actions to take and where to go to for help.

Traumatic injuries to teeth and jaw can occur at any age. They are, however, very common in children. Boys have twice as many injuries as girls in both the primary and permanent dentitions. The majority of injuries affect the maxillary incisors. The most common types of injury are:

- primary dentition: subluxation, luxation
- permanent dentition – crown fractures.

Peak injury times occur at 2–4 years in the primary dentition when a young child is exploring and becoming adventurous and 7–10 years in the permanent dentition owing to falls when playing. At age 5, 31–40% of boys and 16–30% of girls will have injured their teeth. The respective figures at age 12 years are 12–33% and 19%.

Assessment

Classification

Table 17 summarises the classification of dento-alveolar injuries based on the World Health Organization (WHO) system.

History

Dental history

When did injury occur? The time interval between injury and treatment significantly influences the prognosis of avulsion, luxations, crown fractures (with or without pulpal exposures) and dento-alveolar fractures.

Where did the injury occur? May indicate the need for tetanus prophylaxis.

How did the injury occur? The nature of the accident can yield information on the type of injury expected. Discrepancy between history and clinical findings raises suspicion of NAI (non-accidental injury).

Lost teeth/fragments? If a tooth or fractured piece cannot be accounted for when there has been a history of loss of consciousness, then a chest radiograph should be obtained to exclude inhalation.

Concussion, headache, vomiting or amnesia? Brain damage must be excluded and referral to a hospital for further investigation organised.

Table 17 Classification of dento-alveolar injuries

Injury	Description
Injuries to the hard dental tissues and the pulp	
Enamel infraction	Incomplete fracture crack of enamel without loss of tooth substance
Enamel fracture	Loss of tooth substance confined to enamel
Enamel–dentine fracture	Loss of tooth substance confined to enamel and dentine, not involving the pulp
Complicated crown fracture	Fracture of enamel and dentine exposing the pulp
Uncomplicated crown root fracture	Fracture of enamel, dentine and cementum but not involving the pulp
Complicated crown root fracture	Fracture of enamel, dentine, cementum and exposing the pulp
Root fracture	Fracture involving dentine, cementum and pulp; can be subclassified into apical, middle and coronal third
Injuries to the periodontal tissues	
Concussion	No abnormal loosening or displacement but marked reaction to percussion
Subluxation (loosening)	Abnormal loosening but no displacement
Extrusive luxation (partial avulsion)	Partial displacement of tooth from socket
Lateral luxation	Displacement other than axially with comminution or fracture of alveolar socket
Intrusive luxation	Displacement into alveolar bone with comminution or fracture of alveolar socket
Avulsion	Complete displacement of tooth from socket
Injuries to supporting bone	
Comminution of mandibular or maxillary alveolar socket wall	Crushing and compression of alveolar socket; found in intrusive and lateral luxation injuries
Fracture of mandibular or maxillary alveolar socket wall	Fracture confined to facial or lingual/palatal socket wall
Fracture of mandibular or maxillary alveolar process	Fracture of the alveolar process; may or may not involve the tooth sockets
Fracture of mandible or maxilla	May or may not involve the alveolar socket
Injuries to gingiva or oral mucosa	
Laceration of gingiva or oral mucosa	Wound in mucosa resulting from a tear
Contusion of gingiva or oral mucosa	Bruise not accompanied by a break in the mucosa, usually causing submucosal haemorrhage
Abrasion of gingiva or oral mucosa	Superficial wound produced by rubbing or scraping the mucosal surface

Previous dental history? Previous trauma can affect pulpal sensibility tests and the recuperative capacity of the pulp and/or periodontium. In addition, for a child, is the child injury prone or are there suspicions of NAI? Previous treatment experience, age and parental/child attitude will affect the choice of treatment.

Medical history

Congenital heart disease, rheumatic fever or severe immunosuppression are contraindications for prolonged endodontic treatment with a persistent necrotic focus. Endodontic treatment should be under antibiotic cover, at least during extirpation and working length calculation.

Bleeding disorders must be of prime concern if there is soft tissue laceration, avulsion or luxation, or if extractions are required.

Allergies require a suitable alternative antibiotic if necessary.

Tetanus status may lead to referral for tetanus toxoid booster (if no previous infection in the last 5 years).

Extraoral examination

Swelling, bruising or lacerations may indicate underlying bony and tooth injury. Lacerations require careful debridement to remove foreign bodies. Crown fracture with associated lip swelling and a penetrating wound may suggest fragment retention in the lip.

Intraoral examination

Examination must be systematic and include recording of lacerations, haemorrhage and bruising as well as abnormalities of tooth occlusion, displacement, fractures or cracks. Teeth examination should include:

- mobility assessment: possible root fracture, displacement, dentoalveolar fracture
- percussion: duller note may indicate root fracture
- colour: early change seen on palatal or gingival third of crown

- sensitivity tests
  — thermal with warm gutta-percha or ethyl chloride
  — electric pulp tester
  — notoriously unreliable, never use in isolation from other clinical and radiographic data
  — always test contralateral teeth and compare.

Radiographic examination

Periapical radiographs

Reproducible 'long cone technique' periapicals are the best for accurate diagnosis and clinical audit. Two radiographs at different angles may be essential to detect a root fracture. However, if access and co-operation are difficult, one anterior occlusal radiograph rarely misses a root fracture.

Occlusal radiographs

To detect fractures and foreign bodies within the soft tissues:

- upper lip – lateral view using an occlusal film held by patient/helper at side of mouth.
- lower lip – occlusal view using an 'occlusal' film held between teeth.

Orthopantogram

An orthopantogram is essential in all trauma. It may detect unsuspected underlying bony injury. Other views include:

lateral oblique
lateral skull: specialist views for maxillofacial fractures
anteroposterior skull
occipitomental.

Photography

Photographs are useful for clinical records and for medicolegal use.

Primary dentition

During its early development the permanent incisor is located palatally to, and in close proximity with, the apex of the primary incisor. With any injury to a primary tooth, there is risk of damage to the underlying permanent successor.

The most accident prone time is between 2 and 4 years of age. Realistically, this means that few restorative procedures will be possible and in the majority of children the decision is between extraction or maintenance without extensive treatment. A primary incisor should always be removed if its maintenance will jeopardise the developing tooth bud.

A traumatised primary tooth that is retained should be assessed regularly for clinical and radiographic signs of pulpal or periodontal complications. Radiographs may even detect damage to the permanent successor. Soft tissue injuries in children should be assessed weekly until healed. Tooth injuries should be reviewed every 3–4 months for the first year and then annually until the primary tooth exfoliates and the permanent successor is in place.

Crown fractures

Uncomplicated crown fracture This is treated either by smoothing sharp edges or by restoring with an acid-etch restoration if co-operation is satisfactory.

Complicated crown fracture. Normally, extraction is the treatment of choice. However, pulp extirpation and canal obturation with zinc oxide cement, followed by an acid-etch restoration, is possible with reasonable co-operation.

Crown root fracture. The pulp is usually exposed and any restorative treatment is very difficult. The tooth is best extracted.

Root fracture

A root fracture without displacement and with only a small amount of mobility should be treated initially by keeping the tooth under observation. If the coronal fragment becomes non-vital and symptomatic, it should be removed. The apical portion usually remains vital and undergoes normal resorption. Similarly, with marked displacement and mobility, only the coronal portion should be removed.

Concussion, subluxation and luxation injuries

Associated soft tissue damage should be cleaned by the parent twice daily with 0.2% chlorhexidine using cotton buds or gauze swabs until healing is completed.

Concussion. Concussion is often not brought to a dentist until a tooth discolours.

Subluxation. If the tooth has slight mobility, a soft diet for 1–2 weeks is advised, with the traumatised area kept as clean as possible. Marked mobility requires extraction.

Extrusive luxation. Marked mobility requires extraction.

Lateral luxation. If the crown is displaced palatally, the apex moves buccally and hence away from the permanent tooth germ. If the occlusion is not gagged, conservative treatment to await some spontaneous realignment is possible. If the crown is displaced buccally, the apex will be displaced towards the permanent tooth bud and extraction is indicated in order to minimise further damage to the permanent successor.

Intrusive luxation. This is the most common type of injury. The aim of investigation is to establish the direction of displacement through radiographical examination. If the root is displaced palatally towards the permanent successor then the primary tooth should be extracted to minimise the possible damage to the developing permanent successor. If the root is displaced buccally then periodic review to monitor spontaneous re-eruption should be allowed. Review should be weekly for a month then monthly for a maximum of 6 months. Most re-eruption occurs between 1 and 6 months. If this does not occur then ankylosis is likely and extraction is necessary to prevent ectopic eruption of the permanent successor.

Exarticulation (avulsion). Replantation of avulsed primary incisors is not recommended because of the risk of damage to the permanent tooth germs. Space maintenance is not necessary following the loss of a primary incisor as only minor drifting of adjacent teeth occurs. The eruption of the permanent successor may be delayed for about 1 year as a result of abnormal thickening of connective tissue overlying the tooth germ.

Sequelae of injuries to the primary dentition

Pulpal necrosis
Necrosis is the most common complication of primary trauma. Evaluation is based upon colour and radiography. Teeth of a normal colour rarely develop periapical inflammation; conversely, mildly discoloured teeth may be vital. A mild grey colour occuring soon after trauma may represent intrapulpal bleeding with a pulp that is still vital. This colour may recede; if it persists then necrosis should be suspected. Radiographic examination should be 3-monthly to check for periapical inflammation. Failure of the pulp cavity to reduce in size is an indicator of pulpal death. Teeth should be extracted whenever there is evidence of periapical inflammation, to prevent possible damage to the permanent successor.

Pulpal obliteration
Obliteration of the pulp chamber canal is a common reaction to trauma. Clinically, the tooth becomes yellow/opaque. Normal exfoliation is usual, but occasionally periapical inflammation may intervene and, therefore, annual radiography is advisable.

Root resorption
External inflammatory resorption is usually seen after intrusive injuries and internal resorption with subluxation and other luxation injuries. Extraction is advised for all types of root resorption.

Injuries to developing permanent teeth
Injuries to the permanent successor tooth can be expected in 12–69% of primary tooth trauma and 19–68% of jaw fractures. Intrusive luxation causes most disturbances; exarticulation (avulsion) of a primary incisor will also cause damage if the apex moves towards the permanent tooth bud before the avulsion. Most damage to the permanent tooth bud occurs under 3 years of age, during its developmental stage. However, the type and severity of disturbance are closely related to the age at the time of injury. Changes in the morphology and mineralisation of the crown of the permanent incisor are most common but later injuries can cause radicular anomalies. Injuries to developing teeth can be classified as:

- white or yellow-brown discoloration of enamel: injury at 2–7 years
- white or yellow-brown discoloration of enamel with circular enamel hypoplasia: injury at 2–7 years
- crown dilaceration: injury at about 2 years
- odontoma-like malformation: injury at <1–3 years
- root duplication: injury at 2–5 years
- vestibular or lateral root angulation and dilaceration: injury at 2–5 years
- partial or complete arrest of root formation: injury at 5–7 years
- sequestration of permanent tooth germs
- disturbance in eruption.

Most enamel hypoplasia can be treated with a combination of microabrasion or veneers. Most dilacerations and eruption abnormalities require surgical exposure and orthodontic alignment.

Permanent dentition

The aims and principles of treatment are: considered as emergency, intermediate and permanent actions.

1. Emergency
   a. retain vitality of fractured or displaced tooth
   b. treat exposed pulp tissue
   c. reduction and immobilisation of displaced teeth
   d. antiseptic mouthwash, antibiotics and tetanus prophylaxis
2. Intermediate
   a. with or without pulp therapy
   b. minimally invasive crown restoration
3. Permanent
   a. apexification
   b. root filling with or without root extrusion
   c. with or without gingival and alveolar collar modification
   d. semi- or permanent coronal restoration.

Trauma cases require painstaking follow-up to disclose any complications and institute the correct treatment. The intervals between examinations depend on the severity of trauma, but the following schedule is a guide: 1, 3 and 6 weeks then at 3, 6 and 12 months with annual checks for 4–5 years. At these times, colour, mobility, percussion and sensitivity are routinely noted while radiographs are examined for periradicular conditions and changes within the pulp cavity.

Injuries to the hard dental tissues and the pulp

Enamel infraction. These are incomplete fractures and without proper illumination are easily overlooked. Periodic recalls are necessary to review pulpal status.

Enamel fracture. Treatment is usually limited to smoothing any rough edges and splinting if there is mobility. Periodic review is necessary.

Enamel–dentine fracture. Immediate treatment is necessary because of the involvement of dentine. The pulp requires protection against thermal irritation and from bacteria via the dentinal tubules. Restoration of crown morphology also stabilises the position of the tooth in the arch. Emergency protection of the exposed dentine can be achieved by:

- fast-setting calcium hydroxide over dentine followed by an acid-etched dressing of filled or unfilled composite resin or a compomer to protect the calcium hydroxide
- calcium hydroxide and glass ionomer cement within an orthodontic band or incisal end of stainless steel crown if there is insufficient enamel available for acid-etch technique.

These will serve as temporary retainers until further eruption occurs.

Intermediate restoration of most enamel–dentine fractures can be achieved by:

- acid-etched composite or a compomer applied either freehand or utilising a celluloid crown former; at a later age this could be reduced to form the core of a porcelain jacket crown preparation.
- reattachment of crown fragment: now feasible with the development of dentine bonding agents; there is a tendency for the distal fragment to become opaque or require further restorative intervention in the form of a veneer jacket or crown.

If the fracture line through dentine is not very close to the pulp, the fragment may be reattached immediately. If, however, it runs close to the pulp, it is advisable to place a suitably protected calcium hydroxide dressing over the exposed dentine for at least 1 month while storing the fragment in saline, which should be renewed weekly (Box 37).

Complicated crown fracture. The major concern after pulpal exposures in immature teeth is the preservation

Box 37 Technique for refitting a fragment of tooth

1. Check the fit of the fragment and the vitality of the tooth.
2. Clean fragment and tooth with pumice-water slurry.
3. Isolate the tooth with rubber dam.
4. Attach fragment to a piece of gutta-percha to facilitate handling.
5. Etch enamel for 30 seconds on both fracture surfaces and extend for 2 mm from fracture line on tooth and fragment. Wash for 15 seconds and dry for 15 seconds.
6. Apply dentine primer to both surfaces and then dry for 15–30 seconds.
7. Apply enamel–dentine bonding agent to both surfaces then lightly blow away any excess. Light-cure for 10 seconds.
8. Place appropriate shade of composite resin over both surfaces and position fragment. Remove gross excess and cure 60 seconds labially and palatally.
9. Remove any excess composite resin with sandpaper discs.
10. Remove a 1 mm gutter of enamel on each side of fracture line both labially and palatally to a depth of 0.5 mm using a small round or pear-shaped bur. The finishing line should be irregular in outline.
11. Etch the newly prepared enamel, wash, dry, apply composite, cure and finish.

of pulpal vitality in order to allow continued root growth. The injured pulp must be sealed from bacteria so that it is not infected during the period of repair. Partial pulpotomy or pulpotomy is often the treatment of choice.

Uncomplicated crown root fracture. After removal of the fractured piece of tooth, these vertical fractures are commonly a few millimetres incisal to the gingival margin on the labial surface but down to the cementoenamel junction palatally. Prior to placement of a restoration, the fracture margin has to be brought supragingival either by gingivoplasty or extrusion (orthodontically or surgically) of the root portion.

Complicated crown root fracture. As above, with the addition of endodontic requirements. If extrusion is planned, then the final root length must be no shorter than the final crown length, otherwise the result will be unstable. Root extrusion can be successful in a motivated patient and leads to a stable periodontal condition.

Root fracture

Root fractures occur most frequently in the middle of the apical third of the root. The coronal fragment may be extruded or luxated. Luxation is usually in a lingual or palatal direction.

If displacement has occurred, the coronal fragment should be repositioned as soon as possible by gentle digital manipulation and the position checked radiographically. Mobile root fractures need to be splinted to encourage repair of the fracture. Apical third fractures, in the absence of concomitant periodontal ligament injury, are often firm and do not require splinting. They do need to be regularly reviewed to check pulpal status and to be treated endodontically if necessary.

Middle third and coronal third fractures must be splinted, as repair of the fracture is important to the long-term stability and prognosis of the tooth. A functional splint with one abutment tooth on either side of the fractured tooth should remain in place for 2–3 weeks. The splint should allow colour observations and sensitivity testing and access to the root canal if endodontic treatment is required. The splint design and placement techniques are discussed below. In about 80% of all root-fractured teeth, the pulp remains viable and repair occurs in the fracture area. Three main categories of repair are recognised:

- repair with calcified tissue: invisible or hardly discernible fracture line
- repair with connective tissue: narrow radiolucent fracture line with peripheral rounding of the fracture edges
- repair with bone and connective tissue: a bony bridge separates the two fragments.

In addition to these changes in the fracture area, pulp canal obliteration is commonly seen. Fractures in the cervical third of the root will repair as well as those in the middle or apical thirds as long as no communication exists between the fracture line and the gingival crevice. If such a communication exists, splinting is not recommended and a decision must be made to extract the coronal fragment and retain the remaining root, to extract the two fragments or to splint the root fracture internally. The latter can only be regarded as a temporary solution.

If the root is retained, the remaining radicular pulp should be removed and the canal temporarily dressed prior to obturating with gutta-percha. Three options are now available for the root-treated radicular portion:

- post, core and crown restoration if access is adequate
- extrusion of root either surgically or orthodontically if the fracture extends too far subgingivally for adequate access
- cover the root with a mucoperiosteal flap; this will maintain the height and width of the arch and will facilitate later placement of a single tooth implant.

Pulpal necrosis occurs in about 20% of root fractures and is the main obstacle to adequate repair. Most instances of necrosis are diagnosed within 3 months of a root fracture. A persistent negative response to electric stimulation is usually confirmed on radiography by radiolucencies adjacent to the fracture line.

Splinting

Trauma may loosen a tooth either by damaging the periodontal ligament or by fracturing the root. Splinting immobilises the tooth in the correct anatomical position so that further trauma is prevented and healing can occur. Different injuries require different splinting regimens.

Periodontal ligament injuries. Approximately 60% of periodontal ligament healing has occurred after 10 days and it is complete within a month. The splinting period should be as short as possible and the splint should allow some functional movement to prevent replacement root resorption (ankylosis). As a general rule, exarticulation (avulsion) injuries require 7–10 days, luxation injuries 2–3 weeks.

Root fractures. These require 2–3 weeks of functional splinting to encourage a repair. A connective tissue repair may be satisfactory, but if mobility persists the fracture site becomes filled with granulation tissue and the tooth remains mobile.

Dento-alveolar fractures. These require 3–4 weeks of rigid splinting.

Splint construction

The composite resin/acrylic and wire splint uses either a composite resin or a temporary crown material (Box 38). The composite resin is easier to place but the acrylic resin is easier to remove. Although acrylic resin does not have the bond strength to enamel of the composite resin, it is suitable for all types of splinting apart from root fractures. Generally, functional splints should have one abutment tooth each side of the injured tooth and rigid splints two abutment teeth each side.

Box 38 Technique for functional splint

1. Bend a flexible orthodontic wire to fit the middle third of the labial surface of the injured tooth and one abutment tooth either side.
2. Stabilise the injured tooth in the correct position with red wax palatally.
3. Clean the labial surfaces. Isolate, dry and etch middle of crown of teeth with 37% phosphoric acid for 30 seconds, wash and dry.
4. Apply 3 mm diameter circle either of unfilled then filled composite resin or of acrylic resin to the centre of the crowns.
5. Position the wire into the filling material then apply more resin.
6. Use a brush lubricated with unfilled composite resin to mould and smooth the composite. Acrylic resin is more difficult to handle and smoothing and excess removal can be done with a flat plastic instrument.
7. Cure the composite for 60 seconds. Wait for the acrylic resin to cure.
8. Smooth any sharp edges with sandpaper discs.

Table 18 Pulpal survival at 5 years after injuries involving the periodontal ligament

Injury	Open apex (%)	Closed apex (%)
Concussion	100	96
Subluxation	100	85
Extrusive luxation	95	45
Lateral luxation	95	25
Intrusive luxation	40	0
Replantation	30	0

Other types of splint include orthodontic brackets and wire, interdental wiring, foil/cement splint (temporary) and laboratory splints (acrylic or thermoplastic).

Injuries to the periodontal tissues

Figures for pulp survival 5 years after periodontal ligament injuries are shown in Table 18.

Concussion
The impact force causes oedema and haemorrhage in the periodontal ligament and the tooth is tender to percussion (t.t.p.). There is no rupture of periodontal ligament fibres and the tooth is firm in the socket.

Subluxation
In addition to the above, in subluxation there is rupture of some periodontal ligament fibres and the tooth is mobile in the socket, although not displaced. The treatment for both these injuries is:

- occlusal relief
- soft diet for 7 days
- immobilisation with a splint if t.t.p. is significant
- chlorhexidine 0.2% mouthwash, twice daily.

There is little risk of pulp necrosis or resorption.

Extrusive luxation
In extrusive luxation there is rupture of the periodontal ligament and pulp.

Lateral luxation
Lateral luxation involves rupture of periodontal ligament and pulp and compression injury of the alveolar plate. The treatment for extrusive and lateral luxation is:

- local anaesthesia (buccal and palatal)
- atraumatic repositioning of tooth with gentle firm digital pressure
- functional splint 2–3 weeks
- antibiotics: age-related dose of amoxicillin or alternative for 5 days
- chlorhexidine mouthwash
- soft diet 2–3 weeks.

The decision to progress to endodontic treatment depends on subsequent regular clinical and radiographic examination.

With more significant damage to the periodontal ligament, there is an increased risk of root resorption (up to 35% of injuries).

Orthodontic appliances should be used to reduce firm older injuries, as digital pressure could further damage the periodontal ligament.

Intrusive luxation
Intrusive luxation injuries are the result of an axial, apical impact. There is extensive damage to the periodontal ligament and alveolar plate(s). Two distinct categories exist: the open and closed apex. At the outset, both categories should receive antibiotics, chlorhexidine mouthwash and a soft diet as previously described. The risk of pulpal necrosis in these injuries is high, especially with a closed apex. The incidence of resorption and ankylosis sequelae is also high.

Open apex There are two treatment courses for open apex intrusive luxation:

- disimpact (with forceps if necessary) and allow to erupt spontaneously for 2–4 months; if there is no spontaneous movement start orthodontic extrusion
- disimpact and surgically reposition using a functional splint for 7–10 days; then monitor pulpal status clinically and radiographically and start endodontics if necessary.

Non-setting calcium hydroxide in the root canal does not preclude orthodontic movement. Once apexification has occurred and orthodontic movement has ceased, obturate with gutta-percha.

Closed apex The treatment of a closed apex intrusive luxation is:

- elective orthodontic/surgical extrusion immediately
- functional splint for 7–10 days after surgical extrusion
- elective pulp extirpation at 10 days
- maintenance of non-setting calcium hydroxide in the root canal during orthodontic movement
- finally obturation with gutta-percha.

If endodontic treatment is commenced within 2 weeks of an injury to the periodontal ligament, the initial intracanal dressing should be with a polyantibiotic or antibiotic/steroid (Ledermix) paste.

> **Box 39** Technique for replantation of a tooth
>
> *Advice on phone (to teacher, parent, etc.)*
>
> 1. Do not touch the root, hold by the crown.
> 2. Wash gently under cold tap water.
> 3. Replace into socket or transport in milk to surgery.
> 4. If replaced, bite gently on a handkerchief and come to surgery.
>
> The best transport medium is the tooth's own socket. Understandably, non-dentists may be unhappy to replant the tooth and milk is an effective iso-osmolar medium. Saliva, the patient's buccal sulcus, or normal saline are alternatives.
>
> *Immediate surgery treatment*
>
> 1. Do not handle root. If replanted, remove tooth from socket.
> 2. Rinse tooth with normal saline. Note state of root development. Store in saline.
> 3. Local anaesthesia.
> 4. Irrigate socket with saline and remove clot and any foreign material.
> 5. Push tooth gently but firmly into socket.
> 6. Use a functional splint for 7–10 days.
> 7. Check occlusion.
> 8. Take baseline radiographs: periapical or anterior occlusal. Any other teeth injured?
> 9. Antibiotics, chlorhexidine mouthwash, soft diet as previously.
> 10. Check tetanus immunisation status.
>
> *Review*
>
> 1. Take radiograph prior to splint removal at 7–10 days.
> 2. Remove splint at 7–10 days.
> 3. For open apex with an extra-alveolar time of less than 45 minutes simply observe the tooth
> 4. For open apex with an extra-alveolar time greater than 45 minutes or a closed apex, endodontics is commenced prior to splint removal:
> 5. Initial intracanal dressing with polyantibiotic or antibiotic/steroid (Ledermix, Lederle) paste.
> 6. Subsequent intracanal dressing with non-setting calcium hydroxide.
> 7. Treatment then differs for open and closed apex:
>   a. For closed apex, replace calcium hydroxide 3 monthly until apical barrier is achieved and then obturate canal with gutta-percha
>   b. For closed apex, obturate with gutta-percha at 12 months as long as there is no progressive resorption.
> 8. Review radiographically at 1 and 3 months then 6-monthly for 2 years and, finally, annually.
> 9. If resorption is progressing unhalted, keep non-setting calcium hydroxide in the tooth until exfoliation, changing it 6 monthly.

Avulsion and replantation

Replantation of a lost tooth should nearly always be attempted even though it may offer only a temporary solution because of the frequent occurrence of external inflammatory resorption (e.i.r.). Even when resorption occurs, the tooth may be retained for years, acting as a natural space maintainer and preserving the height and width of the alveolus to facilitate later implant placement.

Successful healing after replantation can only occur if there is minimal damage to the pulp and the periodontal ligament. The type of extra-alveolar storage medium and the extra-alveolar time (e.a.t.) (i.e., the time the tooth has been out of the mouth) are critical factors. The suggested protocol for replantation can be divided into advice on the telephone, immediate treatment in surgery and review (Box 39). The immature tooth with an extra-alveolar time of less than 45 minutes may undergo pulp revascularisation. However, these teeth require regular clinical and radiographic review because once external inflammatory resorption occurs it progresses rapidly.

Replantation of teeth with a dry storage time of greater than 1 hour Mature teeth with a dry storage time of greater than 1 hour will have a non-vital periodontal ligament. The periodontal ligament and the pulp should be removed at chairside and the tooth placed for 20 minutes in 2.4% sodium fluoride solution at pH 5.5. The root canal is then obturated with gutta-percha and the tooth replanted and splinted rigidly for 6 weeks. The aim of this treatment is to produce ankylosis, allowing the tooth to be maintained as a natural space maintainer, perhaps for a limited period only. The sodium fluoride is believed to slow down resorptive processes.

Very immature teeth with an extra-alveolar dry time of greater than 1 hour should not be replanted.

Injuries to supporting alveolar bone

The extent and position of the alveolar fracture should be verified clinically and radiographically. If there is displacement of the teeth to the extent that their apices have risen up and are now positioned over the labial or lingual/palatal alveolar plates ('apical lock'), they will first require extruding to free the apices prior to repositioning.

The segment of alveolus with teeth requires only 3–4 weeks of splintage (composite-wire type) with two abutment teeth either side of the fracture, together with antibiotics, chlorhexidine, soft diet and tetanus prophylaxis if necessary.

Pulp survival is more likely if repositioning occurs within 1 hour of the injury. Root resorption is rare.

Child physical abuse (non-accidental injury)

A child is considered to be abused if he or she is treated in a way that is unacceptable in a given culture at a given time. NAI is now recognised as an international issue and has been reported in many countries. Each week at least four children in the UK and 80 children in the USA will die as a result of abuse or neglect. At least 1 child per 1000 in Britain suffers severe physical abuse, for example fractures, brain haemorrhage, severe internal injuries or mutilation. In the USA more than 95% of serious intracranial injuries during the first year of life are the result of abuse. Although some reports will prove to be unfounded, the common experience is that proved cases of child abuse are four to five times as common as they were in the 1980s.

NAI is not a full diagnosis, it is merely a symptom of disordered parenting. The aim of intervention is to diagnose and cure the disordered parenting. Simply to aim at preventing death is lowly ambition. It has been estimated in the USA that 35–50% of severely abused children will receive serious re-injury and 50% will die if they are returned to their home environment without intervention. In some cases, the occurrence of physical abuse may provide an opportunity for intervention. If this opportunity is missed, there may be no further opportunity for many years.

Approximately 65% of cases diagnosed as NAI have extra- and intraoral facial trauma; consequently, the dental practitioner may be the first professional to see or suspect abuse. Injuries may take the form of contusions and ecchymoses, abrasions and lacerations, burns, bites and dental trauma. The incidence of common orofacial injuries are shown in Table 19.

The following 11 points should be considered whenever doubts and suspicions are aroused.

- Could the injury have been caused accidentally and if so how?
- Does the explanation for the injury fit the age and the clinical findings?
- If the explanation of cause is consistent with the injury, is this itself within normally acceptable limits of behaviour?
- If there has been any delay seeking advice, are there good reasons for this?
- Does the story of the accident vary?
- The nature of the relationship between parent and child.
- The child's reaction to other people.
- The child's reaction to any medical/dental examinations.
- The general demeanour of the child.
- Any comments made by child and/or parent that give concern about the child's upbringing or life-style.
- History of previous injury.

Dental practitioners should be aware of any established system in their locality that is designed to address these cases. In the UK, each local authority social services department is required to set up an 'Area Child Protection Committee'. Dental practitioners are advised how to refer and to whom, if they are concerned.

7.2 Dental anomalies

Table 19 The incidence of common orofacial injuries in non-accidental injury

Type of injury	Incidence (%)
Extraoral	
Contusions and ecchymoses	66
Abrasions and lacerations	28
Burns and bites	4
Fractures	2
Intraoral	
Contusions and ecchymoses	43
Abrasions and lacerations (including frenal tears)	29
Dental trauma	29

Learning objectives

You should

- know the types of number and form (morphology) of anomaly and their incidence
- know the types of inherited enamel defect and their incidence
- know the types of inherited dentine defect and their incidence
- know the causes of premature and delayed eruption and exfoliation.

Number and morphology

Hypodontia

Congenital absence of some teeth is common. This can occur sporadically or be inherited. The most common teeth to be absent are the last teeth in each series (i.e. lateral incisor, second premolar and third molar). The presence of conical teeth is often associated with the absence of the same teeth on the opposite side of the arch. Hypodontia arises because of an abnormality in the induction of oral ectoderm by ectomesenchyme.

Anodontia is the term used for the total lack of one or both dentitions. Oligodontia is an older term that has been replaced by hypodontia.

Incidence

Hypodontia in the primary dentition has an incidence of 0.1–0.9%; the gender ratio is not known.

The incidence in the permanent dentition is 3.5–6.5% (excluding wisdom teeth, 9–37%). There is a 1:1.4 male: female ratio.

Permanent anomalies occur in 30–50% of those with hypodontia in the primary dentition.

Hypodontia may be seen in a number of syndromes:

- ectodermal dysplasia
- clefting
- Down syndrome
- chondro-ectodermal dysplasia (Ellis–van Creveld syndrome)
- Reiger syndrome
- incontinentia pigmenti
- orofacial digital syndrome (types I and II).

Management

Management can be complex and requires co-ordination between a number of specialities: paediatric dentistry, orthodontics and prosthodontics.

Supernumerary teeth

Supernumerary teeth can be inherited as an autosomal dominant or X-linked trait and occurs by budding of the dental lamina. The extra tooth can resemble the normal series – supplemental tooth – or, more commonly, it may be conical or tuberculate. Almost all, 98%, occur in the maxilla, mostly in the anterior palate.

Incidence

The incidence of supernumerary teeth in the primary dentition is 0.2–0.8%, with the male:female ratio unknown. In the permanent dentition it is 1.5–3.5% with a male:female ratio of 2:1.

Diagnosis

- failed or ectopic tooth eruption
- routine radiography

- part of a syndrome: cleidocranial dysplasia, Gardner's syndrome, orofacial digital syndrome (type I), clefting.

Management

Conical supernumeraries often erupt and are extracted easily. Tuberculate or inverted conical forms usually require surgical removal.

Macrodontia

Any tooth (or teeth) that is larger than normal for that particular tooth is macrodontic. True macrodontia affecting the whole dentition is rare. More commonly, single teeth are large owing to an isolated disturbance of morphodifferentation.

True generalised macrodontia may occur in pituitary gigantism. Relative generalised macrodontia occurs in orthodontic skeletal base–tooth size discrepancy. True localised macrodontia may be associated with facial hemihyperplasia, hereditary gingival hyperplasia and hypertrichosis.

Incidence

The incidence of macrodontia in the primary dentition is unknown; in the permanent dentition it is 1%.

Management

- Judicious grinding to reduce mesiodistal width
- Build up of antimere to match if only one tooth is affected
- Extraction and replacement with a prosthesis.

Microdontia

Any tooth (or teeth) that is smaller than normal for the tooth type is microdontic. Most commonly, this affects one or two teeth but it can be generalised in syndromes with hypodontia (see above) and in children who have undergone radio- and chemotherapy.

True generalised microdontia may occur in pituitary dwarfism and syndromes with hypodontia. The relative generalised form will occur in orthodontic skeletal base–tooth size discrepancy. True localised microdontia may occur after radio- and chemotherapy.

Incidence

The incidence of microdontia is <0.5% in the primary dentition, 2% in the permanent dentition and it is more common in females.

Management

Management involves build ups with composite resin or porcelain. The mesiodistal width at the ginigival margin will limit the size to which restoration is possible.

Double teeth

Double teeth now embraces the terms fusion and gemination and describes a structure that resembles two teeth that have been joined together. Radiographs are required to determine if there are two pulp systems or if they are joined.

Incidence

The incidence of double teeth is 2.5% in the primary dentition and 0.2% in the permanent dentition. There is a male:female ratio of 1.1 in both. Permanent anomalies occur in 30–50% of those with primary anomalies.

Dens invaginatus

Developmental invagination of the cingulum pit commonly occurs on the maxillary lateral incisors with only a thin layer of hard tissue between the pulp and oral cavity. Pulp necrosis may result in significant facial cellulitis.

Incidence

The incidence of dens invaginatus in the primary dentition is 0.1% and in the permanent dentition it is 4%. It is more common in males than in females.

Management

- Fissure-seal newly erupted tooth
- Root canal therapy if morphology is favourable
- Extraction if internal anatomy is complex.

Dens evaginatus

In dens evaginatus an enamel-covered tubercle projects from the occlusal surface of a usually premolar or sometimes a canine or molar. It is usually bilateral and is more common in the mandible. The tubercle usually contains pulp tissue.

Incidence

The incidence in the primary dentition is unknown but that of the permanent dentition is 4%.

Management

- Composite resin build up to recontour occlusal surface incorporating the tubercle
- Pulpotomy to allow continued radicular growth
- Extraction may be required owing to the immaturity of the root if pulp necrosis occurs.

Talon cusp

A talon cusp is a horn-like projection of the cingulum of maxillary incisor teeth. It may reach and contact the incisal edge.

Incidence

The incidence in the primary dentition is unknown; incidence in the permanent dentition is 1–2%.

Management

- No treatment if there is no occlusal interference
- Enamel reduction
- Pulpotomy/pulpectomy.

Taurodontism

Taurodontism is an enlarged pulp chamber where the distance from the cemenoenamel junction to the bifurcation of the root is greater than the length of the roots. It is caused by a failure of Hertwig's root sheath to invaginate and may be inherited either in a normal individual or as part of a syndrome.

Incidence

The incidence is unknown.

Conditions with enlarged pulp chambers include:

- vitamin-D-resistant rickets (hypophosphophataemic rickets)
- rickets (vitamin-D-dependent)
- hypophosphatasia
- dentinogenesis imperfecta (some cases)
- regional odontodysplasia
- Klinefelter's syndrome
- Shell teeth.

Defects of enamel

Enamel defects may be inherited or acquired. Enamel can exhibit either hypoplasia owing to deficient matrix production or hypomineralisation from imperfect mineralisation of matrix proteins.

Chronological disturbances

Any severe systemic event during the development of the teeth (from 3 months in utero to 20 years) will result in some dental abnormality. Different teeth will show defects at different levels of the crown depending on the stage of crown formation at the time of the disturbance. The enamel may be reduced in quantity or quality and may, therefore, show discoloration, opacities (hypomineralisation) and hypoplasia.

Chronological defects usually affect teeth of the same type on either side of the arch.

Fluorosis

In its mildest form, fluorosis appears as hypomineralisation of enamel causing opacities. These can range from diffuse flecks to confluent opaque patches that lack translucency. At higher fluoride concentrations, hypoplasia occurs with a defect in quantity of matrix. Fluorotic mottling affects the outer third of the enamel.

Amelogenesis imperfecta

Amelogenesis imperfecta (AI) describes hereditary enamel defects resulting from single gene mutations; they follow autosomal dominant, autosomal recessive, or X-linked patterns of inheritance.

Incidence
Incidence is 1 in 10 000.

There are three main types:

- hypoplastic
- hypomineralised: hypocalcified or hypomature
- mixed.

In most, but not all, types of AI, teeth in both the primary and the permanent dentitions are affected.

Hypoplastic AI. There is deficient matrix production but the enamel that is present is normally mineralised. Clinical variants range from the autosomal dominant thin and smooth type of AI to the pitting and grooving of X-linked dominant AI.

Hypocalcified AI. Teeth erupt with enamel that is dull, lustreless, opaque white or honey coloured. Distribution throughout the mouth is not even usually, although there is bilateral symmetry. Soft enamel may wear, leaving rough, discoloured sensitive dentine exposed. The cervical regions of the crowns often have normal enamel.

Hypomaturation AI. This is very similar to hypocalcified AI but with no normal enamel in cervical regions.

Management
Management is discussed together with dentine defects, below.

Defects of dentine

Defects of dentine may be inherited or acquired. Genetic defects can be either limited to dentine or associated with a generalised disorder.

Defects limited to dentine:

- dentinogenesis imperfecta type II (hereditary opalescent dentine)
- dentine dysplasia type I (radicular dentine dysplasia)
- dentine dysplasia type II (coronal dentine dysplasia)
- fibrous dysplasia of dentine.

Defects associated with a generalised disorder:

- osteogenesis imperfecta (dentinogenesis imperfecta type I)

- Ehlers–Danlos syndrome
- brachio-skeleto-genital syndrome
- vitamin D-resistant rickets
- vitamin D-dependent rickets
- hypophosphatasia.

Dentinogenesis imperfecta type II (hereditary opalescent dentine)

In dentinogenesis imperfecta type II both dentitions are usually affected. The teeth are opalescent and on transillumination appear bluish or brownish in colour. Sometimes, later forming permanent teeth are less affected. There is early loss of enamel, exposing underlying dentine that undergoes rapid wear. This is usually most marked in the primary dentition. Radiographically, the crowns appear bulbous and the roots may be short and thin. The pulp chambers obliterate soon after eruption and the root canals are progressively narrowed by deposition of abnormal dentine. Transmission is usually autosomal dominant.

Incidence
The incidence is 1 in 8000.

Dentine dysplasia type I (radicular dentine dysplasia; rootless teeth)

In dentine dysplasia type I, crown colour ranges from normal to bluish or brownish tinge. Radiographs show normal crown morphology but excessively short or blunt roots. Pulp chambers may be small and root canals absent. Primary and permanent dentitions are affected and inheritance is probably autosomal dominant. It is rare.

Dentine dysplasia type II (coronal dentine dysplasia)

Primary teeth in dentine dysplasia type II resemble those in dentinogenesis imperfecta type II, but permanent teeth are clinically normal and radiographs show thistle or flame-shaped pulp chambers partially occluded by pulp stones and narrowing root canals. It is rare and probably autosomal dominant.

Dentinogenesis imperfecta type I with osteogenesis imperfecta

Osteogenesis imperfecta is a heterogeneous group of connective tissue disorders involving inherited abnormalities of type I collagen. Bone fragility, lax joints, blue sclerae, opalescent teeth, hearing loss and a variable degree of bone deformity are features.

Inheritance is autosomal recessive or dominant. Recessive varieties are frequently lethal at or shortly after birth.

Opalescent teeth are commonly observed in the dominant variety. Features are similar to dentinogenesis type II except that the permanent dentition is often less affected and the upper anterior teeth particularly may be clinically normal.

Environmentally determined dentine defects

Local trauma may interfere with dentine formation, and a number of systemic influences can occur, such as nutritional deficiencies (minerals, proteins and vitamins), drugs such as tetracycline and the anticancer drugs (e.g. cyclophosphamide). There is increased formation of interglobular dentine, predentine and osteoid.

Management of enamel and dentine defects

There are four main clinical problems associated with inherited enamel and dentine defects:

- poor aesthetics
- chipping and attrition of the enamel, which may cause reduced face height
- exposure and attrition of the dentine causing sensitivity
- poor oral hygiene, gingivitis and caries.

While it is not possible to draw up a definitive treatment plan for all patients, it is possible to define the principles of treatment planning for this group of patients. It is important to realise that not all children with amelogenesis imperfecta or dentinogenesis imperfecta are affected equally. Many will not have marked tooth wear or symptoms and will not require advanced intervention. Table 20 describes the principles of treatment in terms of the age of the child/adolescent and with regard to the three aspects of care: prevention, restoration and aesthetics.

Eruption and exfoliation disorders

Premature eruption

Premature eruption may be familial. There is a tendency to early eruption in children with a high birthweight. Excessively early eruption is seen in endocrine abnormalities, e.g. precocious puberty, increase of thyroid and growth hormone.

Natal and neonatal teeth
Natal (present at birth) and neonatal (erupts within 30 days of birth) teeth occur in about 1 in 2000–3000 births; the teeth are part of the normal series and development is consistent with age (no root present).

It may be familial but is also associated with some syndromes: pachyonychia congenita, Ellis–van Creveld, Hallermann–Streiff.

Management Teeth are left if possible to allow normal root formation. Extraction may be necessary because of extreme mobility and airway danger, painful suckling or tongue ulceration.

Delayed eruption

In the primary dentition, delayed eruption tends to occur in preterm children or those of very low birthweights. It is also associated with a number of conditions:

- Down syndrome
- Turner syndrome
- nutritional deficiency
- endocrine disorders: hypothyroidism and hypopituitarism
- cleidocranial dysostosis
- hereditary gingival fibromatosis.

Table 20 Principles of treatment for amelogenesis and dentinogenesis imperfecta

	Prevention	Restoration	Aesthetics
Primary dentition (0–5 years)	Diet advice; fluoride supplements; oral hygiene instruction	Adhesive restorations; stainless steel crowns(SSCs) particularly on Es	Minimal intervention,
Mixed dentition (6–16 years)	Diet advice; fluoride supplements; oral hygiene instruction ± chlorhexidine	SSCs on primary molars; adhesive castings or SSCs on first permanent molars; adhesive restorations	Direct or indirect composite veneers
Permanent dentition (16+ years)	Oral hygiene instruction; topical fluoride	Adhesive castings on premolars; full mouth rehabilitation	Porcelain veneers; full crowns, over dentures, complete dentures

In the permanent dentition, localised causes are more frequent: ectopic crypt positions, supernumeraries, odontomes and impaction.

Premature exfoliation

Apart from trauma (accidental or non-accidental), there are a number of rare conditions that may result in premature loss of primary teeth:

- hypophosphatasia
- immunological conditions causing neutropenia
- histiocytosis X.

Delayed exfoliation

Delay in normal exfoliation of primary teeth may be seen in association with:

- double primary teeth
- hypodontia affecting permanent successors
- ectopic permanent successors
- subsequent to trauma or severe periradicular infection of primary teeth
- infraocclusion (preferred term to 'submerged' or ankylosed teeth, which describes teeth that have failed to achieve or maintain their occlusal relationships to adjacent and opposing teeth); on occasion, teeth may be totally reincluded (covered) by surrounding tissues, which is thought to be caused by imbalance in the normal pattern of resorption and repair in primary teeth.

Incidence of infraocclusion

Infraocclusion occurs in 1–9% with an equal incidence in males and females. It is more common in the primary dentition but there is a higher incidence of absent permanent successors.

Treatment of infraocclusion

- onlays
- extraction and space maintenance for permanent successor

Table 21 Prevalence of congenital cardiac disease

Condition	Prevalence (%)
Ventrical septal defect	28
Atrial septal defect	10
Pulmonary stenosis	10
Patent ductus arteriosus	10
Tetralogy of Fallot	10
Aortic stenosis	7
Coarctation of the aorta	5
Transposition of great arteries	5
Rare/diverse conditions	15

- extraction and orthodontic space closure
- extraction and prosthetic restoration of space if successor absent.

7.3 Special needs

Learning objectives

You should

- appreciate the impact of active dental disease on specific medical disorders
- understand the importance of vigorous dental prevention in specific medical disorders
- appreciate the role that the dental practitioner has to play in maintaining the 'whole' patient fit and healthy.

Congenital cardiac disease

Congenital cardiac disease occurs in 8–10 per 1000 live births and has an equal sex distribution. Multifactorial inheritance patterns are responsible and the main types of congenital condition are shown in Table 21. The degree of morbidity is dependent on the haemodynamics of the lesion. Flow disturbances are caused by structural or obstructive defects. For convenience, defects are divided into cyanotic or acyanotic depending on clinical presentation.

Acyanotic defects with shunts. Connection between systemic and pulmonary circulation with a shunt from left to right occurs in:

- atrial septal defect
- ventricular septal defect
- patent ductus arteriosus
- anomalous pulmonary venous return
- atrioventricular canal.

Acyanotic defects with obstruction include:

- coarctation of aorta
- aortic stenosis
- pulmonary stenosis.

Cyanotic defects have right to left shunting of desaturated blood:

- tetralogy of Fallot
- Eisenmenger syndrome (right to left shunt through a ventricular septal defect)
- tricuspid atresia
- transposition of great vessels.

Other cardiac diseases include:

- cardiomyopathies

- cardiac arrhythmias (accessory conduction pathways)
- rheumatic fever.

Dental management

Aggressive prevention regimens including dietary counselling, fluoride therapy, fissure sealants and oral hygiene. Active disease should be treated before cardiac surgery is undertaken.

Antibiotic prophylaxis is required for all dental procedures that are likely to induce a bacteraemia in order to prevent infective endocarditis (Table 22); this includes patients with:

- congenital heart defects
- history of rheumatic fever
- previous infective endocarditis
- previous heart surgery (with exceptions).

If any doubt exists, the cardiologist should be consulted before invasive dental procedures are undertaken.

Other problems may include prolonged bleeding caused by thrombocytopenia and anticoagulant medicine. It is essential to check the platelet count and prothrombin time (INR) if dental extractions are planned. The patient's prothrombin time is compared with normal and called the international normalised ratio (INR).

Bleeding disorders

Primary haemostasis is initiated after injury to a blood vessel and results in the formation of a primary plug. This is mediated by interactions between platelets, plasma coagulation factors and the vessel wall. Secondary haemostasis, with fibrin as the end-product,

Table 22 Prophylactic regimen for dental procedures

Group	Regimen
Under local anaesthesia	
Adults	Amoxicillin 3 g orally 1 hour preoperatively
Children	Amoxicillin 50 mg/kg body weight orally 1 hour pre-operatively (or under 10 years half adult dose; under 5 years quarter adult dose)
Under local anaesthesia and allergic to penicillin	
Adults	Clindamycin 600 mg orally 1 hour preoperatively
Children	Clindamycin 6 mg/kg body weight 1 hour preoperatively (or under 10 years half adult dose; under 5 years quarter adult dose)
Under general anaesthesia	
Adults	Amoxicillin 1 g i.m. or i.v. at induction then 0.5 g amoxicillin by mouth 6 hours later
Children	Under 10 years, half adult dose
	Under 5 years, quarter adult dose
Under general anaesthesia and with an allergy to penicillin or having received penicillin in the previous month	
Adults	Vancomycin 1 g by slow intravenous infusion over 100 minutes plus gentamicin 120 mg i.v. just before induction or 15 min before procedure *or*
	Teicoplanin 400 mg i.v. plus gentamicin 120 mg i.v. at induction or 15 minutes before procedure *or* clindamycin 300 mg i.v. over at least 10 minutes at induction or 15 minutes before procedure then oral or i.v. clindamycin 150 mg 6 hours later
Children under 10 years	Vancomycin 20 mg/kg, gentamicin 2 g/kg *or*
	Teichoplanin 6 mg/kg, gentamicin 2 mg/kg (children under 14 years) *or*
	Clindamycin 150 mg i.v. over at least 10 minutes at induction or 15 minutes before procedure, then oral or i.v. clindamycin 75 mg 6 hours later (children under 5 years half this dose)
	Patients at special risk including a previous history of endocarditis or with prosthetic heart valves and requiring a general anaesthetic
Adults	Amoxicillin 1 g i.m. or i.v plus gentamicin 120 mg i.m. or i.v. at induction; 0.5 g amoxicillin by mouth 6 hours later
Children under 10 years	Amoxicillin, half adult dose, gentamicin 2 mg/kg
Children under 5 years	Amoxicillin, quarter adult dose, gentamicin 2 mg/kg

i.m., intramuscular; i.v., intravenous.

is also triggered by the initial injury and reaches its greatest intensity after the primary platelet plug is formed. It provides the framework for the formation of a stable clot.

Clinical manifestations of a haemostatic disorder vary depending on the phase affected. Defects in primary haemostasis (platelet initiated) generally result in bleeding from skin or mucosal surfaces, while defects in secondary haemostasis (fibrin clot), for example haemophilia, result in deep seated muscle and joint bleeding. Classification of bleeding disorders is shown in Table 23.

Inherited coagulation disorders

The main inherited coagulation disorders are described in Table 24. The severity of haemophilia A depends on the levels of factor VIII: <1% is severe, 1–5% is moderate-to-severe and >25% is mild disease.

Thrombocytopenia

In the thrombocytopenias, there is a reduction in numbers of circulatory platelets (normal is $150 \times 10^9/1$ to $400 \times 10^9/1$).

The minimum for invasive dental procedures is $50 \times 10^9/1$.

Dental management. Good communication with physician/haematologist is essential. Aggressive prevention should be employed from a very early age. Regional anaesthesia should be avoided. Pulp treatment of primary molar teeth may be required to avoid extractions.

Haemophilias

Treatment involves:

- replacement and monitoring of factor VIII and IX levels
- DDAVP (desmopressin) for mild-to-moderate haemophilia A instead of factor replacement
- antifibrinolytics, epsilon-aminocaproic acid (EACA) or tranexamic acid, to prevent clot lysis
- avoid non-steroidal anti-inflammatory agents.

Von Willebrand's disease

Treatment involves:

- DDAVP in combination with EACA or tranexamic acid
- factor replacement in more severe disease.

Red and white cell disorders

Red cell disorders: anaemias

Iron deficiency in children is usually caused by a dietary deficiency or malabsorption. Vitamin B_{12} and folic acid may also be reduced by either mechanism and both are needed for maturation of red blood cells in the marrow.

Glucose 6-phosphate dehydrogenase (G-6-PD) deficiency causes premature haemolysis of red blood cells; it is an X-linked condition.

Table 23 Classification of bleeding disorders

Types	Examples
Coagulation defects	
Inherited	Haemophilia A (factor VIII deficiency), haemophilia B (factor IX deficiency, Christmas disease)
Acquired	Liver disease, vitamin deficiency, anticoagulant drugs (heparin, warfarin), disseminated intravascular coagulation (DIC)
Thrombocytopenic purpuras	
Primary	Idiopathic thrombocytopenic purpura (ITP), pancytopenia, Fanconi syndrome
Secondary	Systemic disease (leukaemia), drug induced, physical agents (radiation)
Non-thrombocytopenic purpuras	
Vascular wall alteration	Scurvy, infections, allergy
Disorders of platelet function	Inherited (von Willebrand's disease), drugs (aspirin, non-steroidal anti-inflammatory drugs, alcohol, penicillin), allergy, autoimmune disease, uraemia

Table 24 Prevalence of inherited bleeding disorders

Type	Missing factor	Inheritance	Prevalence (%)	Incidence
Haemophilia A	VIII	X-linked recessive	80	1:20000
Haemophilia B	IX	X-linked recessive	13	1:1000
von Willebrand's disease	Abnormal VIII	Autosomal dominant		
Haemophilia C	XI	Autosomal	6	(1:1000 in Ashkenazi Jews in Israel)

Sickle cell anaemia is an autosomal recessive disease with substitution of a single amino acid in the haemoglobin chain to produce HBS. Homozygotes have sickle cell disease; heterozygotes have sickle sell trait. Clumping together of red cells under conditions of lowered oxygen tension, such as general anaesthesia, can lead to blockage of small vessels causing pain and necrosis. The trait is carried in 10% of American-Black children and 25% of central African Black children.

Thalassaemia is a homozygous or heterozygous trait resulting in abnormal globin synthesis. It results in a progressive haemolytic anaemia.

Management

A full blood count should be obtained for all anaemic patients especially with reference to general anaesthesia.

Immunodeficiency

Immunodeficiency may be caused by quantitative or qualitative defects in neutrophils, primary deficiencies involving B or T cells or both or by acquired disorders.

Neutrophils

Qualitative neutrophil disorders include:

- chemotactic disorders: Chediak–Higashi syndrome, lazy leucocyte syndrome, leucocyte adhesion defect
- phagocyte disorders: agammaglobulinaemia
- defects in microbial killing: chronic granulomatous disease, recurrent skin infections with *Staphylococcus aureus*.

Quantitative neutrophil disorders include neutropenia, cyclic neutropenia, leukaemic infiltration of bone marrow by other cells, agranulocytosis, aplastic anaemia, drug induced (including induced by chemo- and radiotherapy for neoplasia).

Primary immunodeficiencies

- B cell defects: selective IgA deficiency, agammaglobulinaemia
- T cell defects: DiGeorge syndrome with thymic aplasia, chronic mucocutaneous candidiasis
- combined immunodeficiency: severe combined, Wiskott–Aldrich syndrome, ataxia telangiectasia
- acquired immunodeficiency: HIV, drug induced (cytotoxics, steroids, ciclosporin).

Dental problems in blood cell deficiencies

Neutrophil deficiencies and T cell defects

- candidosis
- severe gingivitis/prepubertal periodontitis
- gingivostomatitis
- recurrent aphthous ulceration

- recurrent herpes simplex infection
- premature exfoliation of primary teeth.

B cell deficiencies

- few oral complications
- recurrent bacterial infections, especially pneumonia and skin lesions.

Dental management

- prevention and regular review
- chlorhexidine 0.2% mouthwashes
- antifungals
- acyclovir
- prophylactic antibiotics
- extraction of pulpally involved teeth.

Leukaemia

Leukaemia is a malignant proliferation of white blood cells. It is the most common form of childhood cancer, accounting for about one-third of new cases of cancer diagnosed each year. Acute lymphocytic leukaemia accounts for 75% with a peak incidence at 4 years of age. The general clinical features of all types of leukaemia are similar as all involve a severe disruption of bone marrow functions. Specific clinical and laboratory features differ, however, and there are considerable differences in response to therapy and long-term prognosis.

Acute leukaemia has a sudden onset but the initial symptoms are usually non-specific, with anorexia, irritability and lethargy. Progressive failure of the bone marrow leads to pallor, bleeding and fever, which are usually the symptoms that lead to diagnostic investigation. The bleeding tendency is often shown in the oral mucosa and there may be infective lesions of the mouth and throat. The dental practitioner may, therefore, be the first to note the condition. Bone pain and arthralgia are also important presenting complaints in about one-quarter of children. On initial haematological examination, most patients will have anaemia and thrombocytopenia. The diagnosis of leukaemia can be suspected on seeing blast cells on the blood smear, confirmed by bone-marrow biopsy, which will show replacement by leukaemic lymphoblasts.

Treatment consists of specific phases:

1. Induction of remission: to remove abnormal cells from the blood and bone marrow; drugs used include vincristine and prednisone
2. Prophylactic treatment to central nervous system; drugs used include intrathecal methotrexate plus irradiation of central nervous system
3. Consolidation; drugs used include cytosine arabinoside plus asparaginase
4. Maintenance; drugs used include methotrexate plus mercaptopurine for approximately 2 years.

On this regimen over 70% of children now survive and can be regarded as cured.

Dental management

Unless there is a major dental emergency, no active dental treatment should be carried out until the child is in remission. Any dental pain should be treated conservatively by the use of antibiotics and analgesics. The drug regimen used to induce remission has numerous side-effects, including nausea and vomiting, reversible alopecia (hair loss), neuropathy and oral ulceration. It can be extremely difficult to carry out normal mouthcare for children at this stage, and many have difficulty with toothbrushing because of acute nausea. Swabbing the mouth with chlorhexidine mouthwash and routine use of antifungal agents are essential. Local anaesthesia preparations such as 20% benzocaine gel or benzydamine hydrochloride (Difflam) applied before mealtimes can help to reduce pain from ulceration or mucositis.

Once the leukaemia is in remission and after consultation with the child's physician, routine dental care can be undertaken with the following adjustments:

- if invasive procedures are planned, current haematological information is required to assess bleeding risks
- prophylactic antibiotic therapy to prevent postoperative infection should be considered; it is given if the functional neutrophil count is depressed
- children who are immunosuppressed are also at risk of fungal and viral infections; fungal infections should be treated aggressively with amphotericin B or fluconazole, and herpetic infections with topical and/or systemic acyclovir
- regional block anaesthesia may be contraindicated because of the risk of deep haemorrhage
- long-term preventive dental care is important.

Respiratory disease

Asthma

Asthma involves hyperactivity of the airway to a variety of stimuli, causing breathlessness, coughing and wheezing. It affects at least 10% of children in UK.

Dental management

- Stress may precipitate an attack in the dental surgery
- Steroids may cause immunosuppression
- Sugared medicines may have caused a high caries rate

- No contraindications to nitrous oxide
- General anaesthesia may require inpatient management.

Cystic fibrosis

Cystic fibrosis is an autosomal recessive multisystem disorder of the mucous secreting exocrine glands. A thick mucous is produced in the lungs, leading to chronic obstruction and recurrent chest infections. Pancreatic exocrine insufficiency will produce malabsorption and failure to thrive.

Dental management

- Previous treatment with tetracyclines may have produced intrinsic staining
- Use of regional or general anaesthetics must be discussed with physician
- Avoid long appointments.

Metabolic and endocrine disorders

Diabetes mellitus

Type I or insulin-dependent diabetes is the most common form in children: 2 per 1000 school-age children will be affected.

Periodontal disease is associated with poor diabetic control. Xerostomia and recurrent intraoral diseases may be present. Enamel hypocalcification and hypoplasia, together with reduced salivary flow, can predispose these patients to an increased frequency of caries. They also have altered flora, with an increase in *Candida albicans*.

Dental management

- Well-controlled diabetics can have routine treatment under local anaesthesia as long as meal times are not interrupted. General anaesthesia, which requires fasting, will need inpatient management
- Healing can be delayed and prophylactic antibiotics are advised in surgical cases.

Adrenal insufficiency

If a child has adrenal insufficiency and/or is receiving steroid therapy, any infection or stress may precipitate an adrenal crisis. For simple extractions and routine restorative care no steroid supplementation is indicated. However, if more extensive oral surgery is indicated or the patient is particularly apprehensive, oral steroid dosage should be increased or parenteral supplementation given (Table 25).

Table 25 Corticosteroid cover for dental procedures

	No steroids in previous 12 months	Steroids given in previous 12 months	Steroids taken currently
Single extraction under local anaesthetic	No cover required	Hydrocortisone i.m. or i.v., preoperatively	Hydrocortisone orally, i.m. or i.v. preoperatively; Normal steroid medication postoperatively
Multiple extractions, minor oral surgery or treatment under general anaesthesia	Consider cover if large doses given previously	Hydrocortisone i.v. preoperatively; oral or i.m. for 24 hours postoperatively	Hydrocortisone i.v. preoperatively; oral or i.m. for normal steroid medication

Doses of hydrocortisone: under 12 years, 50 mg; 12–16 years, 100 mg.
Oral doses given 2 hours preoperatively. Intramuscular (i.m.) and intravascular (i.v.) doses given 30 minutes preoperatively.

Hypopituitarism

Anterior pituitary insufficiency (dwarfism) gives rise to potential risks related to adrenal gland activity and steroid production.

Hyperpituitarism (gigantism)

In hyperpituitarism, there is accelerated dental development and eruption.

Thyroid disorders

Hypothyroidism results in delayed eruption and increased spacing of teeth. Hyperthyroidism is often associated with other immunological deficiencies and results in precocious eruption of teeth, periodontal destruction and osteoporosis.

Dental management

- Principal risks are related to general anaesthesia
- Oral infections should be treated aggressively as they may exaggerate hyperthyroidism
- Antithyroid drugs may produce parotitis and agranulocytosis.

Parathyroid disorders

Hypoparathyroidism gives rise to:

- hypoplasia of enamel, hypodontia and root anomalies
- delayed or arrested tooth eruption
- acute and chronic oral candidiasis
- circumoral paraesthesia and spasm of facial muscles.

Hyperparathyroidism results in bony lesions (brown lesions) containing areas of haemorrhage with multinucleated giant cells, fibroblasts and haemosiderin. Generalised osteoporosis with cortical resorption is the most common bone lesion. The dental effects include:

- increasing mobility and drifting of teeth with no apparent periodontal pocketing
- malocclusion
- metastatic soft tissue calcification
- periapical radiolucencies and root resorption
- loss of lamina dura and generalised loss of radiodensity.

Neoplastic disease

In the UK, 1 in 600 children under the age of 15 years of age develop cancer. There are 1200–1500 new cases each year. Leukaemia is the most common form of cancer (48%); tumours of the central nervous system (16%), lymphomas (8%), neuroblastomas (7%) and nephroblastomas (5%) are the most common solid tumours.

Prognosis varies with the type of tumour, the stage at which it was diagnosed and the adequacy of treatment. The side-effects of treatment have been discussed previously and good oral care is essential.

Dental management
Dental management is similar to that as for all immunocompromised children:

- extraction of teeth with dubious prognosis
- meticulous oral hygiene and 0.2% chlorhexidine mouthwash four times a day
- topical analgesics: 20% benzocaine gel (flavoured) or 2% xylocaine (plain) for mucositis ulceration
- topical fluoride
- topical and systemic antifungals
- prophylactic antibiotics
- systemic antivirals.

Organ transplantation

Kidney, heart, liver and pancreas transplantation

Renal transplantation is the result of end-stage renal disease, heart transplantation is commonly required because of congenital heart disease and myopathy and liver transplantation is commonly required for biliary atresia. Transplantation recipients are prone to infection, bleeding and delayed healing owing to leucopenia and thrombocytopenia.

Dental management

Pretransplant planning. Remove any teeth of doubtful prognosis, treat active caries and institute a full preventive regimen.

Immediate post-transplant. Supportive dental care includes careful oral hygiene utilising chlorhexidine as a mouthwash or spray and a disposable sponge if the mouth is too sore for a toothbrush.

Stable post-transplant period. Reinforce all preventive advice. Antifungal prophylaxis is needed for a few months after transplant. Delayed eruption and exfoliation of primary teeth and ectopic eruption of permanent teeth are related to gingival overgrowth associated with treatment with ciclosporin and nifedipine.

Bone marrow transplantation

Bone marrow transplantation is used to treat first or second relapse of acute lymphoblastic leukaemia, acute myeloid leukaemia in first remission, aplastic anaemia, grade IV neuroblastoma and immunological deficiencies.

Dental management

If possible all treatment should be completed 2 weeks prior to induction chemotherapy or total body irradiation. Following transplant:

- chlorhexidine 0.2% mouthwashes or gels four times a day
- prophylactic systemic acyclovir and antifungals during immunosuppression
- topical fluoride application
- artificial saliva if significant xerostomia
- antibiotic coverage for all procedures.

Graft-versus-host disease

Transplanted T cells recognise host tissues as foreign, a reaction known as graft-versus-host disease. (GVHD). Significant manifestations are present in 50% of patients. Acute GVHD produces fever, rash, diarrhoea, abnormal liver function and jaundice. Chronic GVHD may occur months after transplantation and is characterised by lichenoid or scleroderma-like changes to skin and mucosa, keratoconjunctivitis, pulmonary insufficiency, abnormal liver function and intestinal problems. Oral manifestations often include mild mucosal erytherma, painful desquamative gingivitis, angular cheilitis, loss of lingual papillae, lichenoid maculae and striae, and xerostomia.

Diagnosis

A biopsy is taken of the lower lip to include minor salivary glands. Histological changes will be evident in stratified squamous epithelium with chronic lymphocytic inflammatory infiltrate and in the minor salivary glands with chronic sialadenitis.

Oral disease associated with HIV

Oral diseases are often early warning signs of HIV. Children commonly manifest candidosis, gingivitis and parotid swelling.

Herpes simplex infections occur intraorally and circumorally; recurrences are frequent. Treatment is with acyclovir.

Aphthous-type ulcers are persistent and common. Treatment is palliative.

Salivary gland enlargement is unilateral and bilateral, resulting in xerostomia and pain. Xerostomia can result in candidosis and dental caries. Treatment involves the use of saliva replacements, mouth sprays and salivary stimulants.

Hairy leukoplakia occurs in adults but is rare in children. It occurs on lateral border of tongue and, occasionally, the buccal mucosa and soft palate. No treatment required.

Oral candidosis Acute pseudomembranous candidosis is an early sign and suggests other opportunistic infections. It responds well to treatment with systemic antifungals and oral hygienie improvement.

HIV gingivitis results in red erythematous gingival tissues extending to free gingival margin. There is often spontaneous gingival haemorrhage and petechia at gingival margin, either localised or generalised. Treatment involves improved oral hygiene and 0.2% chlorhexidine mouthwash or gel four times a day.

HIV periodontitis gives rise to deep pain, spontaneous bleeding, interproximal necrosis and cratering, and intense erythema. Treatment is similar to that for acute necrotising gingivitis, with the use of metronidazole.

Kaposi's sarcoma is uncommon in children and adolescents. It affects the palate particularly but can occur on gingivae and tongue. Treatment is by chemotherapy, radiotherapy or laser excision.

Renal disease

End-stage renal failure leads to a fall in the glomerular filtration rate, which results in progressive hypertension, fluid retention and a build up of metabolites, which are not excreted normally. Conditions affecting kidney functions include ureteric reflux, obstructive uropathy, glomerulonephritis and glomerulosclerosis, medullary cystic disease, systemic lupus erythematosus and cystinosis. Renal patients may be anaemic and have a bleeding tendency because of capillary fragility and thrombocytopenia. Those on dialysis will be taking anti-coagulants. Caries rates may be lower, probably because of the ammonia released in saliva. Uraemic stomatitis may develop, with high serum urea. Teeth that are mineralising during renal failure will exhibit chronological hypoplasia or hypomineralisation.

Dental management
Dental problems should be minimised by aggressive prevention; otherwise:

- pulpally involved teeth should be extracted; patients on haemodialysis can have extractions 1 day after dialysis under DDAVP cover; sockets should be packed and sutured
- antibiotic prophylaxis for extractions
- inpatient facilities required for general anaesthesia.

Drug interactions in renal disease. End-stage renal failure is managed with antihypertensives and steroids and these patients are anaemic and immunocompromised. Metabolism of drugs by the kidney as well as renal excretion of drugs is impaired. The following drugs should be avoided:

- paracetamol
- penicillin
- tetracycline.

Hepatic disease

Hepatic disease can affect the metabolism of many drugs. Biliary atresia is congenital obliteration or hypoplasia of bile ducts, resulting in biliary cirrhosis and portal hypertension. It is the most common cause of transplantation in children. Deficiency of α_1-antitrypsin leads to progressive heptomegaly and cirrhosis. It is treated by transplantation.

Dental management
Coagulation problems may occur in hepatic failure because the vitamin K-dependent factors II, VII, IX and X are produced in the liver. Patients will be immunocompromised because of the high dosage of steroids used and will be mildly anaemic through destruction of red blood cells. High levels of unconjugated bilirubin causes a green intrinsic staining of the teeth. Treatment requires:

- aggressive preventive measures
- coagulation problems managed with fresh frozen plasma
- antibiotic prophylaxis.

Hepatitis A, B, C

Hepatitis A is an infectious condition with no carrier state. The transmission period is short (3 weeks).

Treatment is delayed for 4 weeks in patients who are positive for hepatitis A. Hepatitis B is assessed through the hepatitis B antigen (HSsAg) test on serum. Those with a negative test are chronic healthy carriers while those with a positive test are chronic active carriers. In the former, there may be some level of infectivity although less than that in chronic active carriers. Liver function is usually normal. A chronic active carrier has active viral replication and is very infective. They have active liver disease and liver function tests are abnormal.

Hepatitis C (non-A non-B) is usually asymptomatic although liver function tests may be intermittently abnormal. It is transmitted by blood or blood products. Patients are chronic carriers and are potentially infectious.

Dental management requires close liaison with the physician.

Neurological disease
Febrile convulsions

Febrile convulsions affect 5% of children and are associated with illnesses that cause rapid high fevers up to the age of 3 years. It is important to eliminate CNS infection. Febrile convulsions do not commonly result in any permanent damage nor proceed to epilepsy.

Epilepsy

The term epilepsy is applied to recurrent seizures either of unknown origin (idiopathic) or caused by congenital or acquired brain lesions (secondary epilepsy). Epilepsy affects 0.5–1.0% of the population.

Dental management
Phenytoin, used in epilepsy, is associated with gingival overgrowth, and a high standard of oral hygiene is necessary to minimise the development of overgrowth. Gingival surgery should not be contemplated if the oral hygiene is not excellent.

Cerebral palsy

Many patients with cerebral palsy have no mental impairment, and it can take a long time in a patient to assess cognitive ability. Verbal communication requires patience or a communication aid. It is important not to change voice tone or level when speaking to these children.

Dental visits may trigger limb extension especially if transfer to the dental chair occurs. It may be more appropriate to treat in their chair with appropriate pillow support for the head on a special moulded insert on the dental chair.

Gag, cough, bite and swallowing reflexes may be impaired and the position of the child is crucial. They should be upright with slight neck flexion. Rubber dam is especially valuable to reduce the amount of water in the mouth from the air-rotor in those with swallowing problems. Mouth props may be used, but good suction must be available to prevent aspiration. Bite reflex to oral stimulation is difficult to overcome, but sometimes gentle finger pressure on the anterior border of the ascending ramus and retromolar area will help to open the mouth and instruments should be introduced from the side rather than the front.

Some patients who have hydrocephalus will have shunts from the ventricles of the brain to either the vasculature or the periotonal cavity. Current antibiotic prophylaxis guidelines should be followed, but generally ventriculo-atrial shunts will require cover while ventriculo-peritoneal do not.

Visual impairment

A visually impaired person should be allowed to make full use of their tactile sense. Do not lead them roughly to the dental chair but merely guide if required. Allow them also to make full use of their sense of smell when familiarising them to the dental environment and procedures.

Give verbal and physical reassurance once rapport has been established. This is especially important as the patient cannot see your face or your smile.

Constantly describe procedures and the environment to help the patient to relax and feel comfortable in their surroundings.

Photophobia may be a problem in many visually impaired persons. Safety glasses in this situation should be tinted.

Deafness

Establish how the patient communicates. A patient who lip reads will understand if you speak more slowly and make sure your lips and mouth are visible. Basic sign language will certainly improve your rapport with the patient and improve the patient's confidence.

Deaf people are often vibration sensitive; consequently, a full exploration of procedures and slow introduction of the different drill speeds is necessary.

A hearing-aid that is switched on during treatment may produce alarming feedback. It is better to turn it off or reduce the volume.

Developmental disability

The initial consultation is not only important to allow the dentist (and parent) to establish what treatment is required but also to find what is possible. Find out the patient's likes, dislikes and behaviour patterns.

Children with a developmental disability often also have a mental disability, so a full history is important.

Dental management

- aggressive prevention is mandatory
- treatment when required is often under general anaesthesia, which in itself is not without risk especially in the multiple disability syndromic child
- assessment procedures for general anaesthesia require full documentation of all medical complications.

Self-assessment: questions

Multiple choice questions

1. In primary tooth trauma:
   a. Injuries are most common at age 6–7 years
   b. Luxation injuries are commonest
   c. A discoloured upper central without clinical or radiographic evidence of infection can be reviewed
   d. Palatal luxation injuries carry the highest risk to the developing permanent dentition
   e. Dilaceration of the permanent successor tooth is common

2. In permanent incisor trauma:
   a. Luxation injuries require rigid splinting
   b. Immature 'open' apex teeth have a better prognosis for pulp vitality compared with mature 'closed' apex teeth
   c. Avulsion injuries should be splinted for 7–10 days
   d. Open apex teeth replanted within 45 minutes may revascularise
   e. Resorption is greatest in subluxation injuries

3. In intrusion injuries:
   a. Closed apex teeth often retain their vitality
   b. Open apex teeth may re-erupt
   c. Closed apex teeth must be repositioned quickly
   d. Surgical repositioning may be necessary in severe injury
   e. Resorption is a rare complication

4. In avulsion and re-implantation:
   a. Mouthwash is an ideal tooth storage medium
   b. Closed apex teeth may revascularise
   c. Internal resorption is the commonest type of resorption
   d. Ankylosis leads to progressive intrusion of the tooth
   e. Telephone advice is crucial to long-term outcomes

5. Lateral luxation injuries:
   a. Should be left to reposition naturally
   b. May cause occlusal interference
   c. Involving open apex teeth have a better prognosis for pulp vitality than closed apex teeth
   d. Should be extirpated routinely at splint removal
   e. Involve fractures of the alveolar plates

6. Root fractures:
   a. Involving the middle third do not require splinting
   b. Involving the coronal third are easily treated
   c. Usually cause loss of vitality
   d. Can heal by firm union with cementum-like tissue
   e. Are easily diagnosed on radiographs

7. In child abuse:
   a. There are approximately 30 000 children on at-risk registers in England and Wales
   b. The Children Act of 1989 states five categories of abuse
   c. Most 'at risk' children live in rural communities
   d. Males are the most common perpetrators
   e. Disability of a child may be a contributory factor

8. In child physical abuse:
   a. More than 50% of abused children have oro-facial signs
   b. Facial fractures are common injuries
   c. Bruises can have a recognised shape or pattern
   d. Dental trauma has a characteristic appearance
   e. A damaged upper labial frenum can be caused by forcible feeding

9. In dental anomalies:
   a. Hypodontia is familial
   b. Supernumerary teeth may prevent eruption of permanent teeth
   c. Macrodontia occurs in Down syndrome
   d. 'Dens in dente' teeth are easily root filled
   e. Supernumerary teeth are more common than missing teeth

10. In dental anomalies:
    a. Amelogenesis imperfecta may look like fluorosis
    b. Amelogenesis imperfecta may be associated with osteogenesis imperfecta
    c. Teeth with dentinogenesis imperfecta usually undergo pulpal obliteration
    d. Hypoplasia infers deficient matrix with normal mineralisation
    e. Infraoccluded teeth have a higher incidence of absent permanent successors

11. In patients with coexisting disease:
    a. Congenital cardiac defects require antibiotic cover for scaling and polishing
    b. Penicillin is the antibiotic of choice for prophylaxis
    c. Mortality associated with infective endocarditis is about 5%
    d. Cystic fibrosis can result in decreased saliva formation

e. A platelet count of $80 \times 10^9/l$ is safe for invasive procedures in general dental practice

12. In patients with neoplasia or immunodeficiencies:
    a. Neuroblastoma is the most common childhood malignancy
    b. Bone marrow transplant is the preferred treatment for acute lymphoblastic leukaemia
    c. Five-year survival rates for acute lymphoblastic leukaemia are about 60–70%
    d. Candidal infections are common in immunosuppression
    e. Nifedipine and phenytoin can cause gingival overgrowth

13. In patients with renal or hepatic disease:
    a. Renal disease is associated with high caries rate
    b. Penicillin is contraindicated in renal disease
    c. Hepatic disorders can produce coagulation problems because of a deficiency of production of factors V and VIII
    d. Hepatitis C is potentially infective
    e. Renal patients on dialysis receive anticoagulants

14. In patients with coexisting disease or developmental disorders:
    a. Five percent of childhood convulsions are associated with febrile illness
    b. Patients with cerebral palsy are always mentally impaired
    c. Photophobia occurs in the visually impaired
    d. Deafness can result in vibration sensitivity
    e. Developmental disability is not commonly associated with other medical problems

Picture questions

Picture 1

The patient in Figure 92 has had a heart transplant.

1. Which drugs may have caused his mandibular gingival hyperplasia?
2. What other drugs commonly cause the condition?
3. Why does hyperplasia occur?

Picture 2

2. This patient (Fig. 93) has severe wear and discoloration of her teeth.

1. What is the condition?
2. How common is the condition?

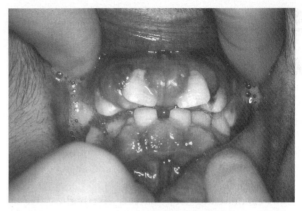

Fig. 92 A patient who has had a heart transplant.

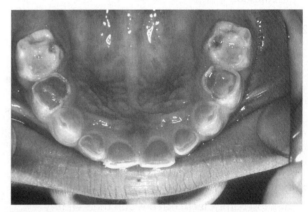

Fig. 93 Patient with severe wear and discoloration.

3. Will the permanent dentition be affected?
4. How would you treat her?

Short note questions

Write short notes on:

1. oral complications that might be expected in a patient undergoing cancer chemotherapy and their prevention
2. the management of an insulin-dependent diabetic who requires an extraction under (a) local and (b) general anaesthesia
3. immediate treatment for a palatally luxated central incisor without a root fracture but with an enamel dentine fracture in a 9-year-old child with no medical illness
4. factors that would make you suspicious of child physical abuse (non-accidental injury).

Self-assessment: answers

Multiple choice answers

1.
a. **False**. Age 2–4 years is the peak age for injuries to the primary teeth.
b. **True**. This is because of the relative elasticity of young alveolar bone.
c. **True**. Extraction need only be contemplated if there is clinical or radiographic infection.
d. **False**. Intrusion injuries carry the highest risk. Palatal luxation carries the root of the tooth away from the developing permanent tooth germ.
e. **False**. Hypoplasias are the most common sequelae. Dilaceration is a rarer complication.

2.
a. **False**. Functional splinting for 2–3 weeks is required.
b. **True**. There is less chance of the neurovascular bundle being compressed by oedema around the developing apex.
c. **True**. Sixty percent of periodontal fibres are reunited within 10–14 days.
d. **True**. Revascularisation proceeds at 0.5 mm a day. This is best assessed by new Doppler technology.
e. **False**. Greatest in intrusion and avulsion injuries where the damage to the periodontal ligament is severest.

3.
a. **False**. There is no evidence that any will retain vitality.
b. **True**. After initial disimpaction, a period of 2–3 months should be allowed for re-eruption.
c. **True**. These teeth will not re-erupt spontaneously, unlike open apex teeth.
d. **True**. This will often be the most practical option.
e. **False**. The incidence of resorption is high because of the severe damage to the periodontal ligament by tearing and crushing.

4.
a. **False**. Saliva, normal saline or milk are the best storage media.
b. **False**. Only open apex teeth replanted within 45 minutes may revascularise.
c. **False**. External inflammatory resorption initiated within the damaged periodontal ligament occurs initially. This will be propogated if non-vital pulp tissue remains in the root canal.
d. **True**. Once the periodontal ligament is lost and bone is fused directly to the tooth tissue, there will not only be progressive loss of root as bone is remodelled but also progressive intrusion.
e. **True**. The immediate management will influence the extra-alveolar time that the tooth is out of the socket and the storage medium that a tooth is kept in.

5.
a. **False**. Require immediate manual reduction if an injury is new, or orthodontic repositioning if an injury is over 2–4 days old.
b. **True**. This is corrected on repositioning.
c. **True**. Evidence after 5 years suggests that while 85% of open apex teeth will retain vitality, only 25% of closed apex teeth will.
d. **False**. This decision should be made after thorough clinical and radiographic examination at regular periods.
e. **True**. Crush fractures will occur on the side of the alveolus to which a portion of root is displaced.

6.
a. **False**. Only apical fractures may not require splinting.
b. **False**. It is difficult to achieve a firm union over the fracture line because of proximity of the periodontal pocket.
c. **False**. Eighty percent of root-fractured teeth retain their vitality.
d. **True**. This requires splinting within 24 hours of injury. Persistent mobility will allow growth of periodontal ligament cells across the fracture line.
e. **False**. Often requires two radiographs at different angles to detect.

7.
a. **True**. Children will remain on registers for 1–2 years.
b. **False**. There are four categories: physical, emotional, neglect, sexual.
c. **False**. Abuse is mainly an urban or metropolitan phenomenon. However, there will be pockets of severe deprivation in some rural areas, where unemployment is high, which will have a high registration rate.
d. **True**. It is often the male member of a household who is responsible.
e. **True**. Crying, soiling of clothes, unwanted pregnancy are also contributary factors on behalf of the child.

8.
a. **True**. A more accurate figure is 60–80%.
b. **False**. Only 2% of oro-facial injuries are fractures. This is because of elasticity of the young facial skeleton.
c. **True**. The pattern of grab marks, pinch marks and slap marks can be recognised.
d. **False**. It would be other factors or marks in association with the dental trauma that would raise suspicion.

e. **True**. This may be associated with a grab mark on the face.

9. a. **True**. Autosomal dominant inheritance.
   b. **True**. In the upper anterior region especially. In clinical practice, if a permanent central incisor has not erupted within 6 months of its antimere, then a radiograph should be taken.
   c. **False**. Microdontia is associated with Down syndrome.
   d. **False**. Unless the invagination is limited to the coronal portion of the crown and can be totally removed with a bur, extraction is usually necessary.
   e. **False**. In the permanent dentition, hypodontia (excluding wisdom teeth) occurs in 3.5–6% of the population, while supernumerary teeth occur in 1.5–3.5%.

10. a. **True**. The 'snow-capped' variety may resemble fluorosis.
    b. **False**. Dentinogenesis imperfecta type 1 is associated with osteogenesis imperfecta.
    c. **True**. They also have bulbous crowns and smaller roots.
    d. **True**. Hypocalcification by comparison infers a normal matrix that is poorly calcified.
    e. **True**. If successors are present, however, then infraoccluded teeth should exfoliate with normal time limits.

11. a. **True**. These are the recommendations in order to prevent infective endocarditis.
    b. **False**. Amoxicillin is the antibiotic of choice. If patients are allergic or have received amoxicillin during the previous month, then clindamycin is the choice.
    c. **False**. The actual figure is 20–30%.
    d. **True**. This can predispose the patient to caries.
    e. **True**. Any injections, scaling or extractions below this at platelet levels should only be done in a hospital department.

12. a. **False**. Leukaemia accounts for 48% of childhood malignancies. Neuroblastoma occurs in only 7% of childhood malignancies.
    b. **False**. Bone marrow transplant is used for relapses of acute lymphoblastic leukaemia and for acute myeloblastic leukaemia, aplastic anaemia and immunological deficiencies.
    c. **True**. This is amazing when you consider the survival rate in 1950 was nil.
    d. **True**. These can be treated with standard agents such as nystatin and amphoteracin.

e. **True**. However, why some patients are better 'responders', i.e. produce more overgrowth, is not known.

13. a. **False**. A low caries rate is thought to be a result of ammonia in the saliva.
    b. **True**. This is because the metabolism of the drug and its renal excretion are impaired. Paracetamol and tetracyline should also be avoided.
    c. **False**. Factors II VII IX X (Vitamin K dependent) are reduced in hepatic disease.
    d. **True**. Infectious and transmitted by blood and blood products.
    e. **True**. Any dental treatment required needs to be discussed with the physicians involved in the renal care.

14. a. **True**. 'Febrile convulsions' rarely occur after age 3 years and any convulsions will be epileptic form.
    b. **False**. A large proportion of patients with cerebral palsy are of normal intelligence.
    c. **True**. Be very careful with bright surgery lights.
    d. **True**. Always explain what instruments you will be using.
    e. **False**. A large proportion have associated syndromes and multiple medical problems.

Picture answers

Picture 1

1. Ciclosporin, nifedipine.
2. Phenytoin.
3. The exact mechanism of drug interaction is unknown. There is proliferation of subgingival collagen, mainly of the interdental papillae, which become grossly swollen, pale and firm. Hyperplasia is more pronounced when oral hygiene is poor.

Picture 2

1. Dentinogenesis imperfecta.
2. Approximately 1 in 8000.
3. Yes, but teeth that develop later may be less affected.
4. Full preventative programme, establishment of posterior occlusion with stainless steel crowns, composite strip crowns or veneers to improve upper anterior aesthetics.

Short note answers

1. These patients will be immunosuppressed and, therefore, will be specifically prone to oral mucosal

disease (ulceration, mucositis), infection (leucopenia) and haemorrhage (thrombocytopenia). These could lead to significant morbidity and even mortality. Removal of teeth of dubious prognosis prior to treatment, restoration of other teeth and aggressive prevention is required. The prevention will include oral hygiene instruction, 0.2% chlorhexidine mouthwash four times a day, topical fluoride application, antifungals and modification of diet (realistic modifications for a child's condition).

2. (a) An early morning or early afternoon appointment, which would be close to their last major meal intake.

   (b) These patients need to be starved prior to a general anaesthetic and, therefore, are not suitable for treatment as outpatients. They need hospital admission to stabilise diabetic control by intravenous drip the night before the extractions and then careful conversion back to their normal regimen postoperatively.

3. Reposition the tooth with gentle finger pressure under local anaesthesia. Splint with a functional splint – composite and ortho wire attached to one abutment tooth either side of the luxated tooth – for 2–3 weeks.

Place a composite or compomer bandage over the enamel–dentine fracture. Record baseline clinical and radiographic data, including vitality tests and radiographs of all teeth in upper labial segment. Prescribe antibiotics (commonly amoxicillin 250 mg twice daily) for 5 days, antibacterial mouthwash (chlorhexidine 0.2% four times a day) and a soft diet for the duration of the splint.

4. Any of the following factors:
- delay in seeking advice or help
- explanation does not fit the age and clinical findings
- story of the accident varies
- child may say something contradictory to parents
- history of previous injury
- history of violence in the family
- child's reaction to any medical/dental examinations
- child's reaction to other people
- nature of the relationship between parent and child
- parent's mood is abnormal and child's needs are not seen as a priority.

Orthodontics I: development, assessment and treatment planning

Overview

Orthodontics relates to facial and occlusal development as well as to the supervision, interception and correction of occlusal and dentofacial anomalies. The practise of orthodontics, therefore, spans from birth into adulthood, with current practice aiming to establish optimal and stable occlusal relationships with dentofacial harmony. An appreciation of facial and occlusal development is fundamental to understanding the possible aetiology of some orthodontic problems as well as being critical for their assessment and the planning of any likely treatment.

This chapter commences with an account of the rudiments of facial and occlusal development. It then details the elements of comprehensive clinical and cephalometric orthodontic assessment. Finally the principles of treatment planning are considered.

8.1 Craniofacial growth and occlusal development

Learning objectives

You should

- understand the pattern of growth of the calvarium, cranial base, the nasomaxillary complex and the mandible

- be aware of what is meant by 'growth rotations' and their impact on the occlusion

- know how occlusal development proceeds in the 'average' child.

An understanding of both craniofacial growth and occlusal development is essential to orthodontic practice as the former has a significant impact on the latter.

Craniofacial growth

Pattern of craniofacial growth

At birth the face and jaws are underdeveloped compared with those in the adult. More growth, therefore, occurs of the facial skeleton than of the cranial structure postnatally. Growth patterns have been established for four major body tissue systems – lymphoid, neural, general or somatic, and genital – and it is important to have an appreciation of these as some patterns are followed by tissues involved in craniofacial growth (Fig. 94). Lymphoid growth is rapid up to about 10 years but undergoes involution as the genital growth is accelerating at puberty. Neural growth, however, is virtually complete by 6 to 7 years, while somatic growth increases in early childhood, then slows, before increasing dramatically at puberty.

The pattern of neural growth affects skeletal growth of the calvarium and orbit, whereas the somatic growth pattern is followed approximately by the mandible and maxilla. More precisely, the jaw growth pattern falls between that followed by the neural and general body tissues, with the mandible aligning itself more to the latter than the maxilla. The spurt in jaw growth at puberty almost coincides with the spurt in height, on average at 12 years in girls and 2 years later in boys, although considerable individual variation exists.

For both the maxilla and mandible, on average, growth in width is completed in advance of that in length, which ceases before growth in the vertical dimension. The lateral dimensions of the jaws and dental arches tend to alter minimally during puberty, as growth in width is largely completed before the growth spurt. Growth in length continues usually until about 14 to 15 years in girls and 17 to 18 years in boys, while vertical growth may extend into the late teens in females and into the twenties in males.

Growth continues into middle age, with changes in the vertical facial dimension predominating over those

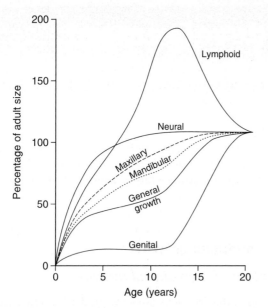

Fig. 94 Postnatal growth curves of various tissue types with superimposed maxillary and mandibular curves.

that occur anteroposteriorly, and least alteration taking place laterally. In the early twenties, growth tends to resume slightly in females, with a backward mandibular rotation being common. Although a late resumption of growth is not witnessed in males, a forward rotating pattern of mandibular growth is usual in adulthood. Irrespective of the direction of mandibular growth rotation, compensatory adjustment occurs in the occlusal relationships. Facial growth should, therefore, be seen as a process that continues well into adult life and not as one that is complete in the late teens.

Control of facial growth

Both genetic and environmental factors impact on the regulation of craniofacial growth but the exact mechanisms are unclear. In theory, genetic control may be expressed primarily via bone, cartilage or the soft tissue matrix. Bone is unlikely to be the primary determinant of its own growth, as sutural growth is reactive rather than inherently programmed. The nasal septum and the synchondroses of the cranial bones probably act as independent growth centres but the cartilage of the mandibular condyle appears to react to, rather than initiate, growth. The present concept is that bone and cartilage respond to soft tissue growth determined by functional needs (the so-called 'functional matrix' theory). While growth of the cranium and of the orbit in direct response to growth of the brain and of the eyes lend support to the theory, no similarly expanding structures exist within the middle and lower facial

thirds. However, growth of the cranial base may be influenced by growth of the brain. The soft tissues, including the facial and masticatory muscles, are also possible contributors to downward and forward maxillary translation.

Growth prediction

At present no method is available to predict accurately the amount, direction and timing of facial growth. Instead, the assumption is usually made that for most patients whose direction and amount of facial growth are about average, the likelihood is that their growth pattern will follow the same pattern through orthodontic treatment.

Methods attempting to predict the pattern of facial growth to assist orthodontic treatment planning include:

- superimposition of a template with average annual growth increments on the patient's cephalometric tracing
- digitisation of a cephalometric film followed by computer addition of average annual growth increments.

These data, however, are derived from children who did not receive orthodontic treatment, and as the amount and direction of growth may not be 'average' in an individual, the possibility of erroneous growth prediction is significant.

Growth of the craniofacial skeleton

Craniofacial growth can be considered conveniently in relation to the calvarium, the cranial base, the nasomaxillary complex and the mandible.

Calvarium
The precursors to the skull bones develop in membrane, and six open spaces (fontanelles) that exist at birth are eliminated by 18 months. Contact between the bones is at sutures. Bone apposition occurs at these periosteum-lined sites in response to brain growth and they fuse eventually in adulthood. The contour of the cranial vault also changes by periosteal remodelling at the inner and outer surfaces.

Cranial base
The cranial base forms initially in cartilage, which is transformed to bone by endochondral ossification. Sutural growth and surface remodelling occur laterally in response to brain growth. Of greater significance are primary cartilageous growth sites: sphenoethnoidal, intersphenoid and most importantly the spheno-occipital synchondrosis. The spheno-occipital synchon-

drosis grows until the mid-teens, having a profound impact on the anteroposterior skeletal pattern; it finally fuses at about 20 years of age. Because of its location in front of the temporomandibular joints but behind the anterior cranial base, both growth in length and in shape of the cranial base affects the maxillary–mandibular relationship. A long cranial base or large cranial base angle is associated with a class II skeletal pattern, while the converse is generally associated with a class III pattern (see Section 8.3 for definitions).

Nasomaxillary complex

The frontal process and a mesenchymal condensation in the maxillary processes of the first pharyngeal arch form the maxilla' which then ossifies intramembraneously starting in the lateral aspects of the cartilagenous nasal capsule. Growth of the maxilla occurs via

- bone apposition at the circum-maxillary suture system
- passive displacement from its articulation with the cranial base
- surface remodelling.

Growth at the maxillary sutures assumes a greater role after age 7, when neural growth is complete and growth at the cranial base synchondroses lessens. As the maxilla moves downwards and forwards in response to growth of the surrounding soft tissues, the space opened at the superior and posterior sutures is obliterated by bone deposition on either side of the suture. Resorption of the anterior maxillary surface occurs simultaneously. Displacement of the maxilla inferiorly is accompanied by bone resorption from the nasal floor and deposition on the palate, while the alveolar process also develops vertically with tooth eruption. Bone is deposited also at the midline suture in response to lateral displacement of the maxillary halves, leading to an increase in midfacial width. Growth is complete by about 17 years in males and on average 2 years earlier in females.

Mandible

Like the maxilla, the mandible is derived from the first pharyngeal arch. It begins development as a mesenchymal condensation just lateral to Meckel's cartilage. Bone formation proceeds intramembraneously, spreading posteriorly along Meckel's cartilage without directly replacing it by newly formed bone. Condylar cartilages are formed distant to the mandibular body but fuse with it at about 4 months. These secondary cartilages are not primary instigators of mandibular growth but respond to other controlling influences. Endochondral ossification at the condyles accounts, in part, for mandibular

growth. Elsewhere, bone apposition and remodelling are responsible for an increase in size and shape. As the mandible is translated downwards and forwards, largely in response to muscular forces, contact with the base of the skull is maintained by cartilagenous growth at the condylar heads, which increases ramal height. The alveolar processes also increase in height with tooth eruption.

Mandibular length is increased by periosteal apposition along the posterior border and simultaneous bone removal from the anterior aspect of the ramus. Increase in mandibular width occurs principally by remodelling posteriorly. The chin is almost passive as a growth area but by the late teenage years it has become more prominent in response to forward mandibular translation. On average, mandibular growth is complete by about 17 years in females and 2 years later in males, but it can proceed for longer.

Growth rotations

The trend is for the facial skeleton to grow downwards and forwards away from the cranial base, although implant studies have indicated that rotations of both the maxilla and mandible occur during growth. These have more marked effects on the mandible than on the maxilla, where remodelling disguises their true impact. Mandibular growth rotations represent a growth imbalance in anterior and posterior facial heights. The direction of condylar growth and the vertical magnitude of growth at the spheno-occipital synchondrosis influence posterior face height. Growth of the masticatory and suprahyoid musculature, including associated fascia and influenced partly by the vertical growth changes in the spinal column, affects the anterior face height together with the eruption of teeth.

While mandibular growth rotations occur in all individuals, these are particularly different where the vertical facial proportions are markedly reduced or increased. A forward rotation, characterised by greater growth in posterior than in anterior facial height, is more common than a posterior growth rotation, where the change in facial height ratio is opposite to that observed in forward rotation (Fig. 95). Where forward rotation of the mandible is extreme

- the lower border is convex with a reduced mandibular plane angle
- the lower anterior face height is reduced
- the overbite is deep.

(a)

(b)

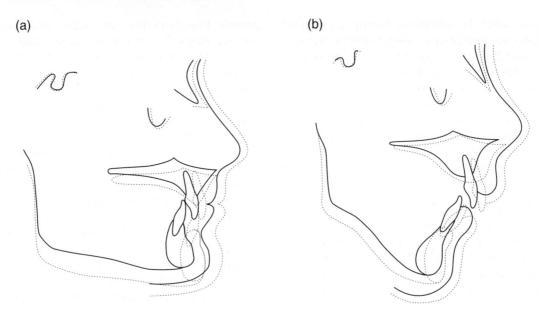

Fig. 95 Growth rotation. (a) Forward growth rotation owing to greater increase in posterior than in anterior facial height, resulting in an increased overbite. (b) Backward growth rotation owing to a greater increase in anterior than in posterior facial height, resulting in a reduced overbite.

Conversely, a backward rotational pattern of mandibular growth results in

- a concave lower border
- a pronounced antegonial notch with a high mandibular plane angle
- increased lower anterior face height
- a reduced or anterior open bite.

Growth rotations also influence the inclination and anteroposterior position of the incisors. Forward maxillary rotation tends to increase upper incisor prominence while a backward rotation has the opposite effect. In the mandible, a marked anterior growth rotation leads to progressive retroclination of the lower incisors and an increase in lower labial segment crowding. With a posterior mandibular growth rotation, the incisors become upright, shortening the dental arch and producing crowding of the lower incisor area.

The pattern of rotation has an impact on treatment. Whereas a forward rather than a backward rotation aids correction of a class II skeletal discrepancy, it also tends to increase overbite. Where the rotation is marked, overbite reduction is more difficult. Furthermore, in the late teens, lower labial segment crowding may result from either an anterior or a posterior growth rotational pattern, and these continue to a lesser extent into the fourth decade.

Soft tissue growth

At birth, the orofacial musculature is well developed to allow suckling and breathing, and it soon responds to other functional demands of mastication, speech, facial expression and changes to the swallowing pattern. The light pressures from the lingual and buccolabial musculature affect tooth position, guiding the teeth towards a functional relationship and compensating, where possible, for any skeletal discrepancy. However, where a severe skeletal discrepancy or abnormal soft tissue behaviour exists, for example a lip trap with a class II division 1 malocclusion, the dentoalveolar compensatory mechanism will be insufficient.

Facial musculature lengthens with facial growth, and these soft tissue influences may be inherently responsible for the skeletal growth processes. The likelihood of lip competence increases during the late stages of facial growth, but soft tissue changes continue into middle age with the chin and nose assuming relatively greater prominence as the lips tend to flatten.

Occlusal development

What follows is an account of normal occlusal development: the changes one would expect to see in the 'average' child. It is important to appreciate the range that exists within normal boundaries, so that developing problems may be recognised early and appropriate orthodontic intervention planned, if required. A thorough knowledge of the calcification and eruption dates of the 20 primary and 32 permanent teeth is essential (see Tables 11 and 12, p. 170). As well as allowing comparison of dental and chronological age, this information also helps to identify the timing of any insult that has led to alterations in the enamel or dentin mineralisation and indicates if a tooth that is absent radiographically is likely to develop.

Development of the deciduous dentition

The gum pads, containing the deciduous teeth, enlarge and widen following birth, with the lower lying slightly behind the upper by the time the first deciduous teeth (lower incisors) start to erupt at about 6 months of age. These are followed closely by the other incisors. The first deciduous molars erupt 3 to 4 months later, followed by the deciduous canines and the eruption of the second deciduous molars at about 3 years. The incisors tend to be upright, and anterior spacing is normal. Spacing is most common mesial to the upper canine and distal to the lower canine – the anthropoid or primate spaces. With 1–2 mm increase in the intercanine distance, spacing between the incisors often increases as the child grows. In the absence of generalised spacing of the deciduous teeth, crowding of the permanent teeth is likely. The overbite, which is often initially 'deep' in terms of lower incisor crown coverage, reduces and by 5 years of age an edge-to-edge occlusion with incisor attrition is common.

Development of the permanent dentition

At about 6 years, the eruption of the first permanent molars, followed by the permanent incisors, signifies the transition from the primary to the permanent dentition, commonly referred to as the 'mixed dentition phase'. The permanent successors are slightly larger than the primary teeth and the first permanent molars need to be accommodated. Existing space is present between the deciduous teeth. Additional space is provided by minor modifications in arch length, arch width and intercanine distance (Table 26). Once the primary dentition is fully erupted, however, the dental arch size remains more or less constant anteriorly apart from a modest change in shape with some growth in the intercanine distance. In addition, growth at the back of the arches is necessary to accommodate the permanent molars and to maintain the arch relationship while the face grows vertically.

The permanent lower incisors develop lingual to their predecessors and are frequently misaligned on eruption, but this usually resolves with intercanine growth. The upper anterior teeth develop palatal to their deciduous predecessors and are accommodated

- by the existing spacing in the arch
- by erupting downwards and slightly forward so that they are placed on a wider arc
- by a small increase in intercanine distance (Table 26).

The upper permanent lateral incisors usually move distally and labially with eruption of the central incisors, but they may be trapped palatally in crowded arches. The upper central incisors are often distally inclined when they first appear. An associated diastema tends to reduce as the lateral incisors erupt. At this time, the upper central and, to a greater extent, the lateral incisors are divergent, the latter because of pressure on their roots from the unerupted canines; this is often referred to as 'the ugly duckling' phase of dental development.

The maxillary canines migrate from their palatal developmental position to lie labially and distally

Table 26 Dental arch development

Characteristic	Measurement	Developmental changes	
Arch length	Perpendicular distance from 1/1 contact point to a line contacting the distal surfaces of e/e or 5/5	Maxilla:	slight increase 6–10 years; followed by a 1–2 mm decrease
		Mandible:	no increase 6–10 years; at 10–17 years 1–2 mm decrease
Arch circumference	Line drawn through the buccal cusps and incisal edges of the teeth from the distal surface of e/e or 5/5	Maxilla:	~1 mm increase in male; ~0.5 mm increase in female
		Mandible:	~3.5 mm decrease in male; ~4 mm decrease in female
Intercanine width	Distance between the cusp tips of c/c or 3/3	Maxilla:	~1–2 mm from 3–6 years; ~3.5 mm from 6–12 years
		Mandible:	~1–2 mm from 3–6 years; ~3 mm from 6–10 years
Arch width	Distance from the palatal/lingual cusps of second molars or 5	Maxilla:	~2–3 mm increase from 3–18 years; greater in males than females
		Mandible:	~3.6 mm increase from 3–18 years in both males and females

above the roots of the lateral incisors, leading to approximation of the incisor crowns as they erupt.

The combined mesiodistal widths of the deciduous canines and molars in each quadrant are slightly greater than those of the permanent canines and premolars. This difference in dimension is known as the 'leeway space' and is about 1 mm in the upper arch and 2.5 mm in the lower arch. The larger leeway space in the lower arch, probably in combination with mandibular growth, allows greater forward movement of the lower first permanent molar, converting a 'flush terminal plane' relationship of the deciduous molars to a class I occlusion (see below).

The static occlusal and functional relations of the normal permanent dentition are:

- the mesiobuccal cusp of the upper first permanent molar lies in the buccal groove of the lower first permanent molar (class I occlusion)
- upper and lower incisors are slightly proclined, with the lower incisors occluding on the cingulae of the upper incisors with an average overjet and overbite of 2–4 mm
- there is no spacing or rotations, and marginal ridges are level
- the occlusal plane is flat or with a slight curve of Spee
- each tooth, with the exception of the lower incisors, is slightly mesially inclined
- the canines through to the molars are inclined lingually
- centric relation should coincide with centric occlusion
- a working side canine rise or group function should be present on lateral excursions with no occlusal contact on the non-working side; the incisors should only contact in protrusion.

Maturational changes in the occlusion

The occlusion of any child must be seen as dynamic and responding to changes in the facial skeleton. As the face continues to grow throughout the late teens and into adulthood, changes in the dentition and occlusion follow.

- There is an increase in lower incisor crowding. This has been observed even in children with previously well aligned, spaced arches and can be regarded as normal. Factors implicated in its aetiology are listed in Table 27.
- There is an increase in the interincisal angle, with uprighting of the incisors.
- A tendency for the overbite to reduce is seen.
- A slight increase occurs in mandibular prognathism in males and in mandibular retrusion in females.

Table 27 Factors implicated in late lower incisor crowding[a]

Factors	Effects/affected tissues
Skeletal	Increase in mandibular prognathism Mandibular growth rotations Minimal forward maxillary growth
Soft tissue	Increase in soft tissue tone of lips and cheeks Transseptal fibre contraction
Dental/occlusal	Lack of approximal attrition Dentoalveolar disproportion Tooth size Mesial drift secondary to anterior component of occlusal force, eruptive force of posterior teeth Uprighting of posterior teeth in response to increase in lower facial height

[a]Tends to be greater in females than males.

8.2 Malocclusion: classification and aetiology

Learning objectives

You should

- be able to classify the first molar and incisor relationship
- know how to apply and categorise malocclusion according to the Index of Orthodontic Treatment Need (IOTN)
- be aware of how the outcome of orthodontic treatment may be assessed.

Malocclusion is an unacceptable deviation either aesthetically and/or functionally from the ideal occlusion. Prevalence of malocclusion varies with age and racial origin as well as according to the assessment methods, but not all malocclusion requires treatment.

Classification of malocclusion

Classification for diagnosis

Angle's classification
Angle's classification is based on the molar relationship (Fig. 96).

Class I (also referred to as normal occlusion or neutrocclusion). The mesiobuccal cusp of the upper first permanent molar occludes in the buccal groove of the lower first permanent molar. Discrepancies no greater than half a cusp width were also regarded as class I by Angle.

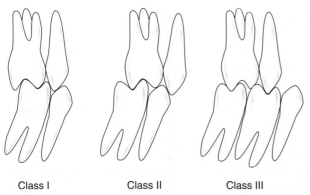

Class I   Class II   Class III

Fig. 96 Angle's classification based on first molar relationships.

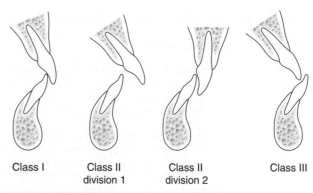

Class I   Class II division 1   Class II division 2   Class III

Fig. 97 British Standard Institute classification based on incisor relationship.

Class II (also referred to as postnormal occlusion or distocclusion). The mesiobuccal cusp of the upper first permanent molar occludes anterior to the buccal groove of the lower first permanent molar. *Class III* (also referred to as prenormal occlusion or mesiocclusion). The mesiobuccal cusp of the upper first permanent molar occludes posterior to the buccal groove of the lower first permanent molar.

Angle believed that the anteroposterior dental base relationship could be assessed reliably from the first permanent molar relationship, as its position, he maintained, remained constant following eruption. As this tenet is incorrect and difficulties arise in classification where mesial drift or loss of a first permanent molar has occurred, other classification systems are now used to categorise the anteroposterior dental base relationship.

British Standard Institute classification

The British Standard Institute classification relates to the incisor relationship (Fig. 97).

Class I. The lower incisor edges occlude with, or lie immediately below, the cingulum plateau (middle third of the palatal surface) of the upper incisors. *Class II.* The lower incisor edges lie posterior to the cingulum plateau of the upper incisors. *Division 1.* There is an increase in overjet and the upper incisors are proclined or of average inclination.

Division 2. The upper central incisors are retroclined; the overjet is usually minimal but may be increased. *Class III.* The lower incisor edges lie anterior to the cingulum plateau of the upper incisors. The overjet is reduced or reversed.

Classification

to assess treatment need

Index of Orthodontic Treatment Need (IOTN)

The IOTN was developed to help to identify those malocclusions most likely to benefit in dental health and appearance from orthodontic treatment. It comprises two components.

The dental health component Malocclusion is categorised into five grades (Table 28) based on the severity of occlusal characteristics that could increase the morbidity of the dentition and impair function. Grading, in relation to treatment need, is according to the worst feature of a malocclusion, as follows:

To facilitate the grading process, a ruler (Fig. 98) has been developed. Occlusal features are assessed in the following order:

- missing teeth (M)
- overjet (O)
- crossbite (C)
- displacement of contact points, i.e. crowding (D)
- overbite (O)

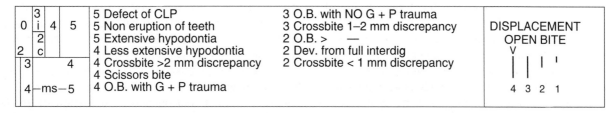

Fig. 98 The IOTN ruler. Occlusal features are assessed in the order given by the acronym 'MOCDO'. M = missing teeth; O = overjet; C = crossbite; D = displacement of contact point (i.e. crowding); O = overbite. (Reproduced by kind permission of the Victoria University of Manchester, England.)

Table 28 The Index of Orthodontic Treatment Need: dental health component

Grade	Characteristics
1 None	Extremely minor malocclusions including displacements <1 mm
2 Little	a. Increased overjet >3.5 mm but ≤6 mm with competent lips b. Reverse overjet >0 mm but ≤1 mm c. Anterior or posterior crossbite with ≤1 mm discrepancy between retruded contact position and intercuspal position d. Displacement of teeth >1 mm but ≤2 mm e. Anterior or posterior open bite >1 mm but ≤2 mm f. Increased overbite ≥3.5 mm without gingival contact g. Prenormal or postnormal occlusions with no other anomalies; includes up to half a unit discrepancy.
3 Moderate	a. Increased overjet >3.5 mm but ≤6 mm with incompetent lips b. Reverse overjet >1 mm but ≤3.5 mm c. Anterior or posterior crossbites with >1 mm but ≤2 mm discrepancy between retruded contact position and intercuspal position d. Displacement of teeth >2 mm but ≤4 mm e. Lateral or anterior open bite >2 mm but ≤4 mm f. Increased and complete overbite without gingival or palatal trauma
4 Great	a. Increased overjet >6 mm but ≤9 mm b. Reverse overjet >3.5 mm with no masticatory or speech difficulties c. Anterior or posterior crossbites with >2 mm discrepancy between retruded contact position and intercuspal position d. Severe displacements of teeth >4 mm e. Extreme lateral or anterior open bites >4 mm f. Increased and complete overbite with gingival or palatal trauma h. Less extensive hypodontia, requiring prerestorative orthodontics or orthodontic space closure to obviate the need for a prosthesis l. Posterior lingual crossbite with no functional occlusal contact in one or both buccal segments m. Reverse overjet >1 mm but <3.5 mm, with recorded masticatory and speech difficulties t. Partially erupted teeth, tipped and impacted against adjacent teeth x. Supplemental teeth
5 Very great	a. Increased overjet >9 mm h. Extensive hypodontia with restorative implications (more than one tooth missing in any quadrant) requiring prerestorative orthodontics i. Impeded eruption of teeth (with the exception of third molars) owing to crowding, displacement, the presence of supernumerary teeth, retained deciduous teeth and any pathological cause m. Reverse overjet >3.5 mm with reported masticatory and speech difficulties p. Defects of cleft lip and palate s. Submerged deciduous teeth

giving the acronym MOCDO. With practice it is possible to ascribe reliably and easily the treatment need category to a given malocclusion.

The aesthetic component The aesthetic component of the IOTN (Fig. 99) uses a set of 10 photographs of anterior teeth in occlusion with increasing aesthetic impairment to grade the dental attractiveness of an individual malocclusion. Colour or black and white photographs can be used to apply a grade to the malocclusion clinically or from study models. The assessment is made by selecting the photograph thought to match the aesthetic handicap of the patient, but judgement is very subjective. The need for treatment is categorised, by score (Fig. 99). Because of the lack of objectivity in assessing the aesthetic component, treatment need is based primarily on the dental health component of IOTN.

To assess treatment outcome Assessment can be carried out objectively by applying the dental health component of IOTN and subjectively by application of the aesthetic component. In addition, the Peer Assessment Rating (PAR) may be recorded. A score is given to the pre- and post-treatment occlusion from the study models. Six aspects are assessed and a weighting given to each, in accordance with their perceived importance as judged by current UK opinion. The components and their weightings (by which the score is multiplied) are: buccal segment alignment (×0), upper/lower anterior segment alignment (×1), buccal occlusion (×1), overjet (×6), overbite (×2) and centreline (×4). Measurement is facilitated by use of a specially designed ruler.

The percentage change in PAR score, obtained from the difference in pre- and post-treatment scores, is a measure of treatment success. A reduction of greater than 70% indicates a 'greatly improved' occlusion while a 'worse/no different' assignment is indicated by less than or equal to 20%.

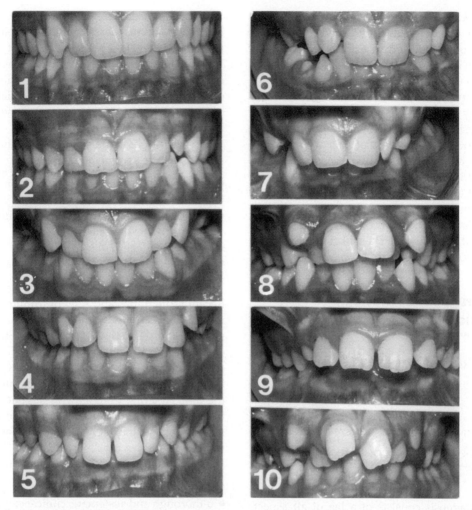

Fig. 99 The aesthetic component of the IOTN. The need for treatment is categorised by subjective judgement based on the photographs: Score 1 or 2 = no need; 3 or 4 = slight need; 5–7 = moderate/borderline need; 8–10 = definite need.

Aetiology of malocclusion

A general overview of the aetiology of malocclusion is presented here while specific aspects related to the aetiology of each malocclusion type are considered in Chapter 9.

The aetiology of malocclusion is often the result of several interacting factors. These are principally genetic and environmental, although the precise role of inherited factors is not fully understood. Whereas the craniofacial dimensions and both size and number of teeth are largely determined genetically, the dental arch dimensions are influenced more by environmental factors.

Specific congenital defects with a genetic basis, which involve the maxilla or mandible, are rare, as is malocclusion caused primarily by trauma or pathology.

Skeletal problems

The majority of anteroposterior skeletal problems are caused by inherited jaw proportions, which are strongly genetically determined. Inherited characteristics, for example mandibular deficiency, account for almost all of moderate class II malocclusion, while the added insult of environmental soft tissue influences is likely in more severe cases. Both maxillary deficiency and mandibular prognathism appear to contribute equally to the aetiology of marked class III malocclusion. In addition, a strong racial and familial tendency to mandibular prognathism exists, although mandibular posturing, possibly caused by tongue size, may stimulate growth and influence jaw size secondarily.

Vertical jaw proportions are also inherited, but soft tissue postural effects, for example anterior tongue position or mandibular postural changes induced by partial nasal obstruction, may contribute in particular to anterior open bite. Other environmental influences such as a high lower lip line may contribute to deep overbite.

Crowding

Crowding is the most common orthodontic problem, and is caused in part by a reduction in jaw and tooth size over the centuries. Also implicated is interpopulation breeding, with independent inheritance of jaw and tooth characteristics. This facilitates the development of crowding as arch width is influenced by jaw size, which is under tight genetic control.

Environmental influences must also be instrumental in the aetiology of crowding, perhaps because a softer diet requires less powerful jaw function, precipitating a reduction in jaw size. Early loss of primary teeth may also increase or create crowding. In particular, soft tissue pressure of sufficient duration in combination with the developmental tooth position may be responsible for a localised crossbite or malalignment. A unilateral crossbite with displacement is often caused by a functional alteration, but it is usual for a skeletal crossbite to have an additional genetic input.

8.3 Patient assessment in orthodontics

Learning objectives

You should

- know what to ask about in the orthodontic history and how to conduct an orthodontic assessment

- be confident in basic cephalometric analysis and interpretation.

Orthodontic diagnosis consists of a list of all aspects that deviate from normal in relation to a particular occlusion. It is a prelude to treatment planning as it allows the relationship between the various factors and their likely impact on treatment and prognosis to be considered. Diagnosis is based on the accurate gathering of information about the patient from a logical case assessment.

Assessment

Timing
At 7 to 8 years, a careful assessment of the developing occlusion should be undertaken to note, in particular, the form, position and presence of the permanent incisors and to plan appropriate intervention should an abnormality be detected that is likely to interfere with the normal eruption sequence. The prognosis of the first permanent molars should be assessed routinely from age 8, and palpation of the maxillary permanent canines is carried out on a regular basis from about 10 years. Early detection of a skeletal discrepancy will allow also for optimal timing of treatment to maximise growth potential, but in most children assessment is delayed until the permanent dentition has erupted.

All general dentists should be able to carry out a basic orthodontic assessment for their patients and recognise when referral to a specialist is appropriate. When dental and/or occlusal development deviates from normal, or when significant discrepancies in established dentofacial or occlusal relationships concern the patient and may compromise dental health long term, referral is indicated.

Apart from basic personal details, the referral letter should include specific reference to:

- the patient's perception of the problem
- their attendance record
- their level of dental awareness including that of their parents (if appropriate)
- the oral hygiene status
- the likely prognosis of restored or traumatised teeth.

Recent radiographs and a set of trimmed current study models registered with the patient in centric occlusion should be forwarded with the referral. Study models are essential for diagnosis; if none are available, two appointments will be necessary to allow collation of the information required to make an accurate assessment of the case. At a first visit, impressions should be taken of the dental arches and the occlusion recorded with a wax registration so that study casts can be available for inspection at the second visit.

Orthodontic assessment comprises three stages:

- a complete history
- a thorough and systematic clinical examination
- collating relevant information from appropriate special investigations.

Demand for treatment
The demand for orthodontic treatment is influenced by two main factors:

- patient/parent factors, which include patient gender, age, level of self-esteem, self- and peer-perception of any occlusal or skeletal discrepancy, social class and parental desires
- awareness by dental professionals and the health care system.

In general, demand for treatment is greatest when the orthodontist:population and orthodontist:general dentist ratios are small. Overall demand is increasing in adults, is higher in females, in those from better socioeconomic backgrounds and when a lower orthodontist:population ratio exists, as appliances become more common and their acceptance increases.

History

Initially the dentist must identify:

- the patient's reason for attendance
- who raised the question of treatment
- the attitude to treatment.

It is important to document if the patient is unconcerned with the appearance of their teeth, particularly in the presence of obvious malocclusion, as any attempt to persuade the patient to undertake treatment is likely to be met with indifference. Attitude to treatment is best assessed from response to enquiries about their perception of orthodontic treatment for their peers, and by observing carefully their reaction when shown photographs or examples of appliances.

Medical history

A health questionnaire should be completed by each patient or their parent, and the findings verified by a clinical interview. A number of conditions may impact on orthodontic treatment.

Rheumatic fever/congenital cardiac defects
Antibiotic cover will be required prior to band placement and extractions in patients with a history of rheumatic fever. For all congenital cardiac defects, it is wise to consult the patient's cardiologist to ascertain the need for antibiotic prophylaxis.

Recurrent oral ulceration
Appliance therapy should be avoided until this condition has been investigated thoroughly. Depending on the frequency and nature of ulceration, limited appliance treatment may be possible.

Epilepsy
Because of the risk of airway obstruction from appliance parts fractured during an epileptic attack and the difficulty with tooth movement in the presence of gingival hyperplasia, no orthodontic appliance should be fitted until the epilepsy is well controlled and the gingival condition healthy.

Diabetes
Diabetic patients are more prone to periodontal breakdown, and active appliance therapy should be withheld until the periodontal condition is sound and the diabetes is stabilised.

Hay fever
Hay fever may interfere with the wearing of functional appliances over the summer months. An alternative approach to treating the malocclusion may be sought.

Nickel allergies
Although rare, patients sensitised to nickel are at risk of developing a severe allergic reaction to appliance components that contain nickel and these must be avoided.

Bleeding diatheses
If extractions are necessary, special medical arrangements will need to be in place.

Severe physical/mental handicap
In selected patients, extractions only may produce an improvement in dental aesthetics and facilitate toothcleaning measures. Appliance therapy is invariably not a viable option.

Dental history

The nature, extent and frequency of previous dental treatment together with the level of patient cooperation should be recorded, along with details of daily oral hygiene practices. A history of early loss of primary teeth or of incisor trauma should be noted. If orthodontic treatment has been carried out previously, details relating to extractions and appliance type should be recorded. If treatment was abandoned, the patient must be questioned carefully for the reasons. For the child patient, enquiries about orthodontic treatment for other siblings, and their co-operation with appliances, may be helpful in indicating the level of family dental awareness and likely support if treatment is offered. It is also wise to ask at this stage if there is any history of temporomandibular joint symptoms including pain, muscle tenderness or difficulty with mouth opening and to record if the patient is aware of any bruxing habit.

Social history

The distance at which the family live and an estimate of travelling time to and from potential appointments should be noted. Access to transport, the ease with which a responsible adult can accompany the child patient, together with information relating to forthcoming events that may influence attendance, are important.

Clinical examination

Before the child patient takes a seat in the dental chair it is often worthwhile to attempt to estimate their chronological age from their height and general level of physical maturity. This may give some indication of future growth potential. If the patient is accompanied by a parent, obvious familial occlusal traits (e.g. upper median diastema) may be observed also. The purpose of the examination is to record and assess facial, occlusal and functional aspects of a patient in order to request appropriate diagnostic aids. An extraoral followed by an intraoral examination should be performed.

Extraoral examination

The skeletal pattern, soft tissues of the lips and tongue, speech, temporomandibular joints and mandibular path of closure should be assessed and the presence of any habits noted.

The relationship of the mandible to the maxilla should be assessed in all three planes of space: anteroposteriorly, vertically and laterally. Before proceeding it is important to ensure that

- the patient is seated upright with the head in the natural postural position or with the Frankfort plane (a line joining the upper border of the external auditory meatus to the inferior aspect of the bony orbit) horizontal. Natural head posture may be obtained by asking the patient to look straight ahead focusing on the horizon
- the lips are in repose
- the teeth are in centric occlusion.

Anteroposterior plane

The relationship of the mandible to the maxilla in the anteroposterior plane is assessed by observing the patient in profile. In most cases, an indication of the skeletal pattern in this dimension may be gained from the soft tissue facial profile allowing the following classification to be made (Fig. 100):

Class I: the mandible lies 2–3 mm behind the maxilla
Class II: the mandible is retruded in relation to the maxilla
Class III: the mandible is protruded in relation to the maxilla.

No indication, however, is given as to where a skeletal discrepancy may lie as the classification reflects solely the position of the mandible and the maxilla relative to each other.

This method is not always reliable because of variation in lip thickness, and palpation of the alveolar bases over the apices of the upper and lower incisors in the midline has been claimed to give a better estimate of skeletal pattern. In essence, any significant discrepancy in the anteroposterior dental base relationship should be investigated more thoroughly by taking and analysing a lateral cephalometric film (see below).

Vertical plane

Two assessments of the vertical relationship of the face should be made (Fig. 101).

Assessment of lower face height In a well-balanced face, the upper face height (distance from the mid-eyebrow level to the base of the nose) should be equal to that of the lower face height (base of the nose to the inferior aspect of the chin). The lower face height may, therefore, be assessed as average (when these measurements are equal), reduced (when lower face height is less than upper face height) or increased (when lower face height is greater than upper face height).

Assessment of the Frankfort–mandibular planes angle (FMPA) With a finger along the inferior aspect of the mandible and a ruler placed along the Frankfort plane, these two lines can be projected backward in the imagination to give an estimate of the FMPA. Where the vertical dimensions of the face are normal, both lines should meet at the back of the skull (occiput) and the FMPA is regarded as average. If the FMPA is reduced the lines will meet beyond occiput and if the FMPA is increased they will meet anterior to it.

Transverse plane

Obvious facial asymmetry may be observed by standing directly behind the patient and looking down across the face, checking the coincidence of the midlines of the nose, upper and lower lips and midpoint of the chin. Alternatively, the face may be assessed from in front. In

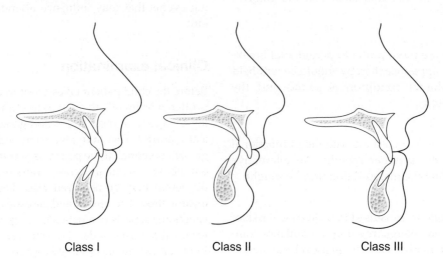

Class I   Class II   Class III

Fig. 100 Classification of the anteroposterior skeletal pattern.

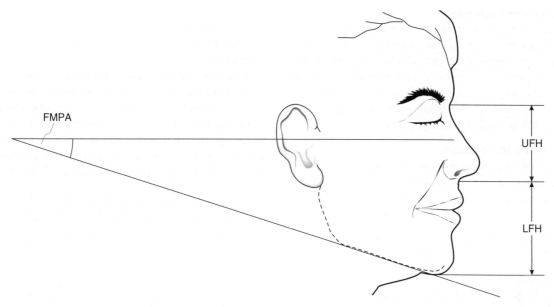

Fig. 101 Assessment of the vertical facial relationships: lower facial height (LFH) compared with upper facial height (UFH) and Frankfort–mandibular planes angle (FMPA).

most people, some degree of facial asymmetry is present and may be regarded as normal. Marked asymmetries, however, require further investigation. The location and extent of any marked asymmetry, e.g. upper, middle or lower facial third, should be recorded.

Soft tissues of the lips and tongue
Seven aspects should be assessed in relation to the lips and tongue:

- lip form and fullness: form may be described as vertical, average or everted, and fullness in terms of whether the lips are full or thin
- lower lip position in relation to the upper incisors: the upper incisors may lie behind, on, or in front of the lower lip
- lower lip coverage in relation to the upper incisors: at rest, on average, the lower lip should cover at least one third to one half of the upper incisor teeth
- upper lip level in relation to the upper incisors: the length of the upper lip and amount of exposure of the upper incisors at rest should be assessed; in males 1–2 mm display of the incisors is average, with slightly more in females
- whether the lips are together (competent) or apart (incompetent) at rest: if lips are apart, it should be noted if they are slightly or wide apart, and if the patient makes any habitual effort to hold them together; markedly incompetent lips confer a poor prospect for stability of a corrected overjet in patients with class II division 1 malocclusion
- tongue position at rest: should be assessed throughout the examination and particular note

made if it lies in contact with the lower lip as this is likely to contribute to an incomplete overbite
- lip and tongue behaviour during swallowing, speech and facial expression: abnormal tongue activity on swallowing, or marked hyperactivity of the lower lip on smiling, should be noted, as should the presence of a marked 'gummy' smile.

Speech
Obvious defects such as a lisp will be noticed during general questioning of the patient, and specific assessment by a speech therapist is rarely indicated in patients referred for orthodontic advice.

Habits
The tell-tale signs of finger- or thumb-sucking habits are generally easy to ascertain:

- proclination of maxillary incisors
- retroclination of mandibular incisors
- incomplete overbite or open bite, often asymmetric
- increase in overjet
- tendency to bilateral buccal segment crossbite, often resulting in a unilateral crossbite with displacement.

Effects vary depending on whether the finger or thumb is placed in a median or paramedian position and on whether one or more digits are sucked. An adaptive tongue thrust is common. Inspection of the hands will usually identify the offender. The patient and their parent should be made aware of the effects of the habit on the dentition and occlusion. Note also if the patient is a nailbiter or bruxist.

Temporomandibular joints

Opening and lateral mandibular movements should be assessed by first observing the patient from in front and second by palpation of the condylar heads while listening for the presence of crepitus, or a joint click. Normal findings should be recorded as a baseline for future reference. Palpation of the masticatory muscles is not required unless symptoms are present.

Mandibular path of closure

The path of closure from rest position to maximum interdigitation should be assessed, noting any anterior or lateral mandibular displacement. This may be difficult to detect in a young and anxious patient where a habitual posture has developed to avoid a premature contact, often from an instanding incisor. Applying gentle backward and upward pressure to the chin while instructing the patient to touch the back of the mouth with the tip of the tongue usually gets around this problem.

Intraoral examination

The soft tissues of the buccal mucosa, floor of the mouth, tongue and the attachment of the maxillary labial frenum should be observed and any abnormality noted. A general dental examination should be carried out prior to assessing the individual arches of teeth and the occlusal relationships. The following should be charted.

- Standard of oral hygiene and caries rate.
- Gingival condition, paying particular attention to any area of gingival recession or attachment loss.
- All erupted teeth, noting those with abnormal shape or size. A quick way to assess if an anterior tooth-size discrepancy exists is to compare the mesiodistal widths of the upper and lower lateral incisors. The upper laterals should be larger than the lower incisors, but only discrepancies of greater than 1.5 mm should be recorded as these are likely to affect treatment planning.
- Teeth with untreated caries, large restorations or previous trauma. The condition of the first permanent molars should be examined, in particular, and a record made of any cervical decalcification (buccally on the uppers or lingually on the lowers), which may indicate a poor prognosis.
- The presence of erosion on the palatal surfaces of the upper incisors. In these cases, the patient should be questioned about frequency of dietary intake of acidic or carbonated drinks.
- Marked attrition of the dentition. This is likely to be present in individuals with a bruxing habit.

The lower arch followed by the upper arch should then be assessed independently. It is very helpful to refer to the study models during this part of the examination.

Assessment of the upper and lower arches
Angulation of the lower labial segment to the mandibular plane. By placing the index finger of the right hand along the mandibular body and gently everting the lower lip, the angulation of the lower incisors may be assessed as average (if they appear to make almost a 90° angle with the mandibular plane), retroclined or proclined.

Angulation of the upper incisors relative to the Frankfort plane. With the patient sitting upright and a finger or ruler placed along the Frankfort plane, the inclination of the upper incisors may be assessed as retroclined, average or proclined.

Presence and site of spacing or crowding including the magnitude of each. The degree of spacing/crowding may be assessed by performing a space analysis on the study models. This only takes account of any space discrepancy anterior to the first permanent molars and is usually carried out as follows:

For each quadrant. Measure with dividers the distance from the mesial surface of the first permanent molar to the distal surface of the permanent lateral incisor, and from there to the midline. Add these measurements for each arch to give the space available.

Measure the mesiodistal width of each tooth and add these together to calculate the space required where the canines and premolars have not erupted, on average 21 mm or 22 mm per quadrant in the lower or upper arch respectively is an estimate of their space requirements.

Quantify any surplus deficit. Subtract the space available from the space required. Individual arches may then be classified as uncrowded, mildly crowded (0–4 mm), moderately crowded (>4 but <7 mm) or severely crowded (>7 mm).

General alignment of the teeth. Include here the presence of rotations (classified by the surface furthest from the line of the arch).

Inclination of the canines. These may be described as upright, mesially inclined or distally inclined.

Assessments with the teeth in occlusion With the teeth in maximum intercuspation, the remaining aspects should be recorded.

Incisor relationship. This may be categorised according to the British Standards Institute classification (see Section 8.2).

Overjet (the horizontal overlap of the upper over the lower incisors). This is usually measured (in millimetres) from the central incisor teeth. If there is a marked difference in the overjet for each maxillary central incisor, both measurements should be noted.

Overbite (vertical overlap of the upper over the lower incisors). This is measured (in millimetres) – an indication should be given as to whether it is complete, incomplete or if there is an anterior open bite or traumatic overbite. The overbite is complete when the lower incisors occlude with the opposing maxillary teeth or with the palatal mucosa; it is incomplete if there is no contact with the opposing surfaces. The extent (in millimetres) of an anterior open bite should be noted and the site of mucosal ulceration recorded (either palatal to the upper incisors, labial to the lower incisors or in both locations) in the presence of a traumatic overbite.

Centrelines. Upper and lower centrelines should be coincident with the midline of the face, and any centreline shift should be recorded (in millimetres) with a note to indicate the direction of the shift.

Molar relationship. Providing a corresponding molar is present in the opposing arch, the molar relationship may be categorised according to Angle's classification (see Section 8.2).

Where the first permanent molar is missing in either arch, the premolar or canine relationship may be assessed.

Canine relationship. This should be recorded in addition to the molar relationship, as although they are often the same, on occasion discrepancies are present.

The presence of anterior or posterior crossbite (buccolingual discrepancy in arch relationship). Is the crossbite buccal or lingual, bilateral or unilateral (Fig. 102)? For the premolar and/or molar teeth, a buccal crossbite exists when the buccal cusps of the lower tooth occlude buccally to the buccal cusps of the upper teeth. A lingual crossbite exists when the buccal cusps of the lower tooth occlude lingually to the palatal cusps of the upper teeth. A unilateral crossbite affects teeth on one side of the arch while teeth on both sides of the arch are affected with a bilateral crossbite. Often a unilateral crossbite is associated with a mandibular displacement (Fig. 103).

Special investigations

Vitality tests

Traumatised incisors or other teeth with suspect vitality should be electric pulp tested and their status recorded.

Radiography

All radiographs should be justified on clinical grounds. Radiographs forwarded by a referring practitioner may provide sufficient information to supplement the clinical findings but often the following views are needed.

A dental orthopantogram (DPT) or right and left lateral oblique views. These are good screening radiographs. The bony architecture of the maxillary and mandibular bases as well as that of the mandibular condyles (if included) should be checked first to exclude any dentally related, or other, pathology. All teeth should be identified and counted. It is a good routine to start in one area, e.g.

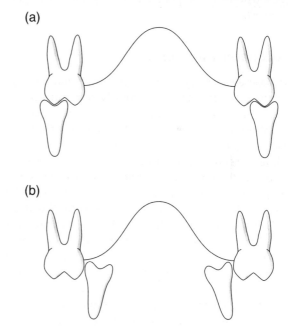

Fig. 102 Bucco-lingual discrepancies. (a) bilateral buccal crossbite. (b) bilateral lingual crossbite.

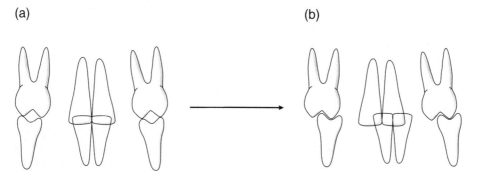

Fig. 103 Unilateral buccal crossbite with mandibular displacement and associated lower centreline shift. (a) Cusp-to-cusp molar contact. (b) Maximum intercuspal position.

upper right third molar area, and follow systematically through the upper left, lower left and finally lower right quadrants to ensure that nothing is missed. Finally, the condition of each tooth should be checked for caries, hypoplasia, or resorption. All unerupted teeth should be charted, noting their developmental stage and position. Teeth previously extracted, those congenitally absent and any pathology should be recorded. Although large carious lesions will be obvious on a panoramic film, a more thorough assessment should be made from bite-wing or periapical films if required.

A maxillary anterior occlusal view. This provides a good view of the upper anterior teeth and is useful to check root lengths of the incisor teeth and to exclude the presence of a supernumerary or other pathology.

A lateral cephalometric radiograph. This film is indicated in the presence of anteroposterior and/or vertical skeletal discrepancies, particularly when incisor movement anteroposteriorly is planned, and prior to implant placement.

Cephalometric analysis

Cephalometric analysis involves the evaluation and subsequent interpretation of both lateral and postero-anterior views of the skull, although in practice it is usually confined to the former because of difficulty in interpreting the posteroanterior view.

To allow comparison of measurements recorded for the same patient at different times, or between patients, attempts have been made to standardise the radiographic technique. Originally developed by Broadbent and Hofrath independently in 1931, the radiograph is taken with the Frankfort plane horizontal, the ear posts positioned in the external auditory meati and the teeth in centric occlusion. The central ray should pass through the ear posts. Importantly, the X-ray source to midsagittal plane distance and the midsagittal plane-to-film distance should be standardised to facilitate reproducibility and to minimise magnification. To allow accurate calculation of magnification, a steel rule of known length should be placed at the midsagittal plane and recorded on each film.

It is now common practice to collimate the X-ray beam, thereby avoiding radiation exposure to areas of the head not required for lateral cephalometric analysis. To enhance the soft tissue profile, the beam intensity can be reduced by placing an aluminium filter between the X-ray source and the patient.

Uses of lateral cephalometric analysis

Lateral cephalometric analysis is used

- as a diagnostic aid

- to check treatment progress
- to assess treatment and growth changes.

A diagnostic aid
Lateral cephalometric analysis sheds light on the dental and skeletal characteristics of a malocclusion, thereby allowing its aetiology to be determined and focusing attention on the aspects that require correction. It also serves as a useful reference of pretreatment incisor position, particularly if anteroposterior movement is intended. In some patients, particularly those with class III skeletal bases, growth may be checked from serial radiographs and treatment commenced at the appropriate time. Unerupted teeth may also be located accurately, soft or hard tissue pathology identified and upper incisor root resorption observed.

A means of checking treatment progress
During treatment with fixed or functional appliances, it is customary to check incisor inclinations and anchorage considerations. Any change in the position of unerupted teeth may be checked also.

A means of assessing treatment and growth changes
If films are to be compared, they must be superimposed on some stable area or points. As orthodontic treatment is generally carried out during the growth period, no natural fixed points or planes exist. The following, however, are reasonably stable areas and are used commonly for superimposition:

- cranial base: after 7 years of age, the anterior cranial base is found to be relatively stable. The S–N (sella–nasion) line is a close approximation to the anterior cranial base (N is not on the anterior cranial base), and holding at sella allows the general pattern of facial growth to be assessed; superimposition on de Coster's line (the anatomical outline of the anterior cranial base) reflects more accurately changes in facial pattern but requires greater skill to carry out
- maxilla: superimposition on the anterior vault of the palate shows changes in maxillary tooth position
- mandible: changes in mandibular tooth position may be assessed by superimposition on Bjork's structures, the most useful of which are the inner cortex of the inferior and lingual aspect of the symphysis and the mandibular canal outline.

Aim and objective of cephalometric analysis

The aim of cephalometric analysis is to assess the anteroposterior and vertical relationships of the upper and lower teeth with supporting alveolar bone to their respective maxillary and mandibular bases, and to the cranial base. The objective is to compare the patient with normal population standards appropriate for his/her racial group, identifying any differences between the two. The technique used is outlined in Box 40.

It is important, however, to remember that irrespective of whether cephalometric measurements are made directly from a digitiser or indirectly from a tracing, the cephalometric technique and its subsequent analysis are open to error. The technique relies on reducing the three-dimensional facial skeleton to a two-dimensional X-ray film. Bilateral landmarks, therefore, are superimposed. The validity of the analysis depends upon the ability of the operator to identify points accurately and reproducibly, which in turn is dependent on the film quality and operator experience.

Box 40 Technique for cephalometric analysis

1. First check the radiograph to ensure that the teeth are in occlusion and that the patient is not postured forward. It may be necessary to refer to clinical measurements to verify the overjet. It is advisable to scan the film for any pathology including resorption of the upper incisor roots, enlarged adenoids or degenerative changes in the cervical spine
2. In a darkened room attach tracing paper or tracing acetate to the X-ray film and secure both to an illuminated viewer ensuring that the Frankfort plane is horizontal and parallel to the edge of the viewing screen
3. With a 4H pencil identify the points (Fig. 104) and planes, the definitions of which are listed in Table 29. By convention, the most prominent incisor is traced and for structures with two shadows (e.g. the mandibular outline), the average is selected for analyses. Alternatively, landmarks may be digitised using a cursor linked to a computer program that allocates x and y coordinates to each point. Angular and linear measurements are calculated automatically. A piece of cardboard with a cut-out area of about 5 cm × 5 cm is helpful in blocking out background light and aiding landmark identification.
4. Record the values for the measurements listed in Table 30.

Table 30 Normal Eastman cephalometric values for Caucasians

Parameter	Value (± SD)
SNA	81 ± 3°
SNB	78 ± 3°
ANB	3 ± 2°
S–N/Max	8 ± 3°
1 to Maxillary PL	109 ± 6°
1 to Mandibular PL	93 ± 6°
Interincisal angle	135 ± 10°
MMPA	27 ± 4°
Facial proportion	55 ± 2%

Table 29 Definition of commonly used cephalometric points and planes (see Fig. 104)

	Definition
Points	
S	sella: midpoint of sella turcica
N	nasion: most anterior point of the frontonasal suture (may use the deepest point at the junction of the frontal and nasal bones instead)
P	porion: uppermost, outermost point on the bony external auditory meatus (upper border of the condylar head is at the same level, which helps location)
O	orbitale: most inferior anterior point on the margin of the orbit (use average of the left and right orbital shadows)
ANS	tip of the anterior nasal spine
PNS	tip of the posterior nasal spine (pterygomaxillary fissure is directly above, which helps location)
A	A point: most posterior point of the concavity on the anterior surface of the premaxilla in the midline below ANS
B	B point: most posterior point of the concavity on the anterior surface of the mandible in the midline above pogonion
Pog	pogonion: most anterior point on the bony chin
Me	menton: lowermost point on mandibular symphysis in the midline
Go	gonion: most poster-inferior point at the angle of the mandible (bisect the angle between tangent to the posterior ramus and inferior body of the mandible to locate)
Planes S–N line	line drawn through S and N
Frankfort plane	line connecting porion and orbitale
Maxillary plane	line joining PNS and ANS
Mandibular plane	line joining Go to Me
Functional occlusal plane	line drawn between the cusp tips of the first permanent molars and premolars/deciduous molars

Cephalometric interpretation

The following aspects may be assessed from the cephalometric analysis.

Skeletal relationships

Maxillary prognathism (SNA). This value is much affected by the cant of the S–N line and the position of nasion.
Mandibular prognathism (SNB).
Skeletal pattern (ANB). The skeletal pattern may be classified broadly according to the ANB value:

Class I skeletal pattern: $2° \leq ANB \leq 4°$
Class II skeletal pattern: $ANB > 4°$
Class III skeletal pattern: $ANB < 2°$.

The ANB value should be considered along with the measurement for SNA, as ANB is affected by variation in both the vertical and anteroposterior position of nasion. In cases where the SNA value is above or below the average value of 81° and provided the S-N/maxillary plane angle is within $8 \pm 3°$, a correction may be employed to the ANB value as follows: for every degree SNA is greater than 81°, substract 0.5° from the ANB value, and vice versa.

The Wits analysis. This is an alternative means of assessing the skeletal pattern in which the distance (in millimetres) is measured between perpendiculars from

A and B point to the functional occlusal plane (a line joining the cusp tips of the permanent molars and premolars or deciduous molars). The average values for males and females are 1 ± 1.9 mm and 0 ± 1.77 mm, respectively. No indication is given, however, of the relation of the dental bases to the cranial base. The functional occlusal plane is also difficult to locate, which casts doubts on any claims made about the skeletal assessment using this method. In some cases, however, it may be a useful check to complement that made from the ANB value alone.

Vertical skeletal relationship (MMPA and facial proportion) (Fig. 105)

The mandibular–maxillary planes angle (MMPA) is often correlated with the amount of overbite and the pattern of mandibular growth – a low MMPA being associated with an increased overbite and a forward pattern of mandibular growth while the converse is often true for those with a high MMPA. The facial proportion should lend support to the value obtained for the MMPA; a reduced facial proportion is usually consistent with a low MMPA and vice versa. Where there is disagreement between these two assessments, the tracing should be checked to identify the cause.

Tooth position

Angle of the upper incisor to the maxillary plane. The inclination of the upper incisors may be assessed as average (109° ± 6°), retroclined (<103°) or proclined (>115°). In class II division 1, it is often helpful to carry out a 'prognosis tracing' to indicate if correction of the incisor relationship may be undertaken by tipping or bodily movement (Fig. 106). An alternative method is to apply the following rule of thumb: for every 1 mm of overjet reduction subtract 2.5° from the upper incisor to maxillary plane angle. Provided the final upper incisor inclination is not likely to be less than 95° to the maxillary plane, tipping rather than bodily movement will be possible.

Angle of the lower incisor to the mandibular plane. This must be looked at in conjunction with the ANB and MMPA angles as the lower incisor inclination may compensate for discrepancies in the anteroposterior and vertical skeletal pattern. Under the influence of the soft tissues, the lower incisors may procline in class II malocclusion while in class III cases they may retrocline. There is also an inverse relation between the lower incisor angulation (LIA) and the MMPA: for every degree the LIA is greater than the average (93°), the MMPA is 1° less than the average (27°); the opposite holds true when the LIA is less than the average.

Inter-incisal angle. Provided the incisors contact, overbite depth is associated with the inter-incisal angle – the greater the angle, the deeper the overbite.

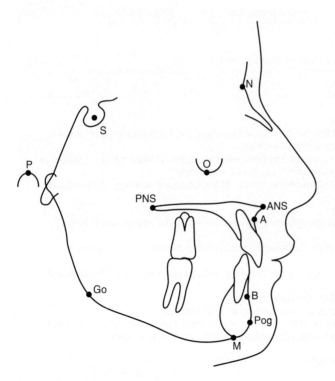

Fig. 104 Standard cephalometric points.

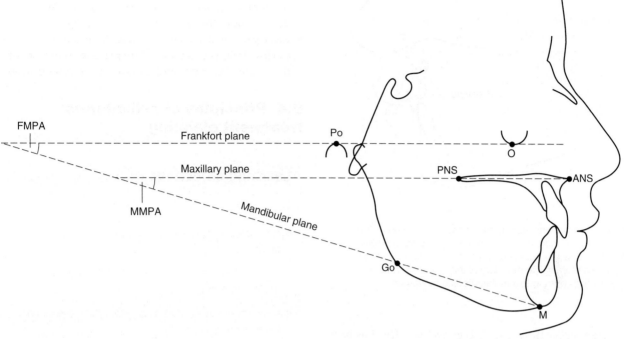

Although measurement of FMPA is favoured by some analyses, MMPA is preferable due to easier and more accurate location of the maxillary plane.

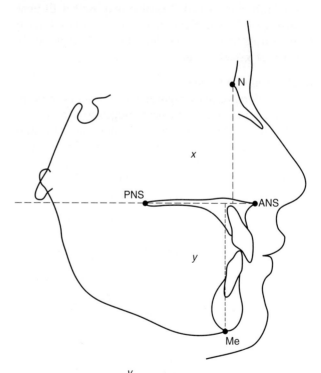

Facial proportion = $\dfrac{y}{x+y} \times 100$

(y = perpendicular distance from maxillary plane to Me
x = perpendicular distance from maxillary plane to N)

Fig. 105 MMPA and facial proportion.

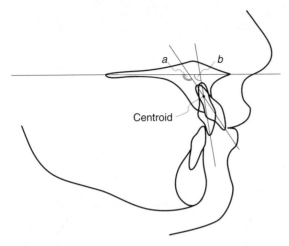

Fig. 106 Prognosis tracing to assess if correction of the incisor relationship can be achieved by tipping or bodily movement. a = presenting angle of 1 to maxillary plane; b = inclination of 1 to maxillary plane following rotation around the centroid to simulate tipping movement.

Lower incisor position to A–Pogonion line. This has been used as an aesthetic reference line for lower incisor positioning (average 0–2 mm) but it is unwise to lend too much credence to this measurement for treatment planning purposes. Both point A and Pogonion may shift with treatment or growth, and orienting the lower incisors correctly with respect to the A–Pog line does not improve the prospect of a stable result.

Analysis of soft tissues
Various reference lines, regarded as indicators of pleasing facial appearance, have been suggested to assess the relationship of the soft tissues of the nose, lips and chin. These lines are more helpful in orthognathic surgical planning than in planning conventional orthodontic treatment. Two lines are shown in Figure 107.

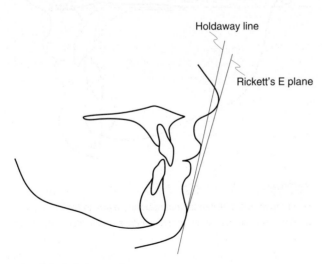

Fig. 107 Soft tissue planes.

- Holdaway line: joins the upper lip and chin; for optimal facial aesthetics the lower lip should lie ± 1 mm to this line
- Rickett's E-line: joins the nasal tip to the chin such that the lower lip is positioned 2 mm (± 2 mm) in front of the E-line, the upper lip lying slightly further behind.

8.4 Principles of orthodontic treatment planning

Learning objectives

You should

- know the potential benefits and limitations of orthodontic treatment

- know and understand the steps generally adopted in treatment planning

- know what factors should be considered in presentation of the final treatment plan

- know how space may be created for desired tooth movement.

Problem list and treatment need

The first stage in treatment planning is to summarise the patient's malocclusion to produce a problem list in order of priority. Then the need for treatment on dental health and aesthetic grounds must be considered (see Section 8.2). Only if appliance therapy and/or extractions can confer significant benefit to dental health and/or appearance of the dentition should treatment be undertaken. If there is any doubt, treatment is best withheld.

Potential benefits and limitations of orthodontic treatment

Dental health and function
Caries. No significant association has been found between crowding and caries, but some severely displaced teeth may be predisposed to decay in individuals with high refined carbohydrate consumption and poor oral hygiene practices.

Periodontal disease. In general, crowding is weakly associated with periodontal disease but where a tooth is severely displaced from its investing bone, periodontal health may be compromised long term. With displacing occlusal contacts, gingival recession and mobility may develop in relation to an incisor in crossbite. Trauma to the palatal or labial gingivae may be associated with a deep overbite. Early recognition and correction of these anomalies in addition to the potential increase in dental awareness following orthodontic intervention is likely to confer long-term benefit to periodontal health.

Incisor trauma. The risk of trauma to the upper anterior teeth peaks at about 10 years and is twice as great when the overjet is increased more than 9 mm. Trauma is more likely in boys and when the lips are incompetent.

Tooth impaction. Unerupted teeth may cause resorption of the adjacent teeth or dentigerous cyst formation but these sequelae are rare.

Speech. Where the incisors do not contact, for example in severe class II or class III malocclusion or anterior open bite, lisping may occur. This may improve with correction of the occlusal relationships.

Masticatory function. In those with marked anterior open bite or reverse overjet, incising food may be difficult or even impossible.

Temporomandibular joint dysfunction syndrome (TMJDS). Research has linked, although weakly, crossbites, class III malocclusion and open bite with TMJDS.

Social/psychological well-being. From the available evidence, it appears that self-esteem and social/psychological wellbeing are not significantly affected by malocclusion. Background facial attractiveness has a greater influence on peer and society acceptance than dental appearance, but marked malocclusion may promote teasing.

Summary
Dental health is likely to benefit long term where any of the following exist: gross displacement of teeth, traumatic overbite, increased overjet, impacted teeth with a risk of resorption, or mandibular displacement in the presence of a crossbite. Long-term social/psychological wellbeing would appear to be affected only to a modest extent by occlusal anomalies.

Limitations of orthodontic treatment

Orthodontic treatment, like all forms of dental treatment, has some limitations, and these should be borne in mind when the aims of treatment and treatment plan are being devised.

- tooth movement is confined to cancellous bone
- the dental bases will not enlarge or widen to provide space for relief of crowding
- limited differential eruption of anterior or posterior teeth may be used successfully to aid correction of malocclusion, but there is limited evidence on the permanency of any alteration in vertical skeletal pattern
- some small restraint or redirection of maxillary and/or mandibular growth is possible, with headgear or functional appliance therapy; with rapid maxillary expansion, some orthopaedic increase in maxillary dental base width is possible
- the effect of tooth movement on the facial profile is modest, with the growth of the nose and chin having a greater effect
- tooth movement is generally more efficient in a growing child but may still be undertaken in the adult
- growth may aid or hinder correction of a malocclusion and attempts to modify its expression must be commenced in the early mixed dentition
- removable appliances tip teeth, whereas fixed appliances may bodily move, tip, intrude, extrude, rotate or torque teeth
- functional appliances alter arch relations through a combination of actions that involves tipping of teeth, differential eruption and possibly some restraint or stimulation of maxillary and/or mandibular growth, depending on the specifics of the design
- headgear restrains or redirects growth of the maxillary complex depending on the force magnitude and direction employed
- treatment success is dependent on:
  — correct diagnosis, treatment planning including assessment of anchorage, and proficiency in whatever appliance system is selected on the part of the operator
  — regular attendance, compliance with all instructions regarding appliance wear, and maintenance of a high standard of oral hygiene by the patient
- a stable result is only possible if the forces from the soft tissues, occlusion and periodontium are in equilibrium and facial growth is favourable.

Aims of treatment

The aims of treatment list in a logical sequence the steps required to achieve the final occlusal result. For example, in a patient with a crowded class II division 1 malocclusion these would often be as follows:

- relief of crowding
- alignment within the arches
- overbite reduction
- overjet correction
- closure of residual spacing.

One should always aim for the ideal plan initially but keep an open mind, as sometimes this plan may require alteration, for instance if the patient does not wish to wear a fixed appliance or headgear. Importantly, where a compromise plan is proposed, the patient must benefit and not suffer long-term.

Treatment planning

In broad terms, the following series of steps will be useful for treatment planning purposes in most malocclusions (refer to the sections covering management of each malocclusion).

Plan the lower arch

In general the lower arch form is to be accepted, in particular the anteroposterior position of the lower labial segment, which lies in a narrow zone of balance between the lips and tongue. Movement beyond this narrow zone is likely to lead to an unstable result apart from in certain circumstances that inevitably require specialist management
   The following factors should be evaluated:

- the presence of crowding/spacing or acceptable alignment: if the arch is spaced or acceptably aligned, attention can be directed to the upper arch; if crowding is present or is likely, it should be assessed in terms of severity and location
- the depth of overbite: levelling an increased curve of Spee requires space, for example about 1–2 mm is required for a 6–7 mm overbite
- midline shift: space will be required to correct a displaced midline, ensuring it is coincident and correct with that of the upper teeth.

These three factors indicate the space requirements in the lower arch. Moderate or severe crowding will require extractions to provide space for alignment of the teeth. For relief of mild crowding, arch expansion may be considered in some circumstances or, very rarely, distal movement of the first permanent molars may be an option (see Section 9.5).
   Imagine $\overline{3}$ repositioned for alignment of the lower labial segment. If the canine is mesially inclined in a crowded arch, it will upright spontaneously following the extraction of a first premolar, thereby providing space for alignment of the lower labial segment. Most improvement occurs within the first 6 months following extraction, and if the premolars are removed as the canines are erupting. If the canine is upright or distally inclined, a fixed appliance will be necessary for its retraction.

Plan the upper arch

Mentally correct $\underline{3}$ position to a class I relationship with the aligned lower canine. This is done assuming that the lower labial segment is not spaced and that the upper incisor teeth are all of normal size and not retroclined. The space needed may come from extractions, arch expansion or distal movement of the buccal segment. Importantly, if all of an extraction space is required to

achieve a class I canine relationship, anchorage will need to be reinforced. The appliance type needed to achieve the desired canine relationship can be assessed also.
   Consideration should be given to relief of upper labial segment crowding, reduction of the overjet and/or overbite and the appliance type necessary to achieve correction. Removable appliances are only capable of tipping movements whereas a fixed appliance may bodily move teeth including intrusion, extrusion, rotation and torqueing.

Plan the final buccal segment relationship and the need for closure of any residual spaces

In general if corresponding teeth have been extracted in each quadrant, the final buccal segment relationship should be class I; however if only upper arch extractions or lower arch extractions have been undertaken, the final relationship will be class II or class III, respectively. The potential for spontaneous space closure depends on

- the degree of initial crowding
- the age of the patient
- the vertical pattern of facial growth (space closure tends to occur more rapidly in patients with increased Frankfort–mandibular planes angle compared to those with a reduced angle).

Alternatively it may be produced mechanically by applying intramaxillary (from within the same arch), intermaxillary (from the opposing arch) or extra-oral traction.

Plan the mechanics and consider the anchorage demands

In general, removable appliances are limited to tipping movements, whereas bodily movement is possible with fixed appliances. Functional appliances are generally confined to correction of class II malocclusion in growing children and mostly produce tipping rather than bodily movement of teeth.
   Tipping movements make only modest demands on the balance between the desired tooth movements and the space available (i.e. anchorage), whereas bodily movements place greater strain on anchorage. Where all the space available from extractions is required to relieve crowding, reduce an overjet or both, anchorage is at a premium and will need reinforcement.

Treatment timing

Intervention in the mixed dentition is advisable in some circumstances (Section 8.3). Some orthodontic treatments rely on growth for success, for example overbite reduction and functional appliance therapy, and treatment is usually best started in the late mixed dentition. In general, most orthodontic treatment is undertaken in the early permanent dentition as this usually coincides with the time when teeth that may be considered for extraction have erupted. Cooperation with treatment, often assisted by peer pressure, tends to be better also at this age than in the mid-teens. This is helped by a more rapid response of the periodontium to orthodontic forces and the potential for enhanced spontaneous tooth movement during the growth period. However, where a severe skeletal problem exists that is likely to be exacerbated by growth, treatment is best deferred until the late teens when a combined orthodontic/surgical approach can be considered.

Retention

A phase of retention is usually required following tooth movement with appliance therapy to allow consolidation of the new tooth positions through adaptation of the alveolar bone, gingival and periodontal tissues. Planning the retention phase of treatment demands on appraisal of the original features of the malocclusion as well as

- the skeletal pattern and growth pattern
- soft tissue and periodontal factors
- the type and duration of treatment.

The likely retention regimen should be individualised for each patient, taking these factors into account, and must be explained to the patient before treatment starts. Specific guidelines in relation to retention are included in the management of each malocclusion type and appliance treatments (Section 10.4). In general, however, following treatment with a removable appliance, 6 months of retention (3 months fulltime with the appliance removed at meals followed by 3 months night only) is recommended and most operators would opt for at least 1 year of retention following fixed appliance therapy. Following functional appliance therapy, it is recommended to retain until growth has reduced to adult levels.

Prognosis

Prognosis is based on an assessment of the problem and the possibility of moving the teeth into a stable position. If the latter is highly unlikely, for example because of very unfavourable soft tissue factors, treatment should be avoided.

Final presentation

The final presentation should outline clearly the objectives of each stage of treatment in a form that is under-standable to the patient and/or parent or guardian. If there is more than one plan possible, the 'pros' and 'cons' of each should be explained. Good colour photographs of any appliance to be used are very helpful. If headgear is required, this must be explained carefully. An outline of the likely appointment intervals and their length, together with an estimate of the overall length of treatment, is also necessary.

The need for maintenance of a high standard of oral hygiene as well as the importance of maintaining regular dental attendance for routine dental care throughout appliance treatment should be emphasised to the patient, together with the level of co-operation expected in relation to wear of specific appliance types, including headgear or intra-oral elastics. The potential risks of each treatment plan (e.g. root resorption, decalcification and alveolar bone loss) should be explained to the patient and parent or guardian, taking care to put them in context and not dramatise sequelae that are usually of minor significance (Table 31). If there is a risk attached to undertaking no treatment, this must also be highlighted.

Informed consent should then be obtained, although this may have to be deferred until a later date if the patient wishes time to consider the options presented. An information leaflet to take away is helpful for the patient.

Creating space for desired tooth movement

Extractions

Extraction of teeth is required to provide space for either relief of crowding and/or to camouflage a class II or class III skeletal discrepancy. In general, to preserve symmetry, teeth are usually extracted on either side of the same arch. The decision to extract teeth is governed by:

- general factors
  — profile considerations
  — incisor relationship
  — appliance to be employed
  — anchorage requirements
- local factors
  — the condition of the teeth
  — the site of crowding
  — the degree of crowding
  — the position of individual teeth.

General factors
Profile considerations. Attempts to expand the arches anteroposteriorly to relieve crowding and improve facial aesthetics are unlikely to be stable long-term. Indeed, the extraction of premolars rather than second permanent molars may produce only 1–2 mm of retraction of the lips. Differences in lip thickness and growth

Table 31 Risks of orthodontic treatment

Adverse effect	Potential problem
Root resorption	0.5–1 mm loss of root length common, but large individual variation Greater resorption with fixed than removable appliances Greater risk with traumatised teeth, previous root resorption, blunt or pipette-shaped roots
Demineralisation	Greater risk with fixed than removable appliances Risk increases with poor oral hygiene and frequent intake of sugary foods/drinks
Periodontal disease	Palatal gingival inflammation common with removable appliances if oral hygiene poor Marginal gingivitis common with fixed appliances; tends to resolve on appliance removal Occasionally 1 mm loss of attachment and 0.25–0.5 mm loss of alveolar bone adjacent to extraction sites
Pulpal/soft tissue damage	Loss of pulpal vitality, particularly if overactivation of appliance and previous history of trauma Abrasion/ulceration of oral mucosa, more common with fixed than removable appliances
Temporomandibular joint dysfunction syndrome (TMJDS)	Orthodontic treatment with or without extractions is not a cause of TMJDS Stress often acts in conjunction with parafunction promoted by occlusal factors TMJDS associated with crossbites, class III malocclusion, open bite
Iatrogenic effects	Greater risk with inexperienced operator, e.g. anchorage loss, inappropriate treatment mechanics

pattern between individuals are likely to have greater bearing on the soft tissue profile than whether or not extractions are employed as part of treatment. However, where there is a marked class II skeletal discrepancy, retraction of the incisors is likely to produce a very unsatisfactory facial profile, and specialist advice should be sought.

Incisor relationships. In class I or class II, it is usual to extract at least as far forward in the upper arch as in the lower, but the opposite holds true in class III. Where the overbite is deep, at least 2 mm of space will be required for its reduction. Centreline discrepancies require greater space on one side of the arch than on the other to facilitate correction. To camouflage a moderate class II or class III skeletal problem, extraction of only upper first or lower first premolars, respectively, may be indicated.

Appliance to be employed. In crowded mouths, extraction of the same tooth from each quadrant encourages mesial drift and spontaneous space closure, but the choice of extraction is not so critical if fixed appliances are to be employed for correction of the malocclusion.

Anchorage requirements. Bodily movement of teeth, particularly apical torque, is more demanding on anchorage than tipping movement, so space near to the site of the intended tooth movement is desirable. In addition, the anchorage balance (best thought of in terms of the combined root surface area posterior and anterior to the extraction site) is unfavourable for aligning crowded incisors the further posterior in the arch extractions are undertaken.

Local factors

The condition of the teeth. Teeth with poor long-term prognosis should be considered for extraction even if

treatment is made more difficult or prolonged as a result.

Site of crowding. Crowding in one part of the arch is more easily corrected if extractions are carried out in, or close to, that part of the arch. This is not true for the incisor areas: extraction of an incisor is not usually undertaken for relief of crowding because of the poor appearance that would result. First premolars, located midway between the front and back of the arches, often provide space for relief of crowding in both locations, whereas second molars may be extracted for crowding confined to the posterior regions.

Degree of crowding. Usually extractions are not indicated when crowding is less than 2 mm in any quadrant. In the mixed dentition, mild crowding may resolve with the leeway space, but after this stage has passed, appliance therapy to either expand the arches or to move the buccal segments distally will be required to provide space. In patients where the apical bases are reasonably long, space shortage of the order of 4 mm per quadrant may be dealt with without extractions, but extractions will be warranted for more severe crowding.

The position of individual teeth. Teeth that are grossly malpositioned and that would be difficult to align are often the choice for extraction. The position of the apex of the tooth must be considered as it is usually more difficult to move the apex than the crown.

Extraction of teeth in the buccal segment
First premolars. These teeth are most commonly extracted for relief of moderate-to-severe labial segment crowding. The second premolar resembles the first premolar in size and shape and usually the resulting contact point between the second premolar and canine is good. Maximum spontaneous labial segment alignment

is likely if first premolars are extracted as the canines are erupting, provided they are mesially inclined.

Second premolars. These teeth are usually chosen for extraction in the following situations:

- mild to moderate crowding, as the anchorage balance favours space closure by mesial movement of the molars; fixed appliances will be required for this
- when the teeth are hypoplastic (usually as a result of an apical infection of the overlying second deciduous molar: Turner's hypoplasia), carious or absent
- in those in whom one or more second premolar is absent and crowding is mild to moderate, the second premolar may be extracted in the other quadrant(s), thereby balancing and/or compensating for the extractions; fixed appliances will be required to align the remaining teeth and close any residual spacing
- where the tooth is completely excluded from the arch either palatally or lingually following early loss of the second deciduous molar; the contact between the first permanent molar and the first premolars should be acceptable.

First permanent molars. See Section 9.1.

Second permanent molars. Extraction of lower second permanent molars may be considered for relief of slight premolar crowding or to compensate for upper second permanent molar extractions, being undertaken to facilitate distal movement of the buccal segments. First permanent molars must have a good prognosis. The best chance of providing space to disimpact a lower third molar successfully occurs when:

- $\overline{8}$ overlaps the distal of $\overline{7}$
- $\overline{8}$ makes <30° angulation to the long axis of $\overline{6}$
- $\overline{8}$ bifurcation is calcified.

However, even when these criteria are met, the final position of $\overline{8}$ is unpredictable. Despite some claims to the contrary, removal of lower second molars has a negligible effect on relief of lower incisor crowding.

Third molars. Removal is only indicated in the presence of pathology and cannot be justified as a means of preventing or ameliorating late lower incisor crowding.

Extraction of teeth in the labial segment

Incisors Rarely extraction of a lower incisor produces an acceptable solution to incisor crowding. It is important to realise that following extraction of a lower incisor, fitting six upper anterior teeth around five lower anteriors may lead to a reduction in the upper intercanine width and upper labial segment crowding. Crowding of three lower incisors may also occur owing to a reduction in the lower intercanine width and a tendency for the labial segment to move lingually. Therefore, extraction of a lower incisor is usually best confined to the following situations:

- where the prognosis is poor because of caries, trauma or gingival recession
- where the crowding is severe, with one incisor excluded labially or lingually
- where the canines are distally inclined with fanning of the lower incisors
- in a mild class III malocclusion with crowded lower incisors
- in an adult patient with class I buccal and incisor relationships and severe lower incisor crowding; here subsequent changes in arch dimensions are likely to be minimal
- where a tooth size discrepancy exists in the upper labial segment, i.e. small upper lateral incisors.

When extraction of a lower incisor is considered, it is wise to see what the final result is likely to be by carrying out a diagnostic set-up on a set of working casts. In each case, a lower fixed appliance is usually required to align and approximate the remaining teeth.

Upper incisors. A permanent central incisor is never a tooth of choice for extraction but may be considered if dilacerated or of poor prognosis owing to trauma. Extraction of an upper lateral incisor is not recommended except in the following circumstances:

- $\underline{2}$ (crown or root or both) abnormally formed
- $\underline{2}$ on opposite side of the arch absent or abnormally formed
- $\underline{2}$ bodily excluded palatally with $\underline{1}$ and $\underline{3}$ in contact
- moderate crowding with $\underline{3}$ distally inclined.

In these cases, the canine should be of good size, shape and colour to allow optimal dental aesthetics in the upper labial segment.

Canines

Lower canines. These should only be removed if the tooth is severely displaced with good contact between $\overline{2}$ and $\overline{4}$.

Upper canines. See Section 9.1.

Interproximal stripping

Removal of 0.25 mm of enamel from each proximal surface of the lower incisors creates 2 mm of space for relief of crowding, but should only be considered in the adult.

Arch expansion

In the upper arch, treatment of a unilateral crossbite with displacement may provide up to 5 mm of space and obviate the need for extractions. In the absence of such a crossbite, arch expansion is unlikely to be stable. Correction of a lingual crossbite by lower arch expansion is possible in some cases but requires specialist skills.

Functional appliances

Some slight increase in arch dimensions may be possible in growing patients treated with a Frankel appliance, providing space to relieve mild potential crowding.

Distal movement of the buccal segments

Space lost to unilateral mesial drift of the molars following early loss of primary teeth may be regained in the upper arch by use of a removable appliance with a screw and headgear support (Fig. 108). Bilateral distal movement of the upper buccal segments is possible in well-motivated individuals, requiring excellent co-operation and usually, with headgear wear. However, without removal of the upper second permanent molars, it is unlikely that more than 2–3 mm of space can be gained.

Distal movement of the lower first permanent molar is more difficult to achieve but may be attempted if the lower second permanent molar is considered for extraction. Treatment is best carried out with a fixed rather than a removable appliance as the latter is usually poorly tolerated in the lower arch.

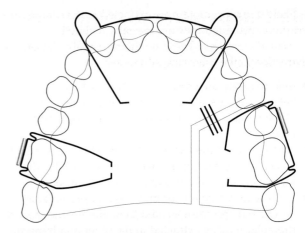

Fig. 108 An upper removable appliance (URA) with screw and headgear support to regain space lost to unilateral mesial drift. URA to move |5 6 distally. Screw section to |5 6; single Adams' clasp 6| and double Adams' clasp |5 6 (both 0.7 mm SS wire); tubes for headgear soldered to clasp bridges; labial bow 2 1 | 1 2 (0.7 mm wire).

Combination of means

In some circumstances, a combination of any or all of the methods listed may be appropriate to create space.

Self-assessment: questions

Multiple choice questions

1. The maxilla:
   a. Is derived from the second pharyngeal arch
   b. Completes growth in length before growth in width
   c. Grows partly by passive displacement of its articulation with the cranial base
   d. Is translated downwards and forwards by the condylar cartilage
   e. On average completes growth by 15 years in males

2. The mandible:
   a. Is derived from the first pharyngeal arch
   b. Ossifies medial to Meckel's cartilage
   c. Has a predictable pattern of growth in each individual
   d. On average follows the growth pattern of the maxilla
   e. Does not grow after age 18 in males

3. Marked anterior mandibular growth rotation:
   a. Occurs when growth in posterior face height is less than in anterior face height
   b. Is more common than backward growth rotation
   c. Is often associated with a deep overbite
   d. Is associated with an increased maxillary/mandibular plane angle
   e. Is associated with a concave lower mandibular border

4. In the dental development of the 'average' child:
   a. Calcification of the primary incisors commences 6–8 months in utero
   b. Root calcification of the primary teeth completes 2–2.5 years after eruption
   c. Primary incisors erupt in contact and proclined
   d. Calcification of the first permanent molars commences at 8–10 months after birth
   e. The 'leeway space' is greater in the upper than in the lower arch

5. Space for the permanent upper incisors:
   a. Is obtained by eruption palatal to their predecessors
   b. Is obtained by use of existing primary labial segments spacing
   c. Is obtained by intercanine width growth
   d. Is likely to be adequate where the primary incisors are crowded
   e. Is affected by the overbite

6. Normal maturational changes in the dentition include:
   a. A reduction in lower labial segment crowding
   b. An increase in upper labial segment crowding
   c. A reduction in lower intercanine width
   d. Increase in overjet
   e. An increase in interincisal angle

7. Clinical assessment of the anteroposterior dental base relationship:
   a. Is undertaken by viewing the patient from in front
   b. Should be undertaken with the teeth just out of occlusion
   c. Is best carried out with the patient supine
   d. Is reflected by the maxillary/mandibular planes angle
   e. Depends on the upper incisor angulation

8. A class II skeletal pattern:
   a. Is present when the mandible is protruded relative to the maxilla
   b. Can be assessed from the SNB angle
   c. Is usually associated with a retrognathic maxilla
   d. Can be assessed from the first permanent molar relationship
   e. Depends on the incisor relationship

9. The maxillary/mandibular planes angle (MMPA):
   a. Can be assessed clinically
   b. Reflects the anteroposterior skeletal pattern
   c. Indicates the vertical skeletal pattern
   d. Reflects posterior lower facial height and anterior lower facial height
   e. Is affected by lower incisor position

10. Class II division 2 malocclusion:
    a. Is defined by a half unit class II buccal segment relationship
    b. Exists when the lower incisor edges occlude anterior to the cingulum of the upper incisors
    c. Is characterised by retroclined upper central incisors
    d. Is usually associated with a minimal overjet
    e. May be associated with an increased overjet

11. A lateral cephalometric radiograph:
    a. Is taken with the head tilted up
    b. Is recorded with tube-to-midsagittal plane distance typically of about 15 cm
    c. Is an exact record of facial dimensions

d. Is essential for orthodontic diagnosis
e. May be useful in localising the position of an unerupted tooth

12. Cephalometrically:
   a. SNA (sella–nasion–A point) angle describes the relationship of the mandible to the cranial base
   b. ANB angle is obtained by subtracting angle SNA from SNB (sella–nasion–B point)
   c. Frankfort plane joins porion and nasion
   d. Mandibular plane joins gonion and menton
   e. Sella is the most anterior point on the cranial base

13. The ANB angle:
   a. Indicates the vertical relationships of the face
   b. Describes the anteroposterior skeletal pattern
   c. Tells about the relationship of the maxilla to the cranial base
   d. Is influenced by variation in the vertical position of nasion
   e. Is affected directly by the position of porion

Case history question

A 13-year-old female patient presents with a class I malocclusion with moderate upper and lower mid-arch crowding on a class I dental base with average FMPA. There is a history of recurrent oral ulceration.

1. What are the priorities in the management of this case?
2. Outline how you would go about orthodontic treatment planning for this patient
3. What orthodontic treatment possibilities may exist?

Picture questions

Picture 1

Examine the records in Figure 109.

1. Classify the incisor relationship
2. Classify the right and left molar relationships
3. Classify the degree of crowding in the maxillary and mandibular arches (all permanent teeth are present)
4. What are the likely causes of this malocclusion?
5. What is the IOTN (DHC) score?
   (Additional information: no mandibular displacement associated with the crossbite; overjet 6 mm; lips competent)

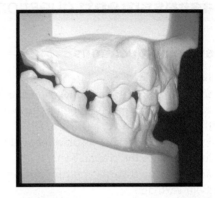
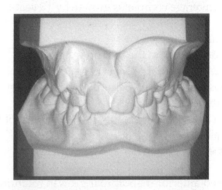
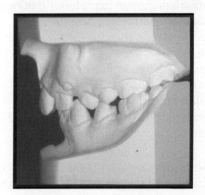
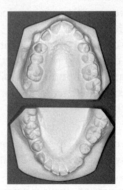

Fig. 109 Records for Picture question 1.

Picture 2

Examine the records in Figure 110.

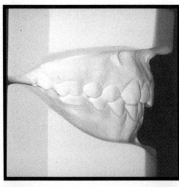

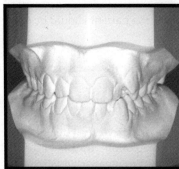

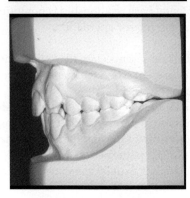

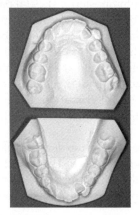

Fig. 110 Records for Picture question 2.

1. Classify the incisor relationship
2. Classify the right and left molar relationships
3. Assess the degree of crowding in the upper and lower arches
4. What is the most likely cause of the upper arch crowding?
5. What is the IOTN (DHC) score? (Additional information: no mandibular displacement associated with /2 or /7 crossbites)

Data interpretation

Given the following cephalometric values: SNA = 78°; SNB = 85°; SN to maxillary plane 7°; MMPA = 30°; $\underline{1}$ to maxillary plane = 130°; $\overline{1}$ to mandibular plane = 75°, answer the following questions, explaining your reasoning.

1. What is the anteroposterior skeletal pattern?
2. Classify the maxillary/mandibular planes angle – explain your classification
3. What feature of the malocclusion is expressed by the incisor angulation?

Short note questions

Write short notes on the following:

1. Angle's classification of malocclusion
2. dental health component of the Index of Orthodontic Treatment Need (IOTN)
3. aesthetic component of IOTN
4. methods of creating space for relief of crowding other than by extraction.

Viva questions

1. What are the potential benefits/risks of orthodontic treatment? How would you assess the need for treatment?
2. Describe the occlusion of an average deciduous dentition in a child aged 5 years. What changes occur up to the age of 14 years leading to the establishment of a 'normal' permanent occlusion?
3. What factors should be considered when obtaining informed consent from a patient prior to orthodontic treatment?

Self-assessment: answers

Multiple choice answers

1. a. **False.** Derived partially from first pharyngeal arch.
   b. **False.** Completes growth in width before growth in length.
   c. **True.**
   d. **False.** Condylar cartilage directs mandibular growth.
   e. **False.** In males, maxillary growth is complete, on average, by age 17 years; it is true in females.

2. a. **True.**
   b. **False.** It ossifies lateral to Meckel's cartilage.
   c. **False.** Pattern of growth is not predictable.
   d. **False.** Growth pattern is independent of maxillary growth pattern.
   e. **False.** Although, on average, mandibular growth will complete by 18–19 years in males, the mandible continues to grow, albeit at a considerably reduced rate, throughout the next three decades.

3. a. **False.** It occurs when growth in posterior face height exceeds that in anterior face height.
   b. **True.** A mild forward growth rotation is normal to produce a well-balanced facial appearance.
   c. **True.** The reduction in the anterior vertical facial proportions will promote overbite increase.
   d. **False.** Reduced maxillary/mandibular planes angle will result from marked anterior mandibular growth rotation, leading to increased overbite. See c.
   e. **False.** It is associated with a convex lower mandibular border.

4. a. **False.** Typically at 3–4 months.
   b. **False.** Typically 1–1.5 years after eruption.
   c. **False.** Typically they are upright and spaced.
   d. **False.** Typically at birth.
   e. **False.** Greater in the lower than in the upper arch.

5. a. **False.** It is provided by their eruption in a more proclined angulation labial to the primary predecessors.
   b. **True.** This will help space requirements.
   c. **True.** Tends to be about 1–2 mm in primary dentition and 2–3 mm in mixed dentition.
   d. **False.** Crowding of the primary incisors is likely to provide insufficient space for the permanent incisors.
   e. **False.** Overbite will have no effect on potential space for the upper permanent incisors.

6. a. **False.** An increase in lower labial segment crowding is normal.
   b. **False.** An increase in lower labial segment crowding is normal.
   c. **True.** This will contribute to lower labial segment crowding.
   d. **False.** This is not a normal finding.
   e. **True.** With uprighting of the lower incisors in response to facial growth changes, the tendency is for the interincisal angle to increase.

7. a. **False.** For anteroposterior assessment of the dental bases, the patient should be observed from the side.
   b. **False.** The teeth should be in maximum indigitation, ensuring that the mandible is not postured forward.
   c. **False.** The patient should be seated upright with the Frankfort plane horizontal.
   d. **False.** This assesses vertical dental base relationship cephalometrically and not clinical anteroposterior dental base relationship.
   e. **False.** Dental base relationship is not influenced by the upper incisor angulation.

8. a. **False.** This represents class III skeletal pattern; class II is present when the mandible is retruded relative to the maxilla.
   b. **False.** SNB angle tells about the relationship of the mandible to the cranial base; ANB angle tells the relationship of the mandible to the maxilla, i.e. the skeletal pattern.
   c. **False.** Class II is usually associated with a normal or prognathic maxilla.
   d. **False.** The anteroposterior skeletal pattern cannot be assessed by examination of the first permanent molar relationship, although Angle believed incorrectly that this was possible. It is possible for the first permanent molar relationship to be class II and the skeletal pattern to be also class II, but where early loss of primary teeth has occurred or if significant hypodontia is present, this will be altered.
   e. **False.** Incisor relationship does not influence the skeletal pattern. A class II skeletal pattern may be *associated* with a class II incisor relationship, but the latter does not have a direct bearing on the former.

9. a. **False.** The maxillary plane cannot be assessed clinically so this angle cannot be calculated. Frankfort/mandibular planes angle is assessed clinically.

b. **False.** It reflects the vertical skeletal pattern. Anteroposterior skeletal pattern is reflected by the ANB angle.

c. **True.** See (b) above.

d. **True.** As it is an angular assessment of vertical skeletal pattern.

e. **False.** It is not affected by lower incisor *position* but MMPA has an inverse relationship with lower incisor *angulation*. As MMPA increases, lower incisor angulation reduces and the converse is also true.

10. a. **False.** Class II division 2 is an incisor classification and is, therefore, not defined by the buccal segment relationship.

b. **False.** This would be present in a class III incisor relationship. For class II malocclusion, the lower incisor edges lie posterior to the cingulum plateau of the upper incisors.

c. **True.** This is a characteristic of this malocclusion type.

d. **True.** This feature is also part of the British Standards Institute definition of this incisor relationship, although the overjet may also be increased.

e. **True.** See (d) above.

11. a. **False.** The radiograph is taken with the Frankfort plane horizontal or the patient in natural head posture.

b. **False.** The tube-to-midsagittal plane distance is usually standardised at the order of about 150 cm.

c. **False.** Because of the magnification factor (which is in the range 8–12%), it is not an *exact* record of facial dimensions.

d. **False.** It is not essential for orthodontic diagnosis, although it may be of benefit in gaining an insight as to the cause of a malocclusion and in treatment planning.

e. **True.** It would not, however, be taken solely for this purpose.

12. a. **False.** It describes the maxillary relationship as 'A' point is on the maxilla.

b. **False.** The ANB angle is obtained by subtracting SNB from SNA.

c. **False.** It joins porion and orbitale.

d. **True.**

e. **False.** It is the midpoint of the sella turcica.

13. a. **False.** It indicates the anteroposterior skeletal pattern.

b. **True.** See (a) above.

c. **False.** This is reflected in the SNA angle.

d. **True.** This affects the angles SNA and SNB, and hence their difference ANB.

e. **False.** The position of porion does not affect the ANB angle.

Case history answer

1. As with all orthodontic referrals, the patient's concern regarding appearance of her teeth as well as willingness to wear any likely appliances should be recorded. Medical history should be checked and a detailed history of the nature of the recurrent oral ulceration should be taken. The patient should be made aware that satisfactory wear of an orthodontic appliance may prove impossible depending on the nature and frequency of the recurrent oral ulceration. Thorough investigation of the ulcers should be undertaken, including referral to a consultant in oral medicine for blood tests if these are deemed necessary. If a systemic cause is identified, orthodontic treatment should be delayed until it is treated as the recurrent ulceration may resolve and allow comprehensive treatment with appliance therapy. If the ulceration is particularly severe, appliance therapy will need to be avoided.

2. Obtain all necessary records – study models recorded in centric occlusion and relevant radiographs (a lateral cephalometric film may be required if comprehensive treatment with upper/lower fixed appliances is likely). Decide on aims of treatment: aim for the ideal outcome but bear in mind the medical history; a plan that avoids the wearing of an orthodontic appliance would be optimal if the ulceration does not resolve. Plan the lower arch first: consider crowding (in this case moderate and midarch), canine inclination, overbite, centreline as well as anchorage requirements for all intended tooth movements. Then proceed to the upper arch and assess crowding, canine inclination, incisor inclination (anchorage requirements). Decide on the type of appliance required to effect tooth movements required and appropriate retention plan.

3. If the ulceration does not resolve, and appliance therapy is still warranted, consider fitting an upper removable appliance and monitor the oral reaction to wear before considering any likely extractions. If the ulceration resolves, upper removable appliance therapy alone or upper/lower fixed appliances may be justified, based on the assessment of the occlusal features.

Picture answers

Picture 1

1. Class II division 1.
2. Almost Class II half unit on the right (mesiobuccal cusp of 6 occludes in a cusp-to-cusp relationship with $\overline{6}$); Class I on the left.
3. Lower arch has mild crowding (note spacing); upper arch has moderate crowding (note spacing).
4. Possible causes are:
   — overjet, possibly mild class II skeletal discrepancy.
   — lower arch crowding: early loss of primary molars: note tilting of 6s and distal drifting and rotation of 4s.
   — upper arch crowding: inherent dentoalveolar disproportion most likely; early loss of primary teeth unlikely (observe the reasonably good alignment of the premolars).
5. 5i because of impaction of lower 5s.

Picture 2

1. Class I: the lower incisors occlude opposite the cingulum plateau of the upper central incisors.
2. Right is class I; left is half unit class II.
3. Lower arch has moderate crowding; upper arch has moderate crowding.
4. Inherent dentoalveolar disproportion.
5. 4d due to contact point displacement between /2 /3.

Data interpretation

1. Class III. Subtracting SNB from SNA gives the ANB angle, a measure of the anteroposterior skeletal pattern. An ANB value of −5.5 after Eastman correction) indicates a marked class III skeletal discrepancy.
2. This angle is average. The maxillary/mandibular planes angle may be classified as average (27 ± 4°); high (>31°) or low (<23°).
3. The upper incisors are very proclined (average angulation 109 ± 6°) while the lower incisors are very retroclined (average angulation 93 ± 6°), indicating dentoalveolar compensation for the class III skeletal discrepancy.

Short note answers

1. Angle's classification is used nowadays to classify the anteroposterior molar relationship, although it was originally intended for classification of the anteroposterior dental arch relationship on the assumption that the first permanent molar erupted into a consistently reliable position in the face.

Three molar relationships exist:
class I: mesiobuccal cusp of the upper first permanent molar occludes in the buccal groove of the lower first permanent molar
class II: mesiobuccal cusp of the upper first permanent molar occludes anterior to a class I relationship
class III: mesiobuccal cusp of the upper first permanent molar occludes posterior to a class I relationship.

2. This records occlusal features of a malocclusion using a MOCDO convention where M is missing teeth, O is overjet, C is crossbite, D is displacement of contact points and O is overbite. A specially designed ruler aids the process. A malocclusion is then ascribed to one of five categories of treatment need: Grades 1, 2, no/slight need; grade 3, borderline; grades 4, 5, great/very great need. Assessment by this means is objective, reliable and rapid.

3. This scores the need for treatment of a malocclusion based on the degree of aesthetic impairment of the anterior teeth. Assessment is made by viewing the anterior occlusion either clinically or from study models and comparing this with a set of ten photographs of increasing aesthetic handicap. Treatment need is accorded as: grades 1–4, no/slight need; grades 5–7, borderline need; grades 8–10, definite need. The set of photographs do not include a full range of malocclusion types and assessment is subjective.

4. Space may be created by each of the following means:
   a. Arch expansion: only indicated where a unilateral crossbite exists, especially if there is an associated displacement.
   b. Distal movement of the buccal segments: may be undertaken in the lower arch if extraction of a lower second permanent molar is considered, but rarely adopted as an approach to relief of crowding. If undertaken, a fixed appliance is invariably required. In the upper arch, bilateral distal movement of the buccal segments using headgear may be undertaken to provide space for relief of mild upper arch crowding or correction of a small overjet. In these patients, the lower arch should be well aligned and the molar relationship no greater than half unit class II. Unilateral distal movement may be undertaken when space is required on one side of the arch only and may be undertaken using a screw section in a removable appliance, although provision for incorporation of headgear in the appliance is advisable. Consider extraction of upper second permanent molar(s) to aid distal movement in the upper arch

provided third molars are present and of good size and position.

c. Interdental stripping: only really a consideration in adults where a small amount of space is required for alignment. Usually confined to the lower labial segment. Involves the removal of ~0.25 mm from the mesial and distal surfaces of each tooth.

d. Any combination of any/all of above.

Viva answers

1. The potential benefits of orthodontic treatment to the patient should outweigh the potential risks and side-effects.

Potential benefits of orthodontic treatment are improvement in dental health through reduction in caries and periodontal potential risks associated with local factors such as severely crowded teeth, traumatic overbite and incisor crossbite with displacement. The risk of incisor trauma or pathological change with possible root resorption is reduced, respectively, where a large overjet is corrected or an impacted tooth is removed. In addition, the risk of developing temporomandibular joint dysfunction is reduced where class III malocclusion, crossbite or anterior open bite are corrected, while the psychological benefits accruing from the correction of severe malocclusion include improved self-esteem and greater social interaction.

The potential risks are failure to achieve the aims of treatment; pulpal, gingival and mucosal damage; root resorption and loss of alveolar crestal height; and possibly instigation or exacerbation of temporomandibular joint dysfunction syndrome (see Section 8.4). With fixed appliances, the risk of decalcification is increased while there is a small but significant risk of facial or ocular damage from headgear.

The need for treatment may be assessed objectively using the Index of Orthodontic Treatment Need (see Section 8.2). This has two components, but the dental health rather than the aesthetic component can only be assessed reliably.

2. In the average deciduous dentition at age 5, abcde have erupted in all quadrants. Although the 'ideal' features have been described as a generalised spaced dentition with specific space mesial to the upper and distal to the lower cs (anthropoid spaces), upright incisors with a relatively deep overbite and flush terminal planes, these rarely occur and great individual variation is encountered.

Where the overbite has been deep initially, it usually reduces by 5 years of age, and an edge-to-edge incisor relationship with attrition is common. From about age 6 onwards, the permanent dentition starts to erupt, usually commencing with the eruption of the lower incisors or of the lower first permanent molars as growth posteriorly in the arch accommodates them. As the permanent incisors erupt lingual to their predecessors, some incisor crowding is often seen, but this generally resolves with growth in the intercanine width.

Order and dates of eruption of permanent teeth are given in Tables 11 and 12 (p. 170). Space for the upper incisors is provided by the deciduous incisor spacing, intercanine growth (1–2 mm in the primary and ~3 mm in the mixed dentition) and the more proclined inclination of the permanent incisors. Commonly, these teeth erupt spaced and distally inclined – referred to as the ugly duckling stage – but this reduces as the permanent canines erupt. These should be palpable in the buccal sulcus at age 10 years and are guided into position by the roots of the permanent lateral incisors.

Space for the premolars and permanent canines is provided by intercanine growth and the 'leeway space', typically 1–1.5 mm and 2–2.5 mm in the upper and lower arches, respectively. The greater space in the lower than in the upper arch also may allow the molar relationship to correct from a possible half a unit class II to a class I relationship.

By 14 years of age, the permanent occlusion should be all but complete apart from third molars, if present. The features of the normal permanent occlusion are given in Section 8.1.

3. All the points listed below should be gone through in a systematic order in a format that is understandable to the patient, with adequate time given to question any item that is not entirely clear.

a. The diagnosis (problem list) should be outlined to the patient and/or parent together with the dental health component of IOTN. The significance of the latter should be explained.

b. If there is more than one possible approach to treatment, the various options should be explained together with the 'pros' and 'cons' of each. If there are risks attached to undertaking no treatment, this must be explained also.

c. Appliances to be used for treatment must be explained and examples demonstrated – colour photographs are a good means of doing this. If headgear is required, this requires special consideration together with an explanation of the specific care required in its use.

d. Likely appointment intervals and an estimate of treatment length are required also.

e. The compliance required from the patient during orthodontic treatment must also be emphasised:

the need for maintenance of a high standard of oral hygiene, regular dental attendance for routine dental care, cooperation required with appliance wear, particularly if headgear or intra oral elastic wear is prescribed, and importance of attendance for appliance adjustment at the appointed times.

f. Importance of risks of each treatment plan (i.e. root resorption, decalcification and alveolar bone loss) should be explained to patient and parent/guardian taking care not to dramatise sequelae, which are likely to be minor.

g. An information sheet may be useful for the patient to take away to think over all the issues related to treatment prior to giving consent for treatment at a subsequent visit.

Orthodontics II: management of occlusal problems

Overview

The management of malocclusion comprises a substantial part of orthodontic practice. It ranges from interception of developing occlusal problems through to comprehensive correction of established malocclusion in the adolescent or adult. It also encompasses the special requirements in orthodontic care of those with cleft lip and/or palate.

This chapter describes the management of the developing dentition and of all major anomalies of established malocclusion, including surgical correction. The occlusal problems particular to cleft lip and/or palate together with their management are also outlined.

9.1 Problem solving in the developing dentition

Learning objectives

You should

- know the problems which are best dealt with in the developing dentition

- be able to classify supernumerary teeth

- know how to localise an unerupted tooth in the anterior maxilla

- understand the principles of management of an unerupted 1, ectopic 3, and first permanent molar with poor long-term prognosis.

Although most orthodontic treatment is undertaken when the permanent dentition is established, some aspects of the developing occlusion may be better dealt with in the mixed dentition. Such interception may eliminate the need for, or simplify, later treatment. Systematic and regular screening of the developing dentition is essential to this process.

Anomalies of eruption and exfoliation

Both eruption and exfoliation of primary and permanent teeth may be premature or delayed.

Natal teeth

Natal teeth are usually lower incisors that are erupted at birth or appear soon after. Removal is indicated only if they interfere with suckling or if they are so mobile as to be at risk of inhalation.

Eruption of teeth

Other than natal teeth, the following points should be borne in mind:

- there is greater variation in the eruption sequence of primary teeth between races than there is in eruption times

- poor diet and chronic ill health in child populations may alter eruption sequence

- eruption times of permanent teeth tend to be later in Caucasians than in Mongoloids, who in turn tend to be later than Negroids

- females tend to erupt their permanent teeth earlier than males, particularly second and third molars.

Factors causing premature exfoliation or delay in the eruption and exfoliation of primary or permanent teeth are given in Table 32.

To ensure that any deviation in the normal eruption sequence is detected early, clinical vigilance is required during the developing dentition, supported by radiographic investigations where necessary. Particular attention should be given to the permanent maxillary incisors and canines, as early recognition of an anomaly in their eruption improves the prognosis.

Table 32 Causes of premature or delayed eruption of primary or permanent teeth

	Causes
Premature eruption	Familial tendency Primary dentition: high birth weight Permanent dentition: early-onset puberty, excess growth or thyroid hormone secretion
Delayed eruption	Primary dentition: very low birth weight, premature birth General causes: Down or Turner syndromes, severe nutritional deficiency, hypothyroidism/hypopituitarism, cleidocranial dysplasia, hereditary gingival hyperplasia, cleft lip and palate Local causes: ectopic crypt position, supernumerary or odontome, congenital absence, retention of primary tooth, dilaceration, primary failure of eruption, crowding
Premature exfoliation	Commonly caries or trauma Rarely hereditary hypophosphatasia, congenital neutropenia, cyclic neutropenia, Chediak–Higashi syndrome, histiocytosis X
Delayed exfoliation	Congenital absence of permanent successor Ectopic position of permanent successor Trauma Severe periradicular infection of primary tooth

Hypodontia

The most common missing teeth are

- third molars (25–35%)
- upper lateral incisors (2%)
- lower second premolars (3%)
- lower incisors.

Absent third molars

Extraction of a second molar either to facilitate distal movement of the upper buccal segments or to relieve posterior crowding should not be considered in the absence of a third molar. These start to calcify any time between 8 and 14 years.

Absent upper lateral incisors

Management options for the space resultant upon absent upper lateral incisors are:

- space opening
- space maintenance
- space closure.

The final decision depends on

- the patient's attitude to orthodontic treatment
- the anteroposterior and vertical skeletal relationships
- the colour, size, shape and inclination of the canine and incisor teeth
- whether the arches are spaced or crowded
- the buccal segment occlusion.

The possible plans are best assessed by carrying out a trial set-up of each using duplicate study models, followed by joint consultation with a restorative colleague.

Space opening In uncrowded or mildly crowded arches, when the buccal segment occlusion is class I or at most half unit class II, or in class III where proclination of the incisors is likely to correct an anterior crossbite, space opening is best. In addition, in patients with low FMPA (Frankfort mandibular plane angle) or where the maxillary canine is considerably darker than the incisors, it may be best to open rather than close the anterior spaces. A fixed appliance may be needed to localise space for the missing units, followed by at least 6 months of removable appliance retention ensuring that the space is maintained by placing wire spurs in contact with the adjoining teeth. If it is possible to reposition the incisors and canines into their desired locations by tipping movements, a removable rather than a fixed appliance may be used. In selected cases, autotransplantation of lower premolars (extracted for relief of crowding) to the upper lateral incisor area may be possible. The prognosis is best when the root of the lower premolars is half to two-thirds formed. More commonly, the missing units may be replaced on resin-retained bridgework, and occasionally by implants at a later date. If bridgework is planned, it is important to ensure that sufficient interocclusal clearance exists for placement of the metal framework; if not, this should be created during appliance therapy.

Space closure In crowded mouths, early extraction of the primary canines should be carried out to encourage mesial drift of the posterior teeth, but a later phase of fixed appliance therapy is usually needed to align and approximate the upper anterior teeth, followed by bonded retention. Recontouring of the canines in addition to composite or porcelain build-up of their mesio-incisal aspects is usually necessary to achieve the optimal aesthetic result. Overjet reduction by space closure may be more favourable than resorting to mid-arch extractions and space opening. Space closure is likely to be facilitated in patients with increased FMPA, crowding and where the buccal segment relationship is a full unit class II.

Second premolars

The primary second molar should be retained where the arch is uncrowded or aligned. If the tooth starts to submerge, an occlusal onlay may be placed to maintain it in function. Removal of the lower second primary molar shortly after eruption of the lateral incisors will encourage spontaneous space closure in mildly crowded mouths, but in those with marked crowding, its extraction should be delayed until orthodontic treatment commences so that the resulting space may be used for arch alignment. In the upper arch, extraction of the second primary molar is again best deferred until orthodontic treatment is about to start. Rarely, a lower second premolar develops late and necessitates an alteration in the original treatment plan.

Lower central incisors

In the absence of permanent lower central incisors, root resorption and progressive incisal wear usually leads to loss of the primary incisors in the later mixed dentition, although occasionally they may last for longer. A fixed appliance may be needed to close incisor spacing in a crowded mouth or to align the lateral incisors prior to placement of resin-retained bridgework in an uncrowded arch. Where one or both lower central incisors is missing and the space is closed orthodontically, mild crowding may result in the upper labial segment as six anterior teeth are arranged around four or five lower teeth.

Supernumerary teeth

Teeth additional to the normal number are termed 'supernumerary'. Most commonly, they occur in the premaxilla (mesiodens) but they often also develop distal to the last tooth in each dental series (lateral incisor, second premolar and third molar) as an exuberant growth of the dental lamina, perhaps representing a tertiary dentition. They are more common

- in males than in females
- in the permanent than in the primary dentition (respective incidences 2 and 1%)
- in cleft and cleido-cranial dyostosis children.

Those in the premaxilla can be categorised into three groups: conical, tuberculate and supplemental.

Conical teeth

Conical teeth occur between the upper central incisors; they are often singular but can sometimes occur in combination with others of similar form. They may have no effect if they are well above the apices of the incisors. If there is no risk of damage to adjacent teeth with tooth movement, they can be left in place and observed. Often,

however, they may displace the adjacent teeth, perhaps creating a large diastema, or they may delay eruption. In these instances, removal is indicated. Occasionally a conical supernumerary tooth erupts and can be extracted.

Tuberculate teeth

Tuberculate teeth are the most common cause of an unerupted incisor. Suspicion should be raised if the lateral incisors erupt in advance of the centrals. In these cases, a radiograph of the premaxilla should be taken to allow early detection and localisation of any supernumerary, which should then be surgically removed. An attachment with gold chain or a magnet should be bonded to the unerupted incisor to allow provision for orthodontic alignment if the tooth fails to erupt spontaneously within 18 months of surgery. Space to accommodate the unerupted tooth must be maintained or opened by appliance therapy, often in upper conjunction with extraction of the primary canines.

Supplemental teeth

The supplemental tooth resembles the normal tooth in morphology and commonly produces crowding or displacement of adjacent teeth. Usually the tooth, which is similar to the contralateral tooth, is better retained (provided it is not severely malpositioned) and the other incisor is extracted.

Anomalies of development

First permanent molars with poor long-term prognosis

The first permanent molar is never the extraction of choice for orthodontic reasons but is invariably enforced because of poor prognosis resulting from caries and/or enamel hypoplasia. Enamel decalcification on the lingual aspect of lower first permanent molars or on the buccal aspect of upper first permanent molars should be treated seriously, as it is often a hallmark of a high caries rate and limited lifespan of these teeth. When a two-surface or deep occlusal restoration is indicated in one molar 2 to 3 years after eruption, careful assessment of the malocclusion and the condition of the other first permanent molars should be made. Timely removal may lead to considerable spontaneous correction of the malocclusion in certain patients but it does little for relief of incisor crowding or correction of an incisor relationship unless appliance therapy is instituted.

A 'cook book' approach to each patient with poor-quality first permanent molars is not possible but some guidelines are listed in Table 33.

Infra-occluded primary molars

Prevalence of submergence of a primary molar is about 8–14%. Submergence results from ankylosis of the tooth

Table 33 Guidelines for management of first permanent molars (FPM) with poor long-term prognosis

- Institute preventive measures including oral hygiene motivation, dietary advice and fluoride therapy
- Evaluate social circumstances, motivation for orthodontic treatment and level of dental awareness
- Ensure (radiographically) that all permanent teeth, particularly second premolars and third molars, are present and that all others are of good prognosis. Avoid extraction of a FPM in a quadrant with an absent tooth, or in uncrowded arches
- Consider balancing or compensating for extraction of a FPM
- Timing of extraction of lower FPM is best when the bifurcation of $\overline{7}$s is calcifying (aged approximately 8.5–9.5 years) and moderate premolar crowding is present
- Timing of extraction of upper FPM is less important because of the distal tilt and downward and forward eruption path of $\underline{7}$s
- Extraction of upper FPM is best delayed
  — in class III until the incisor crossbite is corrected
  — in class II division 1 until $\underline{7}$s erupt
  — in severely crowded mouths until $\underline{7}$s erupt
- Extraction of lower FPM may be deferred in class III with marked incisor crowding until $\overline{7}$s erupt
- Monitor eruption of second and third molars

while alveolar growth and eruption of the adjacent teeth continues. Provided the permanent successor is present, exfoliation will occur eventually, but removal is indicated in its absence and where the submergence is marked, with the crown of the tooth just visible, or where root development of the unerupted premolar is almost complete.

Impaction of the maxillary first permanent molar

Impaction of the maxillary first permanent molar occurs in 2–6% of children. It may correct spontaneously or it may require disimpaction of the molar either by placing a brass wire separator between the adjacent teeth (in mild problems) or by appliance therapy (in more marked impaction). Extraction of the second primary molar is required if the impaction produces symptomatic resorption with pulpal involvement or to facilitate restoration of the first permanent molar. Crowding is exacerbated by the subsequent mesial drift of the first permanent molar, but this can be treated later.

Aberrant position of second premolars

Occasionally the second premolars appear in slightly unfavourable positions when viewed on radiograph, but generally this is of no long-term consequence and their final position is usually satisfactory. A grossly ectopic second premolar is rare and may be observed or surgically removed.

Posterior crossbite with mandibular displacement

Occasionally a unilateral crossbite of the buccal segment teeth with mandibular displacement follows a prolonged finger- or thumb-sucking habit. In some chil-

dren, grinding the primary canines can lead to correction, but usually arch expansion by either a removable appliance and a midline screw or a quadhelix is required; alternatively, correction may be deferred until the premolars erupt (Fig. 111).

Treatment of anomalies by serial extractions

In 1948, Kjellgren, a Swedish orthodontist, ascribed the term 'serial extractions' to the following three-stage procedure:

- extraction of the primary canines at age 8.5–9.5 years to encourage alignment of the permanent incisors
- extraction of the first primary molars approximately 1 year later to encourage eruption of the first premolars
- extraction of the first premolars as the permanent canines are erupting.

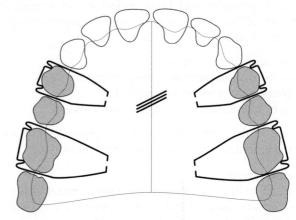

Fig. 111 Upper removable appliance to correct unilateral buccal segment crossbite with associated mandibular displacement. Midline expansion screw; Adams' clasps $\underline{6\ 4}\,|\,\underline{4\ 6}$; buccal capping.

This approach works best in children with class I malocclusion at about 9 years, with moderate crowding, average overbite and a full complement of teeth and where there is no doubt about the long-term prognosis of the first permanent molars. It was originally intended to remove the need for appliance therapy, but in practice this is seldom the case. In addition, extractions under general anaesthesia is an unpleasant and often frightening introduction to dentistry for any child, which may psychologically scar their attitude to subsequent dental treatment. As a result, the full extent of the original technique is never adopted in contemporary orthodontic practice, but consideration is often given to the need to extract the primary canines in the following instances:

- to allow labial movement of a lateral incisor erupting palatal to the central incisors and in potential crossbite
- to create space in the upper labial segment for proclination of an instanding lateral incisor or the eruption of an incisor, where a supernumerary tooth has delayed its appearance
- to promote alignment of a displaced permanent canine; this is particularly beneficial where the maxillary canine is displaced palatally
- to facilitate lingual movement of a labially placed permanent lower incisor with reduced periodontal support or of the lower labial segment to aid anterior crossbite correction in class III malocclusion.

Other developmental problems

Early loss of primary teeth

Early loss of primary teeth is most commonly caused by caries but occasionally it results from premature exfoliation, often when there is severe crowding, or it may be planned, for example to encourage space closure by mesial drift of the buccal segments in children who are missing one or more permanent teeth. In all cases, consideration should be given to balancing (extraction of a tooth on the opposite side of the arch, which may not be the same tooth type) or to compensating (extraction of the equivalent opposing tooth) for an extraction. Premature loss of a primary tooth does not inevitably lead to premature eruption of the permanent successor.

The effects of early loss of a primary tooth depends on several factors including:

- the patient's age
- the degree of crowding
- the tooth extracted
- the arch from which it is removed
- the type of occlusion.

All of these influence the potential for crowding to be concentrated at the extraction site. In general, this potential is greatest in a very young child with pre-existing crowding when a maxillary posterior tooth is removed with poor buccal segment intercuspation.

Incisors. Early loss of a primary incisor tends to have minimal effect as it usually exfoliates in the early mixed dentition. Premature loss of a primary incisor through trauma may, however, lead to dilaceration of the permanent successor.

Canines. Unilateral loss of a primary canine invariably leads to movement of the centreline and should be balanced to prevent this occurring.

First molars. Occasionally, displacement of the centreline follows early extraction of a first primary molar, but the need for a balancing extraction is best assessed by checking the midlines at subsequent reviews.

Second deciduous molars. Where the second primary molar is extracted, the first permanent molar migrates mesially and may lead to considerable space loss if the extraction is carried out before the permanent molar erupts. The second premolar may be excluded palatally and in crossbite. In very crowded conditions, loss of the second primary molar before 7 years of age may promote centreline shift, and the need for balancing or compensating extractions should be considered carefully

Space maintenance for early tooth loss

Space maintenance is indicated

- when premature loss of a tooth promotes crowding in an otherwise acceptable occlusion
- in severely crowded mouths where all of the extraction space is required for alignment of the remaining teeth
- following traumatic loss of an upper incisor.

A removable appliance will usually suffice in the upper arch but a lingual arch soldered to bands cemented to molar teeth is best in the lower.

Upper median diastema

Upper median diastema is a normal phase of dental development and usually reduces as the permanent maxillary canines erupt. It may, however, also result from

- a midline supernumerary tooth
- missing or small upper lateral incisors
- incisor proclination
- a more generalised spacing condition.

A radiograph of the upper incisor area should be taken to exclude the presence of a supernumerary tooth in those with a large midline diastema. The maxillary frenum may contribute to the persistence of a median diastema. Tell-tale signs of fraenal involvement include blanching of the palatal mucosa on stretching the frenum and a 'V' shaped notch interdentally between the upper central incisors on radiograph. The need for fraenectomy is best assessed after eruption of the permanent canines and during subsequent orthodontic treatment. A fixed appliance is usually required to close an upper midline space, with bodily approximation of the incisors followed by palatal bonded retention.

Dilaceration

Dilaceration is a sudden angular alteration in the long axis of the crown or in the root of a tooth. Most commonly it results from intrusion of a primary incisor driving the crown of the permanent successor palatally, and it leads to enamel and dentine hypoplasia. On occasion, dilaceration is developmental in origin, with a characteristic labial and superior coronal deflection of the affected tooth. Usually a dilacerated incisor remains unerupted and requires surgical removal, but if the dilaceration is mild, surgical exposure and orthodontic alignment may be feasible when the root apex is destined not to perforate the cortical plate.

Traumatic loss of an upper permanent central incisor

As the adjacent teeth tend to tilt toward the site of loss in the first days following trauma, the space must be maintained, ideally by immediate reimplantation of the tooth or by fitting a denture carrying a replacement tooth. Later, autotransplantation of a premolar or adhesive bridgework may be considered. This is generally preferable to space closure, as a lateral incisor rarely gives an optimum appearance in a central incisor position, even with coronal build-up and gingival recontouring.

Incisors in crossbite

Early correction of an incisor crossbite is essential to prevent displacing occlusal forces compromising the periodontal support of the lower anterior teeth and to allow the occlusion to develop around an undisplaced condylar position. Provided there is likely to be adequate overbite of 2–3 mm, an upper removable appliance with a double-cantilever spring to procline the instanding incisor will usually suffice. It may be necessary to remove the upper primary canines to facilitate crossbite correction on a lateral incisor or the lower primary canines to allow alignment of a labially placed lower incisor tooth.

Habits

Depending on the positioning of a finger(s) or thumb, the frequency and intensity of a sucking habit may

- procline the upper incisors
- retrocline the lower incisors
- increase the overjet, often asymmetrically
- reduce the overbite
- lead to a crossbite tendency of the buccal segments.

Gentle persuasion to discontinue the habit should be given and simple measures adopted to effect this.

Increased overjet

Where the overjet is greater than 10 mm, the risk of incisor trauma is twice as great as when it is 5 mm or less; the risk is also significantly greater in boys than in girls. An initial phase of functional appliance therapy to retract the incisors is beneficial in these children but seldom produces complete correction of the malocclusion. Often it is necessary to proceed to a second phase of treatment when the permanent dentition is fully erupted. This usually involves fixed appliances to detail the occlusion in combination with premolar extractions for relief of crowding. An early start to overjet correction can lead to protracted treatment, as the functional appliance will need to be worn as a retainer at least until a possible second phase of treatment commences and most likely until growth is complete. As this places considerable demands on patient cooperation, the likely benefits of early treatment must be deemed to outweigh any potential disadvantages before commencing on this course. There is also a potential risk of upper incisor root resorption if these teeth are retracted into the upper canine eruption path.

Ectopic maxillary canines

The maxillary canine is ectopic in approximately 2% of the population, with 15% of these buccal and 85% palatal to the arch. Development of the maxillary canine begins about 4–5 months after birth and the crown is complete around 6–7 years of age. From an initial position high in the maxilla, the tooth moves buccally downwards and forwards to be guided into its final position by the distal aspect of the lateral incisor root. For this reason, absence or diminution in the size of the lateral incisor promotes displacement. There also appears to be a greater incidence of palatal canine displacement where the maxillary arch is spaced or in class II division 2 malocclusion, while buccal displacement is more common in crowded arches. Where routine palpation of the buccal sulcus at 10 years fails to detect a canine prominence, the path of eruption is likely to be abnormal. In addition, considerable delay in the eruption of a canine compared with its antimere points to canine displacement.

Transposition

Transposition is when the position of the canine is interchanged with that of an adjacent tooth. In the upper arch, the maxillary canine and first premolar, or the lateral incisor and canine, are involved, although the former arrangement is more common. In the lower arch, this anomaly affects solely the lateral incisor and canine teeth.

Estimating the maxillary canine position

Clinical estimate. Buccal and palatal palpation along with observation of the lateral incisor inclination give a hint to the canine position. When it is lying low and palatal or high and buccal, the lateral incisor is likely to be labially inclined.

Radiographic estimation. Although a dental panoramic tomogram is helpful in initial assessment of canine position, further radiographic views are needed to locate the position of the tooth. Most commonly a standard maxillary oblique occlusal view or two periapical films taken with a tube shift are needed to allow localisation, using vertical or horizontal parallax respectively. The axial inclination, apex location and the vertical and mesiodistal position of the canine relative to the incisor roots should be assessed. The permanent incisors should be checked carefully to exclude resorption, and the root length of the primary canine noted. If incisor resorption is detected, urgent treatment is indicated. Removal of the impacted canine may arrest the resorption but extraction of the incisor may be required in those with severe resorption.

Management of canine displacement

The management of buccal or palatal maxillary canine displacement including transposition is described in Table 34.

Anomalies of size and form

Size

Teeth of a size that is greater or less than the norms for gender and for a given population are described as 'megadont' or 'microdont' respectively.

Megadontia has a prevalence of 1.1% in the permanent dentition, with maxillary central incisors most frequently affected, although lower second premolars are affected occasionally. The normal shape and absence of incisor notching distinguishes megadont maxillary incisors from 'double teeth'. Megadont teeth may be found unilaterally on the affected side in unilateral facial hyperplasia, but more generalised megadontia is associated with gigantism. A megadont upper incisor may produce crowding, an increased overjet or both. If the tooth is only slightly enlarged, removal of about 1 mm of enamel from each proximal surface and appliance therapy to close the resultant space may suffice. In gross enlargement, extraction of the affected tooth and place-

ment of a pontic following any appliance treatment may be necessary.

Microdontia is frequently seen in association with hypodontia, in Down syndrome and in ectodermal dysplasia. The prevalence is 0.2–0.5% in the primary dentition and 2.5% in the permanent dentition, with diminutive upper lateral incisors accounting for 1–2% of the latter. Short roots are often found on these teeth, which may be a factor in the aetiology of palatally displaced canines. In crowded mouths, where the lateral incisor is peg-shaped on one side of the arch and of normal size on the opposite side, removal of both lateral incisors may be optimal to achieve symmetry in the upper labial segment. If the diminutive lateral incisor is retained, orthodontic treatment should first create sufficient space to ensure that the tooth can be restored to normal dimensions. This space is maintained for at least 3 months with metal spurs on a removable retainer prior to final restoration.

Form

Double teeth

- have a prevalence of 0.1–0.2% in the permanent dentition
- are equally common in males and females
- occur in incisors more frequently than other tooth types.

Clinical appearance can vary from an incisal notch in a tooth of enlarged mesiodistal width to an anomaly resembling two separate crowns. Treatment is best delayed until the pulp has receded. Separation may be possible if there are two separate pulp chambers and root canals, but recontouring of the crown to resemble two separate teeth or reduction of its mesiodistal width may be possible where one pulp chamber exists.

Prevalence in the primary dentition is 0.5–1.6% in Caucasians and it affects teeth mostly in the mandibular labial segment. In the presence of hypodontia, double primary teeth are followed usually by absence of permanent teeth, but supernumerary teeth are more common in the permanent dentition if all of the primary teeth are present. Occasionally eruption of the permanent successor is delayed if a double primary tooth exists, and its removal, possibly in conjunction with that of permanent supernumeraries, may be indicated to allow eruption of the permanent teeth.

Accessory cusps and evaginated teeth

In the primary dentition, the maxillary molars are most commonly affected by additional cusps whereas the incisors, particularly the upper incisors, premolars and molars may be affected in the permanent dentition. An

Table 34 Management of maxillary canine displacement[a]

	Treatment options	Indications	Comments
Buccal displacement	Early removal of 4 before 3 erupts	Moderate crowding	May require removable or sectional fixed appliance to align 3 depending on axial inclination
	Exposure of 3	Delayed eruption of 3	Apically repositioned flap or replaced flap required at surgery Bond bracket, gold chain or magnet to 3 to facilitate alignment
	Removal of 3	Severe crowding with 2 and 4 in contact 3 severely displaced	May require fixed appliance to close any remaining space
Palatal displacement	Early removal of c	Ectopic position of 3 detected at 10 to 13 years of age 3 overlaps up to half width of 2	Extract contralateral c to prevent centreline shift; extraction of c may promote crowding
		3 crown below the apical third of 2 root 3 long axis to midsagittal plane ≤30° Ideally, crowding in arch no greater than mild	Failure of 3 to erupt will leave space
	Exposure of 3	Well-disposed patient	Bond bracket, gold chain or magnet to 3 at surgery
		Good oral hygiene and dentition	May commence alignment of 3 with removable appliance but fixed appliance usually required to align apex of 3
		3 overlaps less than half width of 1 and below the apical third of 2 root 3 root apex is not distal to 5 and 3 long axis ≤ 30° to midsagittal plane Spaced arch or possible to create space	
	Transplantation	Hopeless prognosis for alignment of 3	Prognosis improved if root of 3 is two-thirds formed, minimal handling of the root at surgery and avoidance of rigid splinting
		Adequate space in arch for 3 Intact removal of 3 possible Adequate buccal/palatal bone	Approximately 70% survival rate at 5 years
	Removal of 3	Hopeless prognosis for alignment of 3 Patient not keen for appliance therapy or evidence of incisor resorption or dentigerous cyst 2 and 4 in contact Good root length on c and aesthetics of c acceptable	Prosthetic replacement of c required when lost
	Retain 3	Occasionally in a young patient who is uncertain about treatment at present but may elect to proceed with alignment of 3 later	Periodic radiographic examination of incisors required to exclude resorption
Transposition	Accept	Transposition complete	
	Extraction of the most displaced tooth	If crowding present	
	Orthodontic alignment	Sufficient space in the arch	Apical positions of the transposed teeth will determine whether alignment is carried out in the transposed positions or if these are corrected

[a] In each case, the patient's interest in orthodontic treatment, their level of dental awareness and general features of the malocclusion (including the degree of crowding or spacing and the condition of the primary canine (if present) and adjacent teeth) must be assessed before the final treatment plan can be devised.

additional cusp on a maxillary incisor is termed a 'talon' cusp. As well as being unsightly, it may produce an occlusal interference or predispose to caries between the cusp and the palatal surface of the incisor. Treatment may be either by removal of the cusp and localised pulpotomy or by progressive grinding to encourage secondary dentine formation.

Evagination is characterised by a conical tuberculated prominence on the occlusal surface of a tooth and affects premolars most commonly. Treatment is as recommended for talon cusps.

9.2 Class I malocclusion

Learning objectives

You should

- know the possible aetiological factors in class I malocclusion
- understand the principles of treatment planning.

Aetiology

Skeletal factors

The skeletal pattern may be class I, class II or class III with the incisors compensating for any underlying skeletal discrepancy. An increase in lower anterior face height or a mild transverse skeletal discrepancy may also occur, creating an anterior open bite or buccal segment crossbite, respectively.

Soft tissues factors

Apart from bimaxillary proclination where labial movement of the incisors may result from tongue pressure in the presence of unfavourable lip tone, the soft tissues are not prime aetiological factors.

Dental factors

A tooth/dental arch size discrepancy leading to crowding or spacing is the principal cause of class I malocclusion. Other factors, however, such as early loss of primary teeth, large or small teeth, supernumerary or absent teeth can also influence any inherent dentoalveolar disproportion.

Occlusal features

There are several typical occlusal features.

- 'The lower incisor edges occlude with, or lie immediately below, the cingulum plateau of the upper central incisors' (British Standards Institute classification). Not all of the incisors, however, may relate in this manner. Provided the overall anteroposterior labial segment relationship is normal, even where a crossbite exists on one or two upper incisors, the incisor relationship may be regarded as class I.
- The molar relationship is variable and depends on whether mesial drift has followed any previous extractions.
- Crowding is often concentrated in the upper canine and lower second premolar areas as these teeth often erupt last in each arch.
- Crowding may also displace one or more teeth into crossbite and create a premature contact on closure, with associated mandibular displacement and centreline shift.

Treatment

The need for treatment on dental health grounds is most commonly related to the presence of crowding or displacement of teeth, which may be caused by crowding, although ectopic developmental position, the presence of a supernumerary, retention of a primary tooth or, rarely, a pathological cause may be responsible. Treatment may be indicated also for spacing or for the management of vertical or transverse problems (see Sections 9.1 and 9.5).

Treatment planning

The basic principles of treatment planning have already been outlined in Section 8.4.

Crowding

The possible measures to be considered in relation to the management of crowding have been presented in Section 9.1. Some basic guidelines, however, regarding the management of crowding in class I malocclusion are as follows:

- Mild crowding, often present as the permanent incisors erupt, may resolve with some increase in intercanine width and use of leeway space. If present when the permanent dentition is established, it is best accepted.
- Moderate crowding is usually dealt with by first premolar extractions. Where this is undertaken in a growing patient, considerable spontaneous improvement in labiolingual alignment of the incisors and canines will ensue in the following 6 months provided the canines are mesially tilted and movement is not hindered by the occlusion. Thereafter, the potential for further spontaneous change is much less, and fixed appliances are usually required to correct residual occlusal discrepancies.
- Severe crowding often may be managed expediently by the removal of the most displaced teeth or, on occasion, by the extraction of more than one tooth

per quadrant. Anchorage planning is most critical in this group and the placement of space maintainers prior to any proposed extractions is almost always necessary.

- Late lower labial segment crowding occurs commonly in mid-to late teens and gradually increases throughout the third and fourth decade, representing largely an adaptation to growth changes in the facial skeleton. Other factors have also been implicated (Table 27 in Chapter 8), but the evidence relating the mandibular third molar to late lower incisor crowding is equivocal.

It is important that any possible treatment is considered in the context of overall management of the malocclusion. Mild crowding is best accepted and monitored.

Where the posterior occlusion is class I and the arches otherwise aligned with a mildly increased overbite, moderate-to-severe lower incisor crowding may be dealt with by extraction of one or two incisors folowed by alignment and approximation of the remaining units using a sectional fixed appliance. A bonded lingual retainer is advisable to maintain the result, but lingual movement of the lower labial segment may produce reciprocal palatal movement of the upper incisors and lead to their misalignment. This must be drawn to the patient's attention before treatment starts.

Bimaxillary proclination

Bimaxillary proclination (proclination of upper and lower incisors) is seen typically in Negros, where it can be regarded as normal, but it may occur also in Caucasians in association with class I, class II division 1 or class III maloclusions. In class I, the overjet is increased because of the incisor angulation. Treatment to retract the upper and lower labial segments is generally unstable, as lingual movement of the lower incisors away from their zone of labiolingual balance tends to relapse post-treatment unless retained permanently. The prospect of stability may be improved where the lips have good muscle tone and become competent following incisor retroclination. Where the soft tissue factors are unfavourable, for example grossly incompetent lips, treatment is inadvisable.

Spacing

In Caucasians, a generally spaced dentition is rare and is caused by a disproportion in the size of the teeth relative to the arch size or by absence of teeth. Where the spacing is mild, acceptance is usually best. Alternatively, consideration may be given to composite additions or porcelain veneers to increase the mesiodistal width of the labial segment teeth. In more marked spacing, orthodontic treatment to concentrate the space at specific sites

prior to fitting of a prosthesis or implant placement may be necessary.

Space between the upper central incisors is more common. Although this often exists in the early mixed dentition, it usually reduces considerably as the permanent maxillary canine erupts. An upper median diastema may be caused also by

- an underlying mismatch in tooth/arch size
- small or absent lateral incisors
- a mesiodens
- proclination of the upper labial segment in a class II division 1 malocclusion
- digit sucking.

Rarely a low-lying attachment of the labial frenum is a primary cause, as the attachment usually recedes as the incisors approximate. In a spaced arch, this does not occur, indicating that the frenum is associated with, but not causative of, the diastema.

Where the frenum is implicated in causing a diastema, blanching of the incisive papilla usually occurs when the lip is pulled upwards or outwards, with characteristic 'V'-shaped notching of the alveolar bone between the two central incisors that is visible radiographically. Frenectomy is best carried out during space closure with a fixed appliance as the resulting scar tissue will aid approximation of the central incisors. Palatal bonded retention is essential to prevent relapse. On average, the mesiodistal width of the upper lateral incisor is 80% that of the central incisor. Where the lateral incisor is narrower, it should be enlarged by composite or porcelain additions to assist maintenance of diastema closure.

In patients with missing upper lateral incisors, the resulting space may be opened, closed or accepted.

9.3 Class II malocclusion

Learning objectives

You should

- understand the possible aetiology of division 1 and 2 malocclusions

- appreciate those factors that require special consideration in treatment planning

- know what features are necessary if treatment of division 1 malocclusion is to be undertaken by upper removable appliance therapy alone

- know the treatment possibilities for moderate-to-severe class II skeletal relationship

- understand the principles of management of class II malocclusion.

Class II malocclusions are divided into divisions 1 and 2.

Division 1

Aetiology

The following factors contribute to the production of a class II division 1 malocclusion.

Skeletal relationships

Although the skeletal relationship is usually class II, class II division 1 malocclusion may exist on a class I or mild class III skeletal pattern. Where a class II skeletal pattern is present, mandibular deficiency is almost entirely the primary cause, although excessive maxillary growth or a combination of the two may be factors in other instances. In contrast, the developmental position or inclination of the teeth resulting from soft tissue or digit-sucking influences are to blame where the skeletal pattern is class I or mildly class III. The anterior vertical proportions of the face vary, and where these are greatly increased or reduced treatment is likely to be difficult.

Lips, tongue and habits

The effects of the lips and tongue on the incisor position are determined principally by the skeletal pattern and thereafter by the manner in which an anterior oral seal is achieved. Where the skeletal pattern is class II, an acceptable incisor relationship may be achieved by proclination of the lower incisors under the influence of the tongue. In general, however, the greater the class II skeletal discrepancy, the more likely the lips are to be incompetent and to contribute to upper incisor proclination. Where lip incompetence exists along with a class II skeletal pattern and a reduced lower facial height, an anterior oral seal is likely to be produced by the lower lip lying under the upper incisors. This worsens the overjet by proclining the upper and retroclining the lower incisor teeth. In rare cases, the lower lip may be hyperactive and contribute to a class II division 1 malocclusion by solely retroclining the lower incisors. Where the lower facial height is increased, an anterior oral seal is often produced largely by forward positioning of the tongue, thus tending to reduce the overbite further and compensate for the class II discrepancy by proclining the lower incisors.

In very rare instances, a primary atypical swallowing behaviour will cause an overjet increase, but distinguishing this from an adaptive tongue thrust is difficult.

The effect of a digit-sucking habit is to procline the upper incisors and retrocline the lower incisors although the overjet increase may be asymmetric depending on the positioning of the digit.

Crowding

Labial displacement of the upper or lower incisors caused by crowding may respectively worsen or ameliorate an overjet.

Occlusal characteristics

As forward mandibular posturing to disguise the overjet increase is seen in some patients, it is important to ensure that the mandible is in centric relation before recording the occlusal features.

- 'The lower incisor edges lie posterior to the cingulum plateau of the upper incisors; there is an increase in overjet and the upper incisors are usually proclined.' (British Standards Institute classification.)
- This malocclusion is seen in 25–30% of Caucasians and the upper incisors are often traumatised because of the increased overjet: the likelihood increasing by twofold where the overjet exceeds 9 mm compared with an overjet of 2–4 mm.
- Drying of the gingivae labial to the upper incisors may occur with grossly incompetent lips, and this will aggravate an established gingivitis.
- The overbite varies depending on the skeletal pattern, the presence or absence of an adaptive tongue thrust on swallowing, or the existence of a digit-sucking habit. It is commonly increased and complete, and sometimes traumatic, with the lower incisors impinging on the gingivae palatal to the upper incisors. It may also be incomplete or tend to an anterior open bite.
- Usually the molar relationship is class II, provided mesial drift following early loss of primary teeth has not occurred.

Treatment

There is little need for treatment where the overjet is mildly increased and the arches are aligned (3.5–6 mm with competent lips; IOTN score 2). Here, the facial and dental appearance as well as the risk to dental health are minimal and acceptance of the malocclusion is reasonable.

Treatment is indicated where the overjet increase is greater than 6–9 mm or greater than 9 mm; the need for treatment on dental health grounds is great or very great, respectively.

The factors that must be considered regarding any potential treatment are discussed in Section 8.4.

Special considerations in treatment planning

Skeletal pattern In general, the more the anteroposterior and vertical skeletal relationships deviate from normal, the more likely the profile is to be compromised and the more difficult treatment is likely to be.

Mandibular growth The amount and pattern of mandibular growth can aid or detract from correction of a class II division 1 malocclusion in the growing patient. A forward mandibular growth pattern is favourable and is generally associated with situations where the lower facial height is reduced. A backward pattern of mandibular growth seen in individuals with increased lower facial height is unfavourable because the class II skeletal pattern is aggravated and the likelihood of lip competence post-treatment is reduced. In the non-growing patient, correction of both overbite and overjet of skeletal origin is difficult, and surgical correction may be required.

Form and relationship of the lips and tongue at rest and in function It is important to assess the likely impact of the lips and tongue in the aetiology of the malocclusion and, more importantly, whether a stable correction is possible by altering or correcting their influence. As a digit-sucking habit may affect the swallowing pattern and the incisor position, it should be ceased before treatment commences.

Space requirements Space is required in the lower and upper arches for overbite reduction and overjet correction, respectively, in addition to that needed for possible relief of crowding. On occasion this may necessitate the loss of four units in the upper arch, usually where the lower labial segment is crowded and the buccal segment relationship is more than class II.

Where the lower arch is aligned, the buccal segment relationship typically half a unit class II and the overjet increase modest, space for overjet reduction may be obtained by moving the upper buccal segment distally using headgear. This may be facilitated by removal of the upper second permanent molars once good co-operation with the headgear has been demonstrated.

Overbite and overjet Overbite reduction must always precede overjet reduction.

Treatment in class I or mild class II skeletal relationship

Treatment using upper removable appliances may be considered where

- The FMPA is average or slightly reduced.
- There are no unfavourable soft tissue factors, e.g. grossly incompetent lips or primary tongue thrust.
- The lower arch is uncrowded, has mild acceptable crowding or is moderately crowded with $\overline{3}/\overline{3}$ mesially inclined and no incisor rotations.
- 3/3 are mesially inclined.
- The upper incisors are free of rotations and sufficiently proclined that, when the overjet is reduced, they will form no less than a 95° angle to the maxillary plane.
- The patient is growing, as this will facilitate tooth movement particularly overbite reduction and spontaneous closure of any residual lower arch spacing.

A typical treatment sequence is given in Box 41. The highest quality outcome, however, is to be obtained with fixed appliances. Where occlusal factors (in particular, the inclination of the canines and maxillary incisors)

Box 41 Treatment sequence for class II division 1 malocclusion by upper removable appliance therapy

1. Fit a an upper removable appliance (URA) to retract 3|3 and reduce the overbite (Fig. 112). A suitable appliance design would be as follows (see Section 10.1 for details of components): buccal or palatal springs to retract 3|3 depending on position of 3s; Adams' clasps 6|6 (consider adding EOT tubes if anchorage is at a premium); Southend clasp 1|1; full palatal acrylic coverage with a flat anterior bite plane to half the height of 1|1. A measure of the overjet plus 3 mm must also be sent to the laboratory to ensure the correct horizontal extension of the bite plane.
2. When the patient is wearing the URA satisfactorily on a full-time basis, extract first premolars (assuming first permanent molars are sound and second premolars present) and proceed to retract 3s to a class I relationship with 3s, taking account of any distal movement of 3.
3. Then fit a URA to retract 2 1|1 2 (Fig. 113). A suitable appliance design would be: Roberts retractor to 2 1|1 2; Adams clasps 6|6; flat 'stops' mesial of 3s; full palatal acrylic coverage with a flat anterior bite plane to half the height of 1|1 to maintain overbite reduction. The acrylic must be trimmed back behind the upper incisors but maintain contact with the lower incisors until the final stages of overjet reduction.
4. A retainer should then be fitted (Fig. 114): labial bow 3 2 1|1 2 3; Adams clasps 6|6; full palatal acrylic coverage. Provided favourable factors for stability exist, the patient is instructed to wear it usually full-time for at least 3 months and then at night for a minimum of another 3 months.

---

are not amenable to tipping movements, fixed appliances are indicated (often in combination with extractions to allow relief of crowding) for correction of the incisor and buccal segment relationships. Removal of lower second and upper first premolars often favours the attainment of these occlusal goals.

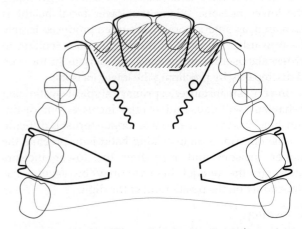

Fig. 112 Upper removable appliance to retract 3|3 and reduce a complete deep overbite (assuming 3|3 are in the line of the arch and 4|4 are to be extracted).

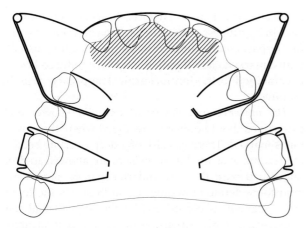

Fig. 113 Upper removable appliance to retract 2 1 | 1 2, while maintaining 3 | 3 retraction and overbite reduction. Teeth 4 | 4 have been extracted.

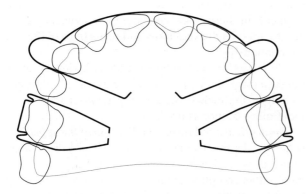

Fig. 114 Retainer to be used following overjet reduction.

In the mixed dentition with a mild/moderate class II pattern, overjet reduction may be carried out using a functional appliance, although this is often followed by a phase of fixed appliance treatment, sometimes in combination with extractions, to optimise the final occlusal result.

Treatment in moderate-to-severe class II skeletal relationship
Three possibilities exist in relation to treatment in moderate-to-severe class II skeletal relationships.

Growth modification Growth modification is only possible in the growing child. Ideally the arches should be uncrowded. Treatment should be undertaken just before and/or during the pubertal growth spurt. Success depends on creating a differential in the rate of growth of the maxilla and mandible. Depending on the relative contribution of maxillary prognathism or mandibular retrusion to the skeletal class II malocclusion, an attempt may be made to restrain horizontal and/or vertical maxillary growth, stimulate mandibular growth or both. While headgear appears to restrain

maxillary growth with forces of up to 1000 g in total, a functional appliance may in addition stimulate mandibular growth. Wear of either or both for 14–16 hours per day, in conjunction with favourable growth, is necessary for a successful outcome.

Wear of the appliance as a retainer until growth has reduced to adult levels is then required, unless a second phase of treatment to align the arches with fixed appliances and possibly extractions are considered.

Orthodontic camouflage The skeletal discrepancy can be disguised by orthodontic tooth movement; this corrects the incisor relationship but the class II skeletal pattern remains. Invariably, treatment involves upper arch extractions, most commonly first premolars, and fixed appliance therapy to retract the incisors bodily. The effect of repositioning the teeth must not have a detrimental effect on the facial profile, otherwise 'camouflage' will have failed. Realistically this option is only acceptable where the class II skeletal pattern is no worse than moderate, the vertical facial proportions are good and the arches are reasonably well aligned so that the extraction spaces can be used for overjet reduction and not for relief of crowding.

Orthognathic surgery Where growth is complete and camouflage would not produce optimal facial and dental aesthetics, surgical correction of the malocclusion is best (see Section 9.6).

Retention and post-treatment stability
The interincisal angle should be within normal limits, the overjet completely reduced with the upper incisors in soft tissue balance (i.e. no tongue thrust) and the lower lip covering at least one third of their labial surface. Where these criteria are met, a few months of retention to allow adaptation of the periodontium and soft tissues will usually suffice, but retention until growth is complete is required following functional appliance treatment.

Division 2

Aetiology

Skeletal relationships
The skeletal pattern in division 2 malocclusion is usually mildly class II, although it may be class I or mildly class III. A reduced or average lower facial height is common, associated with an anterior mandibular growth rotation, which tends to increase the overbite. A relatively wide maxillary base may lead to a lingual crossbite of the first premolars.

Soft tissues
The lips are usually competent and the lower lip line high (covering more than one third of the incisor crown), the most significant factor in the aetiology. The lower lip level depends largely on the lower anterior

facial height. In general, the more reduced the lower anterior facial height, the higher the lower lip line is likely to be. Where the lower lip is also hyperactive, bimaxillary retroclination will result.

Dental factors

The cingulum on the upper incisors is often reduced or absent, which may exacerbate the overbite. In addition, the likelihood of the teeth being smaller than normal is increased, as is the chance of a more acute crown/root angulation. Retroclination of the upper and possibly of the lower incisors also makes existing crowding worse.

Occlusal features

The main occlusal features are:

- 'The upper central incisors are retroclined. The overjet is minimal but may be increased' (British Standards Institute classification)
- the upper lateral incisors are often proclined and mesiolabially rotated but they may also be retroclined
- occasionally upper and lower incisors are retroclined, usually associated with a high lower lip line where the lip is hyperactive
- the overbite may be traumatic: palatal to the upper incisors, labial to the lowers or, in severe cases, in both locations
- because of the discrepancy in arch widths and the class II skeletal relationship, a scissors bite is often present in the first premolar area.

Treatment

Treatment planning

The following factors in particular must be considered in relation to treatment planning.

The underlying skeletal discrepancy, both anteroposteriorly and vertically In general the more class II the skeletal pattern and the lower the FMPA, the more difficult treatment is likely to be to achieve a normal incisor relationship.

The growth potential and pattern of facial growth In a growing patient, correction of both a class II skeletal pattern and deep overbite is facilitated by favourable facial growth. Although a forward mandibular growth rotation aids correction of a class II skeletal discrepancy, it tends to increase the overbite unless the centre of rotation becomes the lower incisor edges by altering the interincisal angle with treatment and creating an occlusal stop.

Profile considerations Occasionally a non-extraction approach may be adopted, usually in those with bimaxillary retroclination, to prevent the proposed risk of adverse profile change that may result from an

extraction-based plan. There is, however, little difference in lip fullness with either approach. When the profile is particularly unfavourable in an adult, usually with a marked class II pattern and very reduced FMPA, a combined orthodontic/surgical approach will be required.

The presence and degree of crowding Lower arch extractions should only be considered where the crowding is marked. There is a risk of a deep overbite becoming traumatic as the lower incisors are allowed to drop lingually if extractions are undertaken in the presence of mild-to-moderate crowding. In addition, as the lower labial segment is constricted by the upper labial segment, some stable expansion of the lower intercanine width and proclination of the lower incisors may be feasible, thereby providing space for relief of mild-to-moderate crowding. Where extractions are necessary, a lower fixed appliance should be used to close residual spacing and prevent retroclination of the lower labial segment. In these cases, consideration should be given also to upper arch extractions and corrections of the incisor relationship.

The lower lip level Where the lower lip level is at the gingival third of the upper incisor crowns or higher, correction of the incisor relationship without recourse to indefinite retention is unlikely.

The depth of overbite and inclination of the upper incisors The depth of overbite and the inclination of the upper incisors determine the two approaches to treatment: either accepting or altering the incisor relationship. *Overbite reduction* may be achieved by various means, including

- molar eruption/extrusion
- upper and/or lower incisor intrusion
- lower incisor proclination
- through a combination of these methods
- by surgery.

In addition, proclination of the upper incisors, followed by a functional appliance to correct the overjet created, will reduce the overbite.

In a growing patient, use of a flat anterior bite plane on an upper removable appliance will retard lower incisor eruption while allowing the lower posterior teeth to erupt, thereby reducing the overbite. Facial growth then accommodates the increase in lower facial height. As this is not possible in the adult, overbite reduction must be by incisor intrusion rather than by molar extrusion. Extrusion of the upper molars by cervical headgear, or of both upper and lower molars using intra-oral elastics attached to a fixed appliance, is only advisable in a growing patient as a means of overbite reduction. Attempts to intrude the incisors by, for example, utility arches produce effects that are more apparent than real, as the incisors are generally held at their original occlusal level while the molars are encouraged to erupt. This, together with the continuing vertical facial growth, leads to overbite reduction. Intrusion of the upper labial segment may be attempted also by attaching high-pull headgear to the anterior part of the archwire incorporated in an upper fixed appliance.

Lower incisor proclination is not usually stable unless the lower incisors have been held in a retroclined position behind the cingulum of the upper incisors. Fitting an upper removable appliance with a flat anterior bite plane will allow spontaneous labial movement of the lower incisors to adopt a position of labiolingual balance. Careful planning by a specialist is required if active proclination of the lower incisors is considered.

A combined orthodontic/surgical approach is best in adults where the overbite is deep and the skeletal pattern is markedly class II.

Treatment in class I or mild class II skeletal pattern

Where the overbite and retroclination of 1/1 or 21/12 are to be accepted Where the upper labial segment crowding and retroclination are mild and the overbite acceptable, it is reasonable that no active treatment be undertaken. If treatment is indicated, however, it is confined to relief of upper arch crowding and alignment of the upper labial segment alone.

Planning starts with the lower arch (see Section 8.4). If the lower arch is acceptable, mild upper arch crowding in the presence of, at most, a half unit class II molar relationship may be dealt with by distal movement of the upper buccal segment using headgear (see Section 10.1) followed by canine retraction just sufficient for upper labial segment alignment. Extraction of upper second permanent molars may be necessary to facilitate buccal segment retraction. Although a series of upper removable appliances may be used where appropriate, class II division 2 malocclusion is rarely amenable to such treatment, the occlusal characteristics dictating the need for fixed appliances in almost all cases. Rather than resort to headgear, an alternative approach is removal of upper second premolars followed by fixed appliance therapy. Where a full unit class II buccal segment relationship exists or extraction of lower second premolars is necessary to relieve crowding, removal of upper first premolars is indicated.

Where the overbite and retroclination of 1/1 or 21/12 are to be corrected Where the overbite is deep and complete on gingival or palatal tissues, with existing or potential trauma, as may occur with lingual tilting of the incisors following lower arch extractions, correction of the overbite and incisor inclination are indicated.

Usually fixed appliances are used to effect palatal root torque and reduce the overbite, sometimes by proclination of the lower incisors. Planning the final incisor positions requires considerable expertise, as proclination of the lower labial segment may stress the labial periodontium and create gingival recession, while the possible degree of palatal/labial root torque required is limited by the thickness of the alveolar processes. Anchorage demands are also increased because of the torquing movements.

Proclining the labial segment or extractions will provide space for relief of mild-to-moderate or severe lower arch crowding, respectively, while in the upper arch, space to correct the incisor relationship may be created by moving the buccal segments distally or by extractions. The interincisal angle must be reduced to at least 135° (preferably less) to give the best prospect of a stable correction. Permanent lower retention may be required depending on the amount of lower incisor proclination, and the addition of a flat anterior bite plane to an upper Hawley retainer is advisable to prevent overbite relapse. This should be worn until at least growth has reduced to adult levels.

Treatment in more marked class II skeletal discrepancy

In more marked class II skeletal pattern, the treatment options are growth modification or orthognathic surgery.

Growth modification In a growing child, with ideally a well-aligned lower arch, a functional appliance may be used to modify growth and correct the incisor relationship. To allow the mandible to be postured forward for the construction bite and to ensure favourable arch coordination post-treatment, the retroclined maxillary incisors must be proclined and the upper arch expanded prior to the functional appliance phase. Alignment is usually completed by fixed appliances, ideally followed by retention until the late teens.

Orthognathic surgery Where the facial profile is poor because of the marked skeletal discrepancy anteroposteriorly and/or vertically, and particularly in the adult with a deep traumatic overbite, a surgical approach in conjunction with orthodontics is best. A class II division 1 incisor relationship is created presurgically but the increased curve of Spee is maintained. Following mandibular advancement to correct the overjet and facial profile, the lower buccal segment teeth are extruded to level the arch and close the lateral open bites.

Post-treatment stability

Two features of class II division 2 malocclusion are particularly prone to relapse:

- the alignment of the upper lateral incisors, particularly where these were rotated pretreatment
- the overbite reduction.

Rotational overcorrection early in treatment and pericision should be undertaken to help to prevent relapse, but as these do not guarantee stability, bonded palatal retention long term is advisable, ensuring that this is supervised appropriately.

Stable overbite reduction requires the interincisal angle to reduce and a cingulum stop to be created where one is reduced or absent. An increase in lower facial height and inferior movement of the lower lip away from the upper labial segment (where these are principal aetiological factors) aids correction of the interincisal angle but is dependent on favourable vertical facial growth. Even where these features are evident, the closing pattern of mandibular growth tends to increase the overbite into adulthood. Following overbite correction, an upper removable retainer incorporating a flat anterior biteplane is recommended until growth is complete, but in many cases permanent retention is advisable.

9.4 Class III malocclusion

Learning objectives

You should

- understand the possible aetiology of class III malocclusion
- account for specific factors in treatment planning
- know the treatment possibilities.

Aetiology

Skeletal pattern

The skeletal pattern is most usually class III although it may be class I with the class III malocclusion due to incisor position or inclination. Mandibular, maxillary and cranial base factors often make a combined contribution to the underlying class III skeletal relationship through

- an increase in mandibular length
- forward placement of the glenoid fossa, positioning the mandible more anteriorly
- a short and/or retrognathic maxilla
- a short anterior cranial base.

The vertical relationship of the skeletal bases varies from increased to average or reduced and is generally reflected in the depth of overbite, which may alter depending on the pattern of facial growth. Where this is vertical rather than horizontal, an anterior open bite is likely.

Commonly, a transverse discrepancy exists in the dental base relationship because of the narrow maxillary and wider mandibular bases, although this is often worsened by the class III skeletal pattern.

Soft tissues

The soft tissues contribute little to the aetiology of the malocclusion. Instead, where the lips are competent, the lips and tongue induce retroclination of the lower and proclination of the upper incisors (dentoalveolar compensation); as a result, the incisor relationship masks the true severity of the skeletal pattern. Where the lower anterior facial height is increased, however, the lips are frequently incompetent, with an adaptive tongue thrust on swallowing which may procline the lower incisors.

Dental factors

Crowding is more common and more severe in the upper than in the lower arch, often resulting from the difference in length and width of the arches: the upper frequently is short and narrow compared with a longer and wider lower arch.

Occlusal features

- 'The lower incisor edges lie anterior to the cingulum plateau of the upper incisors, the overjet is reduced or reversed' (British Standards Institute classification).
- The overbite may be increased, average or reduced. Where the vertical facial proportions are increased, there is often an anterior open bite.
- Frequently, the upper incisors are proclined and the lower incisors retroclined, compensating for the underlying class III skeletal pattern.
- Upper arch crowding is common, often because of a short and narrow dental base, while the lower arch is more commonly aligned or spaced.
- Crossbites of the labial and/or buccal segments are common, resulting from the underlying class III occlusal discrepancy as well as from differences in the length and width of the arches. Crossbites may be associated with a mandibular displacement (see Section 9.5) particularly where a unilateral buccal segment crossbite exists. In the case of an anterior crossbite, the possibility of displacement should be assessed by checking if the patient can occlude in an edge-to-edge incisor relationship. Lower incisor mobility and occasionally gingival recession may be associated with the anterior crossbite. This is more common in class I malocclusion where a single incisor is affected.

Treatment

Treatment planning

Account must be taken of the following factors.

The degree of anteroposterior and vertical skeletal discrepancy

The degree of anteroposterior and vertical skeletal discrepancy is the most important factor in planning treatment and assessing the prognosis. As it is usually directly reflected in the facial and dental appearance, it will influence also the complexity of treatment undertaken through the patient's perception of these characteristics.

The potential direction and extent of future facial growth

The general trend for downward and forward mandibular growth to surpass that of the maxilla is unfavourable for class III correction. Relevant family history, the age and gender of the patient, together with assessment of the vertical facial proportions, may help in making a 'guesstimate' as to the likely changes with growth. A reduced or average anterior vertical face height is often associated with a closing mandibular growth rotation, and a horizontal pattern of mandibular growth worsening the reverse overjet. With an increased vertical face height, there is a tendency for a backward mandibular rotation to increase the likelihood of anterior open bite.

The incisor inclinations

The incisor inclinations indicate the degree of dentoalveolar compensation; if this is already marked, further compensation by orthodontic means is unlikely to be stable or to produce an aesthetic result.

The amount of overbite

It is essential that there is an adequate overbite posttreatment to improve the prospects of stable overjet correction. Where the overbite is average or increased pretreatment, stability is more likely than where the overbite is reduced. Proclination of the upper incisors reduces the overbite while retroclination of the lower incisors increases it. Both movements may be necessary in some cases.

The ability to achieve an edge-to-edge incisor relationship

If it is not possible to achieve an edge-to-edge incisor relationship, correction of the incisor relationship by simple means is unlikely.

The degree of upper and lower arch crowding

The following should be borne in mind. Upper arch extractions should be delayed until a reverse overjet has been corrected. This may provide space for relief of mild-to-moderate upper arch crowding.

Where *extractions are undertaken in the upper arch only*, the reverse overjet may worsen with palatal movement of the upper labial segment.

Where *mid upper arch extractions are necessary*, extraction of lower first premolars is usually advisable to allow correction of the incisor relationship.

Treatment

No treatment is an option when the skeletal pattern is mildly class III and/or the incisor relationship is acceptable, with minimal crowding and no mandibular displacement.

Treatment in normal or mild class III skeletal pattern

Where the lower anterior face height is long, the overbite is usually minimal and the incisor relationship should be accepted. Treatment should focus on aligning the arches, with possible extractions. Upper arch expansion for crossbite correction will create space for relief of crowding. When this is indicated, fixed appliance mechanics must be used to minimise unfavourable dropping of the palatal cusps of the premolars and molars, as this will reduce the overbite further.

Provided the lower anterior vertical face height is average or short, with a normal or increased overbite and upright upper incisors, proclination of the upper labial segment may be undertaken. This is often best carried out in the early mixed dentition before the permanent canines move labial to the lateral incisor roots, thereby increasing the risk of resorption if their proclination is attempted. In such cases, treatment is best deferred until the canines have been retracted, removing the obstruction to crossbite correction of the lateral incisors. An upper removable appliance, incorporating a screw or Z-springs and posterior capping, may be used to correct the anterior crossbite (Fig. 115), but a fixed appliance may be indicated depending on the presence of other occlusal features.

The need for upper arch extractions should be reassessed after the incisor relationship has been corrected, as some additional space for relief of crowding will be forthcoming from anteroposterior expansion. Movement of the upper buccal segments distally is not a favoured option as restraint of maxillary growth is likely. Often, extraction of the lower primary canines in the early mixed dentition, or of first premolars in a crowded lower arch in the permanent dentition, is advantageous in allowing the lower labial segment to drop lingually and increase the overbite.

Treatment in mild-to-moderate class III skeletal pattern

Where the overbite is average or increased, two options exist: growth modification or orthodontic camouflage.

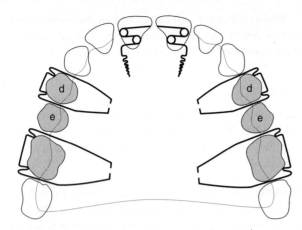

Fig. 115 Upper removable appliance to procline 1 | 1 in the early mixed dentition, assuming all primary teeth are in good condition. Double cantilever springs 1 | 1; Adams' clasps 6 d | d 6; posterior capping 2–3 mm in height to disengage the anterior occlusion.

Growth modification In general, attempts to modify growth in class III malocclusion are disappointing, largely because the inherent tendency for growth is unfavourable. Where the underlying skeletal problem is mild, however, caused by either maxillary deficiency or mandibular excess, an effort may be made in the early mixed dentition to augment forward maxillary growth or 'restrain' mandibular growth. Reverse-pull headgear applies tension to the posterior and superior maxillary sutures via a maxillary splint and is ideal where maxillary retrognathia exists in combination with average or reduced vertical facial proportions, and upright, or slightly proclined, upper incisors. Treatment must be started before 8 years to maximise the chances for successful forward movement.

Compressive forces applied to the condylar area via a chin cup have never been very successful, but if the force is aimed below the condyle, redirection rather than restraint of mandibular growth occurs. In essence, a downward and backward mandibular rotation is effected, which increases the lower anterior face height and reduces chin prominence. Lingual tipping of the lower incisors helps to correct the incisor relationship.

A functional appliance, particularly a Frankel III, may also be used for correction of mandibular prognathism, although only limited posterior mandibular posturing is possible. Mandibular growth is not restrained and the effects are similar to chin cup therapy where the force is directed below the condyle. For both chin cup and functional appliance therapy, the skeletal pattern should ideally be mildly class III with reduced vertical facial proportions, and the ability should exist to achieve an edge-to-edge incisor relationship with upright or proclined lower incisors. In all class III situations where growth modification is attempted, there is a need for prolonged retention of what is almost exclu-

sively a dentoalveolar change, while growth continues. This, coupled with the propensity for further mandibular growth, has tended to lessen the popularity of this approach for skeletal class III correction.

Orthodontic camouflage Orthodontic camouflage may also be considered where the overbite is mildly reduced. Treatment aims to correct the incisor relationship by retroclination of the lower labial segment and/or proclination of the upper labial segment. Lower arch extractions, preferably of first premolars, are usually necessary in conjunction with class III intermaxillary traction to upper and lower fixed appliances. Extrusion of the upper molars must be avoided as this will compromise the overbite. Lower arch extractions must only be undertaken where the likelihood of achieving successful overjet correction is favourable. Should the result relapse with further mandibular growth, surgical correction may be required. Any decompensation will need to be undone as part of presurgical orthodontics, which will result in opening up of the extraction spaces.

In some cases, proclination of the upper labial segment may be aided by reverse-pull headgear to the upper fixed appliance. More commonly this technique is reserved for use in cleft lip and palate or maxillary hypodontia to augment anchorage during upper arch space closure.

Treatment in severe class III skeletal pattern
Orthognathic surgery Where the skeletal discrepancy is moderate or severe, and therefore not amenable to satisfactory correction by orthodontic camouflage, the arches may be aligned and the incisor relationship accepted, or correction may be brought about by orthognathic surgery. The latter is usually preceded by fixed appliance therapy to decompensate the arches. Then, often a combination of maxillary advancement and/or posterior impaction with mandibular set back, and possibly a reduction genioplasty, is necessary to attain the optimal profile change.

9.5 Open bite and crossbite

Learning objectives

You should

- be aware of the aetiology of open bite and crossbite
- appreciate treatment possibilities and limitations of open bite management
- be able to classify crossbite
- know how to manage anterior crossbite correction with an upper removable appliance in favourable cases.

Open bite

An open bite may exist anteriorly or posteriorly in the arch.

Anterior open bite

The incisors do not overlap vertically when the posterior teeth are in occlusion.

Aetiology

Skeletal pattern An increase in lower facial height and high FMPA leads to an increase in the distance between the upper and lower incisors. Where it is not possible for the incisors to erupt sufficiently to compensate for the increased interocclusal distance, an incomplete or anterior open bite results. This is worsened by the downward and backward pattern of mandibular growth, which contributes to the likely additional class II skeletal pattern.

Soft tissues Rarely an open bite is caused by the action of the tongue. The forward positioning of the tongue to achieve an anterior oral seal is usually adaptive in those with increased vertical skeletal proportions, as there is a greater tendency for the lips to be incompetent. A similar swallowing pattern is often observed in children with an anterior open bite caused by a digit-sucking habit. Where a tongue thrust is endogenous/primary (which is rare), there is often a lisp and some proclination of upper and lower incisors.

Habits A persistent digit-sucking habit inhibits eruption of the incisors, often producing an asymmetric anterior open bite. Occasionally a posterior crossbite is produced through unopposed action of the cheek muscles as the tongue is lowered by the presence of the digit during sucking.

Localised failure of alveolar development A localised failure of alveolar development can occur in those with clefts of the lip and palate, but it can also occur where no cause is readily discernible.

Treatment

With the exception of when an anterior open bite is caused by a habit, treatment is complex and is best managed by a specialist.

Treatment in open bite caused by skeletal factors The open bite may be accepted if it is mild or where the prospect of stability is poor because of adverse skeletal and/or soft tissue factors, notably grossly incompetent lips and/or the suspicion of a primary tongue thrust.

Orthodontic management of anterior open bite The aim is to increase or at least maintain the overbite. Extrusion of molars, which may occur through use of a flat anterior bite plane on an upper removable appliance or cervical-pull headgear, must be avoided. Expansion of the upper arch, which is likely to extrude the palatal cusps and 'prop open' the bite, should also be avoided.

Assuming that there are no adverse growth or soft tissue factors, growth modification may be possible using high-pull headgear to the upper molars in mild open bite, or by attaching high-pull headgear to a removable or functional appliance with buccal capping where a class II skeletal pattern and a more marked anterior open bite exists. Where an anterior open bite is associated with a 'gummy smile', high pull headgear to a full-coverage maxillary splint is indicated. As extrusion of the incisors to close an anterior open bite is unstable, the aim in all cases is to attempt to maintain the vertical position of the maxilla while preventing eruption of the upper posterior teeth. Attempts to intrude the maxilla and modify growth require excellent patient cooperation, with a minimum of 14–16 hours per day wear of the headgear and any other appliance. Following correction of the anterior open bite, fixed appliances are often required, sometimes in conjunction with extractions, to detail the occlusion.

Occasionally, camouflage by incisor retraction following relief of crowding can be stable if the lips become competent post-treatment. The contention that extraction of molars may aid overbite increase is unproven.

Where the anterior open bite is severe, a combined orthodontic/surgical approach is best when growth is complete.

Treatment in open bite caused by habits Gentle discouragement of a digit-sucking habit in the early mixed dentition often leads to spontaneous correction of an anterior open bite, although it may take up to 3 years for the overbite to be regained. Fitting an upper removable appliance may act as a habit breaker and allow incisor retraction once the habit has ceased.

Treatment of open bite with aberrant soft tissue factors Where an endogenous tongue thrust is suspected or the lips are grossly incompetent, treatment is best withheld, as relapse of any treatment is guaranteed.

Posterior open bite

Posterior open bite exists where there is no contact between the buccal segment teeth when the remainder of the dentition is in occlusion.

It is very rare and the exact aetiology often incompletely understood. Causes include unilateral condylar hyperplasia. Here removal of the condyle is required if growth is excessively active. It is also caused, rarely, when the molar teeth fail to erupt despite apparent bone resorption in advance of the tooth, or eruption is arrested at a certain occlusal level while adjacent teeth maintain contact with the opposing teeth. In both cases, a posterior open bite will result and extraction of the molar is the only treatment option. A lateral open bite is occasionally seen in the buccal segments with submergence or following early loss of primary molars. In the latter situation, lateral tongue spread has been proclaimed as a cause, but it is likely that other factors operate. Any attempt to extrude the teeth into occlusion usually relapses. Lateral open bites usually occur bilaterally as a transient feature during twin block therapy but resolve as the buccal blocks are trimmed and the posterior teeth erupt into occlusion.

Crossbite

A crossbite is a buccolingual malrelationship of the upper and lower teeth. It can be anterior or posterior, unilateral or bilateral and may be associated with a mandibular displacement on closing. That is, an occlusal contact deflects the mandible laterally or anteriorly to allow maximum interdigitation. With a lateral displacement there is often a centre-line shift. By convention, the lower teeth are described relative to the upper so where the lower teeth occlude buccal to their opponents a buccal crossbite exists. Conversely, where the lower teeth occlude lingual to the palatal cusps of the upper teeth, a lingual (scissors) crossbite exists.

Aetiology

Skeletal factors
A mismatch in the widths of the dental arches or an anteroposterior skeletal discrepancy may produce a crossbite of a complete arch segment – a lingual crossbite commonly found in class II – while a buccal and/or anterior crossbite is often associated with a class III malocclusion.

Growth restriction of the maxilla following cleft repair or of the mandible secondary to condylar trauma can lead also to buccal segment crossbite.

Soft tissue factors
With a digit-sucking habit, the tongue is lowered and the cheeks' contraction during sucking is unopposed. This displaces the upper posterior teeth palatally and often creates a crossbite.

Crowding
Where the arch is inherently crowded, the upper lateral incisor may be displaced palatally and the upper second or third molar pushed into a scissors bite.

Local causes
Retention of a primary tooth or early loss of a primary second molar in a crowded arch can lead to the permanent successor erupting in crossbite.

Treatment

It is important to realise that where a crossbite is associated with a mandibular displacement, there is a functional indication for its correction, as displacing occlusal contacts may predispose to temporomandibular joint problems in susceptible individuals. In addition, a traumatic displacing anterior occlusion may deflect a lower incisor labially and compromise periodontal support.

Treatment of anterior crossbite
Where one or two incisors are in crossbite there is usually a mandibular displacement, and correction early in the mixed dentition is advisable provided adequate overbite exists to maintain correction. Space must be present in the arch (or can be created by extraction) to allow alignment of the tooth. If the tooth inclination is amenable to tipping, an upper removable appliance with buccal capping to free the occlusion and a Z-spring for proclination may be used. Anterior retention must be good to resist the displacing force caused by the action of the spring. Alternatively, an appliance with a screw section, clasping the teeth to be moved, overcomes this problem. Where insufficient overbite is likely to exist post-treatment, or the incisor is bodily displaced, treatment is better carried out with a fixed appliance in the permanent dentition. Treatment of anterior crossbite involving two or more incisors is considered in Section 9.4.

Treatment of unilateral buccal crossbite
An upper removable appliance incorporating a T-spring or screw section may often be considered for correcting a crossbite on a premolar or molar, respectively (Figs 116 and 117). However, where reciprocal movement of opposing teeth is needed, fixed attachments should be placed and cross-elastics used to achieve the desired movement. Where a single tooth is mildly displaced from the arch, relief of crowding may be necessary to aid crossbite correction. In those with more marked tooth displacement, extraction rather than orthodontic alignment may be a better option.

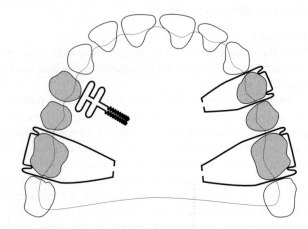

Fig. 116 Correction of crossbite on a premolar – upper removable appliance to move 4| buccally. T spring (0.5 mm stainless steel wire) to 4|: Adams' clasps 6|46; buccal capping, with acrylic relieved over 41.

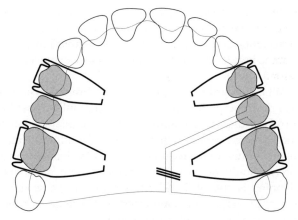

Fig. 117 Correction of crossbite on a molar – upper removable appliance to move |6 buccally. Screw section to move |6 buccally; Adams' clasps 6 4 | 4 6; buccal capping.

Where a unilateral buccal segment crossbite is associated with a mandibular displacement, this usually results from a mild mismatch in widths of the dental bases, often as a result of narrowing of the upper arch caused by digit sucking. Upper arch expansion using an upper removable appliance with midline expansion screw and buccal capping to disengage the occlusion, or by a quadhelix appliance, may be used for correction provided the teeth are not tilted buccally already. The quadhelix consists of a 1 mm stainless steel wire with four coils in the shape of a 'W'; it is attached to bands cemented to a molar tooth on each side of the arch. Alternatively, a preformed appliance may be slotted into welded attachments on the palatal aspect of the molar bands. Differential slow arch expansion anteriorly and/or posteriorly may be achieved following customary activation of 1.5 and 2 cm, respectively.

Treatment of bilateral buccal crossbite
A bilateral buccal crossbite is seldom associated with functional problems. Generally, as its existence indicates an underlying symmetrical transverse skeletal discrepancy, it is best accepted unless correction is planned as part of overall treatment, when rapid expansion of the midpalatal suture should be attempted only by a specialist. This is achieved by turning a midline screw, connected to bands cemented on first premolar and molar teeth, twice daily for 2 weeks. Expansion of the suture must be carried out no later than in early teenage years but dental relapse of 50% promoted by cheek pressure, is common.

Treatment of lingual crossbite
Crowding may displace a single tooth into lingual crossbite. Once the crowding is relieved, the crossbite may be corrected, often by palatal movement of the upper unit using a buccally approaching spring on a removable appliance, provided the occlusion is disengaged. Where

a complete unilateral lingual crossbite is associated with a mandibular displacement, lower arch expansion and upper arch contraction with either removable or fixed appliances can produce a stable result provided a good buccal intercuspation is achieved. Surgical correction may be indicated to correct a complete bilateral lingual crossbite or unilateral lingual crossbite with no displacement.

9.6 Adult and surgical–orthodontic treatment

Learning objectives

You should

- be aware of special considerations in undertaking orthodontic treatment in adults
- know the indications for surgical–orthodontic treatment
- understand how surgical–orthodontic treatment is planned and executed
- be aware of common orthognathic surgical procedures.

Adult orthodontics

Orthodontic treatment in adults is the most rapidly expanding area of contemporary orthodontic practice because of an increased availability of services, greater acceptability of appliances and increasing awareness of the potential of orthodontic tooth movement.

Special consideration in adults

There are a number of factors that are specific for orthodontic procedures in adults.

- Adults are generally highly motivated orthodontic patients, able to specify their concerns, but they tend to have higher expectations of the final result than younger patients.
- The dentition may be compromised because of periodontal disease, tooth loss or extensive restorative treatment. Careful pre-treatment assessment is required and all systemic and dental disease must be controlled before orthodontic treatment starts. Occasionally existing bridgework may need to be removed to allow tooth movement to proceed. Often, input from a variety of disciplines (restorative, periodontal, prosthodontic, orthodontic and surgical) are necessary to achieve the best result, and integrated treatment planning must be coordinated in a logical sequence.

- There is also a greater likelihood of systemic illness impacting on the treatment plan in adults.
- There is a lack of growth, so skeletal discrepancies (other than mild) are best dealt with by orthodontics in combination with surgery rather than by camouflage.
- Where camouflage is considered, overbite reduction by intrusion of the incisors rather than by extrusion of the molars is necessary.
- Anchorage planning is often more demanding than in the younger patient because of previous tooth loss and the possibility of reduced bony support of the remaining teeth. Headgear is not a realistic treatment option.
- Because of reduced cell population and often reduced vascularity of the alveolar bone, the initial response to orthodontic forces is slow; however, once tooth movement starts it tends to progress as efficiently as in adolescents.
- Some pain is common for 3–4 days following appliance adjustment, and light forces should be applied initially in all cases and throughout treatment where periodontal support is compromised.
- Retention may be lengthy or permanent.
- Aesthetic brackets may be required to improve the appearance of the appliance.

Adjunctive or comprehensive orthodontic treatment in the adult

Adjunctive treatment
Adjunctive treatment involves carrying out tooth movement to correct one aspect of the occlusion to improve dental health or function, although the final occlusal result may not be necessarily ideal or class I. Treatment duration is usually about 6 months and typically is integrated with periodontal or advanced restorative procedures. Uprighting of teeth that have tilted into an extraction space prior to bridgework, extrusion of teeth with a subgingival fracture margin to allow placement of a coronal restoration on sound root surface, and anterior alignment to facilitate the best appearance of restorative work are examples of some adjunctive treatments.

Comprehensive treatment
The aim of comprehensive treatment is to achieve the optimal aesthetic and functional occlusal result. Where the skeletal discrepancy is mild, camouflage by dentoalveolar movement is possible using fixed appliances. The principles of treatment planning and practical treatment follow similar lines to those adopted for class I, class II division 1 and division 2 and class III malocclusions (see Sections 9.2–4) but overbite reduction must be

achieved by intrusion rather than by extrusion. In those with a more marked skeletal discrepancy, a combined orthodontic and surgical approach is required to ensure that the best facial and occlusal results are achieved (see below).

Where significant periodontal breakdown has occurred, comprehensive treatment may still be possible provided disease is controlled and a regular maintenance scheme operates throughout orthodontic treatment. Because of the reduced periodontal ligament area, forces should be as light as possible, and anchorage planning is critical. Fixed appliances using a sectional arch approach are often indicated, and permanent retention with a bonded retainer is usual.

Surgical–orthodontic treatment

Surgical–orthodontic treatment involves correction of dentofacial deformity through a combined surgical and orthodontic approach. In contemporary practice, surgery to correct a jaw deformity (orthognathic surgery) is rarely undertaken independent of concurrent orthodontic treatment, as the final result is likely to be compromised otherwise.

Timing of treatment
Treatment is usually deferred until growth is essentially completed, which is generally in late teens in males and slightly earlier in females. This delay is most important where growth is excessive, particularly in class III cases, as it safeguards against relapse brought about by further growth. Where the temporomandibular joint is ankylosed or the dentofacial deformity is causing severe psychological distress, earlier intervention can be undertaken.

Indications
Surgical–orthodontic treatment is indicated where the problem cannot be dealt with satisfactorily by orthodontics alone. This includes moderate-to-severe anteroposterior, vertical and lateral skeletal discrepancies as well as craniofacial anomalies, including cleft lip and palate.

Planning surgical–orthodontic treatment

A team approach is required, involving the orthodontist and oral and maxillofacial surgeons. Input from a plastic surgeon, restorative specialist, speech therapist or a clinical psychologist may be required.

First, the patient's complaint must be ascertained. This may relate to their dental and/or facial appearance, masticatory function, speech or a combination of these. Occasionally a patient may be overly concerned about some relatively minor skeletal or dental anomaly, which is blamed for lack of success in some aspect of life. In these instances, there is often a deep-rooted psychological problem and referral to an appropriate counsellor may be indicated.

A detailed medical and dental history together with a thorough examination must then be performed, including an analysis of facial form in full face and profile. The height and width proportions of the face, interalar distance, nasolabial angle, upper incisor exposure, relation of the upper dental midline to the other facial midlines, and the location of any cranial, maxillary, nasal, mandibular or chin deformities should be noted. Temporomandibular joint signs or symptoms must be documented.

Facial and dental photographs, panoramic and lateral cephalometric films and dental casts should be obtained. A postero-anterior cephalometric film is indicated if facial asymmetry is apparent.

Record analysis and planning

The patient's cephalometric film should be traced or digitised and then a 'standard' skull template (e.g. Bolton standard, representing the norm) is superimposed to indicate sites of discrepancy. These templates, however, are composites for males and females. Planning can involve enlargement of the photographic-negative profile to match 1:1 with the cephalometric film and then 'cutting and pasting' to simulate the desired surgical changes.

A simpler method is via a computer program that allows movements to be planned and visually displayed on a screen before printing. Newer video-imaging techniques allow superimposition of the patient's profile on the cephalometric tracing and the video image is adjusted in line with changes in the tracing.

Surgical movement may also be simulated on a duplicate set of dental casts. Where a maxillary procedure is planned, however, the casts should be mounted on a semi-adjustable articulator.

The final plan should be explained to the patient, ensuring that they are aware of the likely final changes to the facial appearance. As presurgical decompensation usually worsens facial appearance, this should be explained also. It may, on occasion, be helpful for a prospective patient to have an opportunity to discuss the process with another individual where a successful outcome has been achieved.

Orthodontic management

Presurgical orthodontics and at surgery

Presurgical orthodontics allows the jaws to be positioned in their desired location without interference from tooth positions. This phase of treatment should rarely take longer than 1 year. It aims to align and co-ordinate the arches or arch segments as well as to establish the vertical and anteroposterior position of the incisors. Usually, this involves placing the incisors at a normal inclination to their respective bases, decompensating for any existing dentoalveolar compensation (nature's attempt to camouflage a skeletal discrepancy). The full extent of the skeletal problem is thus revealed so maximum surgical correction can then be achieved. Intermaxillary traction for class III or II cases is often used to aid decompensation. Depending on the crowding and space requirements, extractions may be necessary to allow the tooth movements required. Consideration should also be given to removal of impacted third molars at this stage.

In some cases, it is not possible or advisable to decompensate fully for the incisor position because of anatomical constraints, for example a narrow symphysis or thin labial gingival tissue in a class III malocclusion. Marked gingival recession is likely in the latter if the lower incisors are proclined.

Space must be created interdentally to allow access for surgical cuts when a segmental procedure is planned. Some tooth movements (e.g. levelling of a curve of Spee in patients with a short face) are managed in a more expeditious manner postsurgically while other movements (e.g. correction of a bilateral skeletal crossbite of the upper arch) can be managed simultaneously with Le Fort I correction for other skeletal problems at the time of surgery.

When presurgical orthodontics is nearing completion, impressions should be taken to check arch co-ordination. Providing this is satisfactory, rigid rectangular stabilising archwires with ball hooks, to allow for intermaxillary fixation, should be placed. Final presurgical records, including a cephalometric film, are taken. An interocclusal acrylic wafer, made from casts positioned to simulate the desired occlusal result, is recommended routinely to ensure accuracy of the postsurgical result. At surgery, the interocclusal wafer is used to locate the jaws or jaw segments accurately; these are then usually fixed semi-rigidly in position by either miniplates in the maxilla or lag screws in the mandible. Intermaxillary fixation may also be required.

Surgical procedures

Surgery may be carried out on the maxilla, mandible or on both jaws depending on the nature and severity of the skeletal problem.

Maxilla

Le Fort I osteotomy The Le Fort I osteotomy is the most common maxillary orthognathic procedure. Access is usually provided by an incision in the buccal sulcus from left to right first molar areas, or by vertical incisions and tunnelling of the mucosa in those for whom the adequacy of the palatal blood supply may be in doubt. The maxilla is sectioned above the apices of the teeth so that it can be 'downfractured' from its anterior wall, tuberosities, lateral nasal walls and nasal septum but remain pedicled on the palate. Superior, inferior or forward movement of the maxilla is then possible; posterior repositioning is not realistic.

Le Fort II osteotomy With the Le Fort II procedure, the incisions pass through the bridge of the nose and lower border of the orbit, allowing the correction of marked maxillary retrognathism and nasal retrusion.

Le Fort III osteotomy Via a bicoronal flap, the whole mid-face including the zygomas is separated from the cranium. This is most frequently employed in correction of rare craniofacial anomalies (e.g. Crouzon's syndrome where the coronal and orbital sutures fuse early, leading to cessation of forward maxillary growth).

Segmental procedures The Wassmund osteotomy involves separating the premaxilla by vertical cuts distal to the canines; the cuts are then extended horizontally across the palate. It was popular for overjet correction in the presence of premaxillary prominence but is now rarely used. Lack of interdental space for surgical cuts and damage to the adjacent teeth are potential problems with this procedure.

Mandible

Sagittal split osteotomy A sagittal split osteotomy is the most frequently undertaken mandibular procedure. The inner and outer parts of the ramus are split through a cut made horizontally above the lingula and obliquely across the retromolar area. These cuts are extended vertically through the buccal cortical plate to the inferior aspect of the mandible. The tooth-bearing part can then be moved forwards or backwards or rotated slightly, but inferior alveolar nerve damage is a common complication.

Vertical subsigmoid osteotomy The mandible is sectioned via an extra-or intraoral incision by a vertical cut through the sigmoid notch, passing behind the lingula, to the mandibular angle. This procedure is used for correction of mandibular prognathism.

Body osteotomy Surgical cuts are made in the mandibular body, ideally where a space exists. Otherwise space is created orthodontically or by removal of teeth. This operation is valuable in those with marked mandibular prognathism and asymmetry.

Subapical osteotomies Subapical osteotomies are confined to patients in whom the dentoalveolar segment(s) alone need to be moved. They are usually confined to the anterior segment, allowing it to be repositioned inferiorly or superiorly, but may involve the complete arch if necessary. Vitality of the teeth may be compromised.

Genioplasty Using a horizontal sliding osteotomy and muscle pedicle, with/without bone removal or bone grafting, the chin can be repositioned in a variety of locations, often producing dramatic profile changes. In some cases it may be used alone as a masking procedure.

Postsurgical orthodontics
Once adequate bone healing and a satisfactory range of mandibular movement has been achieved, the wafer is removed and light round archwires placed to allow occlusal settling. Light elastic traction is used to guide the teeth into the desired position and ensure that good interdigitation is achieved so the appliances can be removed within 6 months of surgery. This is followed by a retention regimen that usually follows standard fixed appliance therapy. Surgical follow-up should be for a minimum of 2 years.

Stability and relapse

In general, stability is enhanced and relapse minimised when

- surgical and orthodontic plans are correct and realistic, well-integrated and executed competently
- surgical movement is modest – no greater than 5–6 mm vertically or anteroposteriorly in the maxilla or 8 mm in the mandible – does not place the soft tissues under tension and the condyles are not distracted at surgery
- abberant soft tissue factors are absent, e.g. tongue thrust or previous surgical scarring, as may occur in repaired cleft palate
- patient is compliant with all aspects of treatment, particularly postsurgical wear of elastic traction
- fixation is adequate.

9.7 Cleft lip and palate

Learning objectives

You should

- know the likely aetiological factors in oro-facial clefting
- be aware of the common clinical features
- understand how care is managed and the role of the general dental practitioner.

Management of patients with cleft lip and palate is best undertaken in special centres. The general practitioner should, however, understand the timing and sequence of treatment for these patients and the importance of providing a high standard of preventive and routine dental care for them.

Aetiology

Whether a cleft occurs in isolation or as part of a syndrome, both genetic and environmental factors interact in its aetiology. A distinct family history exists in 40% of those with cleft lip (with or without palate involvement) and in 20% of those with cleft palate only. Environmental factors such as folic acid deficiency, maternal infections, anticonvulsant drug therapy, aspirin, and cortisone may act synergistically in a susceptible, genetically predisposed individual to promote clefting. Clefting of the lip and primary palate follows from failure of fusion of the medial nasal, lateral nasal and maxillary processes at around the sixth week of intrauterine life. Clefts of the secondary palate follow failure of fusion of the palatal shelves from 8–10 weeks. Elevation of the palatal shelves from a vertical to a horizontal position occurs later in females than males, allowing for more lateral facial growth, which possibly contributes to the greater prevalence of isolated cleft palate in females.

Classification

Several classification systems exist, but the cleft is easiest described as involving the primary (lip and alveolus to the incisive foramen) and/or secondary palate (hard palate from incisive foramen back and soft palate), as being unilateral or bilateral, complete or incomplete (Fig. 118). A submucous cleft may not be detected for some time as the overlying mucosa is unaffected, but it is usually noticed when speech development is poor.

Prevalence

Clefts of the lip and/or palate occur in 65% of all craniofacial deformities, with a prevalence of 1 in 750 live births for cleft lip and palate in Caucasians, and 1 in 2000 live births for isolated cleft of the secondary palate. Cleft lip and palate more frequently affects males and is more common on the left than on the right side, while females are more often affected by cleft palate alone. Occasionally the latter is a feature of other syndromes such as Pierre Robin, Treacher Collins and Down.

Common clinical features

Skeletal features
- Both the maxilla and mandible tend to be retrognathic relative to non-cleft individuals; the maxillary position is possibly a result of growth restriction post surgically.
- Upper face height tends to be reduced but the lower face height increased, with an excess freeway space.
- Class III skeletal relationship often results from the retrusion of maxilla and mandible but is aggravated by mandibular overclosure to allow posterior tooth contact.

Dental and occlusal features
On the side of the cleft the following anomalies often exist:

- the lateral incisor is absent, of abnormal size and/or shape, hypoplastic or appears as two conical teeth on the medial or lateral side of the cleft
- a supernumerary or supplemental tooth may be present on either side of the cleft
- the central incisor is often rotated and tilted toward the cleft and may be hypoplastic, particularly in bilateral clefts
- eruption is delayed.

Elsewhere in the mouth, tooth size tends to be smaller, with a greater prevalence of hypodontia, enamel hypoplasia and abnormal tooth shape than in unaffected individuals.

A class III incisor relationship is common with a crossbite of one or both buccal segments and occasionally a lateral open bite.

Growth
Postsurgical scarring in those with cleft lip and palate restricts anteroposterior, vertical and transverse growth

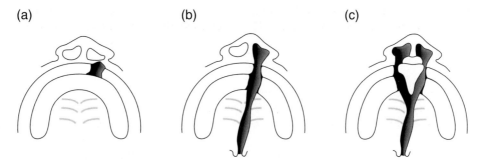

Fig. 118 Classification of cleft lip and palate. (a) Left incomplete cleft of primary palate. (b) Left unilateral complete cleft of primary and secondary palate. (c) Bilateral complete cleft of primary and secondary palate.

of the midface. These changes do not seem to occur to any significant extent in unrepaired clefts.

Hearing and speech

Where the cleft involves the posterior palate, the action of tensor palati on the Eustachian tube is impaired, often leading to hearing difficulties. This, in addition to palatal fistulae and adverse palatopharyngeal function, means that speech is often defective. Regular assessment of hearing and speech is essential before and during school years.

Anomalies of other body tissues

Cardiac and digital anomalies are found in one fifth of those with clefts and are most common in those with clefts of the secondary palate only.

Care management

Care management is best coordinated in a specialised centre by a team usually comprising an orthodontist, speech therapist, health visitor, plastic, ear–nose–throat and maxillofacial surgeons. General dental care must be monitored regularly by a caring and interested general dental practitioner.

Neonatal period

Parental counselling and reassurance should be given by an orthodontist, with emphasis on the importance of a high standard of dental care for later treatment. The mother must be instructed in feeding using special bottles and teats (e.g. Rosti bottle and Gummi teat). A specialised health visitor should be available for provision of ongoing advice and support.

Repositioning of the displaced cleft segments by removable appliances, often with extraoral strapping to facilitate surgical repair (presurgical orthopaedics), is now undertaken less frequently than before owing to its dubious benefits.

Lip closure is usually undertaken at around 3 months, with the Millard technique (often with modifications) adopted most commonly. The extent of alar cartilage dissection and the simulataneous use of the Vomer flap are disputed. In bilateral clefts, the lip may be repaired in one or two stages. Repair of the hard and soft palate is usually carried out between 9 and 12 months, most commonly by means of a von Langenbeck procedure.

Deciduous dentition

Preventive advice including dietary counselling and possibly provision of fluoride supplements is essential. Speech should be assessed formally at about 2 years and speech and hearing assessed regularly. Speech therapy can be instituted as necessary. Pharyngoplasty and/or lip revision may be required prior to starting school.

Mixed/permanent dentition

Correction of an incisor crossbite may be necessary early in the mixed dentition or may be postponed until preparation for alveolar bone grafting at 8–11 years of age. Alignment of the upper incisors and arch expansion is usually undertaken prior to grafting to facilitate access. Extraction of any primary teeth in the upper arch should take place at least 3 weeks prior to surgery to allow healing. Bone is harvested from the iliac crest or the chin, placed in the cleft site and the wound closed with keratinised flaps. The graft, in addition to allowing eruption of the permanent canine and space closure, supports the alar base and helps to close oronasal fistulae.

Once the permanent canine has erupted, further treatment usually involves centre-line correction and space closure by mesial movement of the buccal segment teeth so that the canine replaces a missing or diminutive lateral incisor. Crowding should be relieved in the non-cleft quadrant if necessary, and in the lower arch if orthodontic correction of the malocclusion is likely. Otherwise lower arch extractions should be delayed until surgical correction of the malocclusion is planned.

Where gross mid-face retrusion is present in late teenage years, a Le Fort I or II surgical advancement is likely, with possible mandibular setback and/or genioplasty depending on the severity of the skeletal problem. Presurgical orthodontics proceeds along conventional lines (see Section 9.6). Rhinoplasty may be required as a later procedure to optimise the facial profile.

Retention

Because of scar tissue in the cleft area, bonded permanent retention is necessary in all cases.

Self-assessment: questions

Multiple choice questions

1. Hypodontia:
   a. Affects the upper permanent lateral incisors in 20% of cases
   b. Affects lower second premolars more so than upper second premolars
   c. Is more common in males than females
   d. Has not a familial link
   e. Of third molars can be determined definitively by 8 years of age

2. Supernumerary teeth:
   a. Occur in about 10% of the population
   b. Are more common in females than males
   c. May occur in the lower incisor area
   d. May cause spacing of $\underline{1/1}$
   e. May have no effect on the dentition or occlusion

3. Removal of a $/\overline{6}$ deemed of poor prognosis in a class I (incisors and molars) malocclusion with generalised moderate premolar crowding where all other teeth are sound:
   a. Is advisable when the bifurcation of the $/\overline{8}$ is calcifying, to maximise the potential for spontaneous correction of malocclusion in that quadrant
   b. Should be compensated
   c. Should be balanced
   d. Is likely to lead to overjet increase
   e. Is likely to lead to 3 mm overbite increase

4. Extraction of $\underline{c}$s may be indicated:
   a. To allow spontaneous correction of potential crossbite on erupting $\underline{2}$s
   b. To allow space to be created for an unerupted upper central incisor whose eruption has been inhibited by the presence of a supernumerary
   c. To allow the lower incisors to drop lingually in a developing class III malocclusion
   d. To encourage improvement in the position of a displaced $\underline{3}$
   e. Along with $\underline{b}$s in early mixed dentition to encourage space closure in children in whom $\underline{2}$s are absent

5. Extraction of a lower right first primary molar:
   a. Is described as balanced when extraction of the upper left first primary molar is requested also
   b. Is described as compensated when extraction of the lower left first primary molar is requested also

   c. Should be compensated to prevent a centre-line shift
   d. Should be balanced to prevent overbite reduction
   e. Should be requested if the crown of the tooth is submerged level with the gingival margin

6. A persistent thumb-sucking habit may produce:
   a. An increased overbite
   b. An asymmetric increase in overjet
   c. A buccal segment crossbite
   d. An adaptive tongue thrust
   e. Upper incisor root resorption

7. Buccal displacement of $\underline{3}/$ may be contributed to by:
   a. Crowding in the arch
   b. Retention of $\underline{c}/$
   c. An increased overbite
   d. Early loss of lower primary molars
   e. Absent $\underline{2}/$

8. Bimaxillary proclination:
   a. Represents inclination of the upper/lower incisors less than the mean for Caucasians
   b. Is common in Caucasians
   c. Results when lip pressure is higher than tongue pressure
   d. May exist with incisor relationship class I
   e. Has a high chance of stability when corrected

9. Factors that may aggravate an already increased overjet include:
   a. A persistent thumb-sucking habit
   b. Upper arch crowding
   c. A bilateral buccal segment crossbite
   d. An anterior mandibular growth rotation
   e. Proclination of the lower incisors

10. Prognosis for stable correction of a 10 mm overjet in a 12-year-old female patient with normal overbite is enhanced when:
    a. The underlying anteroposterior skeletal pattern is class I
    b. There is a backward pattern of mandibular growth
    c. The lower lip lies under the upper incisors post-treatment
    d. A thumb-sucking habit persists
    e. A buccal segment crossbite is present pretreatment

11. A functional appliance for correction of a class II division 1 malocclusion:
    a. Works by maintaining the mandible in its rest position
    b. Is least effective during active growth
    c. Is ideal for treating irregularities in tooth alignment
    d. Requires 14–16 hours per day wear to be effective
    e. Requires post-treatment retention until growth has ceased

12. Deep overbite in class II division 2 malocclusion is associated with:
    a. A reduced interincisal angle
    b. A high lower lip line
    c. Normal cingulum thickness on the upper incisors
    d. A forward pattern of mandibular growth
    e. Early loss of a mandibular primary first molar

13. Relative to class I malocclusion, cephalometric features of class III malocclusion may include:
    a. A short maxillary length
    b. A more posterior position of the glenoid fossa
    c. A reduced mandibular length
    d. A more protrusive position of the maxilla
    e. Retroclined lower incisors

14. An anterior open bite may be caused by:
    a. A low Frankfort mandibular planes angle
    b. An endogenous tongue thrust
    c. A cleft of the lip and alveolus
    d. A digit-sucking habit
    e. A horizontal pattern of facial growth

15. A buccal crossbite on 5/ may result from:
    a. Early loss of e/
    b. Submergence of ē/
    c. A repaired cleft palate
    d. A prolonged thumb-sucking habit
    e. A class III malocclusion

16. In a 30-year-old adult male patient:
    a. Overbite reduction is generally easier than in an adolescent
    b. Molar extrusion is the approach of choice for overbite reduction orthodontically
    c. Lighter forces are desirable for tooth movement if the dentition is periodontally compromised
    d. Anchorage demands may be less if teeth have been lost
    e. Significant skeletal discrepancies may be addressed by growth modification

17. Factors associated with dental and/or skeletal relapse following mandibular advancement osteotomy include:
    a. Mandibular advancement greater than 8 mm
    b. Condylar distraction during surgery
    c. Adequate fixation
    d. Poor cooperation with wear of intermaxillary elastics
    e. Tongue thrust

18. Common dental anomalies in a 10-year-old child with a left unilateral cleft of lip and palate include:
    a. Enamel hypoplasia of /1
    b. Delayed eruption of the permanent dentition
    c. Absent /2
    d. A lingual crossbite of the buccal segments
    e. Anterior crossbite

19. Alveolar bone grafting in patients with cleft lip and palate:
    a. Is best undertaken before age 8 years
    b. Improves alar base support
    c. Provides bone through which 6 can usually erupt
    d. Stabilises a mobile premaxilla in a bilateral cleft
    e. Should be undertaken simultaneously with any extractions on the cleft side

Case history questions

Case history 1

An 8-year-old girl presents with her mother, who is very concerned about her daughter's large (5 mm) upper median diastema.

1. What are the causes of an upper median diastema in an 8-year-old?
2. What are the management options?

Case history 2

A 10-year-old child presents with an anterior open bite.

1. What are the possible causes of the open bite?
2. What treatment options may be considered?

Case history 3

A 7-year-old boy presents with 1/1 in crossbite but otherwise has features of a class I malocclusion.

1. What is the possible aetiology of the crossbite?
2. When is early treatment advisable?
3. What factors must be considered regarding treatment possibilities?
4. List the desirable features in the design of an upper removable appliance to correct the incisor relationship.

Picture questions

Picture 1

Figure 119 is a radiograph.

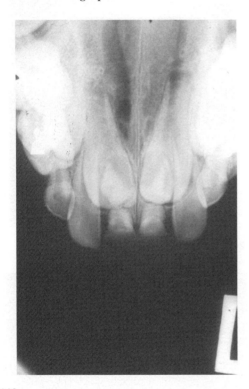

Fig. 119

1. What features are visible?
2. What other common factors or conditions may produce a similar effect?
3. How would you manage the case?

Picture 2

Figure 120 shows the anterior occlusion of a 13-year-old female.

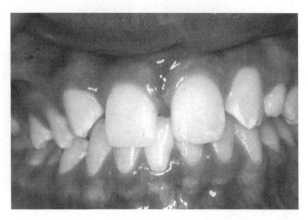

Fig. 120

1. What anomaly is visible?
2. What is its likely aetiology?
3. What are the management options?
4. What factors would dictate your decision regarding treatment?

Picture 3

Figure 121 shows an intraoral view of an 8-year-old girl.

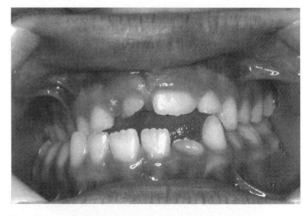

Fig. 121 Intraoral view in an 8-year-old girl.

1. What occlusal anomaly is visible?
2. What clinical assessment would you wish to perform and why?
3. What is the possible aetiology?
4. What are the treatment options?

Picture 4

Figure 122 is a dental panoramic tomogram.

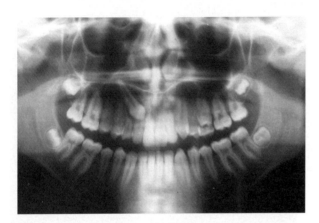

Fig. 122

1. What anomaly is visible?
2. What factors may account for this?
3. How would you aid localisation?
4. What interceptive method may have helped to avoid this problem developing
5. What factors determine whether orthodontic alignment is possible?

Picture 5

Figure 123 is a lower intraoral occlusal view in a 19-year-old male patient.

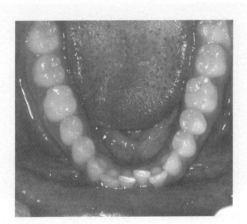

Fig. 123

1. What anomaly is present?
2. How may this arise?
3. What advice would you give?
4. What management possibilities exist?

Picture 6

Figure 124 shows the frontal view of a 22-year-old female who presented for orthodontic treatment with an obvious facial anomaly, which she reported to be gradually worsening.

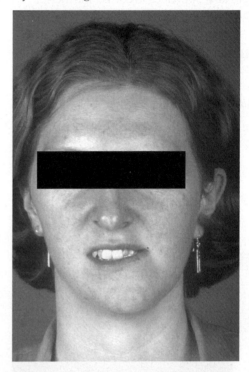

Fig. 124

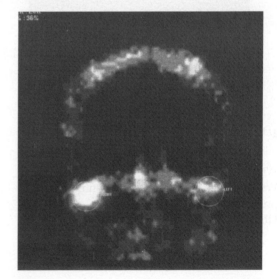

Fig. 125

1. What obvious facial anomaly is present?
2. What investigation is shown in Figure 125? What does this show?
3. What occlusal features would you expect?
4. How would you manage the patient?

Picture 7

The intraoral views (Fig. 126) are of a 2-day-old infant with a cleft.

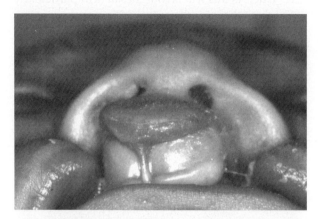

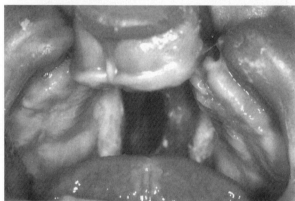

Fig. 126

1. Classify the cleft and outline the anatomical aetiology.
2. What would be the initial management (first weeks)?
3. When would surgical intervention usually be considered?
4. What would be your management during the primary dentition?

Short note questions

Write short notes on the following:

1. Infraoccluded primary molars
2. Impacted <u>6</u>s
3. Serial extractions
4. Transposition
5. Space maintenance
6. Methods of overbite correction
7. Growth modification for class II correction
8. Camouflage therapy for class II correction
9. Bilateral buccal crossbite
10. Differences in orthodontic treatment in adults compared with adolescents
11. Maxillary osteotomies
12. Aetiology of clefting.

Viva questions

1. What are the possible effects of early loss of primary teeth on the permanent dentition? What factors determine the severity of these effects and how may the impact of any undesirable effect be minimised?

Self-assessment: answers

Multiple choice answers

1. a. **False.** Affects upper lateral incisors in 2% of cases.
    b. **True.** Affects lower second premolars (3%) more so than upper second premolars (less than 2%).
    c. **False.** Hypodontia and microdontia are more common in females than males.
    d. **False.** Hypodontia has a strong tendency to run in families.
    e. **False.** Third molars start to calcify any time between 8 and 14 years so one must wait until age 14 before making a definite diagnosis of hypodontia of third molars.

2. a. **False.** Occur in about 2% of the population in the permanent dentition (~ 1% in primary dentition).
    b. **False.** More common in males.
    c. **True.** Typically as a supplemental lower incisor.
    d. **True.** Typically by a conical mesiodens.
    e. **True.** For example, a conical mesiodens high above the apices of 1/1.

3. a. **False.** Timing of removal is best when the bifurcation of /7̄ is calcifying (aged ~8.5 to 9.5 years) and not when bifurcation of /8̄ is calcifying.
    b. **True.** In a class I malocclusion with a Class I molar relationship, a compensating extraction (i.e. removal of /6̱) is advisable to prevent the 'plunger cusp' effect of overeruption of /6̱ into the lower extraction site.
    c. **False.** There is no need to balance for the extraction with removal of 6̄/ as all other teeth are sound; however, an extraction from the lower right quadrant will be necessary to relieve the moderate premolar crowding.
    d. **False.** Removal of one lower first permanent molar is not likely to lead to an overjet increase.
    e. **False.** There is likely to be no overbite increase.

4. a. **True.** Timely removal of c̱s may allow this to occur.
    b. **True.** Extraction of c̱s will provide space to allow for 2s to be moved distally with appliance therapy, thereby creating space for alignment of an unerupted upper permanent incisor.
    c. **False.** Extraction of c̱ will have no effect on the position of lower incisors.
    d. **True.** Displaced 3̱ may align spontaneously with timely extraction of c̱ (usually about age 10) provided position of 3̱ and space conditions in the arch are favourable.

    e. **True.** As this will favour mesial drift particularly where there is inherent crowding.

5. a. **False.** A balancing extraction would involve extraction of a lower left primary molar.
    b. **False.** A compensating extraction would involve removal of the upper right first primary molar.
    c. **False.** Extraction should be balanced to prevent centre-line shift.
    d. **False.** Balancing extraction will not prevent overbite reduction.
    e. **True.** Early removal is advisable to prevent adjacent teeth tilting into its space and making removal more difficult.

6. a. **False.** An open bite is characteristic.
    b. **True.** The upper incisors are proclined and lower incisors retroclined, often in an asymmetric manner through positioning of the thumb.
    c. **True.** The action of the cheek musculature is unopposed in sucking because the tongue is displaced out of the palatal vault by the insertion of the thumb.
    d. **True.** Because of the anterior open bite, this is necessary to achieve an anterior oral seal for swallowing.
    e. **False.** No evidence to support this.

7. a. **True.** Buccal displacement is likely in a crowded arch as 3s are the last teeth to erupt in the buccal segments with exception of second and third molars and therefore may be displaced buccally if the arch is intrinsically crowded.
    b. **True.** This will deflect the eruption path of 3/.
    c. **False.** This will have no effect on position of 3/.
    d. **False.** Early loss of primary molars in the lower arch will not affect crowding in the upper arch.
    e. **False.** This will not produce buccal displacement of 3/.

8. a. **False.** Inclination of upper/lower incisors is more proclined than the Caucasian means.
    b. **False.** It is more common in Negroes.
    c. **False.** Typically lip pressure is less than tongue pressure.
    d. **True.** Overjet may be slightly increased because of the incisor inclination, although the incisor relationship may be class I.
    e. **False.** Stability is generally poor and at best guarded as any retroclination of upper/lower incisors is prone to relapse owing to encroachment on tongue space.

9. a. **True.** This will procline upper incisors and retrocline lower incisors, worsening the overjet.
   b. **True.** If the upper arch is inherently crowded, the upper incisors may be displaced labially making the overjet worse.
   c. **False.** This will have no effect.
   d. **False.** This will tend to reduce the overjet; a backward mandibular growth rotation will tend to make the overjet worse.
   e. **False.** This will tend to mask an increased overjet.

10. a. **True.** The greater the class II skeletal pattern, the more difficult stable correction is likely to be.
    b. **False.** A backward pattern of mandibular growth will tend to worsen the prognosis.
    c. **False.** Coverage of one third to one half of the labial surface of the upper incisors by the lower lip confers a better prognosis.
    d. **False.** This will promote overjet increase.
    e. **False.** This will not affect the prognosis for overjet correction.

11. a. **False.** The mandible is held in a forward postured position.
    b. **False.** The appliance is most effective during the growth spurt.
    c. **False.** Typically the appliance has no components to treat irregularities in tooth position; these are best dealt with by other appliance systems, particularly fixed appliances.
    d. **True.** Full-time wear is generally not required but at least 14–16 hours wear per day is required to give the best chance of success.
    e. **True.** Wear of the appliance on a night-only basis until the late teens is advisable to minimise overjet relapse.

12. a. **False.** A high interincisal angle would produce a deep overbite.
    b. **True.** This will retrocline upper incisors.
    c. **False.** Maxillary incisor cingulae tend to be poorly developed.
    d. **True.** This will tend to increase overbite.
    e. **False.** No evidence to support this.

13. a. **True.** This leads to maxillary retrusion.
    b. **False.** The condylar head is in a more anterior position producing mandibular prognathism.
    c. **False.** Increased mandibular length leads to mandibular protrusion.
    d. **False.** More retruded position of the maxilla leads to maxillary retrusion.
    e. **True.** Because of dentoalveolar compensation for the skeletal pattern.

14. a. **False.** A low angle would tend to produce a deep overbite and a high angle an anterior open bite.
    b. **True.** This will procline upper and lower incisors and reduce the overbite.
    c. **True.** As this would inhibit vertical alveolar growth.
    d. **True.** As upper incisors are proclined, and eruption of lower incisors is inhibited.
    e. **False.** A vertical pattern of facial growth would lead to anterior open bite.

15. a. **True.** As this will allow 6/ to migrate forward in a crowded arch displacing 5/ palatally.
    b. **False.** This will not produce a buccal crossbite but perhaps allow over eruption of 5/.
    c. **True.** As transverse maxillary growth is likely to be restricted.
    d. **True.** See (6c) above.
    e. **True.** As a wider part of the lower arch opposes a relatively narrower part of the upper arch.

16. a. **False.** As successful overbite reduction depends on favourable growth and growth can be regarded as ceased in the adult, treatment is generally more difficult than in the adolescent.
    b. **False.** Incisor intrusion rather than molar extrusion is the preferred approach for overbite reduction. Molar extrusion will increase the vertical posterior face height, which will be unstable.
    c. **True.** As the pressure (force per unit area) on the periodontium will be greater for a given force in a periodontally compromised dentition, forces need to be lighter than where there has been no loss of periodontal support.
    d. **False.** Anchorage demands are likely to be greater where teeth have been lost as there are fewer teeth to incorporate in the anchor unit.
    e. **False.** Although small increments in growth occur in adulthood, for the purpose of any orthodontic treatment adults can be regarded as non-growing. Growth modification is, therefore, not a viable treatment option.

17. a. **True.** Movement greater than 8 mm is likely to place the soft tissues under tension and tend to induce relapse.
    b. **True.** Distraction of the condyles will lead to relapse when they return to the condylar fossae.
    c. **False.** This is likely to promote stability.
    d. **True.** Non-compliance with elastic wear is likely to lead to relapse in the occlusal result.

e. **True.** Tongue thrust would tend to lead to relapse of the incisor occlusion, particularly an overjet increase and an incomplete overbite.

18. a. **True.** As the enamal organ in the site of the cleft is affected.
    b. **True.**
    c. **True.** Teeth are often absent in the line of a cleft as all tissues (dental as well) are affected.
    d. **False.** A buccal crossbite is common following postsurgical restriction in transverse growth of the maxilla.
    e. **True.** Collapse and inward rotation of the cleft segment commonly leads to anterior crossbite.

19. a. **False.** If grafting is undertaken before 8 years, it may interfere with transverse anterior maxillary growth.
    b. **True.** The added bone improves alar base support.
    c. **False.** It provides bone through which $\underline{3}$ usually (not $\underline{6}$) may erupt.
    d. **True.** A bony bridge will reduce mobility of the premaxilla.
    e. **False.** Extractions should be undertaken at least 3 weeks prior to bone grafting to allow keratinised mucosa to heal.

Case history answers

Case history 1

1. An upper median diastema occurs as a normal developmental stage of dental development (sometimes called the 'ugly duckling' stage), which tends to reduce as the permanent maxillary canines erupt. It can also be caused by:
   - missing or small upper lateral incisors
   - generalised spacing in the upper arch
   - proclination of the upper incisors in a class II division 1 malocclusion or digit sucking
   - supernumerary tooth, ie mesiodens.
   - low lying frenal attachment may be associated with a midline space; blanching of the incisive papilla when the frenum is put under tension and a characteristic 'V'-shaped notch in the alveolar bone between the incisors indicate possible involvement of the frenum.
2. There are a number of treatment options if this is more than a normal stage.
   - If a supernumerary tooth is interfering with approximation of the incisors, removal is indicated ensuring no damage to the adjacent teeth. Otherwise wait until $\underline{3}$s erupt before considering treatment.

- Where the lateral incisors are absent, space opening or space closure are options. If the latter is the preferred option, consider early extraction of primary teeth to encourage mesial drift of the buccal segments. Fixed appliances are usually required later to complete alignment and space closure, followed by recontouring of the cusp tips of $\underline{3}/\underline{3}$ and composite additions to their mesial aspects (or veneers) followed by bonded retention to $\underline{31}/\underline{13}$.
- If space opening is deemed a better option, wait until $\underline{3}/\underline{3}$ erupt and then create space for $\underline{2}/\underline{2}$, followed by their replacement initially on a partial denture/removable retainer followed at a later stage by either resin-retained bridgework or implants.
- In class II division 1, or crowded maxillary arches where $\underline{3}$ is upright/distally inclined and of favourable colour and form, space closure is generally preferable to space opening. Conversely where a class III incisor relationship or spacing exists, space opening is usually the option of choice.
- If spacing is generalised and mild, advise the patient to accept it or consider composite additions or veneers to close the anterior spaces. Where the spacing is more marked in those with severe hypodontia, orthodontic treatment is usually required to reposition the teeth and localise space prior to prosthetic or implant replacement.
- Correction of a class II division 1 malocclusion should eliminate the midline diastema; early treatment with a functional appliance may be indicated. If the space is caused by digit sucking, the patient should be advised to stop. In some instances fitting an upper removable appliance to act as a reminder may be useful.
- If a frenal involvement is suspected, fraenectomy prior to completion of space closure will be advantageous, the scar tissue encouraging incisor approximation.

Case history 2

1. There are a number of possible causes:
   - skeletal: an increased FMPA and anterior lower facial height
   - soft tissues: an endogenous tongue thrust (often difficult to distinguish from an adaptive tongue thrust), although lisping and proclination of both upper and lower incisors are thought to be characteristic
   - digit-sucking habit: this arrests eruption of the incisors
   - cleft of the lip and primary palate: this may

produce a local failure of development of the alveolus.

2. If the open bite is caused by digit sucking, gently persuade the child to stop. Otherwise wait until the permanent dentition is fully established. Ensure that the habit is stopped before considering correction of an overjet, otherwise relapse is likely, although occasionally the habit may stop if appliance therapy is instituted.

   If it is not caused by digit sucking, monitor, and where growth is likely to be favourable with no adverse soft tissue factors consider growth modification with a maxillary intrusion splint and high-pull headgear. Accept the open bite if it is mild or if the soft tissue factors are adverse (endogenous tongue thrust or grossly incompetent lips). Crowding may, however, be relieved and the arches aligned accepting the vertical discrepancy.

   Orthodontic correction may be possible in a limited number of children, particularly where the arches are crowded with bimaxillary proclination and the lips are likely to become competent post-treatment.

   Orthognathic surgery is required in severe anterior open bite and is best carried out when growth is complete.

Case history 3

1. Retention of a/a may deflect the path of eruption of the permanent successors into crossbite. A mild class III skeletal pattern may also produce an incisor crossbite, even though the malocclusion is otherwise class I. In those with repaired cleft lip and palate, scar tissue contraction may restrain maxillary growth, producing an incisor crossbite.

2. Early treatment is advisable if the crossbite is associated with a mandibular displacement on closure, as this may predispose to temporomandibular joint dysfunction syndrome. In addition, displacing occlusal contacts may push the mandibular incisors labially and compromise periodontal health.

3. • The inclination of the upper incisors: this will determine if tilting or bodily movement will be necessary.
   • The inclination of the lower incisors: lingual movement of the lower incisors in addition to labial movement of the upper incisors may be needed.
   • The amount of overbite likely: a positive overbite is necessary for stability.
   • The amount of space available for 1/1 proclination.

4. Desirable features include:
   • activation: two Z-springs may be used to procline the incisors but activation may displace the baseplate away from the palate; use of a screw section clasping the teeth to be moved will overcome this problem
   • retention: typically 6/6 – or a screw section clasping the teeth to be moved
   • anchorage: from all teeth other than 1/1, and the palate contacted via the baseplate
   • baseplate: posterior capping is necessary to disengage the anterior teeth by about 2 mm, thereby facilitating crossbite correction.

Picture answers

Picture 1

1. Unerupted 1/1 owing to the presence of two supernumerary teeth with retained a/a.
2. Delayed eruption of 1/1 may also occur through ectopic position of the tooth germs, dilaceration, delayed exfoliation of a/a, crowding or a cleft lip and palate.
3. Remove the supernumerary teeth and bond gold chain to the unerupted 1/1; maintain or create space to accommodate the unerupted 1/1. This will involve fitting an upper removable appliance with palatal finger springs to move 2/2 distally. It may be necessary to extract cs also. If 1/1 do not erupt spontaneously, then traction can be applied to the gold chain to extrude them into alignment.

Picture 2

1. Absent 2/2.
2. Strong genetic link and is more common in females than males (overall prevalence about 6%). The 2s may also be absent in cleft lip and palate owing to absence of the tooth-forming tissues in the line of the cleft.
3. Management options include accept, open spaces for prosthetic replacement (possibly by implants) of missing units, close spaces orthodontically, restorative build-up of the teeth on either side of the space with either composite or veneers or crowns.
4. Consider what the patient wishes, level of oral hygiene, dental status, interest and likely cooperation with orthodontic treatment/complex restorative treatment. Space closure is best considered where the upper arch is crowded, FMPA is increased, an overjet exists, size/shape/colour of 3s will give satisfactory aesthetics beside 1s and the buccal segment relationship is a full unit class II. Space opening is best considered where there is no crowding/spacing in the

arch, FMPA is average or reduced, morphology of 3s will not give good aesthetic result when approximated to 1s, buccal segment relationship is class I/half unit class II and/or there is a class III incisor relationship where proclination of incisors will correct an anterior crossbite.

Picture 3

1. A crossbite of the right buccal segments.
2. It would be essential to determine if there is a mandibular displacement associated with the crossbite. This may be assessed by asking the child to touch the back of her hard palate with her tongue and to maintain this while gently closing her mouth. It is wise to correct a crossbite with an associated mandibular displacement sooner rather than later to allow the remaining occlusal development to occur in an undisplaced position.
3. This may result from a thumb-sucking habit (although in this case none of the other features associated with such a habit are visible; the anterior open bite is due to partial eruption of the permanent incisors rather than to a digit-sucking habit). It may also be skeletal resulting from a mismatch in the width of the upper and lower dental arches. Condylar hypoplasia and hemimandibular hypertrophy are rarer causes.
4. If there is an associated mandibular displacement, expansion of the upper arch either by a midline screw incorporated in an upper removable appliance with buccal capping to disengage the occlusion or by a quadhelix may be undertaken. If no displacement is present, the crossbite may be accepted unless correction as part of more comprehensive treatment is considered at a later stage. Should hemimandibular hypertrophy be the cause, then either condylar or ramus surgery should be considered depending on the outcome of a technetium-99 m bone scan. For condylar hypoplasia, distraction ostogenesis, costochondral graft or ramus osteotomy with a bone graft, are options.

Picture 4

1. Ectopic position of 3/.
2. The following factors have been implicated in the aetiology of maxillary canine impaction:
   - recent evidence suggests a strong genetic influence
   - 3 has the longest path of eruption of any tooth in the dental arches and has therefore a greater likelihood of becoming displaced

- absent or short-rooted 2. 3 is guided into position by the root of 2 and where 2 is absent or has a short root there is a twofold increase in the incidence of palatal displacement of 3.
- a higher incidence of palatal canine ectopia has been identified also in class II division 2 malocclusion, where small teeth in well-developed arches have been noted
- absence of crowding: palatal impaction of 3 is more likely in a spaced rather than a crowded arch.

3. Clinical palpation of the buccal sulcus and palatal mucosa should have been undertaken before any radiographic investigation.

   A dental panoramic tomogram will give an indication as to the position of 3: if the image is enlarged relative to its antimere, the tooth is likely to be palatal in 80% of cases. However, two views are required to localise the position of 3; the panoramic view may be supplemented with a standard oblique occlusal view (Fig. 127) or by two periapical films. Parallax is then employed to locate the tooth: if the tooth moves in the same direction as the tube shift it is palatal, if it remains stationary it is in the line of the arch, if it moves in the opposite direction to the tube shift it is buccal.

4. Removal of c/ (and balancing extraction of c/) at age 10 may have helped to encourage improvement in the position of 3/.
5. Exposure and orthodontic alignment of 3/ depend on the following:
   - general factors: motivated patient with a well-maintained mouth
   - local factors: adequate space for 3/, or likely from extractions

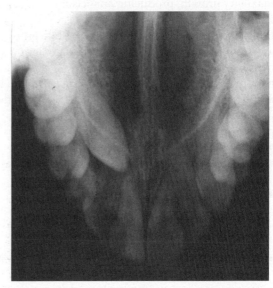

Fig. 127 Localisation of 3/ position, standard oblique occlusal view.

- 3/ below apical third of incisor roots, overlapping less than half the mesiodistal width of 1, less than 30° to the midsagittal plane and the apex not distal to 5.

Picture 5

1. Late lower labial segment crowding.
2. Normal developmental anomaly. This has a multifactorial aetiology including uprighting of lower labial segment (possibly owing to increased tissue tone in the lips with maturation and in response to mandibular growth rotation), tendency for intercanine width to reduce in late teens, mesial drift and anterior component of force. Third molar eruption has been implicated in its aetiology but is unlikely to exert any great impact.
3. Explain that it is a normal maturational change in the occlusion. Study models should be taken to act as a baseline record from which to monitor any further change. The patient may be seen again if the crowding worsens considerably.
4. Management option initially is to accept and monitor. If crowding worsens, consider interdental stripping in moderate cases or extraction of a lower incisor in severely crowded mouths and alignment with a fixed appliance followed by bonded retention.

Picture 6

1. Marked facial asymmetry with chin point displaced about 1 cm to the left.
2. An image (anterior Towne's view with the mouth open) from a bone scan with technetium-99 m. It shows a 'hot spot' in the right condylar area and the difference in isotope uptake between the right and left sides.
3. One would expect a buccal crossbite of the left buccal segments with the lower centre-line displaced to the left.
4. Management. If the referring practitioner or the patient has previous dental casts, the magnitude of any occlusal change in the intervening period can be assessed. Similarly the degree of facial change can be assessed from previous facial photographs. As the condyle is still actively growing, producing hemimandibular hypertrophy, this will require a high 'condylar shave'. When the condition has stabilised, orthodontic treatment – in combination with orthognathic surgery – will be required then to ensure a satisfactory facial appearance and occlusion.

Picture 7

1. Complete bilateral cleft of lip and palate. Failure of fusion of the medial nasal process on each side with the corresponding maxillary process produces the bilateral cleft lip (probably at about 6 weeks of intrauterine life). Failure of fusion of the palatal shelves, which form the secondary palate at about 8 weeks of life, leads to the cleft palate.
2. Initial management. The weeks following the birth of a child with a cleft are very difficult for the parents, who invariably feel somewhat shocked and disappointed at the birth of an abnormally looking child. Great sensitivity on the part of the nursing staff and support from family and other members of the cleft team is required. Instruction in bottle feeding with the aid of special teats is necessary and introduction to a support group, such as the Cleft Lip and Palate Association, who can provide counselling, is invaluable. The likely future management should also be explained by a member of the cleft team and a contact person identified who can provide advice as required. In some centres, feeding plates are made and presurgical orthopaedics commenced with the intention of reducing the size of the cleft to make surgical closure easier. The benefits of this intervention are disputed and it is not so widely practised nowadays.
3. Usually lip closure is undertaken at about 3 months of age. With a bilateral cleft one side may be repaired at a time. Palatal repair is usual at about 9–12 months.
4. During the primary dentition the following is advisable:
   - regular care by the general dental practitioner and prescription of fluoride supplements if required
   - speech assessment at 2 years and speech therapy as required; regular monitoring of speech and hearing should be carried out during childhood
   - lip revision, closure of palatal fistulae and possible pharyngoplasty may be undertaken at about 4–5 years of age if required.

Short note answers

1. Infraoccluded primary molars occur in about 8–14% of children. They arise because of ankylosis of the primary molar while alveolar bone growth and development of the adjacent teeth continues. Exfoliation will occur eventually if the permanent successor is present and not in an ectopic position. Removal, however, is indicated where the submergence is marked, with the crown of the tooth

just visible, or where root development of the unerupted premolar is almost complete.

2. This occurs in 2–6% of children but its prevalence is ~25% in cleft lip and palate. A number of factors have been implicated in its aetiology, including a more mesial eruption path of 6, a larger mean size of primary first and second molars and a retruded maxilla. Impaction may be reversible and self-correct, although this is uncommon after 8 years. In mild cases, placement of a brass wire separator for a few months may allow disimpaction, but appliance therapy to move 6 distally may be required in more marked cases. Removal of e may be required if symptomatic resorption has occurred or to allow restoration of 6. Extraction of e will aggravate existing crowding by facilitating mesial drift of 6 but can be managed at a later stage.

3. This was advocated by Kjellgren in 1948 as an interceptive procedure in a developing malocclusion to eliminate the need for any further intervention later. It involves removal of cs at age 8.5–9.5 years to encourage relief of incisor crowding; removal of ds at about 1 year later to encourage 4s to erupt; removal of 4s as 3s are erupting. A class I malocclusion with generalised moderate crowding is required for this to have the best chance of success, but even where these features are present there is no guarantee that appliance therapy will not be required later. For this reason and because three episodes of dental extractions, often requiring three episodes of general anaesthesia, are required, the full extent of serial extractions is not practised nowadays. Rather extraction of cs alone may be considered in some circumstances: removal of cs to allow the position of ectopic 3s to improve in the early mixed dentition; to allow a 2, which is likely to erupt in crossbite, to move labially; to create space for crossbite correction on 2 or for alignment of 1 following removal of a supernumerary which has impeded its eruption. Removal of c̄s may be considered to facilitate lingual movement of a lower incisor that is being displaced labially by a crossbite relationship with the upper incisor teeth, or of the whole lower labial segment lingually in a class III malocclusion.

4. Transposition is a positional interchange of two adjacent teeth (particularly of their roots) or the development of a tooth in a position occupied normally by an adjacent tooth. It is an uncommon dental anomaly (0.1–0.2% prevalence). It affects 3/4 and 2̄,3̄ most commonly. Management involves acceptance of the transposition if it is complete, extraction of the most displaced tooth if crowding is present or orthodontic alignment where sufficient space exists in the arch. The apical positions of the transposed teeth will determine whether alignment

is carried out with the teeth in their transposed positions or if these can be corrected.

5. Space maintenance is indicated:
   - typically in the late mixed dentition where there is likely to be no crowding in an arch, if mesial drift can be withheld and the leeway space used to provide space for arch alignment
   - where there is moderate/severe crowding in an arch such that there will be just sufficient space for the remaining teeth following removal of a unit/units. In the upper arch, it involves fitting either a removal appliance or palatal arch, whereas a lingual arch is best in the lower arch.

6. An increased overbite may be reduced by several means. In a growing child, a flat anterior bite plane on a removable appliance restrains vertical eruption of the lower incisors while allowing the lower molars to overerupt, thereby reducing the overbite. Lower incisor capping on a functional appliance will effect overbite reduction by similar means. Extrusion of the upper molars by cervical headgear to upper molar bands in a growing patient will also reduce overbite. In the child patient, facial growth then compensates for the increase in vertical face height. Where the overbite increases through overeruption of the upper labial segment, often with an associated 'gummy' smile, intrusion of the upper incisors either by high-pull headgear to a full-coverage maxillary splint or by a fixed appliance is indicated. In the adult, overbite reduction must be by incisor intrusion with a fixed appliance rather than by molar extrusion as there is no favourable vertical facial growth. In adults where the overbite is greatly increased, overbite reduction by orthognathic surgery will be required. Presurgical orthodontics does not involve overbite reduction. Rather, where class II correction is undertaken by mandibular advancement, overbite is reduced postsurgically by extrusion of the buccal segment teeth into occlusion to close the lateral open bites. In some patients, segmental osteotomies to 'set down' the lower labial segment and/or impact the upper labial segment may be indicated.

7. Growth modification is indicated in moderate-to-severe class II malocclusion in the mixed dentition when the child is growing. Treatment should commence just prior to the pubertal growth spurt so that maximum advantage is taken of the growth potential. Depending on the contribution of maxillary prognathism or mandibular retrusion to the aetiology of the malocclusion, treatment attempts to restrain maxillary vertical and forward growth and/or encourage mandibular growth. In doing so, the growth expression of the maxilla and/or mandible is altered but the amount of

growth of both is unaffected. This is carried out by either a functional appliance or headgear (1000 g required to restrain maxillary growth), or by a combination of the two. At least 14 hours per day wear is required of any appliance trying to modify growth. After occlusal correction, the appliance should be worn until growth is reduced to adult levels in late teens or until a second phase of treatment commences, possibly with extractions and fixed appliances.

8. Where growth modification is no longer a viable treatment option, the skeletal discrepancy can be disguised by tooth movement so that the incisor relationship is corrected, but the class II skeletal discrepancy remains. The skeletal pattern should be no worse than moderate and the vertical facial proportions good. Upper arch extractions are required (usually first premolars) to provide space for overjet correction by bodily retraction of the incisors. Importantly, the profile must not be worsened by this tooth movement, otherwise camouflage will have failed. The arches should be reasonably well aligned so that the extraction spaces are used for overjet reduction and not for relief of crowding.

9. Bilateral buccal crossbite exists where the lower buccal segment teeth occlude buccal to the opposing upper teeth. It indicates underlying symmetrical transverse skeletal discrepancy. It is common in class III malocclusions, often resulting from the anteroposterior skeletal discrepancy. It may also result from growth restriction laterally in a patient with repaired cleft palate. Rarely is there a functional problem associated, so it may be accepted unless being corrected as part of comprehensive treatment in a cleft patient. Where correction is considered, it may be undertaken by rapid maxillary expansion: turning a midline screw connected to bands cemented to premolar and molar teeth, twice daily for 2 weeks. This must be undertaken before early teens and overcorrection is advisable.

10. Adults are usually very specific about their complaint and have high expectations of treatment. The dentition may be compromised by periodontal disease or it may be heavily restored with perhaps apical pathology or retained roots. All dental disease must be controlled before orthodontic treatment can be considered. Anchorage may be a problem because of loss of bony support and previous tooth loss. Headgear is not realistic to reinforce anchorage, and alternatives such as palatal arches may be needed. Aesthetic brackets are often required to improve the appearance of the appliance. Initial response to tooth-moving forces is generally slower, but subsequent progress is as efficient as in the adolescent. Lighter forces should be used in the periodontally compromised dentition. Retention is often for longer as periodontal and alveolar bone remodelling takes longer. Permanent retention is essential in the periodontally compromised dentition. The absence of growth has two implications: overbite reduction should be by incisor intrusion rather than by molar extrusion and skeletal discrepancies other than mild are best dealt with by orthognathic surgery.

11. The type of maxillary osteotomy undertaken depends on the nature and severity of the skeletal problem. Maxillary osteotomies are described according to the fracture lines described by Le Fort or they may be segmental. Le Fort I is the most common osteotomy and allows the maxilla to be repositioned superiorly, inferiorly or anteriorly. Posterior movement is not realistic. The maxilla is disarticulated from its anterior wall, tuberosities, lateral nasal wall and nasal septum but pedicled on the palate to retain its blood supply. Le Fort II osteotomy is used for correction of marked maxillary retrognathia and nasal retrusion. Le Fort III osteotomy is employed for correcting rare craniofacial anomalies including Crouzon's syndrome. The Wassmund osteotomy separates the premaxilla with cuts distal to the canines, which are then extended horizontally across the palate. Although previously popular for overjet correction where premaxillary prominence exists, it is used rarely nowadays. Lack of interdental space and damage to adjacent teeth from the interdental cuts are potential problems.

12. Genetic and environmental factors interact to produce clefting. Positive family history exists in 40% of cleft lip (with or without palate) and in 20% of cleft palate only. Environmental factors (e.g. folic acid deficiency, maternal infections, anticonvulsant drug therapy, aspirin and cortisone) may act in a genetically susceptible individual to promote clefting. Cleft of lip and primary palate results from failure of fusion of medial nasal and maxillary processes by around the sixth week of intrauterine life. Failure of the palatal shelves to fuse at about 8–10 weeks leads to cleft palate. As palatal shelf elevation is later in females, it may promote cleft palate as there is greater potential for more lateral facial growth.

Viva answers

1. Early loss of primary teeth may have no effect (for example, early loss of a primary incisor rarely has an effect on the permanent dentition) or it may cause:
   - dilaceration of the root of the permanent successor or hypoplasia of its crown if the loss results from trauma
   - mesial drift: leading to worsening of inherent crowding, which may displace the permanent successor into crossbite and create a premature contact with associated mandibular displacement, or to tooth impaction or complete exclusion of a tooth
   - centreline shift if the loss is asymmetric
   - temporary relief of labial segment crowding.

The following five factors determine the effects:
- Which tooth is lost: loss of a or b rarely has any detrimental effect, although dilaceration of the permanent incisor root or hypoplasia of the crown may follow trauma; loss of c or d tends to improve labial segment crowding, often temporarily; unilateral loss of c or d will result in a centreline shift; loss of e facilitates mesial drift of the first permanent molar, which may lead to impaction of the second premolar but has minimal effect on the centreline

- age at which the tooth is lost: in general the earlier a tooth is lost, the greater the impact on the occlusion
- the arch from which it is lost: as there is a greater tendency to mesial drift in the upper arch, the effects of early loss are generally more marked in the upper than in the lower arch
- the occlusion: provided good interdigitation exists of the teeth on either side of the extraction site, minimal mesial drift is likely where a tooth is lost early from one arch
- other losses: the potential for space loss is enhanced where a tooth is lost from the opposing arch also
- the presence/absence of underlying crowding: where the arches are spaced, there is little untoward effect but where crowding is inherent or likely, this is exacerbated by early loss.

Undesirable sequelae may be minimised by:
- retaining a primary molar where possible by root treatment and placement of a stainless steel crown; this necessitates a co-operative child with a high level of dental motivation and very supportive parents
- considering the need to balance or compensate if an extraction is deemed necessary
- space maintenance (see Short note question 5 above).

10 Orthodontics III: appliances and tooth movement

Overview

Central to the success of any orthodontic treatment is selection of the appropriate appliance and competence in its handling. It is, therefore, necessary to be aware of the scope and limitations of each appliance system and the care required with its use.

In this chapter, removable, fixed, functional and headgear appliances are discussed. Histological aspects of tooth movement are then addressed and the factors that must be considered in planning retention are presented.

10.1 Removable appliances

Learning objectives

You should

- know the composition of stainless steel and acrylic resin used in appliance construction
- know the indications for removable appliance therapy
- know how to design, fit and adjust an upper removable appliance
- understand what is meant by anchorage
- be aware of those factors that influence anchorage loss
- realise the potential hazards and safety requirements with headgear.

Removable appliances consist primarily of wire and acrylic components and can be removed from the mouth. They are used almost exclusively in the upper arch. Lower appliances are poorly tolerated because of encroachment on tongue space and are usually used for the sole purpose of retention post-treatment. Although functional appliances are composed of the same materials, they have a different mode of action and are dealt with in Section 10.3.

Material composition

Wire

Adams' clasps, bows and springs are made from 18:8 austenitic stainless steel, so-called because of the content (18% chromium, 8% nickel) and the face-centred cubic crystal structure. The passive surface oxide layer produced by chromium and the resistance to corrosion conferred by the addition of nickel gives the steel its 'stainless' characteristic. Greater than 0.5% carbon reduces corrosion resistance as chromium carbide is deposited at grain boundaries on heating. Blue Elgiloy (cobalt chromium nickel alloy) may be used in the construction of Southend clasps. This wire has the advantage of being formed in the soft state and is then hardened by heat treatment. Work hardening of stainless steel wire occurs with repeated manipulation, and fracture is likely if the wire is adjusted where it has been bent previously. Soldering and welding of stainless steel are possible.

Soldering. The procedure should be carried out as follows:

- thoroughly clean the wires to be soldered
- mix a fluoride-containing flux with water to form a thick paste and apply it to the areas to be soldered; the flux removes the passive oxide layer
- heat a low-fusing silver solder in a gentle blue flame and apply to the joint area, ensuring that the wires are in close contact
- rapidly remove the flame to avoid annealing and softening the wire adjacent to the joint.

Welding. With the components to be welded held under pressure, fusion by melting is achieved on passing a 100 A, 5 V current for 0.01 seconds.

Acrylic resin

Acrylic resin is a polymethylmethacrylate (PMMA) formed from a chain of methacrylate molecules. It may be presented either as a liquid and powder (self-cure and heat-cure) or as a gel (light-cure). For self-cure and heat-cure resins, the liquid contains methylmethacrylate monomer, a cross-linking agent, an inhibitor (e.g. hydroquinone) and, in the case of self-cure resins only, an activator. The powder contains PMMA beads, an initiator (e.g. benzoyl peroxide), colour pigments and possibly fibres.

For baseplate construction, a separator should be applied to the working model after the wire components have been positioned. Incremental addition of powder and liquid, or of a gel, until the desired thickness is reached usually works satisfactorily after some practice. Removal of excess resin is easier when a gel is used rather than a powder/liquid combination. The powder/liquid ratio of the mixed resin should ideally be 2.5:1 by weight. Progressive setting occurs through sandy, string, dough, rubbery and hard phases in the mix.

Self-cure resins are usually satisfactory for orthodontic purposes: curing taking on average 20 minutes. Heat-cure appliances take 10 hours to cure, 7 hours at 70°C in a hot-water bath followed by 3 hours at 100°C and a slow cooling process to reduce stresses in the acrylic. Light-cure resins take 5 minutes to cure in a microwave.

Heat-cured appliances are more robust, less porous, more resistant to abrasion and contain less unreacted monomer than self-cured acrylics, but production cost and technician time are increased. The self-cured acrylics are also more prone to water absorption, and the residual monomer may cause a sensitivity reaction.

Indications for removable appliance therapy

The role of removable appliances in the contemporary management of malocclusion is much more restrictive than it has been in the past principally because of the more widespread use of fixed appliances and a greater awareness of the limitations of removable appliances. Removable appliances are best used in the following situations:

- where tilting movement of teeth is desirable and acceptable
- to maintain space in the mixed or early permanent dentition
- to help to transmit forces to groups of teeth (e.g. for arch expansion or distal movement of buccal segments)
- to free the occlusion and facilitate crossbite correction or other tooth movement
- to produce overbite reduction

- when minor rotation of an incisor or extrusion and rotation (with a fixed attachment) is required
- as a retainer following removable or fixed appliance treatment.

Designing a removable appliance

Some important points should be remembered in relation to appliance design:

- always design the appliance with the patient in the dental chair; this helps to avoid design errors
- keep the design as simple as possible: aim to carry out a few tooth movements with each appliance
- use the acronym ARAB to help to design the appliance in a logical sequence, ensuring nothing is overlooked: A, activation; R, retention; A, anchorage; and B, baseplate.

Active components

Springs The force (F) delivered by a spring is expressed by the formula $F \propto dr^4/l^3$, where d is the deflection of the spring, r is the radius of the wire and l is the length of the spring. Radius and wire length, therefore, have most effect on wire stiffness.

Screws Where the teeth needed for retention of the appliance are those to be moved, a screw rather than springs may be useful. However, screws are more expensive than springs and also make the appliance bulky. They also exert large intermittent forces, but this is tolerable because of the small (0.2 mm) activation with each quarter turn.

Elastics Elastic traction from intraoral elastics designed for orthodontic purposes should be avoided for overjet reduction with removable appliances as it tends to flatten the arch; in addition, the elastics may slide up the tooth surface and impinge on the gingivae. Elastic traction is best used with fixed appliances.

Retention component

The retention component maintains the appliance in the mouth, and it is generally advisable to have the clasps located to optimise retention. The following components are commonly used.

Adams' clasp Fixation is achieved by the arrowheads, which engage about 1 mm of the mesial and distal undercuts on the tooth. This clasp is the most common means of gaining posterior retention. For molars 0.7 mm wire is used, but 0.6 mm wire is advisable for premolars and deciduous molars. The clasp is easily modified to incorporate hooks for elastics, or tubes may be soldered for extraoral anchorage. Adjustment where the wire emerges from the baseplate is necessary if the 'flyover' is out of contact with the marginal ridge and/or close to the arrowhead to move it towards the tooth.

Southend clasp This 0.7 mm clasp is recommended anteriorly with the U-loop engaging the undercut between the incisors. Pushing the loop towards the baseplate is the only adjustment usually required.

Long labial bow This bow is constructed from 0.7 mm (0.8 mm if designed with reverse loops) wire and is useful in preventing buccal drifting of teeth during mesial or distal movement. Alternatively it may be fitted to the teeth as a retainer.

Adjustment depends on the design, but for a U-looped bow it is usual to squeeze the legs of the U-loop, followed by an upward adjustment anteriorly to restore its optimal vertical position.

Anchorage

Anchorage provides the resistance to the force of reaction generated by the active components and is best thought of in terms of the available space for the intended tooth movement. The anchorage demands should be assessed before treatment commences and may be classified as:

low: where the space from an extraction will provide more than sufficient space to achieve the desired result

moderate: where some residual extraction space is likely to remain following the intended tooth movement

high: where all the space from an extraction is needed to align the remaining teeth or reduce an overjet; anchorage must be reinforced from the start of treatement

very high: the extraction space will not allow successful achievement of the desired tooth movement and either additional extractions or extraoral traction is required to gain further space.

Patients for whom anchorage demands are high or very high are best treated by a specialist.

The tendency for space (anchorage) to be lost is related to:

- the force applied: greater forces place greater demand on anchorage; bodily movement requires greater force than tipping movement and hence the former is more 'anchorage straining'
- the root surface area (RSA): teeth with larger RSA or a block of teeth with a large RSA will resist anchorage loss more than those with a smaller RSA
- mesial drift tendency: this is greater in the upper than in the lower arch
- FMPA (Frankfort mandibular planes angle): space loss is easier with increased than with reduced FMPA
- occlusal interdigitation: where this is good, mesial drift is less likely.

To minimise anchorage loss, the correct force should be used for the movement required (~30 to 60 g for tip-ping; ~100 to 150 g for bodily movement), the minimum number of teeth should be moved at one time and the resistance of the anchor teeth should be increased. It is possible to ensure that only bodily movement of the anchor teeth is permissible with a fixed appliance but this is difficult to achieve with a removable appliance.

Intraoral reinforcement of anchorage Anchorage may be reinforced:

- intramaxillarily using teeth in the same arch by incorporating the maximum number of teeth in the anchorage unit; this is applicable to fixed appliances also
- by mucosal coverage: the palatal coverage of the baseplate provides greater anchorage in removable than in fixed appliances
- intermaxillarily using teeth in the opposing arch; this is not recommended with removable appliances as elastic traction tends to displace the appliance, but it is suitable with fixed appliances, the direction of the elastic traction depending on the malocclusion: class II traction pulls backward on the upper labial segment and forward on the lower buccal segment; class III traction pulls forward on the upper molars and backward on the lower labial segment.

Extraoral reinforcement of anchorage Anchorage may be reinforced by using headgear, pulling upward and backward on a facebow attached to a removable or fixed appliance against the cranial vault. Forces of 200–250 g for 10 hours per day are necessary. If distal movement of the buccal segments is required, extraoral traction is indicated with forces of 500 g for 14–16 hours per day.

Safety with headgear Safety is a priority because of the potential hazards to the eyes and face. Two safety mecha-nism should be fitted to each headgear assembly, prefer-ably a facebow with locking device (e.g. Ni Tom®) and a safety release spring mechanism attached to the headcap. Verbal and written instructions must be issued to the patient and parent or guardian emphasising that:

- the headgear is only to be assembled and removed in the way demonstrated by the orthodontist
- no horseplay is permissible when the headgear is attached
- it is never to be worn outside the house or while engaged in contact sports
- if anyone tries to pull the facebow out of the mouth with the headgear attached, firmly grab hold of their hand to prevent this
- if the headgear ever comes out at night, discontinue wear and contact the orthodontist as soon as possible
- if it ever damages the face or eyes contact your local hospital immediately; discontinue wear and contact your orthodontist.

Baseplate

The baseplate connects the other components of the appliance and may be passive or active.

Anterior bite plane An anterior bite plane is required when overbite reduction is necessary or when removal of an occlusal interference is required to allow tooth movement. Three essential elements must be addressed:

- the bite plane should be flat: if inclined it may procline or retrocline the lower incisors
- it must contact two and preferably three of the lower incisors; to ensure this, a measurement of the overjet (+ 3 mm) should be forwarded to the technician at the time of appliance fabrication
- it should separate the molar teeth by 2–3 mm; it will be necessary, in most cases, to add cold cure acrylic to the flat anterior bite plane during treatment to continue overbite reduction.

Posterior bite planes Posterior bite planes are required to remove occlusal interferences and facilitate tooth movement when overbite reduction is unnecessary. This is commonly the case when correcting a unilateral buccal crossbite with mandibular displacement or an incisor crossbite. The acrylic coverage should be just sufficient to disengage the occlusion but must be adjusted to give even contact of the posterior teeth. The bite planes should be removed when the malocclusion is corrected and the appliance should then be worn as a retainer while the posterior occlusion settles.

Common tooth movements required

Table 35 on page 305 summarises the common desired tooth movements and the active components to achieve this. Box 42 on page 306 describes the technique involved in fitting a removable appliance.

Managing problems during treatment

The common problems that arise during treatment are listed in Table 36 on page 307 together with the common causes and necessary treatment.

10.2 Fixed appliances

A fixed appliance is attached to the teeth and is, therefore, not usually removable by the patient!

Components

The appliance is composed of three elements: the brackets/bands, the archwires and the accessories.

Learning objectives

You should

- be aware of the components of a fixed appliance
- know the indications for a fixed appliance
- be aware of how management of fixed and removable appliances differ
- be aware of different fixed appliance types.

Brackets and bands

Brackets are bonded to all teeth, with the usual exception of molars, via composite resin following acid etching of the enamel; some resin-modified glass ionomer cements, (e.g. Fuji Ortho LC) may be used for this purpose also and have the advantages of not requiring etching of enamel, the capacity to bond in the presence of saliva and release fluoride, which may reduce enamel decalcification. The bracket allows the tooth to be directed by the active component comprising the archwire and/or accessories. Brackets may be made from stainless steel, polycarbonate, ceramic or a combination of polycarbonate/ceramic. Polycarbonate and ceramic brackets are more aesthetic than metal but have disadvantages. Polycarbonate brackets soften in saliva, leading to tie-wing fracture, discolour and have poor torque control without a metal insert in a bracket slot. Ceramic brackets are hard and brittle so may wear the opposing teeth, increase friction with the archwire and can cause enamel fracture at debond (common with the early-marketed types). These problems have now been overcome by a polycarbonate base on a ceramic-faced bracket with a metal insert in the bracket slot.

Bands are usually cemented to molar teeth only using a glass ionomer cement. They may be considered where repeated bond failure occurs on other teeth or when a lingual attachment is required to aid derotation. Separation of the teeth, usually with elastomeric rings, is required for up to 1 week to facilitate band placement and guarantee best fit.

Archwires

Archwires may be round or rectangular.

Stainless steel is the most commonly used archwire material, but nickel–titanium, cobalt–chromium and beta-titanium – all with greater flexibility than stainless steel – have gained increasing popularity in contemporary practice. Nickel–titanium has two unique properties – shape memory and superelasticity – that relate to phase transitions between the mastensitic and austenitic

Table 35 Common tooth movements and related active components

Tooth movement required	Component and wire diameter	Activation
Retraction of 3 Buccal	Buccal canine retractor: 0.5 mm sleeved with coil or 0.7 mm with U-loop	For 0.5 mm spring, bend anterior leg about 2–3 mm around the round beak of a spring-forming plier
		For 0.7 mm spring, cut 1 mm of wire from the free end, ensuring that the spring is curved into contact with the mesial surface of the canine
Palatal	Palatal finger spring 0.5 mm	Ensure that spring is just above the gingival margin on the tooth and that movement tangential to the point of contact will keep the tooth in the line of the arch
		Bend in the free arm in the area between the coil and guardwire
Buccal movement of 3, 4, 5 or 6	Single tooth: 'T' spring, 0.5 mm Two or more teeth: screw	Pull spring away from the baseplate ~2 mm Instruct the patient to turn screw once or twice per week
Palatal movement of single tooth other than 3	Buccal retractor either 0.5 mm sleeved with coil or 0.7 mm with U-loop	As per buccal canine retractor but activation may be greater or less depending on root surface area of the tooth
Mesial/distal movement of teeth other than 3	Palatal finger spring: 0.5 mm for incisors or premolars; 0.6 mm for 6	For 0.5 mm, activation 2–3 mm, For 0.6 mm, activation 1–2 mm
Distal movement of upper buccal segments	Screw appliance or appliance with coffin spring (1.25 mm) with provision for EOT	Either instruct patient to turn screw, one turn per week, or pull the two parts of the appliance apart by 2–3 mm if a coffin spring is used
		Also EOT to be worn 14–16 hours/day with a force ~500 g per side
		Must fit EOT with two safety mechanisms (e.g. 'Ni Tom' ® facebow and 'Snap-away' headcap, ensuring direction of pull is above the occlusal plane)
Proclination of incisors	Z-spring 0.5 mm	First adjust spring close to coil at the fixed end and then at the other limb end to give 1–2 mm of activation
	Double cantilever springs 0.7/0.8 mm	As for Z- spring
	Screw appliance	Instruct patient to turn screw one or two turns per week
Retraction of incisors[a]	Roberts retractor, 0.5 mm with coils and sleeved distal to coils	3 mm in the vertical limb below the coil
	Labial bow with U-loops, 0.7 mm	1 mm by squeezing the U-loops; may increase flexibility by splitting the bow. If overjet >4 mm, use Roberts retractor

[a]Overbite reduction must precede overjet reduction always. Trim the flat anterior bite plane in the horizontal plane *and* from behind 21/12 to allow overjet reduction, ensuring that $\overline{2\,1}$ / $\overline{1\,2}$ maintain contact with the biteplane until the last 2 mm of movement is required.

alloy forms. Even with a large deflection, a relatively constant low force is applied, making these archwires an excellent choice for initial alignment. They are, however, more expensive than stainless steel archwires.

Cobalt–chromium alloy (Elgiloy) may be shaped while in a soft state and then hardened by heat treatment.

Beta-titanium has excellent strength and springiness, midway between nickel–titanium and stainless steel, making it ideal for intermediate and finishing stages of treatment.

Accessories

Elastics or elastomeric modules/chain/thread Latex elastics produced for orthodontic purposes may be used for intra- or intermaxillary traction. A range of sizes is available. Elastomeric modules are used to maintain an archwire in an edgewise bracket slot (see below) while elastomeric chain or thread is usually used to move teeth along an archwire, or for derotation.

Springs Uprighting or rotation of teeth may be carried out by uprighting or whip springs, respectively, while space opening or closure may be undertaken by coil springs.

Indications for fixed appliances

Indications include

- bodily movement of incisors to correct mild-to-moderate skeletal discrepancies
- overbite reduction by incisor intrusion

Box 42 Fitting a removable appliance

1. Check that the working model and appliance are those of the patient and that the appliance has been well made to your design.
2. Check the fitting surface for roughnesses and any sharp edges of wire tags. These should be smoothed off with an acrylic bur or green stone, respectively.
3. Try the appliance in the patient's mouth. If any teeth have been lost or extracted since the impression was taken, some adjustment is likely to be required to get the appliance to fit well.
4. Adjust the posterior and then the anterior retention until satisfactory.
5. Trim any anterior or posterior biteplane to the correct height.
6. Leave all springs passive for the first 2 weeks until the patient has adapted to wearing the appliance.
7. Show the patient in a mirror how to insert and remove the appliance, stressing that it is important not to damage any springs. Let the patient practise this several times under your supervision.
8. Instruct the patient and parent or guardian in wear and care of the appliance, emphasising the following:
   - full-time wear, including mealtimes, is essential; it will take a few days to get used to eating with the appliance in, but you must persevere
   - sticky and hard foods, particularly toffees and chewing gum, must not be eaten
   - the appliance must be taken out after meals for cleaning and for contact sports (when it should be stored in the strong plastic container provided)
   - speech is likely to be affected for the first week but will be normal thereafter
   - if the appliance cannot be worn as instructed or causes discomfort or breaks, you must contact the clinic immediately. A list of written instructions should be issued.
9. Explain that the appliance has been fitted passively

and that any extractions will be requested once there is evidence of full-time wear.
10. Make a review appointment for 2–3 weeks.

Subsequent visits
1. Check that the appliance is being worn full-time; if so
   - speech should be normal with no lisp
   - the patient should be able to remove and insert the appliance unaided by a mirror
   - the baseplate should have lost its shine
   - if there is an anterior or posterior bite plane on the appliance, there should be occlusal markings from the opposing teeth
   - mild gingival erythema and a slight mark across the posterior extent of the appliance on the palate should also be present
2. If full-time wear is not apparent, the patient should be questioned as to why and informed that treatment will be terminated unless total compliance is forthcoming.
3. Check oral hygiene
4. Check for anchorage loss by recording the buccal segment relationship and the overjet. If headgear is being worn, ask if there have been any problems. These must be documented, and if none are apparent this should be noted. Check for evidence of headgear wear and for how long it is worn by assessing the time sheet. Check the headgear safety mechanisms.
5. Assess the intended tooth movement; record any change with dividers and punch this in the patient's records.
6. Adjust the retention of the appliance if necessary.
7. Check the baseplate so that there is no impediment to the intended tooth movement and/or that its height is satisfactory for overbite reduction or to prevent occlusal interference.
8. Adjust the active component if necessary.
9. Indicate in the patient's records the action plan for the next visit.

- correction of rotations
- extensive lower arch treatment
- alignment of grossly misplaced teeth particularly those requiring extrusion
- closure of spaces
- multiple movements required in either one or both arches.

Tooth movement

As with a removable appliance, a fixed appliance may also tip teeth but has the additional possibilities of producing bodily movement (crown and root apex move in the same direction), uprighting, torquing, rotation, intrusion and extrusion of teeth.

Anchorage control

Because the palate is not covered by a baseplate, anchorage control is more critical with a fixed than

with a removable appliance. In addition, bodily rather than tipping movement places greater strain on anchorage.

Anchorage may be reinforced by:

- increasing the anchorage unit by bonding more teeth and ligating them together
- preventing forward tipping of the molars by anchor bends in the archwire (placed between premolar and molar at 30° to the occlusal plane)
- placing torque in the archwire ensuring that the anchor teeth can only move bodily, thereby increasing resistance to unwanted movement
- palatal and/or lingual arches: prevent molar tipping
- intermaxillary traction (see Section 9.5): as well as reinforcing anchorage, the incisor relationship (either increased or reverse overjet) may be corrected

Table 36 Problems during treatment

Problem	Cause	Management
Baseplate fracture	Existing crack Baseplate too thin Damage by patient out of the mouth Clicking habit Eating sticky/hard foods	Check co-operation; caution the patient if necessary If small fracture, cold cure acrylic repair; if large fracture, consider remake with heat-cured acrylic Discourage habit Reinstruct the patient regarding avoidance of inappropriate foods
Wire fracture	Work hardened from repeated bends or occlusal loading Damaged while trimming baseplate Clicking habit Eating sticky/hard foods	If arrowhead fracture on Adams' clasp use solder; otherwise replace component; ensure component is not loaded by the occlusion Discourage any 'clicking' habit with the appliance Dissuade from eating inappropriate foods
Rapid deterioration in retention	Clicking habit	Discourage
Palatal hyperplasia	Failure to trim baseplate during overjet reduction Poor oral hygiene	Ensure baseplate trimmed and shelved behind incisors before retraction and that overbite reduction is adequate Oral hygiene instruction/application of antifungal agent (e.g. nystatin) to the fitting surface
Slow progress	Lack of full-time wear Active component not being adjusted as instructed or spring overactivated/passive/distorted Incorrect positioning of springs by patient Acrylic, wire or the opposing occlusion preventing movement Retained root fragment/anxylosis	Caution the patient and encourage to wear the appliance full time Reinstruct or adjust/reposition spring correctly Reinstruct in appliance insertion and removal Remove acrylic/adjust wire/increase height of any biteplane Arrange for removal of root fragment; if tooth anxylosed, reassess and consider other treatment options
Lack of overbite reduction	Appliance not worn at meals Adult patient	Caution and reinforce importance of full-time wear Fixed appliance may be a better option to expedite treatment
Marked tipping of tooth	Incorrect spring positioning Excess force	Relocate spring to just above gingival margin Reduce force
Anchorage less	Appliance not being worn full-time Anchorage demands exceed those required	Reinforce importance of full-time wear Reassess anchorage need carefully; consider revised treatment plan, appliance design, anchorage reinforcement

- placement of an implant
- extraoral means, including reverse headgear (see Sections 9.4 and 10.1).

Appliance types

Edgewise Edgewise appliances use attachments with a rectangular slot and round flexible wires for initial alignment. Rectangular wires are required for precise apical control.

Begg The Begg appliance uses a bracket with a vertical slot and round wires exclusively held in place loosely with brass pins. Tipping movement is facilitated and auxiliaries are necessary for rotational and apical movement.

Pre-adjusted appliances
Edgewise. The edgewise pre-adjusted appliance uses an individual bracket for each tooth to give it 'average'

inclination and angulation and allow the placement of flat archwires. Bracket prescriptions described by Andrews and Roth are available. Clinical time is saved and good occlusal results are achieved with greater consistency with these techniques, but cost is greater than with the 'standard' edgewise appliance technique because of the larger inventory of brackets and bands required.

Tip-edge appliance. This technique uses special brackets with rectangular slots. Although round wire is used for most of the treatment, as with the Begg technique, the facility exists to place rectangular wire in the final stages.

Lingual appliance. This uses brackets bonded to the lingual or palatal surfaces of the teeth and specially configured archwires. Although the ultimate in terms of aesthetics, it is uncomfortable for the patient and difficult to adjust.

Sectional appliance. This comprises components attached to teeth in usually one segment of the arch; it is used for localised alignment as part of adjunctive treatment, particularly in adults.

Fixed–removable appliances An upper removable appliance may be used with the following fixed components:

- bands cemented to <u>6</u>s for extraoral traction
- a bracket with elastomeric chain or a gold chain bonded to a surgically exposed incisor and extruded via a labial arm
- a bracket bonded to a favourably inclined palatal canine, and traction applied from a buccal arm on the appliance to the bracket via an elastic module.

Appliance management

An excellent standard of oral hygiene is essential prior to and during fixed appliance treatment. All patients must be instructed specifically in relation to diet and optimal oral hygiene practices following placement of the appliance to minimise the risk of enamel demineralisation. Mucosal ulceration is common in the early stages of treatment and it is wise to give the patient some soft ribbon wax to place over any components that are causing minor trauma. Adjustment visits are usually at intervals of 4 to 6 weeks. Repairing fixed appliances occupies more chairside time than does removable appliances. Mild discomfort is normal for a few days following adjustment and is usually overcome by mild analgesics.

10.3 Functional appliances

Learning objectives

You should

- have an appreciation of how functional appliances work

- know the indications for functional appliance therapy

- be familiar with the practical management of a patient with a functional appliance

- be aware of differences between functional appliance types

- know the skeletal and dental effects of functional appliance therapy.

Functional appliances correct malocclusion by using, removing or modifying the forces generated by the orofacial musculature, tooth eruption and dentofacial growth.

Mechanism of action

How functional appliances work is not completely understood. They are generally devoid of active components such as springs and are incapable of moving teeth individually. Instead they operate by applying or eliminating forces that are generated through the facial and masticatory musculature and by harnessing those that occur through natural growth processes. They are, therefore, only effective in growing children, preferably just prior to their pubertal growth spurt. The specific force system set up by any appliance will depend on its particular design. Essentially, forces are developed by posturing the mandible – either downward and forward in class II or downward and backward in class III. This applies intermaxilliary traction between the arches, as can be produced by elastics with fixed appliances. As the scope for posturing the mandible backward is far less than for posturing it forward, functional appliances are more successful in, and are indicated almost exclusively for class II malocclusion. For this reason, the possible mechanisms of action will only be considered for class II malocclusion. In these cases, the result is a forward tipping of the lower incisors and the entire mandibular dentition, with acceleration of mandibular growth, as well as a backward tipping of the upper incisors and restraint of maxillary growth. Overall mandibular growth is modified – the total amount is unaffected but the expression of growth is altered.

Indications

Where the appliance is the sole means of correcting the malocclusion in a growing child, the following features should be present:

- mild skeletal class II owing to mandibular retrusion or mild skeletal class III owing to mandibular protrusion
- average or reduced FMPA
- uncrowded arches
- lower incisors upright or slightly retroclined in class II, and proclined in class III; proclined lower incisors in class II usually contraindicates functional appliance therapy.

In severe class II malocclusion, a preliminary phase of functional appliance therapy in the mixed dentition may be useful to aid overbite reduction and occlusal correction prior to proceeding to further treatment with fixed appliances and possible extractions.

Practical management of patients with a functional appliance.

Box 43 outlines the general steps involved in using a functional appliance. The orthodontist must be confi-

Box 43 Management technique for a patient with a functional appliance

1. Ensure that the patient is keen for treatment and is growing.
2. A lateral cephalometric film, in addition to the normal diagnostic records, is essential before treatment starts.
3. In some patients, a preliminary phase of arch expansion and/or alignment is necessary before proceeding to functional appliance treatment. This is particularly so in class II division 2, where the upper incisors must be proclined and aligned to allow a forward posturing of the mandible to obtain the construction bite. The appliance used for the first stage of treatment may then be worn as a retainer at all times when the functional appliance is out of the mouth.
4. Obtain well-extended upper and lower impressions and a construction bite, the specifics of which depend on the functional appliance chosen.
5. Record the patient's standing height at the appointment when the appliance is fitted.
6. With most appliances (except the Twinblock and Herbst appliances), wear should be built up gradually until the appliance is worn for a minimum of 14 hours per day and preferably more. A time sheet should be used to record the number of hours of wear and should be brought along for inspection at each review visit.
7. Warn the patient that minor discomfort is common initially, particularly muscular and temporomandibular joint tenderness, but this usually subsides after 1–2 weeks. Mild analgesics may be taken as required. If an area of mucosal ulceration develops, the patient must return for appliance adjustment.
8. Review 1–2 weeks after appliance fitting to check appliance wear, to make any necessary adjustments and, most importantly, to encourage compliance. Then recall at intervals of 6–8 weeks.
9. Measure the overjet and check the buccal segment relationships at each recall visit, ensuring that the patient's mandible is retruded maximally – otherwise a false indication of any progress will arise. Check the time sheet at each visit and encourage if progress is good; about 1 mm of overjet reduction per month is usual in co-operative, growing individuals. If the appliance is not being worn as instructed, careful counselling, highlighting that this form of treatment is only effective for a finite time while the patient is growing, may improve co-operation.
10. Depending on the initial construction bite, at 4 to 6 months in treatment, reactivation of the appliance (or a new appliance) may be necessary, with further posturing of the mandible to achieve the desired incisor relationship.
11. If there is no discernible progress in six months, stop treatment and reassess.
12. Slight overcorrection of the occlusion is advisable and then the appliance should be worn as a retainer at nights until growth reduces to adult levels. It may be necessary to make a new appliance for this purpose.
13. In some patients, a second phase of treatment will be required, with possible extractions and fixed appliance therapy. Occlusal correction may be retained with the functional appliance until this gets under way.

dent about the ability of the appliance to work and relay this enthusiastically to both the patient and parent.

Types of functional appliance

The following account describes some standard functional appliances. However, current thinking regarding design is to 'pick and mix' the components that are necessary for the specific correction of a particular malocclusion. Such a 'components approach' to design requires considerable insight into the working of these appliances and requires specialist knowledge and expertise.

Bite planes

By using the action of the masticatory musculature, both anterior or posterior bite planes may intrude teeth in the corresponding parts of the arch. They are, however, not conventionally thought of as 'functional appliances' as this term is generally confined to appliances that effect anteroposterior correction of malocclusion.

Andresen activator

The Andresen activator is constructed to a bite giving 2–3 mm of incisal opening, usually with an edge-to-edge incisor relationship. A second advancement may be necessary with a large overjet. Specific design aspects include no clasps, a passive labial bow and upper and lower acrylic baseplates fused together. Acrylic capping extends over the lower incisors to allow overbite reduction while the buccal interocclusal acrylic is trimmed to direct mesial movement of the lower teeth and distal and buccal movement of the upper teeth.

Harvold Harvold is a bulky appliance derived from the Andresen activator but differs from the latter in that

- the working bite is typically 8–10 mm greater than the freeway space and slightly behind the maximum protrusive position
- the occlusal shelves contact the upper posterior teeth only.

Wear for 14–16 hours per day is recommended, but as there are no clasps on the appliance, retention is sometimes a problem.

Bionator The bionator is a less bulky (therefore more popular) derivative of the Andresen activator. In addition the construction bite is taken edge to edge. The labial bow is extended back to hold the cheeks out of contact with the buccal segment teeth and allow arch expansion, while a thick palatal loop takes the place of acrylic. Full-time wear is advisable except for meals.

Medium opening activator This is a substantially 'trimmed down' variant of the Andresen activator, with molar clasping to aid retention, minimal acrylic extensions lingual to the lower incisors and no buccal acrylic capping. Heat-cured acrylic is recommended to minimise the likelihood of fracture of the lingual extensions. Often arch expansion is required prior to proceeding with treatment. The construction bite is generally 3–4 mm open in the premolar areas with forward posturing of 6 mm. Full-time wear with the usual exceptions is possible.

Frankel appliance

The Frankel appliance was originally termed a 'function regulator' and has particular use in the management of abnormal soft tissue pattern, for example hyperactive mentalis muscle, which is often associated with partial or complete lip trapping and retroclination of the lower labial segment. Buccal shields hold the cheeks away from the teeth and stretch the mucoperiosteum at the sulcus depth, intending to expand the arches and widen the alveolar processes. Stability of such changes are doubtful long term.

There are four subtypes:

- Fr I is used to correct class I and class II division 1 malocclusions
- Fr II is used for correction of class II division 2 malocclusion
- Fr III is used for correction of class III malocclusion
- Fr IV is used for correction of anterior open bite.

Fr I is the most popular and includes acrylic pads labial of the lower incisors to encourage development of the mandibular alveolar process. Although lower incisor capping is not traditionally prescribed, it may be incorporated to aid overbite correction. The construction bite is usually as in the medium opening activator. Wear is gradually built up from 2–3 hours per day in the first few weeks, to night-time and then full-time apart from sports and while eating.

Fr III has labial pads in the upper labial sulcus, and heavy wires palatal to the upper and labial to the lower incisors. For the construction bite, the mandible is postured down and slightly backward to achieve an edge-to-edge incisor relationship. Instructions regarding wear are as for the Fr I.

Frankel appliances are complex in design, expensive to make and repair and easy to damage and distort. They can, however, be reactivated by sectioning the buccal shields and repositioning them forward.

Twin block appliance

The twin block appliance consists of upper and lower appliances incorporating buccal blocks, with interfacing inclined planes that posture the mandible forward on closure (Fig. 128). Often, headgear is added to the upper appliance at night. The construction bite is taken with the mandible postured forward comfortably, with about 6 mm separation in the molar region. Those with normal or reduced overbite are most suited to this appliance. Full-time wear is facilitated by the two-part design. Overjet reduction tends to be rapid, but either trimming of the buccal blocks is required later or a modified retainer with a steep inclined plane is required anteriorly to close the lateral open bites that develop. The incorporation of repelling magnets in the inclined planes leads to faster overjet reduction. Variants for treatment of class II division 2 and class III malocclusions also exist.

Herbst appliance

A Herbst appliance consists of splints cemented to the upper and lower arches joined by pin and tube telescopic arms that determine the amount of mandibular posturing. Full-time wear is guaranteed!

(a)

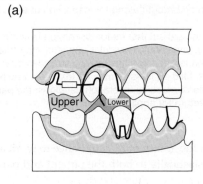

(b)

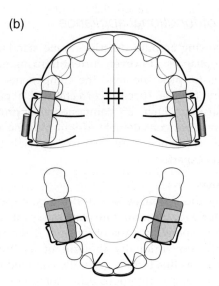

Fig. 128 The twin block appliance. (a) Profile. (b) Occlusal views.

Headgear addition to functional appliances

In cases where maximal anteroposterior and vertical maxillary restraint is desirable, occipital-pull headgear may be added to tubes incorporated in the acrylic or soldered to the clasp bridges. Forces of about 500 g should be used for 14–16 hours per day and the usual headgear safety precautions and instructions should be followed (see Section 10.1). If the FMPA is increased, molar capping is essential to promote a closing rotation of the mandible and prevent molar eruption, thereby facilitating an increase in overbite. The addition of high-pull headgear to the appliance will facilitate this process.

Effects of functional appliances

For class II with deep overbite
Dental effects

- Retroclination of the upper incisors and proclination of the lower incisors are usual, although the latter is not found consistently and is best minimised by placing acrylic capping on the lower anterior teeth.
- Inhibition of lower incisor eruption and promotion of eruption of the posterior teeth leads to levelling of the curve of Spee. This process is facilitated by lower incisor capping on the appliance.
- Guidance of eruption of the lower posterior teeth in an upward and forward direction while preventing eruption and forward movement of the upper posterior teeth encourages correction of a class II buccal relationship.
- Arch expansion is intended through the buccal shields of the Frankel appliance and the buccal wire of the Bionator. Long-term stability of these changes is unsubstantiated.

Skeletal effects

- Enhancement of mandibular growth is brought about by movement of the mandibular condyle out of the fossa, promoting growth of the condylar cartilage and forward migration of the glenoid fossa. This effect is very variable.
- Inhibition of forward maxillary growth occurs.
- An increase in lower facial height is mediated by the alterations in the eruption of the posterior teeth, as described above.

For class III
Dental effects

- Proclination of the upper and retroclination of the lower incisors can be achieved.

- The appliance facilitates downward and forward eruption of the upper posterior teeth while inhibiting eruption of mandibular teeth.

Skeletal effects There is no evidence to substantiate an anteroposterior skeletal effect, but lower face height is increased.

10.4 Orthodontic tooth movement and retention

Learning objectives

You should

- know the histological response in areas of pressure and tension with orthodontic tooth movement, and how tipping differs from bodily movement
- be able to give the range of force required for each type of tooth movement
- know the undesirable sequelae of orthodontic forces
- understand the rationale for retention and factors to be considered in planning retention.

Orthodontic tooth movement

The biological response to a sustained force is determined mainly by the force magnitude and duration, which generate zones of pressure and tension within the periodontal ligament, their extent and location depending on the intended movement.

Pressure zones

The cellular response relates to whether a light or heavy force is applied. With a light sustained force, movement occurs within a few seconds as periodontal ligament fluid is squeezed out and the vascular supply is compressed, setting off a complex biochemical response. Osteoclastic invasion occurs within 2 days and frontal resorption follows.

When a heavy sustained force is applied, the periodontal ligament is compressed to such a degree that the blood flow is cut off completely, producing an area of sterile necrosis (hyalinisation). Small zones of hyalinisation are inevitable even with light forces, but the area of hyalinisation is extended with forces of greater magnitude. Osteoclastic differentiation is impossible within the necrotic periodontal ligament space, but after several days osteoclasts appear adjacent to and within the adjacent cancellous spaces. From there they invade the bone adjacent to the hyalinised area and tooth movement eventually occurs by undermining resorption.

Tension zones

Following initial application of a light force, the blood vessels vasodilate and the periodontal ligament fibres are stretched, while fibroblast and preosteoblast proliferation occurs. The stretched fibres become embedded in osteoid, which later mineralises. The normal periodontal ligament width is eventually regained by simultaneous collagen fibre remodelling.

With heavy forces, rupture of blood vessels and severing of the periodontal ligament fibres are likely, but these are restored with the remodelling processes.

Mechanisms of tooth movement

Although the histological response to an applied orthodontic force has been investigated extensively, the mechanism by which a mechanical stimulus effects a cellular response is complex and at present unclarified. It is likely that vascular changes in the periodontal ligament in areas of pressure and tension, electrical signals generated in response to flexing of alveolar bone following force application, prostaglandins and cytokine release interact in the process.

Types of tooth movement, force magnitude and duration

Although it was previously thought that tipping of a single-rooted tooth (Fig. 129) occurred about a point almost midway along the root, rotation now appears to take place near the apical third within an elliptically shaped area. Half of the periodontal ligament is stressed, with maximum pressure created at the alveolar crest in the direction of movement and at the diagonally opposite apical area. For bodily movement and rotation, a force couple must be applied, loading uniformly the whole of the periodontal ligament in the direction of translation so both crown and root move in the same direction by equal amounts (Fig. 130). With extrusion, all of the periodontal ligament is tensed, but when a tooth is intruded the force is concentrated at the apex. An element of tipping is unavoidable with extrusion, intrusion and rotation.

For tooth movement to occur optimally, the force per unit area within the periodontal ligament should ideally not occlude the vascular supply yet be sufficient to induce a cellular response. A force should, therefore, be as light as possible for the movement intended, taking into account the root surface area over which it is spread. Optimal force ranges for various tooth movements are:

- tipping 30–60 g
- bodily movement 100–150 g
- rotation or extrusion 50–75 g
- intrusion 15–25 g.

Although tooth movement can occur in response to heavy forces, these should not be applied continuously;

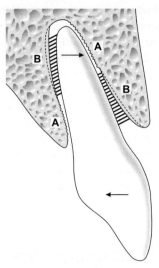

Fig. 129 The effect of tipping movement. A = area of periodontal ligament compression/alveolar bone resorption; B = area of periodontal ligament tension/alveolar bone deposition.

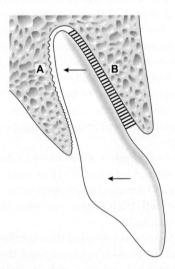

Fig. 130 The effect of bodily movement. A = area of periodontal ligament compression/alveolar bone resorption; B = area of periodontal ligament tension/alveolar bone deposition.

intermittent application may be clinically acceptable. Not only must a force be of sufficient magnitude to effect the movement desired but it must also be sustained for sufficient time. For successful movement, a force must be applied for at least 6 out of 24 hours, and continuous application of light forces is optimal. This is favoured, because control of tooth movement and anchorage is facilitated while the risks of pulpal and radicular damage are minimised. Excessive mobility is avoided and movement is more efficient with less discomfort. Movement of the order of 1 mm in a 4-week period is regarded as optimal, with faster progress recorded in children than in adults. This is largely a consequence of the greater cellularity of the periodontal ligament, more cancellous alveolar bone and faster tissue turnover in a growing patient, which ensure a more rapid response to an applied force.

Undesirable sequelae of orthodontic force

Pulpal damage

A mild pulpitis following initial force application is common, but has no effect long term. Where the apical blood vessels are severed by the use of heavy continuous force or by injudicious root movement through the alveolar plate, pulp death is likely, although this is usually associated with previous trauma.

Root resorption

Areas of cementum resorbed during tooth movement are usually repaired. Some permanent loss of root length is found, however, on nearly all teeth following bodily movement over long distances. This occurs primarily in the apical or apicolateral regions of maxillary incisors and mandibular first permanent molars. Fortunately, in most instances, loss of 0.5–1.0 mm of root length is of no long-term significance. The risk is increased where

- root resorption is present before treatment
- there is a history of previous trauma irrespective of whether endodontic treatment was undertaken
- the root is pipette shaped, blunt or demonstrates a marked apical curvature.

Torquing movements and apical contact with cortical bone are also significant risk factors.

Loss of alveolar bone height

With fixed appliance treatment, 0.5 to 1 mm loss of crestal alveolar height is common, with the greatest loss occurring at extraction sites. In the presence of good oral hygiene, this appears of little concern.

Pain and mobility

Even with appropriate force magnitude, ischaemic areas develop in the periodontal ligament after activation of an orthodontic appliance, leading to mild discomfort and pressure sensitivity. These usually last for 2–4 days and return when the appliance is reactivated. Some increase in mobility is common, as the periodontal ligament space widens and the fibres reorganise in response to the applied force. With heavy orthodontic forces, however, the likelihood of almost immediate onset of pain and marked mobility is increased, as the periodontal ligament is crushed and further undermining resorption occurs.

Retention

Following tooth movement, a period of retention is usually required to hold the teeth passively, preventing them returning to their pretreatment position while the periodontal fibres and alveolar bone adapt to their new locations. The retention phase should be planned and discussed fully with the patient before treatment starts. The following factors are likely to destabilise the final result.

Forces from the supporting tissues

Reorganisation of the principal periodontal ligament fibres and supporting alveolar bone occurs within 4 to 6 months, but at least 7 to 8 months is required for the supracrestal fibres to reorganise because of the slow turnover of the free gingival fibres. Rotational correction is, therefore, liable to relapse, but this tendency may be reduced by surgical sectioning (pericision) of the supracrestal fibres. Overcorrection of the rotation early in treatment may help to minimise relapse; however, irrespective of strategy, bonded retention is required to guarantee alignment.

Where periodontal support is compromised, indefinite retention will be necessary following orthodontic treatment. When the maxillary labial frenum is suspected in the aetiology of a diastema (see Section 9.1), a fraenectomy is recommended. This is best undertaken during space closure so incisor approximation is aided by scar formation, although indefinite retention is required.

Soft tissues

Following appliance therapy, the teeth should be in a position of soft tissue balance. The original mandibular archform should remain unchanged, as markedly altering the inclination of the lower incisors will promote relapse. Limited proclination of the lower labial segment may be stable, however, where the lower incisors have been retroclined by a thumb-sucking habit, a lower lip trap or by retroclined upper incisors. In addition, some retroclination of the lower incisors may be stable in class III correction where the upper incisors have been proclined and, as a result, the labiolingual position of the incisors is, in effect, interchanged. Assessing the amount by which the lower incisors may be moved without being unstable is a matter of fine judgement and is definitely in the realm of the specialist.

In class II division 1, a pretreatment assessment of the degree of lip incompetence and mechanism of achieving an anterior oral seal should be made, followed by an estimate of the likely post-treatment coverage of the upper incisors by the lower lip. One-third to one-half of the labial surface of the upper incisors should be covered to give the best chance of stable overjet correction.

Occlusal factors

A good buccal segment interdigitation without displacing contacts and a satisfactory interincisal angulation promote stability. In addition, a positive overbite is necessary following incisor proclination to prevent relapse.

Facial growth

Continuing growth in the original pattern that contributed to the malocclusion is particularly likely to occur post-treatment in class III, open bite and deep bite cases. Some overcorrection of these incisor relationships is recommended, and retention should be continued until growth is complete. To prevent facial growth impacting on the development of late lower incisor crowding, permanent retention to the lower labial segment is now widely advocated.

Retention strategies

There are no specific rules as to the most appropriate retention strategy for each patient; this must be devised on an individual basis. The following guidelines are useful.

- After crossbite correction, where there is adequate overbite or good buccal segment interdigitation, no retention is necessary.
- On completion of removable appliance therapy, with the exception of space maintenance, a period of 3 months full-time followed by 3 months nocturnal wear of a Hawley retainer or a passive existing appliance is usually sufficient.

- At least 1 year of retention, 6 months full-time followed by 6 months of night-only retainer wear, is required following comprehensive treatment with fixed appliances. Although upper and lower Hawley retainers may be used, often this retainer type is prescribed for the upper arch only and a bonded retainer placed lingual to the lower labial segment. Because of the tendency for lower incisor crowding to occur, even when orthodontic treatment has been undertaken, prolonged retention to the lower labial segment by leaving the bonded retainer in place is recommended. Lengthy retention by a bonded retainer is advisable also following correction of rotations.
- Where growth modification has been used to correct a malocclusion, retention should continue until growth has ceased.
- In periodontally compromised dentitions, indefinite retention is recommended.
- In adults, the duration of retention should be longer than in adolescents because of the slower nature of the remodelling processes.
- Guidance in relation to the retention strategy following correction of other occlusal anomalies is given in the relevant sections.

Self-assessment: questions

Multiple choice questions

1. A removable appliance:
   a. Is indicated for bodily tooth movement
   b. Is particularly effective as a lower arch space maintainer in the mixed dentition
   c. May act as a retainer following active tooth movement
   d. Provides less anchorage than a fixed appliance
   e. Is indicated for correction of premolar rotations

2. When designing an upper removable appliance:
   a. It is not recommended to do so with the patient in the dental chair
   b. It is advisable to incorporate as many active components as possible
   c. Using the acronym ARAB is helpful
   d. The overjet measurement minus 2 mm gives an accurate indication of the required extent of a flat anterior bite plane
   e. It is advisable to specify the wire dimensions of the appliance components

3. A flat anterior bite plane:
   a. Is indicated for lower incisor proclination
   b. Is an aid to correction of anterior open bite
   c. Should contact at least two lower incisors
   d. Should separate the molar teeth by 5 mm
   e. Should allow the lower incisors to occlude posterior to it

4. Fixation of an upper removable appliance may be improved by:
   a. A T-spring
   b. An Adams' clasp
   c. A Southend clasp
   d. Palatal finger springs
   e. Minimal extension of the baseplate

5. The following removable appliance components are usually made from 0.6 mm stainless steel wire:
   a. A Z-spring to procline 1/
   b. A coffin spring
   c. An Adams' clasp on d
   d. A T-spring
   e. A Southend clasp

6. The force exerted by a typical 0.5 mm palatal finger spring to retract a maxillary canine is:
   a. Directly proportional to the length of the wire
   b. Inversely proportional to the wire diameter
   c. Inversely proportional to the deflection of the spring at activation

   d. Directly proportional to the thickness of acrylic covering the terminal end of the spring in the baseplate
   e. Inversely proportional to the number of retention components on the appliance

7. A fixed appliance is indicated for:
   a. Correction of rotations
   b. Space closure
   c. Bodily retraction of upper incisors for overjet reduction
   d. Alignment of grossly misplaced teeth
   e. Overbite reduction by incisor intrusion

8. Active components on a fixed appliance may be:
   a. The molar bands
   b. The archwire
   c. Elastomeric chain
   d. The baseplate
   e. A Nance palatal arch

9. The following are types of functional appliance:
   a. Begg
   b. Frankel
   c. Tip-edge
   d. Bionator
   e. Edgewise

10. The twin block appliance for class II correction:
    a. Cannot be worn while eating
    b. Has buccal shields to allow arch expansion
    c. Has six subtypes
    d. Is usually constructed using a wax registration with the patient opened 2 mm in the first permanent molar region
    e. May have headgear added to the lower appliance

11. There is a greater likelihood of anchorage loss:
    a. When light forces are used to move teeth
    b. On average, in the upper than in the lower arch
    c. When few teeth are being moved in an intact arch
    d. When the buccal interdigitation is good
    e. In the upper arch with a full arch fixed appliance than with a removable appliance

12. Anchorage may be reinforced with an upper removable appliance by:
    a. Extending the baseplate maximally
    b. Using intermaxillary traction
    c. Addition of headgear
    d. Using a close fitting labial bow
    e. By minimising the number of clasped teeth

13. Application of excessive force for tooth movement:
    a. Leads to loss of pulp vitality
    b. Hastens tooth movement
    c. Conserves anchorage
    d. Is likely to evoke a pain response
    e. Has no effect on root length

Case history questions

Case history 1

> A 14-year-old male patient presents complaining of slow progress of upper removable appliance therapy to retract 3/3 following extraction of 4/4. Treatment commenced 8 months ago and the canine teeth are still not in a class I relationship. On examination, 3/3 only appeared to have moved 3 mm in the past 8 months.

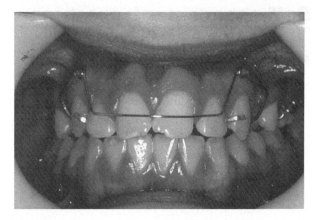

Fig. 131

1. What are the possible reasons for slow treatment progress?
2. What investigations would you undertake?
3. How would you manage treatment from now on?

Case history 2

> A 16-year-old female patient presents complaining of increase in the prominence in her upper incisor teeth following twin-block functional appliance therapy, which was concluded 14 months previously.

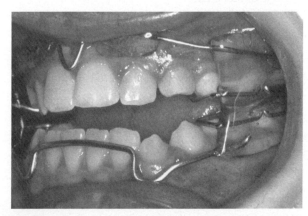

Fig. 132

1. What may account for the overjet increase?
2. How may it have been prevented?
3. What management options are there?

Picture questions

Picture 1

Figure 131 shows a patient wearing an upper removable appliance.

1. What is the active component?
2. What is it used for?
3. What are its wire dimensions?
4. What problems may arise with its use?

Picture 2

Figure 132 shows an appliance.

1. Specify the appliance type
2. What are the indications for its use?

3. How does it work?
4. What factors determine whether the occlusal correction achieved will be stable long term?

Picture 3

Figure 133 shows components of an orthodontic appliance.

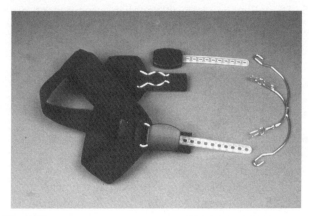

Fig. 133

1. List the components shown
2. What functions are served by the two components shown in the upper and lower middle section of the figure?
3. When would you use this appliance?
4. What instructions would you issue with it?

Picture 4

Figure 134 is an occlusal view of the lower arch.

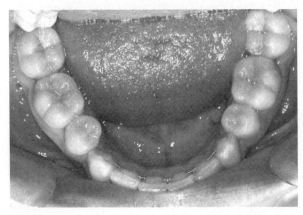

Fig. 134

1. What is visible lingual to the lower anterior teeth?
2. What is its purpose?
3. When would you consider its use?
4. What alternative approaches are there to treatment?

Short note questions

Write short notes on each of the following:

1. Adams clasp
2. Disadvantages of removable appliances
3. Orthodontic screws
4. Preadjusted edgewise fixed appliances
5. Optimal force range for tipping, bodily movement, rotation, intrusion
6. Intermaxillary traction
7. The histological effects that occur with a tipping movement to retract a maxillary canine
8. Retention procedures to minimise/prevent rotational relapse

Viva questions

1. What instructions would you give a patient who was issued with an upper removable appliance to procline /$\underline{1}$?
2. How would you know if a passive removable appliance you had issued 4 weeks previously was being worn full-time?
3. a. Classify functional appliances.
   b. Outline your management of a class II division 1 malocclusion to be treated by a functional appliance.
   c. Explain the mode of action and effects of a functional appliance in such a case.
4. Define what is meant by the term 'anchorage'. Classify anchorage and describe how anchorage can be preserved and monitored during removable appliance therapy. What special measures may need to be taken with anchorage reinforcement?

Self-assessment: answers

Multiple choice answers

1. a. **False.** It is only capable of a tipping tooth movement, not bodily tooth movement.
    b. **False.** Removable appliances are generally poorly tolerated in the lower arch as they encroach on tongue space. In addition, retention is not as good as in the upper arch because of the lingual tilt of the lower molars, which makes clasping difficult.
    c. **True.** It is indicated most commonly for retention following active tooth movement.
    d. **False.** A removable appliance provides greater anchorage than a fixed appliance owing to palatal coverage by the baseplate.
    e. **False.** Rotational correction is best carried out by a fixed rather than a removable appliance.

2. a. **False.** The appliance should be designed with the patient in the dental chair to avoid errors.
    b. **False.** The number of active components should be kept to a minimum.
    c. **True.** ARAB stands for activation, retention, anchorage, baseplate; this sequence is useful when designing a removable appliance.
    d. **False.** The overjet plus 3 mm should be forwarded to the laboratory at the time of fabrication to ensure accurate extension of the flat anterior bite plane.
    e. **True.** This reduces the likelihood of error in wire selection particularly for components that may be fabricated in one of two wire diameters, e.g. a buccal canine retractor may be made as 0.5 mm sleeved or in 0.7 mm wire.

3. a. **False.** A flat anterior bite plane is indicated for overbite reduction.
    b. **False.** See (a) above. An anterior bite plane would worsen an anterior open bite.
    c. **True.** This will distribute the occlusal load. Contact on one incisor may lead to periodontal trauma and mobility.
    d. **False.** Molar separation of about 3 mm is sufficient initially. Addition of cold cure acrylic to the bite plane can be made, as required, to reduce the overbite further.
    e. **False.** It should be constructed so that the lower incisors occlude on the anterior bite plane. If the lower incisors occlude posterior to the flat anterior bite plane overbite reduction will not ensue.

4. a. **False.** This is an active component and hence will not improve retention.

b. **True.** This is a retentive component.
c. **True.** This is a retentive component.
d. **False.** These are active components.
e. **False.** Maximal extension of the baseplate would improve retention; minimal extension would not aid retention.

5. a. **False.** This is usually made from 0.5 mm wire.
    b. **False.** This is usually made from 1.25 mm wire.
    c. **True.** This is usually made from 0.6 mm wire; clasps on 6s may be made in 0.7 or 0.8 mm wire.
    d. **False.** This is usually made in 0.5 mm wire.
    e. **False.** This is usually made in 0.7 mm wire.

6. a. **False.** Inversely proportional to wire length to the power of three.
    b. **False.** Directly proportional to the radius to the power of four.
    c. **False.** Directly proportional.
    d. **False.** Not relevant.
    e. **False.** Not relevant.

7. a. **True.**
    b. **True.**
    c. **True.** Bodily movement is necessary in all cases (a–e).
    d. **True.**
    e. **True.**

8. a. **False.** On their own, these are not active components but become active through the interaction of the archwire with the slot in the molar attachments.
    b. **True.** The archwire may be active or passive.
    c. **True.** This is used for space closure or to aid correction of rotations.
    d. **False.** Fixed appliances do not have a baseplate; this is a component of a removable appliance.
    e. **False.** This is used to support anchorage.

9. a. **False.** This is a type of fixed appliance.
    b. **True.**
    c. **False.** This is a type of fixed appliance.
    d. **True.**
    e. **False.** This is a type of fixed appliance.

10. a. **False.** It is issued to be worn full time and the patient is instructed to wear it while eating.
    b. **False.** These are incorporated in the Frankel appliance.
    c. **False.** There are two principal subtypes.

d. **False.** The bite should be open 4–5 mm in the first permanent molar region.

e. **False.** Headgear may be added to the upper appliance, not the lower appliance; sometimes elastic traction may be added from the lower appliance to the facebow attached to the upper appliance.

11. a. **False.** Lighter forces are less likely to produce anchorage loss.
   b. **True.** As there is a greater tendency to mesial drift.
   c. **False.** There will be less total force than when a larger number of teeth are being moved.
   d. **False.** As this will resist mesial drift.
   e. **True.** A fixed appliance does not have a baseplate, so resistance to unwanted movement is less; a few teeth will only be moved by tipping movements with a removable appliance, both factors tending to reduce the likelihood of anchorage loss.

12. a. **True.** As this will spread the reaction force over a greater area.
   b. **False.** This is not appropriate with an upper removable appliance as it will tend to dislodge the appliance.
   c. **True.** As will prevent or minimise mesial drift.
   d. **True.** This will prevent the overjet increasing in response to any forward reaction force from the active components.
   e. **False.** This will tend to make the appliance loose and encourage mesial drift of the posterior teeth if the fit then becomes poor.

13. a. **True.** As apical blood flow is compromised.
   b. **False.** As extensive hyalinisation of the periodontal ligament takes place followed by undermining resorption, tooth movement is slowed.
   c. **False.** Anchorage is likely to be lost as the reaction force to the active force may be sufficient to make the anchor teeth move.
   d. **True.** Likelihood of pain is greater as extensive areas of the periodontal ligament will be compressed.
   e. **False.** Likelihood of root resorption is increased.

Case history answers

Case history 1

1. Possible reasons for slow progress include the patient not wearing the appliance full time, not placing the springs in the correct position, underactivation/overactivation or distortion of the springs, movement impeded by acrylic/wire/opposing occlusion/retained root of $\underline{4}$.

2. Ask the patient about the length of time the appliance is worn on a daily basis. Check that the springs are positioned correctly and are not overactivated, underactivated or distorted. Check if acrylic/wire/opposing occlusion is impeding tooth movement. Enquire from the patient if there was any mention from the practitioner who carried out the extraction as to whether any root fragment was retained. Radiograph the extraction sites of $\underline{4}/\underline{4}$ to ensure that there is no root remnant of the extracted units if any doubt exists and to check if the bone density and periodontal architecture are normal.

3. If the appliance has not been worn as instructed, discuss this with the patient and warn him that if full-time wear is not forthcoming, treatment will be terminated. Reinstruct the patient in correct positioning of the springs if this is the problem. Check the activation is correct; if the springs are distorted it may be possible to improve this. However, in some instances it may be necessary to construct a new appliance. Remove acrylic if it is preventing tooth movement; if a wire component is preventing movement, it can be removed if possible or it may be necessary to remake the appliance with a slightly different design to allow movement to proceed. Acrylic addition to the bite plane or to posterior capping may be required if the occlusion with the opposing arch is impeding movement. If a retained root is identified on radiograph, arrangements should be made for its removal and tooth movement then recommenced after a period of healing.

Case history 2

1. Overjet increase following functional appliance therapy represents relapse. This may result from insufficient wear of the appliance as a retainer following correction of the occlusion. Ideally, it should be worn until growth is almost complete, in the late teens. A poorly interdigitating occlusion, persistent thumb/finger-sucking habit, lip trap or tongue thrust may also account for overjet relapse, as may a posterior mandibular growth rotation.

2. Prevention could involve the following:
   - checking that the final occlusion was well interdigitating and ensuring that there was slight overcorrection
   - reducing wear of the appliance to night-time only, and then maintaining wear at that level until late teens. Alternatively an upper removable appliance

with steeply inclined anterior bite plane may be constructed and worn for a similar duration
- ensuring that digit/thumb-sucking habits had ceased before commencing treatment
- if the lower lip coverage of the upper incisors was not at least one-third to one-half of the upper incisor crowns at completion of overjet reduction, the patient should have been informed that retention may be lengthy and perhaps require the placement of a bonded retainer at a later stage.

A tongue thrust should also have been checked for and if present (it may be adaptive if the lips are incompetent) retention carefully monitored. A pretreatment cephalometric radiograph would have given an indication of the growth pattern, and if this is likely to be more backward and vertical than forward and horizontal then prolonged retention is likely to be required as the former is likely to be less favourable for overjet stability.

3. Management options are as follows. As a 16-year-old female patient will be beyond her pubertal growth spurt, recommencing functional appliance therapy is not a realistic option. If the overjet relapse is only minimal (of the order of a few millimetres), with the patient's consent it could be monitored by recording the occlusion on study casts and reassessing it in 6 months when further treatment could be embarked on should there be evidence of further relapse. Further treatment options are orthodontic camouflage with, most likely extraction of the upper first premolars and upper/lower fixed appliance therapy. Alternatively, if the relapse is significant and the underlying skeletal pattern/facial profile unlikely to benefit from camouflage treatment, orthognathic correction when growth is complete is the only other satisfactory solution.

Picture answers

Picture 1

1. A Roberts retractor.
2. It is used for overjet reduction.
3. Its wire dimensions are 0.5 mm wire sleeved in 0.5 mm internal diameter stainless steel tubing.
4. If the coils are positioned too high in the buccal sulcus, ulceration is likely. Also where the acrylic is not relieved sufficiently behind the upper incisors, the gingivae will become heaped up between the baseplate and the palatal surfaces of the upper incisors during overjet reduction.

Picture 2

1. Frankel III appliance.

2. Indications are a growing child in the early mixed dentition (preferably 7–8 years) with a mild class III skeletal discrepancy and reduced FMPA who is able to achieve an edge-to-edge incisor relationship. Dentoalveolar compensation should be minimal, or ideally lower incisors proclined and upper incisors upright.
3. The appliance is constructed to a wax registration recorded with the mandible postured open slightly and backwards as much as possible. The wire labial to the lower incisors is fabricated to a groove cut into the teeth on the work casts so it is active at insertion. A wire palatal to the upper incisors pushes them labially. The buccal shields allow upper arch expansion and maintain lower arch width. Other components aid retention of the appliance.
4. Stable correction of the class III incisor relationship is enhanced by achieving adequate overbite and by favourable mandibular growth.

Picture 3

1. Headcap, safety release spring mechanism (in two parts) and a facebow with locking device.
2. The spring mechanism connects the headcap to the facebow and controls the amount of force applied.
3. Headgear is used either to reinforce anchorage or for extraoral traction. For anchorage, wear of the appliance for 10 hours per day with 200–250 g force is required; for extraoral traction the appliance should be worn for at least 14 out of 24 hours and force magnitude is 400–500 g. Forces over 500 g with even longer wear prior to and during the pubertal growth spurt are necessary to restrain maxillary downward and forward growth.
4. Headgear must be fitted with two safety mechanisms and safety instructions issued. The following instructions are necessary: wear the appliance as instructed; it must never be worn without the safety mechanisms attached. Do not adjust the force yourself at any time. The headgear should not be worn during sports or other activity. If it ever becomes detached from the appliance, discontinue wear and return to the orthodontist. If the headgear ever becomes detached and rubs your face or eyes, go immediately to your doctor or hospital; cease appliance wear and report to your orthodontist.

Picture 4

1. A bonded canine to canine lower retainer.
2. It is used to maintain alignment of the lower labial segment following orthodontic movement.

3. As the lower labial segment will tend to crowd with time in all cases irrespective of the original malocclusion and the type of orthodontic treatment undertaken, it is now advocated by many that some form of permanent retention be used, particularly following fixed appliance therapy, to prevent relapse. This may involve placing a bonded retainer as seen here. Bonded retention is particularly indicated where rotations are present, where the lower labial segment has been proclined intentionally and in periodontally involved dentitions.

4. A lower removable (Hawley) retainer may be issued instead but these are not good at maintaining rotational correction and may not be well tolerated. An alternative is a clear vacuum-formed retainer with full occlusal coverage.

Short note answers

1. An Adams clasp is used to provide retention for a removable appliance. Designed for this purpose to engage the mesiobuccal and distobuccal undercuts on a first permanent molar, it may be used also to provide retention on primary molars or incisors. It is usually made from 0.7 mm hard drawn stainless steel wire but 0.6 mm wire is used for incisors and primary molars. Tubes may be soldered for extraoral anchorage or the clasp may be modified to incorporate hooks for elastics. To adjust the clasp, it is necessary to bend it where it comes out of the acrylic or closer to the arrowhead to move it toward the undercut.

2. Disadvantages of removable appliances include: appliance is removable and can be taken out of the mouth by the patient; lower appliances are not well tolerated; speech is affected; limited to tipping movements only and not efficient where multiple tooth movements are required; intermaxillary traction cannot be used and good technical support is required.

3. A screw may be used as the active component rather than a spring where several teeth need to be moved or where these also are required for retention of the appliance. There are two types: a Landin screw, which has a piston-like action and is used for movement of a single incisor tooth, and a Glenross screw, which has two interlocking pieces and is generally used to move several teeth. The disadvantages of screws are that they make the appliance bulky as well as being more expensive and less versatile in action than a spring. Activation is dependent on the patient remembering to adjust the screw as instructed – each turn producing about 0.2 mm of movement.

4. This appliance uses individual attachments with a rectangular slot for each tooth with 'average' inclination and angulation. Brackets are available in a range of prescriptions including those of Andrews and Roth. Flat archwires may be placed. Clinical time is saved and a high standard of occlusal finish is achieved more consistently with these techniques than with standard edgewise techniques.

5. For tipping movement, forces in the range 30–60 g are appropriate; for bodily movement 100–150 g; for rotation 50–75 g; for intrusion 15–25 g.

6. Intermaxillary traction is a means of producing tooth movement in one arch using teeth in the opposing arch as anchorage. It is the means of tooth movement employed by functional appliances but may be applied also with fixed appliances. It is not practical to employ intermaxillary traction with removable appliances as it will dislodge the appliance. With fixed appliances, intermaxillary traction takes the form of either class II or class III traction with application of interarch elastics; the force necessary is decided by selecting elastics of appropriate size and weight. For class 11 traction, the elastics are stretched from posteriorly in the lower arch (usually the hook attached to the buccal molar tube) to an attachment anteriorly in the upper arch, commonly to either a hook on the canine bracket or a soldered hook on the archwire. For class III traction, the elastics run from posteriorly in the upper arch (usually first permanent molar area) to anteriorly (canine area) in the lower arch. Class II elastics may be used to reduce an overjet while simultaneously closing space posteriorly in the lower arch. Both types of traction may extrude molar teeth and increase the vertical facial proportions, which would be undesirable in individuals where this is already increased. Proclination of lower incisors is a possible side-effect of class II traction and may be best avoided depending on the objectives of treatment.

7. A tipping force applied to a maxillary canine will induce areas of pressure and tension within the periodontal ligament space: pressure at the alveolar crest margin distally and at the apical area diagonally opposite; tension at the other sites. In the pressure areas, the blood vessels are compressed and osteoclasts invade within 4–5, days leading to frontal alveolar bone resorption. In the tension sites, the blood vessels are dilated and the periodontal ligament fibres are stretched, with osteoblast invasion leading to osteoid deposition along the fibre bundles in the direction of tooth movement. Eventually this is mineralised. All of the socket is remodelled in response to the tooth movement.

8. Once the rotation has been corrected, percision to sever the free gingival fibres may be undertaken to reduce the amount of relapse. However, prolonged retention is also necessary with a bonded retainer to prevent relapse.

Viva answers

1. a. The appliance should be worn full time with the exception of after meals (when it should be removed for cleaning) and also for contact sports. Please place it in the hard plastic container provided when it is removed for contact sports.
   b. The main difficulties you will experience are likely to be in the first week, particularly during eating and speaking but these should resolve after that.
   c. You may experience mild discomfort related to /1 for a few days. Take a mild analgesic, if necessary.
   d. You should not eat sticky or hard foods, so chewing gum is to be avoided.
   e. The appliance should be removed after meals for cleaning, when you should also brush your teeth.
   f. If there are any problems with appliance wear, or if the appliance breaks, return immediately.

2. a. The patient's speech should be normal.
   b. The patient should be able to insert and remove the appliance unaided by a mirror.
   c. The baseplate should have lost its shine and there may be bite marks on a biteplane if this is part of the appliance.
   d. There is likely to be mild gingival erythema in relation to the baseplate adaptation to the gingival margins and across the palate.
   e. The appliance will have lost some of its retention through being inserted and removed.

3. a. Classification could be tooth borne passive (e.g. Andresen), tooth borne active (e.g. Bionator), tissue borne (e.g. Frankel appliance).
   b. Obtain full diagnostic records, including a lateral cephalometric film. Take well extended upper and lower impressions. With the patient sitting upright, instruct them in posturing the mandible to the desired position. Place a roll of softened wax over the lower arch avoiding the lower incisors and gently instruct the patient to close into the rehearsed postured position – the exact extent of the forward posturing and mandibular opening will depend on the appliance chosen. Chill the wax registration and check it in the mouth, ensuring that the centre-lines are not displaced if they were already coincident. When the working casts have been constructed, mount them on an articulator using the construction bite

to allow appliance fabrication. Wear of any appliance should be generally increased slowly over the first few weeks until it is being worn for at least 14 out of 24 hours. This is with the exception of the twin block appliance, which should be worn full-time from the start. A time chart should be issued for recording wear. It is wise to see the patient 2 weeks after fitting the appliance to discuss any problems and to encourage cooperation with wear. Thereafter, an interval of 6–8 weeks between review appointments is usual. At each visit, with the mandible fully retruded, the overjet and buccal segment relationship should be recorded; the appliance adjusted for comfort and to facilitate eruption of permanent teeth, if necessary; the standing height checked; and the time chart checked and encouragement given regarding wear. Overcorrection is advisable. The appliance should be worn as a retainer until growth is ceased unless a further phase of treatment is planned with fixed appliances, and possible extractions to detail the occlusion.

   c. The mode of action of a functional appliance is incompletely understood, but its primary function is to posture the mandible downwards and forwards, displacing the condyles out of the glenoid fossae. This stretches the orofacial musculature and generates a force vector that tends to procline the lower incisors, while the reaction force is transmitted backwards through the appliance to the upper teeth and maxilla. The effects, therefore, are to procline the lower incisors (which in most cases is undesirable and can be resisted by capping of the incisal edges) and to retrocline the upper incisors. Condylar growth is stimulated and the glenoid fossae may be positioned more anteriorly, while downward and forward maxillary growth is restrained. Overbite reduction occurs by restraining eruption of the lower incisors while the posterior teeth are allowed to erupt.

4. Anchorage is the resistance to the force of reaction generated by the active components. It may be classified as intra-or extraoral anchorage. Intraoral anchorage can be simple, where movement of one tooth is pitted against that of several others for which movement is not desired, or reciprocal, where movement of one group of teeth is used as anchorage for movement of another group of teeth in the opposite direction; for example closure of a median diastema or upper arch expansion. Extraoral anchorage is anchorage obtained by wearing headgear.

Anchorage may be preserved by:

- moving a few teeth at a time
- control of the force magnitude to 0.3–0.5 N for tipping
- maximum baseplate extension
- clasping additional teeth to increase resistance to movement
- preventing the incisors from tipping labially by placing a close-fitting labial bow
- fitting headgear.

Anchorage may be monitored by:

- careful measurement of the space required for the intended tooth movement at each visit
- measurement of the overjet in class II division 1 and/or the buccal segment relationship is useful.

If extraoral anchorage is fitted, two safety mechanisms must be added to the headgear: a locking device on the facebow (Ni Tom®) and a safety release headcap with spring mechanism. Specific instructions regarding wear (10–12 hours), placement and removal, as well as warnings regarding possible facial and eye injuries, must be given together with a contact number should any problems arise. Patient and parent must understand these.

Contents

Overview

As members of a healing profession, dental surgeons are expected not only just to obey the law of the land but also to abide by ethical principles in their professional and personal life. Ethics are moral principles or rules of conduct expected in the professional and personal conduct of someone practising a profession. To assist dental surgeons in ethical matters, the General Dental Council recently updated its advisory booklet.

The new booklet, *Maintaining Standards* (*Guidance to Dentists on Professional and Personal Conduct*) was issued in November 1997. This booklet was sent to all dentists on the Dental Register of the United Kingdom and distributed to the Dental Schools to be given to dental students during their course on ethics and jurisprudence.

11.1 The General Dental Council

Learning objectives

You should

- understand the roles and functions of the General Dental Council
- be aware of its membership.

The General Dental Council (GDC) is the regulatory body of the dental profession. It protects the public by means of its statutory responsibilities for dental education, registration, professional conduct and health. It supports dentists and dental auxiliaries in the practice of dentistry and encourage their continuing professional development. (GDC's Mission Statement).

The GDC exists to protect the general public by ensuring that only qualified, competent and ethical people practise dentistry; it is a statutory body that was set up when Parliament passed the Dentists' Act (1956). Prior to this, the registration and regulation of the dental profession was carried out by the Dental Board of the General Medical Council.

The composition of the GDC is currently under review and in the future there may be more lay members and less nominated academic members. Changes can only made by Act of Parliament.

In 1998 the Membership of the General Dental Council comprised:

- the President (a registered dentist elected from and by the Council)
- 18 dentists elected by Registered Dentists 14 from England, two from Scotland and one each from Northern Ireland and Wales
- 17 dentists nominated by universities who issue dental degrees and the Royal Surgical Colleges
- four Chief Dental Officers of the countries in the UK
- three nominees of the General Medical Council, who participate in educational matters only
- one enrolled dental auxiliary
- six members who are not registered dentists but appointed by Her Majesty the Queen on the advice of her Privy Council.

As well as the elected registered dentists and the Chief Dental Officers, the appointed lay members reflect the four Countries making up the UK.

Registration with the GDC

Only dental surgeons registered with the GDC and medical practitioners registered with the General Medical Council are entitled to practise dentistry. Graduates and licentiates in dentistry of universities and Royal Surgical Colleges of the UK may be registered on completion of the appropriate form and payment of the prescribed registration fee. The universities and Royal Colleges in the UK provide the GDC with lists of their dental graduates or licentiates. Registration has to be renewed annually as long as a dentist is practising in the UK.

Holders of an appropriate European Dental Diploma who are nationals of member states of the European Union (EU) are also entitled to register, as are Icelandic and Norwegian graduates, since Norway and Iceland are members of the European Economic Association (EEA). Any European dentist applying for registration requires documentary evidence of identity, academic attainment, good standing and good health. Disqualification from practise in any EU/EEA member state automatically bars a dentist from registering with the GDC.

Dentists holding a primary dental diploma from certain overseas universities that the GDC has visited to check educational standards may also register. These universities are in former Commonwealth or Commonwealth countries where dental education is similar to that in the UK. No other qualifications are accepted by the GDC for full registration and, therefore, the right of undertaking independent dental practice in the UK.

There are two ways by which dentists with qualifications that do not fit into the above categories can register with the General Dental Council.

Temporary registration

Temporary registration is available to allow such dentists to teach, do research work or obtain postgraduate instruction in certain approved hospital posts for a limited period. Temporary registration only lasts for the period of a particular post or employment and can be renewed normally up to a maximum of 4 years. Applicants for temporary registration must personally attend the GDC offices with:

- proof of identity (a passport)
- their original qualifying degree or diploma plus a certified true translation if it is not in English
- evidence of good character
- proof of a necessary knowledge of English
- proof of good mental and physical health.

People with temporary registration can only practise dentistry under the supervision of a named, fully registered dentist of consultant status in the UK.

After 2 years of temporary registration and subject to satisfactory reports from the consultant(s) supervising the temporary registrant, a 'Temporary Registration with Limited Supervision' may be granted. This will

allow, for instance, the temporary registered dentist to undertake out of hours on-call duty when the supervising consultant will probably not be on the premises but only available by telephone or some form of paging.

Statutory Examination

Until 2001 the GDC regularly arranged the Statutory Examination for dentists whose qualifications were not recognised for full registration by the GDC. The Statutory Examination is in two parts; should a temporary registered dentist fail either part on more than one occasion, the temporary registration will be immediately withdrawn. Many people intending to sit the Statutory Examination do so after a period of temporary registration in order to increase their understanding of dentistry as it is practised in the UK and, if necessary, to improve their ability to communicate in English. When both parts of the Statutory Examination have been passed, the dentist is entitled to full registration with the GDC.

The Statutory Examination has now been replaced by the International Qualifying Examination. At the same time the GDC has ceased to recognise the primary dental diplomas from certain universities overseas. From 2001, all dental surgeons who do not have a primary dental qualification gained through a dental school or Royal Surgical College in the UK, the EU or the EEA will have to sit the International Qualifying Examination.

Also it should be noted that dentists from outside the EU require a work permit to undertake any form of employment in the UK. It is recommended that the application for a work permit is made in the country of residence and is available to be shown to an immigration officer on arrival in the UK.

11.2 Titles and descriptions

Learning objectives

You should

- understand what dental specialties are available

- know the scope and limitations of the tasks that auxiliaries are allowed to undertake.

Dentists

Registration with the GDC allows the use of the title Dentist, Dental Practitioner or Dental Surgeon. Also, since November 1995, the GDC has accepted the use of the courtesy title Doctor, provided that it is not used in a way to suggest that the user is anything other than a dentist. Before 1998 no other title was permitted, but the GDC is now empowered to set up and maintain specialist lists of practitioners who can show they have received sufficient postgraduate training to be considered specialists in a particular field. Practioners on these lists are permitted to use the appropriate titles, eg. 'Specialist in XXXXX'.

There are two methods of entry to these specialist lists:

- at the end of the appropriate time in a recognised training post the appropriate postgraduate diploma and an assessment by the Specialist Advisory Committee (SAC) for the specialty
- by virtue of current specialist practice and previous training. This pathway is open for two years following the establishment of each individual specialist list only and is referred to as transitional arrangements.

The GDC have established 13 specialist lists. These are:

Specialty	End of transitional entry period
Dental and maxillofacial radiology	31 May 2002
Dental public health	15 April 2000
Endodontics	31 May 2000
Oral medicine	30 June 2001
Oral microbiology	31 May 2002
Oral pathology	31 May 2002
Oral surgery	15 April 2000
Orthodontics	30 June 2000
Paediatric dentistry	30 June 2000
Periodontics	31 May 2000
Prosthodontics	31 May 2000
Restorative dentistry	15 April 2000
Surgical dentistry	31 May 2000

The specialty of restorative dentistry involves training in endodontics, periodontics and prosthodontics; it, therefore, involves a longer training period than that required for specialisation in only one of the three recognised restorative specialties. Surgical dentistry is confined to dentoalveolar surgery, whereas oral surgery encompasses surgery to surrounding structures and the treatment of maxillofacial injuries. Maxillofacial surgery is considered to be a medical specialty by the EU, and maxillofacial surgeons are registered with the General Medical Council.

Dental auxiliaries

The GDC is also responsible for maintaining a register of dental hygienists and dental therapists. These auxiliaries can undertake a limited form of dental practice under the supervision of a registered dentist.

Dental hygienists

Dental hygienists are permitted to scale, clean and polish teeth and also to apply certain prophylactic materials to the surface of teeth. They may only provide treatment when under the direction of a registered dentist who has examined the patient and prescribed the course of treatment to be provided. If the hygienist is not under the personal supervision of the dentist when carrying out prescribed treatment, the dentist must be satisfied that the hygienist is competent to carry out that treatment. Hygienists who qualified prior to 1992 and who administer local anaesthetic infiltration analgesia must have attended a course and received a certificate in administration of local infiltration analgesia, or hold the Diploma of Dental Therapy.

Dental therapists

Dental therapists are permitted to extract deciduous teeth, undertake simple fillings, scale, clean and polish teeth and apply certain prophylactic materials to the surface of teeth. They are also permitted to give advice on dental matters within the limits of the treatments mentioned above and to administer local infiltration analgesia. They are also able to carry out work under regional block analgesia that has been administered by a registered dentist. At the present time dental therapists are only allowed to work in Health Authority services to provide treatment that has been authorised and prescribed in writing by a registered dentist who has examined the patient. A registered dentist does not have to be on the premises but should be readily available should an emergency arise.

New classes of 'Professionals Complementary to Dentistry'

If, in the future, dental auxiliaries are allowed to perform additional duties, it is essential that they attend for appropriate courses of instruction on these additional duties and techniques before undertaking them.

The Dental Auxiliaries Review Group of the GDC published a report in November 1996. This report recommended that in future dental auxiliaries should be known as Professionals Complementary to Dentistry (PCD) and that all classes should be statutorily registered with the GDC. Only those in training and with appropriate qualifications would be eligible for registration. Several new classes of registered PCDs are envisaged and 'grandparenting' arrangements are likely to be agreed for several classes, but not for clinical dental technicians. A number of classes of registered PCD have been suggested.

Dental nurses

Only qualified dental nurses will be allowed to register and undertake additional duties such as removing sutures and packs and taking impressions for study models on the written instruction of a dentist who is on the premises. Following appropriate additional instruction dental nurses will also be allowed to take radiographs and give oral hygiene advice.

Dental hygienists

The duties of dental hygienists will be expanded to allow them to place temporary fillings in an emergency, re-cement crowns with temporary cement and remove excess cement from around restorations. They will also be able to take impressions for study models, give infiltration local anaesthetics and possibly inferior dental blocks in the future. Additional training will be required for all these new duties.

Dental therapists

Dental therapists will be able to carry out the same additional procedures as dental hygienists following appropriate training. They will also be allowed to work in all sectors of dentistry.

Orthodontic auxiliaries

Orthodontic auxiliaries will be trained to carry out orthodontic duties to a previously agreed treatment plan and under the direct supervision of the dentist. In the first instance, only dental hygienists and therapists will be able to undertake additional training in orthodontics. Their duties will include taking impressions, fitting removable appliances and headgear, fitting separators and orthodontic bands, placement of direct bonded orthodontic attachments and the ligation and removal of arch wires previously fitted by a dentist and the removal of orthodontic bands and excess cement.

Dental technicians

Only qualified technicians will be allowed to register and to call themselves dental technicians. In addition to the construction of appliances, they will be able to take tooth shades of patients for the construction of prostheses and impressions for study models on a written prescription, but only on the dentist's premises.

Maxillofacial prosthesis and technologists

Suitably qualified persons will be able to register and only they will be able to use this title.

Clinical dental technicians

Clinical dental technicians would be limited to the fitting and insertion of complete upper and/or lower dentures. They will only be able to treat patients referred to them by a dentist who has examined the patient. Clinical dental technicians working within a dental practice will also be allowed to provide partial dentures.

This is a completely new class of PCD and they will require new training programmes and examinations that will have to be approved by the GDC. The Dentists' Act needs to be amended for this group to be recognised as it is currently illegal for dental technicians to insert dentures into patients' mouths. Also the resistance of the dental profession will need to be overcome before clinical dental technicians are trained and then registered!

The GDC has proposed three new Boards that will be responsible for registration, standards of education and training, health and conduct of PCDs. These are for:

- dental nurses
- hygienists and therapists
- technicians, maxillofacial technologists and clinical dental technicians.

11.3 Requirements for the practice of dentistry

Learning objectives

You should

- understand how the GDC carries out its regulatory tasks and how disciplinary matters are dealt with

- understand the educational and indemnity requirements of being a member of a profession.

Regulation by the General Dental Council

It is the GDC's duty to maintain the Dentists' Register and the Rolls of Dental Auxiliaries. The Registrar and Chief Executive of the GDC is responsible in ensuring the accuracy of the Register and the Rolls. The Register must remove the name of any dentist or dental auxiliary who fails to pay the annual retention fee. A name can only be restored to the register by formal application and the payment of a restoration fee in addition to the annual retention fee.

Education

The Dentists Act (1984) gives the GDC the responsibility to supervise all stages of dental education, postgraduate as well as undergraduate. The GDC determines minimum standards as set out in its *Recommendations Concerning the Dental Curriculum*. The GDC sends visitors to dental schools to check on standards of teaching and of examination of students. It has the power to recommend that the recognition of a dental qualification by the GDC is withdrawn should the Council consider that the training or examination no longer secures sufficient knowledge and skill to practise dentistry.

Conduct

The GDC also has a duty to remove from the Dentists' Register any member who is shown to have behaved in a manner unsuitable for continued registration. From time to time, the GDC has issued booklets entitled *Professional Conduct and Fitness to Practise*, the last edition of which was May 1993. This booklet was replaced in 1997 by a new style booklet entitled *Maintaining Standards (Guidance to Dentists on Professional and Personal Conduct)*. This new publication is a loose leaf document designed to be put in a file. This will allow it to be updated or added to quickly and economically. All senior dental students and registered dentists are advised to read this document and have it readily available for reference.

At all times the dentist's conduct must be of the high standard that the public and the profession expect. The dentist's first priority is a responsibility to patients. If a dentist's conduct falls below this high standard, the GDC has the power to suspend or remove the dentist's name from the register. Conviction for a criminal offence or serious professional misconduct can be grounds for refusal, erasure or suspension from the Dental Register. Conduct or behaviour prior to qualification is also considered by the GDC, therefore, this power applies to dental students as well as qualified dentists.

Serious professional misconduct cannot be precisely defined. However, it is considered to be conduct by a dentist that falls short of the standards of conduct expected amongst dentists and that this should be a serious omission/commission. The GDC's publication *Maintaining Standards* gives clear guidance on standards expected of a practising dentist; failure to maintain these standards could lead to a charge of serious professional misconduct. Also any criminal conviction in the UK of a dentist is automatically forwarded to the Council by the police, who may also inform the GDC of formal cautions and other matters of concern. The GDC accepts a court conviction as conclusive proof. A later claim of innocence to the GDC cannot, therefore, be made in mitigation!

Disciplinary procedure

In addition to criminal convictions, a patient, a member of the public or another dentist may make a formal complaint to the GDC. The GDC's solicitors or a person acting in a public capacity (e.g. an officer of a health authority or similar body) can inform the Council of any matter that they feel should be considered under the GDC's disciplinary procedure. There may be up to three stages in this procedure.

Preliminary screening
Preliminary screening is undertaken by the President of the GDC, who may decide that there is no case to answer or refer the complainant on to the appropriate committee. If it is decided that there is no case to answer, the complainant is informed of that decision. If it is considered that there may be a case to answer, this is referred to the Preliminary Proceedings Committee.

Preliminary Proceedings Committee
The Preliminary Proceedings Committee sits in private and normally considers documentary information only, unless interim suspension may be considered. It comprises the President and five other Council Members including one lay member; there is also a legal assessor when required. A dentist is informed on any matter being referred to the committee and sent a copy of the information/complaint. Written comments or observations from the dentist are invited generally at least 28 days prior to the committee meeting. If the committee decides there is no case to answer, the matter proceeds no further. However, should the committee decide there is evidence to support an allegation of serious professional misconduct, the matter will be referred to the Professional Conduct Committee for enquiry or, if appropriate, to the Health Committee of the GDC. The dentist and complainant are normally notified of the committee's decision. In those cases that the committee does not refer on, it may give advice on behaviour to the dentist concerned. It can also warn the dentist that this matter may be reconsidered if, in the future, further information is formally brought to the attention of the GDC. Should the Preliminary Proceedings Committee feel that members of the public may be at risk, it can order the immediate suspension of a dentist's registration pending the outcome of the enquiry by the Professional Conduct Committee. In this case, the dentist is immediately advised of this decision and offered the opportunity to make representations to the committee concerning the proposed suspension. Interim suspension can only be considered when the committee has decided to refer a matter to the Professional Conduct Committee and on the advice of a legal assessor.

Professional Conduct Committee
The Professional Conduct Committee comprises the President and 10 other members of Council (including five elected and two lay members). A legal assessor sits with the committee to advise on matters of law and procedure. The committee sits in public; evidence is taken on oath and either party may subpoena witnesses. This is similar to a court of law and matters must be proved 'beyond reasonable doubt' as in criminal proceedings.

A notice of the enquiry, including the charge to be faced, is sent to the dentist by the GDC's solicitors at least 28 days before the date of enquiry.

The committee's first duty is to determine whether the facts in the charge have been proved. Only after some or all of these facts have been proved, does the committee consider whether this amounted to serious professional misconduct.

If a dentist has been found guilty of serious professional misconduct or convicted in a criminal court the committee may:

- admonish the dentist
- postpone judgement to a future meeting with consideration of the dentist's conduct meanwhile; judgement is generally postponed for 1 year
- order the suspension of a dentist for a specific period up to 12 months
- direct that the dentist's name be erased from the Dentists' Register
- refer the matter to the Health Committee.

In the case of suspension or erasure, the committee may authorise suspension with immediate effect to protect the public or in the best interests of the dentist. In other cases, there is a period of 28 days during which the dentist may lodge an appeal with judicial committee of the Privy Council, against his suspension or erasure before this comes into effect. Should an appeal be lodged, the dentist may continue to practise until the outcome of that appeal is known.

In the case of suspension, the dentist's name is automatically restored to the Dentists' Register at the end of that period. Following an erasure, a dentist may apply to the Professional Conduct Committee for his name to be restored to the Dentists' Register. This may not be made until at least 10 months after the date of erasure. The Committee will consider the circumstances leading to the erasure and the dentist's behaviour during the intervening period, including evidence of professional rehabilitation. If successful, the dentist's name may be restored to the Dentists' Register on payment of the appropriate registration fee. If restoration is refused, the dentist must wait at least a further 10 months after the hearing before submitting another application.

Health and fitness to practise

If a formal complaint is made to the GDC, the President again acts as the preliminary screener. If it is considered that the dentist's fitness to practise is seriously impaired, the dentist is sent a copy of the information and invited to submit to medical examination. Response by the dentist is requested within 14 days and must be made within 28 days.

Medical examiners are asked to report on the fitness of a dentist to engage in practice generally or on a limited basis. They are also asked for recommendations on the management of the case. Additionally, the dentist may nominate a medical examiner to examine him (or her) and provide a separate report at his/her own expense. The dentist can also submit observations on the matter under consideration. On receipt of the report, the President will decide whether or not the matter should be referred to the Health Committee; if not the dentist is notified accordingly and sent a copy of the reports. Should a dentist fail to respond or refuse to be medically examined, the President may still refer the matter to the Health Committee.

Health Committee

The Health Committee comprises a Chairman, who must be a registered dentist, and 10 other members of Council (including five elected and two lay members). The Committee is assisted by a legal assessor and one or more medical assessors. The dentist being considered will be sent a formal notice at least 28 days before the date of the hearing. The hearing is of a judicial nature but rather less formal than the Professional Conduct Committee. The committee's first duty is to decide whether or not a physical or mental condition has seriously impaired the dentist's fitness to practise. If not, the matter is then concluded. If it is, the committee has the following powers.

- if the case was referred by the Preliminary Proceedings Committee or the Professional Conduct Committee, the matter is referred back to that committee
- the dentist's registration can be suspended for a period up to 12 months
- conditions imposed on the dentist's conditional registration may be made for a period not exceeding 3 years.

After the initial period of conditional registration, the committee may direct a further period of conditional registration of up to 12 months. Also the dentist remains under the review of the Health Committee until the committee feels that fitness to practise is no longer seriously impaired. Following this, any previously imposed conditions will be revoked.

Professional competency and performance

The GDC is concerned about those dentists whose clinical skills and performance are seriously and chronically deficient, thereby constituting a risk to the public. Such dentists may not fall within the remit of the Professional Conduct or Health Committees. A consultation paper was published by the GDC in May 1998 recommending the formation of a *Performance Review Committee*. It is envisaged that the Performance Review Committee will take referrals from the Preliminary Proceedings Committee, Professional Conduct Committee or Health Committee, who will arrange an assessment of the dentist and, if necessary, recommend a programme of re-education. If on re-assessment, the dentist's professional performance is considered satisfactory (s)he will be referred back to the appropriate committee.

The Performance Review Committee may also consider complaints that originate from a member of the public, a professional colleague or an organisation. It is expected to have the following powers:

- to appoint a panel of screeners, who will be members of the GDC
- appoint a team of assessors who are not members of GDC but are chosen because of their expertise and experience
- to impose conditions on continuing registration of a dentist
- to suspend a dentist
- to erase a dentist's name from the Dentists' Register.

The proposed membership of the Committee will be nine members of GDC and must include three lay members and three elected dentists.

Following a complaint or referral, the matter will be assessed by two screeners. The screeners will consider whether it is appropriate that the matter should be considered by the Performance Review Committee or whether it is more appropriate for consideration as a conduct or health matter by the appropriate committees. If the screeners consider that there may have been a consistently poor standard of performance or a serious level of failure implying serious risk to the public, the case will be referred to the Performance Review Committee for investigation and assessment. This Committee may make recommendations for remedial education and refer the dentist to the local Postgraduate Dental Dean or Director. Following appropriate further education and a report from the Postgraduate Dental Dean to the committee, re-assessment can be undertaken. If the dentist's performance is considered adequate, the Performance Review Committee will withdraw any limitations on his practice. However, if it becomes evident that the dentist is not likely to benefit sufficiently from further training, the dentist will be allowed to apply for voluntary withdrawal from the Dentists' Register. If a dentist refuses to comply or cooperate with this committee, it will have the power to immediately suspend them from the Dentists' Register.

The appeals mechanism for this committee is likely to be similar to that of the Professional Conduct and Health Committees. Changes in the Dentists' Act will be required before a statutory performance review scheme for the dental profession can be implemented. A similar scheme is already in operation by the General Medical Council to deal with poorly performing doctors.

Although a dentist may come under the jurisdiction of any of the committees mentioned above, it should be stressed that (s)he cannot be under the jurisdiction of more than one of these committees at any one time!

Other requirements for the practice of dentistry

Following qualification, a dental surgeon is immediately eligible for full registration with the GDC. However, before commencing the practice of dentistry, there are several requirements or recommendations that should be carried out in addition to registering with the GDC.

Professional indemnity

There are three organisations in the UK that provide indemnity for dentists and doctors. These are mutual organisations, which mean that the organisation belongs to the members and all profits made by these organisations have to go to the benefit of the members (unlike a limited company where owners or shareholders reap the benefit of any profits). These organisations are:

- Dental Defence Union (a subsidiary of the Medical Defence Union)
- Dental Protection (a subsidiary of the Medical Protection Society)
- the Medical and Dental Defence Union of Scotland.

These organisations provide members with indemnity against any legal action brought by patients; advice and assistance on medico/legal matters; legal representation at courts, tribunals or professional committee hearings on disciplinary matters; and general advice on professional conduct. Hospital trusts and health authorities who employ salaried practitioners have corporate indemnity should a patient sue the organisation or individual employees. However, this cover does not include representation of a practitioner at tribunals or disciplinary hearings of any sort. Therefore, it is advisable to belong to one of the professional protection organisations; these organisations offer lower rates of subscription for those practitioners who have indemnity from their employers.

Professional indemnity is also available on the commerical market, but this normally has a maximum limit of indemnity and only provides cover within the time of the insurance contract. This is an important factor, recognised by the professional protection organisations, as there may be a delay of several years between an incident occurring and a patient bringing an action for damages.

The first steps

There is nothing to prevent a dental surgeon on qualification and initial registration from setting up in single-handed private practice, but the benefit of a period of a supervised practice cannot be overemphasised. The majority of UK dental graduates undertake a year of vocational training in general practice on qualifying. Vocational training, which is under the supervision of regional Postgraduate Dental Deans, provides a very good introduction to the practice and business of dentistry. Without satisfactory completion of a year of vocational training, no dentist can now have their own contract to provide dental treatment under the General Dental Services' part of the National Health Service. Newly qualified entrants to the Community Dental Service are also required to undergo vocational training. In the hospital service, there is supervision from more senior dental staff; the training aspect of junior hospital staff is overseen by the regional Postgraduate Dental Dean.

Continuing education

There are five important aspects to postgraduate training and education.

General professional training
General professional training is a broad-brush training in all aspects of dentistry to consolidate what was learnt as an undergraduate. It should encompass more than one branch of dentistry, and to this end there are several 2-year general professional training schemes in operation that include a year in general practice necessary for the completion of vocational training in general practice and a year spent in the hospital and/or community dental service. These 2-year training schemes are voluntary at present. Another form of general training that is frequently undertaken is a year in each of vocational training in general practice and the hospital service, carried out as two separate periods of employment. Several Dental Postgraduate Deans have organised further professional training for the year following vocational training, which involves 30–50 hours of formal teaching while working in practice as an assistant or associate.

Specialist training
Following a period of at least 2 years general professional training and obtaining any necessary postgraduate qualification (e.g. MFDS), specialist training may be undertaken to qualify a dental surgeon to become a specialist in one of the fields mentioned above. On suc-

cessful completion of the appropriate period of higher professional training and obtaining any required postgraduate qualifications a certificate of completion of specialist training (CCST) will be issued and that person will be eligible to apply to join a specialist list held by the GDC.

There is no exact postgraduate equivalent training in general dental practice, but general practitioners can undertake further study to sit for various diplomas awarded by the Royal Surgical Colleges:

- MFGDP (formerly DGDP): this is the initial postgraduate qualification, which is in two parts; The first part has equivalence with the first part of MFDS, both of which can be taken 15 months after qualifying
- MGDS: dentists with a minimum of 4 years' experience can sit for this diploma, which is designed for experienced practitioners showing excellence in clinical practice with a bias towards restorative dentistry
- FFGDP: this is only open to principals in general dental practice of 10 years' standing who are full members of the Faculty of General Dental Practice. It consists of a formative assessment of 12 modules covering all aspects of primary dental care. Some exemption from the clinical module is permitted for those holding MGDS.

Continuing professional education
It is essential that dental surgeons, or members of any other profession, continue to update their knowledge and expertise throughout the whole of their professional practising life. Learning more about dentistry should continue until at least retirement to provide the best for one's patients. The Royal Surgical Colleges expect that specialists keep a record of their continuing professional/medical education and (CPE or CME) recommend a minimum of 250 hours CME every 5 years. The GDC published a discussion document in July 1997 entitled *Re-accreditation and Recertification for the Dental Profession*, which recommended that all registered dentists should submit evidence of CPE undertaken in the previous 5 years in order that their name can remain on the Dentists' Register. If this re-accreditation process is to be mandatory, it will require amendments to the Dentists' Act 1984. The recommendation is for a core component of 15 hours of formal CPE per year and a further 35 hours that could be either formal or informal. This minimum recommendation amounts to approximately 1 hour per week.

Professional organisations and societies
It is not compulsory to join any organisation or society connected with dentistry, but all dentists practising in

the UK are recommended to join the British Dental Association (BDA). The BDA is the official negotiating body with the government on matters concerning general dental practice and the community dental service. It also contracts with the British Medical Association to negotiate on bahalf of the hospital dental service and clinical academic staff.

Advice on all aspects of dental practice are available to members from the BDA and it has a large library available to members. The BDA publishes many advice booklets, which are regularly updated, as well as giving individual advice on request. As it is a registered trade union, it can assist members who have problems relating to their employment.

There are also many specialist dental societies, and it is worthwhile joining those related to any special interest one may have. Dental surgeons undergoing higher professional training are strongly recommended to join the appropriate specialist society or societies pertaining to their specialty.

Ability and experience

Ability and experience are essential matters of self-regulation throughout one's professional life, not just at the beginning. Prior to undertaking any particular item of treatment for a patient, a dental surgeon must be certain that (s)he has both the ability and the experience to complete the treatment successfully in the patient's best interest, as well as having the necessary equipment and materials available to complete the task.

11.4 Records and documentation

Learning objectives

You should

- realise the importance of neat contemporanious records detailing all aspects of patient care

- have a clear understanding of informed consent prior to undertaking any treatment

- be aware of the importance of a chaperone.

Records

The patient's records do not just consist of clinical notes but also include radiographs, referral letters and replies, study models, occlusal recordings, photographs, dental laboratory cards and investigation results. Consent forms, copies of treatment plans and cost estimates should also be retained with patients' records. If patients are receiving treatment under NHS regulations,

NHS documentation should also be retained. Appointment books and day sheets may be useful should any query arise concerning the timing and extent of a particular patient's treatment; consequently, their long-term retention can be extremely helpful. Telephone messages and any other memoranda concerning patients should be stored with their records. Finally, all records should be stored in a safe place where they are easily retrievable when next required.

Retention of records

Records should be retained for as long as possible, as patients who have received treatment over many years, or only discover negligence at a later date, may take court action. Allegations have been made by patients concerning treatment carried out over 20 years previously!

Records of dental treatment carried out in general practice under NHS regulations have to be retained for a minimum of 2 years after the completion of any course of treatment or period of care. This gives the Dental Practice Board the time to check that treatment and payment coincide, but this is insufficient for reasons of law.

Any action for personal injury (e.g. negligence) or breach of contract has to be started within 3 years of the incident causing the action, or within 3 years of the plaintiff (patient) being aware that something has gone wrong. Courts have the power to extend these limits if good reason can be shown. Therefore, it is recommended that records are kept for a minimum of 7 years from the completion of the last course of treatment. Records of treatment of children should be kept until they are 25 years of age (18 + 7) because their 'legal awareness' that something may have gone wrong does not start until they reach the age of majority (18 years). Prior to this, parents or guardians have to commence action in a court on behalf of the minor concerned. If they decide to take no action, on becoming an adult the patient can undertake legal proceedings in their own right. At the other end of the scale, trustees or beneficiaries can take action on behalf of someone deceased. If records are kept on computer, the practitioner must ensure that there is adequate back-up of the records to prevent any risk that the records become lost or irrecoverable. The printing of hard copies of radiographs and clinical photographs is recommended.

It cannot be overstated that records should be:

- accurate
- complete
- comprehensive
- contemporaneous
- legible
- retrievable

• retained for as long as possible, but at least 7 years after completion of treatment.

Medical history

It should never be forgotten that medical history is an essential part of medical records. Medical history should always be taken at the initial visit of a patient and re-checked and updated at every subsequent course of treatment to prevent inappropriate treatment or harm befalling a patient.

Confidentiality and disclosure

All medical and dental records are confidential between the patient and the dentist or doctor and should not be disclosed to a third party without the patient's permission. This confidentiality normally extends to withholding records and information from both the police and the courts of law. If either police or the courts have good cause to request patients records, a formal request should be made, stating the circumstances. Disclosure is then a matter for the dentist's conscience; in the investigation of a serious crime, for instance, the dentist may agree to disclosure. However, the High Court has certain powers to insist on the production of documents in a person's possession or custody. As the rules governing disclosure vary according to the circumstances, the advice of the dentist's defence/protection organisation should be sought on this matter. It is essential that all staff employed by a dentist are aware of patient confidentiality and do not break any confidences. Any breach of confidentiality by a member of staff is the responsibility of the dentist both legally as an employer and ethically as a member of a caring profession.

If patients' records are maintained on a computer, the dentist must register as a data user with the Data Protection Registrar under the Data Protection Act of 1984. It is a criminal offence not to do so. Application forms and details of registration are available from the Data Protection Registrar and main post offices in the UK. Anyone considering using a computer for patients' records is advised to seek further information from their defence/protection organisation or the BDA.

Consent and related matters

No treatment can be carried out on a patient without that patient's or their legal guardian's valid informed consent for that specific treatment to be undertaken. Undertaking treatment without consent is an assault on the patient. Consent can be implied, verbal or written.

Implied consent
Examples of implied consent:

• if a patient has previously been presented with a treatment plan and arranges further appointments for this treatment plan to be carried out, implied consent can be assumed
• if a patient requests local anaesthetic for fillings and opens his mouth to allow local anaesthetic to be administered.

Verbal consent
For instance a dentist may say:

• 'Would you like a local anaesthetic for me to put the filling in your tooth?'
• 'I am going to give you local anaesthetic for this filling/extraction'
• 'I think that the most urgent treatment you need is a filling in this tooth.'

The patient either verbally agreeing to the above or opening his mouth to allow the dentist to proceed would be valid consent providing the dentist is confident that the patient understands what is going to happen. If there is any doubt regarding the patient's mental ability to understand the treatment fully, no treatment should be undertaken.

Implied or verbal consent is frequently sufficient for treatment without any form of anaesthetic or when treatment is undertaken with local analgesia, as the patient can request that the treatment is stopped at any time they may wish to withdraw consent.

Written consent
Written consent must be obtained if the patient is having treatment under sedation or general anaesthesia when they are not fully conscious of the treatment being carried out and are, therefore, in no position to ask for the treatment to be stopped should they wish to withdraw consent. Written consent is also advisable for any complicated and/or expensive treatment even when this is carried out without any form of anaesthetic or with local analgesia.

Written consent is advisable when carrying out a procedure that carries one or more specific risks. For instance, prior to the removal of an impacted lower wisdom tooth, a patient should be warned of the possibility of swelling, trismus and the risk of trauma to the inferior dental nerve, which would lead to labial anaesthesia/paraesthesia, or trauma to the lingual nerve, which would cause similar problems with the tongue. The mnemonic STALL (swelling, trismus, anaesthesia of lingual or labial nerves) may ensure that appropriate warnings are given. These warnings should be entered in the patient's record. It is essential that written consent should contain details of the procedure, the type of anaesthetic or analgesic that will be used and any complications that may occur during treatment. Without being patronising, consent should be worded in a language that a particular patient can understand, avoiding the use of jargon and abbreviations to describe a particular clinical procedure.

Because of the nature of dentistry in the UK at the present time, it is essential that the patient is aware of whether they are consenting to treatment under the NHS or by private contract before treatment commences.

Special cases

Age of the patient. The minimum age for valid consent is considered to be 16 years; however, if a practitioner is satisfied that someone of less than 16 years of age fully understands the treatment to which they are consenting, their consent may be valid. Particularly in the case of sedation or general anaesthesia, the consent of a parent or guardian or someone over 18 should be obtained as well as from the patient themself for those between 16 and 18 years of age.

Mentally impaired adults. These patients may be unable to give informed consent and the consent of the patient's carer should be obtained plus the second opinion of a colleague that the proposed treatment is the most suitable for the patient. For any major treatment, it is normal practice for the agreement of two practitioners of consultant status to be obtained prior to treatment.

Patients with specific ethnic customs or religious beliefs. Practitioners should always be sympathetic to specific patient beliefs and requests, for instance the avoidance of blood transfusions to Jehovah's Witnesses, the avoidance of materials derived from any animals for vegetarians and from certain animals for religious or cultural reasons. It should also be remembered that certain cultures object to women receiving treatment from male practitioners.

Life-saving procedures. Occasionally, it may be necessary to carry out a life-saving procedure on an unconscious person. Under these circumstances, informed consent is normally unobtainable, but any treatment under these circumstances should be limited to that which is life-saving. Non-life-saving treatment should be delayed until consent is obtained.

Chaperones

It is always advisable to have a chaperone present for all patient contact even if active treatment is not involved. The presence of a third person can be useful in confirming consent and may be required to avoid any allegation of impropriety. It is custom and practice in the UK to have a female chaperone (either a member of staff or an accompanying person) when treatment is being carried out by a male practitioner. For female practitioners, the convention of opposite sex chaperonage is less rigid.

When carrying out treatment, the dentist should normally be assisted by a dental nurse, who can also act as a chaperone. It should be remembered that whether attending a patient in the dental surgery or on a domiciliary visit, another member of the dental team or another person should be present at all times.

11.5 General anaesthesia and sedation

Learning objectives

You should

- know who can administer general anaesthesia and sedation to your patients
- understand the role of the dental operator under these circumstances.

When patients are receiving treatment under general anaesthesia or sedation, it is essential that written informed consent is obtained prior to the procedure being undertaken. Whenever possible, this consent should be obtained at a consultation and treatment planning appointment, as signing the consent from when the patient arrives for this treatment and immediately before the anaesthetic and sedation is administered could be considered as signing under duress.

Any patient who is to receive treatment under general anaesthesia or sedation must be accompanied by a friend or relative who can take responsibility for the patient's care following treatment. The presence of this accompanying person, and confirmation of their availability for the time required for the patient to recover sufficiently to not need support, must be established prior to administering any general anaesthesia or sedation.

Prior to November 1998, dental surgeons who had received the appropriate training were allowed to administer general anaesthesia to patients. The new ethical guidance on general anaesthesia from the GDC clarifies the roles and responsibilities of those involved in carrying out dental treatment under general anaesthesia and now precludes dentists from administering general anaesthesia.

General anaesthesia

The referring dentist

Any dental surgeon who refers a patient for treatment under general anaesthesia must:

- take a full medical history
- explain to the patient the risks involved

- offer alternative methods of pain control
- obtain consent.

When sending a patient for treatment under general anaesthesia, the dentist's referral letter should contain full justification for the use of general anaesthesia and proper records must be kept by the referring dentist.

The dentist treating a patient under general anaesthesia

The dentist treating a patient under general anaesthesia must:

- repeat the history taking
- repeat the explanations concerning risk and the alternative methods of treatment and pain control
- obtain the patient's or the parent's written consent
- give written pre- and postoperative instructions
- keep careful records.

Treatment under general anaesthesia

For treatment of a patient under general anaesthesia it is essential that:

- the dentist/surgeon has an appropriately trained dental/general nurse available for assistance
- the anaesthetic is administered by an anaesthetist on the General Medical Council's Specialist Register; if a trainee anaesthetist/non-consultant career-grade anaesthetist gives the anaesthetic, that doctor must be working under a named consultant anaesthetist
- the anaesthetist is supported by someone experienced in monitoring the patient's condition and able to assist the anaesthetist in an emergency
- the anaesthetist and the dental surgeon have an agreed written protocol for the provision of advanced life support, including agreed arrangements for the immediate transfer of a patient to a critical care facility
- recovery and discharge is the responsibility of the anaesthetist, and recovery nurses must be properly trained and responsible to the anaesthetist
- all personnel involved in anaesthetics train together.

The GDC make it clear that it is the responsibility of the treating dentist to ensure that these protocols for general anaesthesia are adhered to.

Sedation

Conscious sedation is defined as a technique in which the use of a drug or drugs depresses the central nervous system, thus enabling treatment to be carried out, but during which communication with the patient can be maintained. The modification of the patient's state of mind should be such that the patient will respond to command throughout the period of sedation. Techniques used should carry a margin of safety wide enough to render unintended loss of consciousness unlikely.

A suitably experienced and trained dental surgeon can administer sedative drugs as well as operating on the patient providing at least one other appropriately trained person is present throughout the procedure. This other person must be capable of monitoring the clinical condition of the patient and of assisting the dental surgeon in the event of an emergency. An appropriately trained dental or general nurse can fulfil this duty, ideally this person should be present in addition to the dental nurse providing close support for the dental treatment.

The GDC recommend that normally a single drug should be used for intravenous sedation; if more than one sedative drug is utilised, the provision of advanced life support must be immediately available. Whatever sedation techniques are used, contemporary appropriate standards of patient monitoring should be adopted during conscious sedation. As intravenous sedation is unpredictable in children, it is recommended that this technique is used only under very special circumstances.

Before undertaking treatment under sedation a dental surgeon must:

- carefully assess the patient, including a full medical and dental history
- explain the sedation technique proposed
- advise on appropriate alternative methods of pain and anxiety control
- provide clear and comprehensive pre- and postoperative instructions in writing
- obtain written informed consent for the sedation and treatment proposed
- ensure that proper equipment for the administration of the sedation technique is available
- ensure that the facilities are adequate
- adopt contemporary standards of monitoring the patient
- ensure that appropriate drugs for resuscitation of the patient are readily available
- ensure that the dentist and staff are trained in the sedation procedure being used and resuscitation techniques; it is essential that all those involved in the provision of sedation and/or the supervision of recovery of sedated patients should train together as a team to deal with any emergencies and that this training should include frequent practise of resuscitation routines in a simulated emergency

- ensure that patients recovering from sedation should be appropriately supervised, protected and monitored in adequate recovery facilities.

Monitoring of patients should be undertaken either by the sedationist or by an appropriately trained person responsible to the sedationist. When the sedationist considers the patient is sufficiently recovered to leave the premises, they must be accompanied by a responsible adult. Where nitrous oxide/oxygen sedation alone has been used for an adult patient, a dental surgeon may exercise discretion as to whether that patient is fit enough to be discharged unaccompanied.

Chaperones

During treatment under general anaesthesia or sedation and in the recovery room following general anaesthesia or sedation, the presence of a third person is mandatory. It is advisable that either the dentist or another person present is of the same sex as the patient.

11.6 Complaints procedure and negligence

Learning objectives

You should

- understand how the health complaints procedure works in UK so that you are able to deal with any complaints expeditiously

- understand the meaning of negligence

- be aware of how best to avoid an accusation of negligence.

Under the UK Patients' Charter, all health care organisations must have a complaints procedure. This applies to all branches of dentistry, including general dental practice. There has to be a designated person/persons in the organisations to accept complaints, acknowledge the receipt of all complaints and keep the complainant informed of how the complaint is progressing. Complaints should be answered in writing within a reasonable time of the complaint being made. Mediation between the parties, rather than confrontation, is encouraged to allow the resolution of any grievance the patient may have.

An apology for lateness or an explanation of a particular difficulty occurring during treatment will often avoid formal complaints being made. If the dentist and his/her staff always deals with patients in a polite caring way, this will go a long way to minimise the number of formal complaints received.

'Mixing'

Mixing is the term used for providing some treatment under the NHS for a patient and other treatment for the same patient privately. It is a situation frought with difficulties and is best avoided if at all possible. Wherever possible, any course of treatment should be undertaken entirely under NHS regulations or entirely under a private contract. If this is not possible it is important that:

- it is not implied to the patient that NHS treatment is inferior to private treatment
- the patient fully understands which items are being carried out under NHS regulations and which privately and consents to this, preferably in writing.

If possible the NHS-funded treatment should be completed prior to undertaking items of treatment that will be charged privately.

Dealing with complaints

Under the Patients' Charter, every provider of the health care is obliged to set up a system for dealing with complaints from patients. Although this applies to NHS treatment, in addition an in-house protocol for dealing with patient complaints concerning any treatment carried out under private contract is advisable.

Encouraging comments and suggestions from patients can decrease the risk of formal complaints being made. Suggestions and comments should not be ignored, a verbal or written thank you with a mention of any changes made as a result of the comment or suggestion should always be given. Every practice, clinic or hospital should have a specific person nominated to deal with comments, suggestions or complaints. This is particularly important when dealing with complaints, to help to ensure that they are managed adequately and within the time scales laid down. In general practice, the practice manager or a senior dental surgeon should undertake this duty. In hospitals and clinics, a senior member of the administrative staff normally undertakes this responsibility.

Every effort should be made to deal with complaints as quickly as possible, as the longer a feeling of dissatisfaction or aggravation continues, the more entrenched the parties become, which makes the problem more difficult to solve. The Patients' Charter sets out the formal stages in the resolution of patient complaints.

Local resolution

It is hoped that the vast majority of complaints will be dealt with in-house. If a patient makes a verbal complaint, the designated person should endeavour to discuss the nature of the problem with the patient and/or their relative or carer at the time the complaint is made. Any discussion should take place in a private office to protect patient confidentially and give an atmosphere conducive to resolution of the complaint. The term 'Complaints Manager' is probably best avoided, but the person designated to deal with complaints should inform the complainer of their name and status in the practice or organisation.

If complaints are received in writing, they should be acknowledged within 2 working days of their receipt. This acknowledgement should state how soon a full response can be expected. NHS practitioners (doctors, dentists, opticians or pharmacists) are expected to respond to a complaint within 10 working days. NHS trusts are expected to respond within 4 weeks of receiving a complaint by way of a written reply from the chief executive. Where there are good reasons why these time limits cannot be achieved, there is a duty to inform the complainer of what progress is being made.

The majority of complaints can be resolved locally, and every effort must be made to ensure that this is achieved whenever possible. Anyone who has received NHS treatment or services has the right to complain, and a relative or close friend may complain on behalf of anyone unable to do this for themselves. Complaints should be made within 6 months of the event or 6 months of realising that there is something to complain about, provided that the latter is no longer than 12 months after the event itself. However, these time limits can be waived if there are good reasons why the complaint could not be made sooner.

A courteous and efficient system for dealing with complaints should lead to their resolution in most cases.

Conciliation and mediation

If a complaint cannot be resolved in-house, it will normally pass to the appropriate local Health Authority. Some Health Authorities in consultation with local dental committees have established lay conciliators for informal resolution of problems. Some Health Authorities also employ trained mediators for this purpose.

Independent review

If a patient is not satisfied with the outcome of local resolution, conciliation or mediation they can write to the appropriate Health Authority requesting an independent review. This request should be made within 4 weeks of the date of the letter sent to the patient concerning the outcome of the action taken in attempting local resolution. This letter also has to inform the patient how to request an independent review.

Every NHS Trust or Health Authority has to appoint a convenor who will ask the patient to explain exactly in writing why they are still dissatisfied, unless they have already done so in requesting the independent review. With the aid of an independent lay person, the convenor will enquire whether any other form of local resolution action can resolve the problem. If not, the convenor has to decide whether or not there should be an independent review of the complaint by a special panel. The convenor does not have to set up a panel on request, but only if he/she feels that a panel investigation is likely to resolve the problems that have been identified by the patient. In any case, the convenor has to inform the complainer of his/her decision in writing within 4 weeks of receiving the request for an independent review. If an independent review panel is set up, the convenor has to set out what particular matters of the complaint the panel will investigate.

The independent review panel consists of three people, an independent lay person acting as chairman, the convenor and one other person. This panel has to re-examine fully the concerns referred to it by the convenor, talking to everyone involved and getting any special advice it needs. The panel then prepares a report setting out the result of its investigations, its conclusions and any appropriate comments or suggestions. Copies of this report will be sent to all parties. The practice manager or a senior person in the practice (or the chief executive in the case of health authorities and NHS trusts) has to write to the complainee informing them of any action being taken as a result of the panel's recommendations.

There are certain matters that cannot be dealt with by the NHS complaints system above. These include:

- complaints about private treatment
- complaints about local authority social services
- events requiring investigation by a professional disciplinary body
- events about which the patient is already taking legal action.

The Health Service Commissioner ('Ombudsman')

Any patient still dissatisfied after the NHS complaints procedure has been completed may ask the Health Service Commissioner to investigate the case. This ombudsman is completely independent of both the NHS and the government and can investigate complaints about NHS services and how the complaints procedure is working. The Health Service Commissioner is not obliged to investigate every complaint and will not generally consider any case that has not first been through the NHS complaints procedure, nor a case which is being dealt with by the courts.

Negligence

In the treatment of patients, the following may be considered negligent:

- failure to exercise reasonable skill and care
- omitting to do something that a reasonable person would do, considering what normally regulates the conduct of human affairs
- doing something that a prudent reasonable person would not do.

Every dentist is expected to exercise reasonable skill and care in every treatment she/he carries out by virtue of the dental qualification; this is, a similar degree of skill and care as exercised by the majority of colleagues. A general practitioner would be compared with other general practitioners, and a specialist with other specialists in the same field. Also, no dentist should undertake treatment for which he/she is not trained and competent to undertake; consequently failure to refer to a specialist when appropriate could be considered negligent.

A practitioner is expected to exercise reasonable skill and care whether a patient is being treated privately, under the NHS, as an act of friendship, or even as a 'good Samaritan act' in an emergency.

To recover compensation for negligence it is necessary:

- to prove that the practitioner owed a duty of care to the patient at the time
- that there was a breach of that duty
- that damage occurred as a result of the action of the practitioner.

If the patient suffered no harm or damage as a result of the practitioner's action, there is nothing for the patient to be compensated for, so no compensation will be paid.

A dentist cannot guarantee that all treatments provided will be uneventful or free from accident even if there is no lack of care and skill. To prove negligence, the patient (plaintiff) has to prove that harm has been caused as a result of lack of care and/or lack of reasonable skill that the practitioner (defendant) had a duty to apply. Unless the plaintiff can satisfy the court of this, the claim will fail.

If a very obvious mistake or damage has occurred to a patient, the patient's legal adviser will make a plea of *res ipsa loquitur*. This legal term basically means 'the thing speaks for itself'. Carrying out treatment on the wrong tooth, or treating the wrong patient could be considered as examples.

Contributory negligence

If something occurs or is made worse by an action or failure by the patient, the defendant can plea contributory negligence, which may reduce or negate any damages that are awarded. An example of this would be failure on the part of the patient to follow pre- or postoperative instructions or grabbing the dentist's arm when he was using a sharp instrument or a dental handpiece.

Unsuitable treatment

Dentists should always resist being talked into undertaking treatment by a patient that is unsuitable or of very poor prognosis, e.g. advanced restorative treatment on teeth with gross periodontal disease. Carrying out treatment that is very likely to fail or cause severe problems is as much negligent as any other professional act a dentist performs.

Vicarious liability

As an employer, a dentist can be held responsible for any acts or omissions of his/her staff. This applies to all grades of staff, whether or not that member of staff was or was not acting in accordance to instructions. At the same time, however, the employee is responsible for his/her own acts. Therefore, a claim for negligence could be brought against the employer, employee or (as is more commonly the case) against both. In the case of partnership agreements, each partner is individually and jointly liable for the actions of other partners. Therefore, it is essential that all partnership agreements include the provision to provide indemnity for the partnership as a whole.

The Bolam principle/test

The Bolam principle has been used as the bench mark in the assessment of professional negligence. In 1957, Judge McNair in the High Court directed the jury in the case of *Bolam* v. *Friern Hospital Management Committee* that 'a doctor is not guilty of negligence if he has acted in accordance with the practise accepted as proper by a reasonable body of medical men skilled in that particular art'. This means that if there is more than one respectable body of professional opinion concerning diagnosis or treatment, there is no negligence should a practitioner choose one protocol in preference to another.

The Bolam principle was re-examined in 1997 in an appeal to the House of Lords (*Bolitho* v. *City and Hackney Health Authority*). This particular case involved an omission to carry out a procedure on a patient that several experts supported but others did not. Their Lordships opined that the use of the adjectives 'responsible, reasonable or respectable' concerning a body of opinion may not be sufficient, but that experts' views should include scientific evidence on the comparative risks and benefits to decide whether or not an act or omission is defensible. With the advent of clinical governance and evidence-based medicine leading to clinical guidelines, the Bolitho judgement may replace the Bolam principle as the benchmark for negligence.

Time limits

Claims for negligence normally have to be made within one of the following time limits:

- within 3 years of the plaintiff becoming aware of having suffered damage
- within 6 years of the incident occurring
- within 6 years of reaching the age of majority (18 years) in the case of alleged negligence occurring in a minor.

At the Court's discretion, claims can be brought outside these limits if the plaintiff can persuade the Court that there is a good reason for ignoring them. Because of these time limits, it is advisable that all patient records are retained for at least 7 years following any treatment, or until the age of 25 years in the case of treatment being carried out on patients under the age of 18 (see above).

In 1999, two important legal changes have occurred affecting all claims for compensation, not just medical and dental claims: legal aid/contingency fees and the Woolf report.

Legal aid/contingency fees

The government has introduced further limits to the payment of legal aid so that fewer plaintiffs will be eligible to receive legal aid. By way of compensation for this restriction of legal aid, solicitors are now able to work on a contingency fee basis. Contingency fees, which have been accepted in USA for many years, involve the lawyer only receiving a fee if the client's claim is successful. As this system is just starting, it is too early to judge its success. It has the advantage that if the plaintiff/client does not have sufficient capital available to pay legal fees, these will not be charged should the case be unsuccessful This gives an additional impetus to the lawyer to make certain of success. Disadvantages may include lawyers charging higher fees, which may be fixed or a percentage of the total compensation obtained, and a reluctance of lawyers to take on any cases except those with an almost certain chance of success. Even with this system, there may be some cost to the claimant, as solicitors may be unwilling to fund such fixed costs as specialist medical reports necessary to support a claim – unless, that is, they can find dental/medical experts who are also willing to work on a contingency fee basis.

The Woolf report

In July 1996, Lord Woolf published his report to the Lord Chancellor on proposed reforms of the Civil Justice System for England and Wales. These recommendations came into effect on 26 April 1999 and affect the legal profession more than the dental and medical professions in that a very strict timetable is laid down for each stage of the procedure. These new rules are detailed in the Civil Procedure Rules published in January 1999. The overriding objective of these new rules is to enable the courts to deal with cases justly. This includes:

- ensuring that the parties are on an equal footing
- saving expense
- dealing with the case in ways that are proportionate to
  — the amount of money involved
  — the importance of the case
  — the complexity of the issues
  — the financial position of each party
- ensuring that the case is dealt with expeditiously and fairly
- allotting to a case an appropriate share of the court's resources, while taking into account the need to allot resources to other cases
- requiring the parties involved to help the court in the furtherance of the above objectives
- restricting expert evidence to that which is reasonably required to resolve the proceedings; this means that whenever possible a single joint expert is appointed to act on behalf of the court, rather than the plaintiff/claimant or the defendant. This can occur either by agreement with the parties involved or, if necessary, an expert can be appointed by the court
- the plaintiff/patient will in future be called the claimant.

Claims will be divided into three types:

- *small claims track*: this is for claims of compensation of up to £5000 in most cases but is limited to £1000 in personal injury
- *fast track*: this is for claims of up to £15 000; complicated claims of under £15 000 may not be considered suitable for the fast track system; dental/medical negligence claims may often come into this category and have to be dealt with under the multitrack system
- *multitrack*. this is for cases which are complicated or where claims are in excess of £15 000.

On occasions, potential claims may start as a complaint. In this case, dealing with the complaint fairly and expeditiously with a clear explanation, as recommended above, may mean that a claim does not arise. However, should the patient be dissatisfied she/he may consult a solicitor for advice regarding whether or not a claim for damages should be made. The solicitor may request a copy of the patient's health records from the health care provider (HCP) and these should be disclosed within 40 days. If this time limit is not kept, the patient's solicitor can apply to the court for an order for pre-action disclosure and the HCP will be responsible for any costs involved in this. Should the patient or their legal adviser decide there are grounds for a claim, a detailed letter of claim should be sent to the HCP. This letter should contain:

- a clear summary of the facts of the case
- the main allegations of negligence
- the injuries incurred, present condition and future prognosis
- any financial losses and damage
- reference to any relevant documents.

The HCP then has 3 months to respond to this letter of claim before court proceedings are issued. During this period, either side may negotiate or offer to settle the claim. Either side may support its position with an appropriate dental/medical report. Should this not lead to the resolution of the matter, there are strict protocols and timetables that have to be observed, or the defaulting party may be liable to any additional costs of the other side.

Fast track timetable

It is intended that any fast track cases will come to trial within 30 weeks of the court issuing a Notice of Allocation following the submission of a claim. In fast track cases, the trial is expected to last a maximum of 1 day. The timetable following the date of the Notice of Allocation is:

- 4 weeks for the disclosure of documents by both parties
- 10 weeks for the exchange of witness statements between the parties
- 14 weeks for the exchange of expert reports between the parties
- 20 weeks for sending a list of questions to the court and the other party for clarification
- 22 weeks for response to questions from the other side or the court (note: each side is limited to one request for clarification and cannot delay matters by asking further questions at a later date).
- 30 weeks for the court hearing, unless the case has been previously resolved.

Under the Civil Procedure Rules, there is an appendix setting out the fast track standard directions, which it is expected that the parties will use to ensure that the timetable is adhered to.

Multitrack timetable

It is expected that the majority of clinical negligence claims will be dealt with by the multiple track system even if they are below £15 000 in value. This is because they are regarded as too complex for the fast track. The multitrack timetable is not as tight as the fast track, but the Court will have far greater control of cases than previously. Once a case has been allocated, a case management conference will be called. At the case management conference:

- both parties and/or their legal representatives will be expected to be present
- a substantial amount of information will be expected from all parties, including details of witnesses to be called and experts whose evidence will be heard; this means that parties must have their case in order at a very early stage and this may facilitate settlement in some cases
- the timetable for the case will be set, which will be closely controlled by the court, who will not allow delay
- trial dates will be fixed at, or soon after, the case management conference and these dates will be immovable.

To ensure that the case is dealt with expeditiously, the courts have power to impose sanctions should, for example, either party fail to comply with the pre-action protocol. These sanctions include costs, penalties and the disallowing of evidence.

To further speed resolution of a case, the court may suggest mediation, and it is expected that courts will build up a list of mediators suitable for different categories of claims. In addition, the trial judge will hold a pre-trial review of the case. Normally, additional evidence or reports cannot be submitted following the case management conference without the permission of the court and the other parties.

These changes basically mean that the court will control the timetable and scrutinise the progress of the case. The court will now act without prompting by one of the parties, which means that the lawyers will no longer be able to determine the timetable of the case.

11.7 Laws and regulations

A dentist may be an employer and/or an employee, both of which involve a myriad of legislation. The Dentists' Act of 1984, which has had several minor amendments over the years, makes the practice of dentistry illegal other than by registered practitioners and enrolled auxiliaries. It is this Act that gives the GDC the powers that have already been discussed.

A summary of other important legislation is listed below, as it is so extensive and complicated, appropriate professional advice should always be sought. This list should be used only as a guide to those situations or occasions when further details should be sought and/or appropriate professional advice obtained. Ignorance of the law is not acceptable for defence or mitigation.

Employment

All employees should have a written contract of employment. There is a nationally agreed contract for the employment of vocational trainees and the BDA offers specimen contracts for various types of employee and working agreements to its members on request.

Termination. There is specific legislation regarding the termination of employment, redundancy and unfair dismissal. Legal advice should be sought on this matter.

Employees cannot be discriminated against on account of either their race or sex. This may also extend to age in the fairly near future.

Employer's liabilities. These include the safety of employees, customers and the general public, as well as the collection of income tax and National Insurance contributions.

Premises and working environment

Legislation involving factories, offices and other work places prescribes standards of cleanliness, levels of occupation and the provision of sanitary facilities of any work place. Specific legislation concerning, for instance, eye protection, air compressors, autoclaves and the safety of all electrical appliances are amongst those applicable to dental practice. For instance, autoclaves should be inspected by a competent person at least once every 14 months.

Health and Safety at Work legislation states that every employer has a general duty to ensure the health,

safety and welfare at work of all employees. There are many general and specific regulations under this umbrella. Every employer has to:

- provide and maintain safety equipment and systems of work
- ensure safe handling and storage of any potentially harmful substances
- maintain entrances and exits in a safe condition
- provide a working environment for employees that is no risk to their health
- provide instruction, training and supervision necessary to ensure health and safety.

The Health and Safety Executive has the duty to enforce legal requirements and provide advisory services. Its inspectors have the power to enter premises and carry out investigations.

If an inspector notes a risk to health and safety, she/he can issue a Prohibition Notice preventing the continuance of that risk activity until remedial action as specified has been taken. In the case of a less severe risk, an Improvement Notice may be issued, which requires action within a specified time to remove that risk. Failure to comply with either of these notices within a specific time can lead to prosecution of the offender (employer).

Under the health and safety umbrella there are several specific regulations that are particularly important to dentistry.

Ionising Radiations Regulations 1999 & 2000 The Ionising Radiations Regulations [1999] replaced IRR [1985], and came into force on 1st January 2000. These regulations are concerned with the safety and maintenance of X-ray equipment, quality assurance, and the health and safety of employees.

The protection of patients is covered by the Ionising Radiations [Medical Exposure] Regulations [2000] (IRMER). These regulations replaced the 1988 Ionising Radiation [Protection of Persons Undergoing Medical Examination or Treatment] Regulations (POPUMET). The IRMER came into force on 13th May 2000. They are mainly concerned with the protection of patients and specify the responsibilities of those ordering and taking radiographs to ensure that only necessary examinations are undertaken and that the dose of radiation that the patient receives is kept to a minimum.

As there is no doubt that dental radiography is included in medical exposures, these regulations have to be fully covered in all undergraduate dental courses in the UK. Additionally, all dentists and ancillary staff involved in ordering and/or taking radiographs for patients must undertake a formal radiation protection course of at least 5 hours' verifiable CPE covering these regulations every 5 years.

Control of Substances Hazardous to Health Regulations 1988 (COSHH). Within these regulations are occupational exposure limits (OEL) and maximum exposure limits (MEL). In dental practice, substances such as glutaraldehyde, mercury, methylacrylate, phenol and trichloracetic acid are common and could cause hazard if mishandled. The employer has the duty to make a risk assessment on all hazardous substances and to reduce any identifiable risk as much as possible.

Notification of Accident and Dangerous Occurrences Regulations 1980. These regulations require employers to notify the Health and Safety Executive of any dangerous occurrences and any accidents causing death or major injury. This notification must be made with the minimum of delay and the employer is required to keep a record of all such occurrences and make it available to the Executive.

General Liability. Owners of property and/or land have a general liability concerning safety to the general public, and prudent owners take out insurance to cover this liability.

Legislation involved in dental treatment

National Health Service Acts and Regulations. Naturally these only cover patients receiving NHS treatment. Copies of the appropriate rules and regulations should be issued to all independent practitioners undertaking treatment under Health Service Regulations by the appropriate Health Authority. In the case of employees, the appropriate Health Authority or NHS Trust has this responsibility.

Data protection. Personal data on patients, and anyone else, are covered by the Data Protection Act of 1984. No personal data should be disclosed to a third party without the permission of the person whose data has been recorded. Should any personal data be held on computer, the computer user must register this with the Data Protection Registrar and inform him of the purpose for which the data is kept.

The Consumer Protection Act 1987. The provision of dental treatment may be considered as the provision of goods or services under this Act. However, the vast majority of actions in dental and medical matters are dealt with via the negligence route.

Social Security Acts. Certain patients on low income are able to have the patient's contribution to NHS dental treatment paid for by the State. Employees applying for Statutory Sick Pay, Statutory Maternity Pay or various other allowances come within the umbrella of Social Security.

Agreements and contracts of employment

There is a nationally agreed contract concerning vocational training. Health Authorities have standard agreements on terms and conditions of service. The majority of these follow national guidelines and if there are any parts of the employment contract that are not understood, or appear to be contrary to national guidelines, advice from the BDA or a dental/medical protection organisation should be sought. The contract to provide treatment under the general dental services of the NHS is subject to national negotiation and cannot be changed by the individual.

Other contracts of employment are between the employee and employer. For these contracts, each party is advised to obtain its own legal and professional advice prior to signing the contract. Once a contract has been signed it is too late.

Awareness of the law

The field of law and ethics is subject to change, and all dentists have a duty to keep up to date on these matters. For instance the GDC *Guidance to Dentists on Professional and Personal Conduct (Maintaining Standards)* was published in November 1997; several amendments to this document were approved by the GDC in November 1998 and sent to all dentists in December 1998. These amendments involved the reprinting of over half the pages of this document! The next amendment occurred in May 1999; this mainly affected the section concerning treatment under sedation and reorganising the order of certain sections. Because the changes also involved renumbering of many sections, over a third of the pages had to be replaced on this occasion.

In September 1999, a separate *Maintaining Standards* was produced for dental hygienists and dental therapists.

At the November 2000 meeting of the GDC, recording of continuing professional development/education (CPD/CPE) was made compulsory from April 2001, when the next amendment was published. A new introduction and minor changes were published in June 2001.

The up-to-date version of *Maintaining Standards* is also available on the GDC website (www.gdc-uk.org).

The Revised Civil Procedure Rules for the courts will necessitate a major change in attitude by both the caring and the legal professions.

There are several differences between the Scottish legal system and the legal system applying to England and Wales as well as Northern Ireland: for instance the category of cases seen in the various levels of courts and the naming of those levels. This applies to both civil and criminal cases. Whichever jurisdiction is involved, it is essential to obtain legal advice from someone trained in that jurisdiction.

Self-assessment: questions

Multiple choice questions

1. The General Dental Council (GDC):
    a. Was set up in 1956
    b. Its membership comprised of more elected than appointed dentists
    c. Includes five members of the General Medical Council
    d. Includes one enrolled dental auxiliary
    e. Its six lay members are appointed by Parliament

2. The following are eligible for full registration with the GDC:
    a. Dentists who qualified in the USA
    b. Dentists who qualified in India
    c. Dentists who qualified in Norway
    d. Dentists who have not completed vocational training
    e. Dentists who only have a Licentiate of Dental Surgery from a Royal College, not a Bachelor of Dental Surgery from a UK university

3. Dentists with temporary registration:
    a. Can take the statutory examination
    b. Can work in an oral surgery unit in a UK hospital
    c. Are automatically permitted to undertake 'on-call' duties in a UK hospital
    d. Can work in the Community Dental Service
    e. Are automatically entitled to a 'work permit' for the UK

4. The statutory examination of the GDC:
    a. Is in three parts
    b. Each part can only be attempted once
    c. Has to be passed by French dentists for full registration
    d. Has to be passed by Greek dentists for full registration
    e. Has to be passed by Israeli dentists for full registration

5. A dentist is entitled to use the following titles:
    a. Dental Practitioner
    b. Doctor
    c. Dental Surgeon
    d. Dentist
    e. Orthodontist

6. The following specialties are recognised by the GDC for specialist registration:
    a. Community dentistry
    b. Endodontics
    c. Oral surgery
    d. Surgical dentistry
    e. Crown and bridge

7. All registered dental auxiliaries, in 1999:
    a. Can administer local anaesthetic
    b. Can extract permanent teeth
    c. Can extract deciduous teeth
    d. Can scale, clean and polish teeth
    e. Can work in general dental practice

8. Professions complementary to dentistry will include:
    a. Dental nurses
    b. Maxillofacial prosthetists and technologists
    c. Dental health educators
    d. Dental practice managers
    e. Dental therapists

9. The GDC review group recommends that dental technicians:
    a. Can fit and insert full dentures
    b. Can fit and insert partial dentures
    c. Can take tooth shades for the construction of prostheses
    d. Can take impressions
    e. Will all be able to register with the GDC

10. The GDC can remove a dentist from the Dentists' Register if:
    a. (S)he is addicted to prescribed drugs or alcohol
    b. (S)he has not paid the annual registration fee
    c. (S)he has been found guilty of 'serious professional misconduct'
    d. (S)he has been refused/removed from the equivalent register in another country
    e. (S)he has been convicted of a criminal offence prior to qualifying as a dentist

11. The following may initiate the GDC's disciplinary procedure:
    a. A formal complaint by a member of the public
    b. A formal complaint from a person acting in a public capacity
    c. The GDC's solicitors
    d. Notification by the police
    e. Notification by a criminal court

12. GDC disciplinary procedures:
    a. Are all screened initially by the President of the GDC
    b. A dentist's name can be erased from the register for a maximum of 12 months only

c. The Professional Conduct Committee is the first committee that can sanction a punitive action
d. A dentist can be suspended for a maximum of 6 months
e. Lay members of the GDC cannot sit on disciplinary committees

13. A dentist found guilty of 'serious professional misconduct' may:
    a. Have his or her name erased from the Dentists' Register
    b. Be referred to the Health Committee
    c. Be admonished
    d. Be suspended from the Dentists' Register for a specified period
    e. Have judgement postponed for a period to allow his or her conduct to improve

14. Following suspension or erasure from the Dentists' Register:
    a. A dentist can be re-registered at the end of a period of suspension
    b. Suspension or erasure always takes place immediately
    c. A dentist cannot apply for restoration to the Register until 2 years after being erased
    d. Further applications for restoration to the Register cannot be made for 1 year
    e. No fee is payable for restoration to the Dentists' Register

15. In matters of a dentist's health, rather than conduct, the GDC:
    a. Does not have 'preliminary screening' by the President of the GDC
    b. Medical examination is compulsory
    c. Allows the dentist 2 months to respond to an enquiry on health matters
    d. Allows the dentist to submit a report by his own medical examiner
    e. The Preliminary Proceedings Committee decides if a dentist should be referred to the Health Committee

16. The Health Committee of the GDC:
    a. Can impose conditions to a dentist remaining on the Register
    b. Can suspend a dentist from the Register
    c. Keep a dentist under review for an indefinite period
    d. Must refer all cases of suspension to the Professional Conduct Committee
    e. Impose conditional registration for up to 3 years

17. The powers of the proposed Performance Review

Committee are expected to include:
    a. Suspension from the Dentists' Register
    b. Erasure from the Dentists' Register
    c. The application of conditions to continuing registration
    d. Recommend remedial education
    e. Appointment of assessors, who must be members of the GDC

18. It is expected that the Performance Review Committee will be able to take referrals from:
    a. A professional colleague
    b. An organisation
    c. A member of the public
    d. Other GDC committees concerned with professional conduct
    e. The President of the GDC acting as preliminary screener

19. To practise dentistry in the UK, you must:
    a. Be a citizen of an EU or EEA country
    b. Register with the GDC
    c. If a new graduate, have completed a vocational training year
    d. Be of sound mind
    e. Hold a university degree in dentistry

20. To practise dentistry in the UK, you are strongly advised to:
    a. Have professional indemnity
    b. Have undertaken vocational or general professional training after qualifying
    c. Continue with training and education until you retire from dentistry
    d. Realise your limitations and not undertake any treatment beyond them
    e. Join one or more dental professional associations

21. Records of a patient's treatment:
    a. Must be hand written
    b. Should be kept for 5 years
    c. Must include a medical history
    d. Can be destroyed if the patient dies
    e. Should be written up at the end of each month

22. Records can be shown to:
    a. The patient
    b. The patient's spouse
    c. A police officer
    d. A specialist who the patient is referred to
    e. A court of law

23. Consent to treatment:
    a. Can be verbal
    b. Can be written

c. Can be implied

d. Is not required for patients under 16 years of age

e. Can be withdrawn by the patient

24. At the present time, the following can administer general anaesthesia for dental treatment:
    a. A doctor
    b. A suitably trained dentist
    c. A consultant anaesthetist
    d. A trainee anaesthetist
    e. A staff-grade anaesthetist

25. A dentist referring a patient for general anaesthesia must:
    a. Fully justify why a general anaesthetic is required
    b. Take a full medical history
    c. Explain to the patient the risks involved
    d. Obtain consent from the patient or their guardian
    e. Offer alternative methods of pain control in order to complete treatment for the patient

26. When treating a patient under general anaesthesia the dentist must:
    a. Repeat the history taking
    b. Repeat the explanations concerning risk, alternative treatments and pain control
    c. Obtain verbal consent
    d. Keep careful records of the treatment
    e. Give written pre- and postoperative instructions

27. When carrying out dental treatment under general anaesthetic:
    a. The dentist is responsible for the recovery of the patient
    b. The dentist is responsible for the discharge of the patient
    c. There must be a protocol for providing advanced life support
    d. There must be arrangements in hand to transfer a patient to a critical care facility
    e. There must be three appropriately trained personnel present

28. Sedation for dental treatment:
    a. Depresses the nervous system
    b. Can be administered by an appropriately trained dental nurse
    c. Requires the presence of three trained personnel
    d. Should be administered intravenously in children
    e. Must not involve the use of more than one drug

29. Before undertaking treatment under sedation, the dentist must:
    a. Assess the patient
    b. Take a full medical history
    c. Obtain written informed consent
    d. Ensure that equipment and facilities are adequate
    e. Advise on alternative methods of completing treatment

30. When treating a patient under sedation:
    a. A chaperone must be present
    b. The patient should be monitored only during the sedation
    c. Drugs must be available for resuscitation
    d. The patient's recovery must be supervised
    e. The patient must be accompanied by a responsible adult

31. Complaints from patients:
    a. Every dental practice should have a complaints procedure
    b. Only dentists and doctors can deal with complaints from patients
    c. Every dental hospital should have a complaints procedure
    d. Every dental department in a hospital or clinic should have a complaints procedure
    e. Should be answered in writing

32. When dealing with complaints:
    a. These should be undertaken by an outside body or organisation
    b. Acknowledgement should be sent within 1 week
    c. Dental practitioners should respond within 3 weeks
    d. NHS Trusts should respond within 3 weeks
    e. Only complaints in writing can be accepted

33. Making a complaint:
    a. It can only be made by the patient
    b. It must be made within 3 months of the incident
    c. The complainant can request an independent review of an unresolved complaint
    d. The complainant can ask the Health Service Commissioner (Ombudsman) to investigate
    e. Health Authorities must have a convenor and a lay assessor to deal with requests for independent review

34. The following would *not* be considered negligent:
    a. Something going wrong when treating a friend out of hours
    b. Not treating a patient as a specialist would

c. If the patient did not suffer harm or damage from a dentist's error

d. If the dentist had a duty of care at the time

e. If the dentist did not exercise reasonable skill and care

35. A claim for compensation for negligence against a dentist is *unlikely* to succeed:

   a. If the patient pleads 'res ipsa loquitor'

   b. If the dentist carried out reasonable treatment

   c. If the patient persuaded the dentist to undertake treatment that the dentist was doubtful would be successful

   d. If the damage occurred as a result of the patient grabbing the dentist's working arm

   e. If the negligent act or omission was carried out by an employee

36. The dentist (defendant) can use the following in his defence:

   a. The Bolam principle/test

   b. The Bolitho judgement/test

   c. The fact that the patient was under 18 years

   d. That the incident occurred 10 years ago

   e. That (s)he was carrying out a 'Good Samaritan' act

37. The 'Woolf' reforms for civil justice:

   a. Give the courts, rather than the parties' legal advisors control of the timetable

   b. Allocate an appropriate time for each case

   c. Set strict timetables

   d. Affect all civil courts in the UK

   e. Are designed to save expense

38. Medical and dental negligence cases under the 'Woolf' system:

   a. Must have disclosure of patients medical/dental records within 40 days of a solicitor's request being made

   b. Following a letter of claim, a defendant has 40 days to respond before court proceedings are issued

   c. Will have a single joint expert acting for the court whenever possible

   d. A case management conference will be held before the case comes to court to present information and try to resolve matters

   e. The court may suggest mediation

39. The following laws affect the practise of dentistry:

   a. COSHH Regulations (1998)

   b. The Dentists' Act

   c. Health and Safety at Work Acts

   d. Data Protection Act

   e. Financial Services Act

40. It is illegal to discriminate against people because of their:

   a. Race

   b. Dietary habits

   c. Colour

   d. Sex

   e. Age

Essay questions

1. Discuss consent in relation to a 15-year-old Girl Guide at a camp close to your practice who requires treatment for a dental abscess.

2. How would you deal with a complaint from a patient whom you treated a few months earlier?

Self-assessment: answers

Multiple choice answers

1. a. **True**.
   b. **False**. 17 elected and 21 appointed, plus the President.
   c. **False**. 3 members of GMC.
   d. **True**.
   e. **False**. They are appointed by the Queen on the advice of her Privy Council.

2. a. **False**.
   b. **False**.
   c. **True**.
   d. **True**.
   e. **True**.

3. a. **True**.
   b. **True**. But only under supervision.
   c. **True**. 'On call' duties are only allowed after 2 years of temporary registration and subject to satisfactory reports.
   d. **False**.
   e. **False**. Work permits are part of immigration and have to be applied for separately.

4. a. **False**. In two parts.
   b. **False**. Failure after two attempts leads to immediate removal of temporary registration.
   c. **False**. Providing that dentist has a qualification from an EU or EEA country.
   d. **False**. Providing that dentist has a qualification from an EU or EEA country.
   e. **True**.

5. a. **True**.
   b. **True**.
   c. **True**.
   d. **True**.
   e. **False**. Unless (s)he is on the orthodontic specialist list.

6. a. **False**.
   b. **True**.
   c. **True**.
   d. **True**.
   e. **False**.

7. a. **False**. Unless they have received the appropriate training before or after qualification.
   b. **False**.
   c. **False**. Only registered dental therapists can extract deciduous teeth.
   d. **True**.
   e. **False**. At present dental hygienists can, but dental therapists cannot.

8. a. **True**.
   b. **True**.
   c. **False**.
   d. **False**.
   e. **True**.

9. a. **False**.
   b. **False**.
   c. **True**.
   d. **True**. But only for study models, on written prescription, on the dentist's premises.
   e. **True**. But only if qualified.

10. a. **True**.
    b. **True**.
    c. **True**.
    d. **True**.
    e. **True**.

11. a. **True**.
    b. **True**.
    c. **True**.
    d. **True**.
    e. **True**.

12. a. **True**.
    b. **False**. Erasure is permanent, unless the dentist applies for restoration.
    c. **False**. The Preliminary Proceedings Committee can suspend registration immediately if members of the public are considered at risk.
    d. **False**. The maximum is 12 months.
    e. **False**. Lay members sit on all of these committees.

13. a. **True**.
    b. **True**.
    c. **True**.
    d. **True**.
    e. **True**.

14. a. **True**.
    b. **False**. Unless the public are considered at risk, the dentist can appeal to the Privy Council.
    c. **False**. Can reapply after 10 months.
    d. **False**. Can reapply after 10 months.
    e. **False**.

15. a. **False**. The President does undertake preliminary screening.
    b. **False**. It is not compulsory, but refusal will not stop the investigation proceeding.

c. **False**. 28 days are allowed.

d. **True**. But in addition to GDC's appointed medical examiner.

e. **False**. The President refers directly to the Health Committee.

16. a. **True**.
   b. **True**.
   c. **True**.
   d. **False**.
   e. **True**. At any one time, but conditions can be imposed for a further 12 months after review by the Health Committee.

17. a. **True**.
   b. **True**.
   c. **True**.
   d. **True**.
   e. **False**. The screeners will be members of GDC, but assessors will not.

18. a. **True**.
   b. **True**.
   c. **True**.
   d. **True**.
   e. **False**. Not directly, only via other GDC disciplinary committees.

19. a. **False**. Citizens from any country who hold a UK dental qualification can register.
   b. **True**.
   c. **False**. Vocational training is only necessary to hold a contract to provide NHS primary dental care.
   d. **True**.
   e. **False**. A licentiate of a Royal Medical College or from an appropriate EU, EAA country body is admissible.

20. a. **True**.
   b. **True**.
   c. **True**.
   d. **True**.
   e. **True**.

21. a. **False**. They can be typed or on computer.
   b. **False**. They should be kept for at least 7 years or until the patient is 25 years old.
   c. **True**.
   d. **False**.
   e. **False**. Should be written up during or immediately after each item of treatment.

22. a. **True**. Although the patient can be charged a reasonable fee.
   b. **False**.

c. **False**. But in cases of serious crime, seek advice from a dental defence organisation

d. **True**.

e. **False**. Unless there is a specific court order.

23. a. **True**.
   b. **True**.
   c. **True**.
   d. **False**. Required for all patients, in loco parentis if necessary.
   e. **True**.

24. a. **False**.
   b. **False**.
   c. **True**.
   d. **True**. But only under the direction of a named consultant anaesthetist.
   e. **True**. But only under the direction of a named consultant anaesthetist.

25. a. **True**.
   b. **True**.
   c. **True**.
   d. **True**.
   e. **True**.

26. a. **True**.
   b. **True**.
   c. **False**. Written informed consent is essential.
   d. **True**.
   e. **True**.

27. a. **False**. That is part of the anaesthetist's responsibility.
   b. **False**. That is part of the anaesthetist's responsibility.
   c. **True**.
   d. **True**.
   e. **False**. The dentist must have an appropriately trained assistant, as must the anaesthetist (four people).

28. a. **True**.
   b. **False**. Only an appropriately trained dentist or doctor.
   c. **True**. The dentist, his assistant and a dental or general nurse trained in patient monitoring is advised.
   d. **False**. Intravenous sedation is generally unsuitable for children; relative analgesia is preferred.
   e. **False**. One drug is preferred. Also, if using more than one drug, advanced life support must be immediately available.

29. a. **True**.
 b. **True**.
 c. **True**.
 d. **True**.
 e. **True**.

30. a. **True**.
 b. **False**. The patient must also be monitored during recovery.
 c. **True**.
 d. **True**.
 e. **True**.

31. a. **True**.
 b. **False**. Every practice or health organisation should have someone nominated to deal with complaints, but they do not have to be a doctor or dentist.
 c. **True**. Unless it is part of a larger unit.
 d. **False**. It is the responsibility of the organisation (e.g. NHS Trust) to deal with complaints.
 e. **True**.

32. a. **False**. Complaints should be dealt with internally in the first instance.
 b. **False**. Within 2 working days.
 c. **False**. Within 10 working days.
 d. **False**. Within 4 weeks.
 e. **False**. Complaints can be verbal or written.

33. a. **False**. As well as the patient, a parent, guardian or a friend can make a complaint.
 b. **False**. Normally within 6 months of problem or realising there was a problem; normal maximum 12 months.
 c. **True**.
 d. **True**. But he is unlikely to before attempts at local resolution and independent review.
 e. **True**.

34. a. **False**. Liability is present whenever treating any patient.
 b. **False**. Unless you are a specialist in the same or a related field.
 c. **True**.
 d. **False**.
 e. **False**.

35. a. **False**.
 b. **True**.
 c. **False**. A dentist should refuse to treat in this case.
 d. **True**.
 e. **False**. A dentist is liable for acts and omissions of employees.

36. a. **True**. If it supports his case.
 b. **True**. If it supports his case.
 c. **False**. The patient or their parents/guardians can sue.
 d. **True**. Unless the patient only became aware of the negligence less than 6 years ago.
 e. **False**.

37. a. **True**.
 b. **True**.
 c. **True**.
 d. **False**. Only England and Wales.
 e. **True**.

38. a. **True**.
 b. **False**. 3 months.
 c. **True**.
 d. **True**.
 e. **True**.

39. a. **True**.
 b. **True**.
 c. **True**.
 d. **True**.
 e. **False**.

40. a. **True**.
 b. **False**.
 c. **True**.
 d. **True**.
 e. **False**. But this may change in the near future, and guidelines have been drawn up.

Essay answers

1. As this patient is under 16 years of age, consent from a parent or legal guardian is normally required. However, as the patient is away from home on a group activity, one of the following may be used to obtain consent, which should be in writing if possible.
 • Contact a parent or guardian by telephone to explain the treatment and ask for consent. It is advisable to have a second person listen to the telephone call, and to write notes of the call in the patient's records.
 • Check if the patient's parents or guardian have signed a letter giving a group leader 'in loco parentis' rights. If so this person can consent. A copy of the 'in loco parentis' document should be taken.
 • If you feel that the patient fully understands the proposed treatment, then she can consent herself. This is sometimes referred to as 'Gillick

Competent' following a UK court case concerning consent. It would be advisable to get a colleague to approve your treatment plan and the patient's understanding of it in this case.

- Treatment should be limited to the relief of pain (by the most appropriate method) and reviewing progress if necessary. Definitive treatment and any other non urgent matters should be referred to the patient's own dentist.

2. Under the Patients' Charter, every health organisation must have a system for dealing with complaints. Although this charter applies to National Health Service treatment, it is advisable to have a parallel arrangement for private patients.

Always treating patients politely, and apologising when necessary for such things as lateness or unexpected difficulties will minimise complaints. In dental practise, written treatment plans and estimates of costs should be provided to patients as these are also helpful. In all organisations it is essential that everyone in that organisation is aware of how complaints are dealt with.

All health care organisations, however small, must have a nominated person to deal with complaints. If the complaint is verbal, the complainant should be asked to go to a place where the problem can be discussed with the nominated person confidentially. If the complaint is in writing, its receipt should be acknowledged within two working days.

The nominated person should:

- Try to resolve the problem as soon as possible.
- Make a response to the complaint within 10 working days.
- Keep the complainant informed of progress
- Tell the complainant the outcome of their investigation and inform them of any remedial

measures that the organisation has instituted to minimise the chance of a similar problem occurring in the future.

If the complaint cannot be resolved, then for:

NHS patients

- There may be a local conciliation service available from the local Health Authority.
- If the complainant is not satisfied, the local Health Authority or NHS Trust has to appoint a convenor to collect information and try to resolve the matter with the aid of an independent lay person.
- Should the second point not be successful, the convenor will decide whether or not an Independent Review Panel should be set up to investigate the complaint. If there is an independent review, all parties receive a copy of the review and the nominated person has to inform the complainant of any action taken.
- Finally a dissatisfied complainee may ask the Health Service Commissioner (Ombudsman) to investigate if they are still not satisfied.

Private patients

If the complaint cannot be resolved in-house, it may be necessary to employ an independent mediator/arbitrator. Alternatively, the complainant may sue the practitioner for negligence or the practitioner may attempt recovery of fees as a method of resolution.

The practitioner should consult his or her professional indemnity organisation for advice as soon as it appears that in-house resolution may not be possible.

Index

Note: Question and Answer sections are indicated in the form of 54Q/58A. The answer may include detailed mention of the subject.